Practical Radiother

Good and effective treatment in radiotherapy requires careful consideration of the complex variables involved along with critical assessment of the techniques. This new edition of an established classic takes into account advances in imaging and treatment delivery and reflects the current state of the art in the practice of radiotherapy, emphasising the underlying principles of treatment that can be applied for conventional, conformal and novel treatments.

From reviews of previous editions:

'Beautifully illustrated, adequately referenced [...] and written in plain English ... buy it and don't lose it'
RAD Magazine

'I strongly recommend this book as essential reading for trainees in clinical oncology as well as radiographers … a useful book for anyone involved in the planning and delivery of radiotherapy'
Oncology News

'Both trainees and practitioners of radiotherapy will find this a useful and quick guide to radiotherapy planning and treatment'
Doody's Book Review

About the Authors

Dr Stephen Morris is a Consultant Clinical Oncologist at Guy's and St Thomas' Hospital Cancer Centre. He graduated from Guy's and St Thomas' medical school and trained in clinical oncology at the Royal Marsden Hospital and at the Guy's and St Thomas' Cancer Center. He was appointed as a consultant in 2005. He specialises in the management of prostate cancer and skin cancer. He has a special interest in prostate brachytherapy and skin lymphoma.

Dr Tom Roques is a Consultant Clinical Oncologist at Norfolk and Norwich University Hospitals NHS Foundation Trust. He joined the trust in 2004 as a consultant having trained in Cambridge, Oxford, London and Vancouver. He specialises in head and neck, upper gastrointestinal and hepatobiliary cancers and is Vice President, Clinical Oncology at the Royal College of Radiologists.

Dr Shahreen Ahmad, MRCP, FRCR, MD(Res), is a Consultant Clinical Oncologist at Guy's and St Thomas' Cancer Centre, London. She graduated from University College London Medical School and trained in clinical oncology at St Bartholomew's Hospital, London and Guy's & St Thomas' Hospital. She treats lung and breast cancer, and her research interests include imaging & radiotherapy and cardiac SABR.

Dr Suat Loo, MRCP, FRCR, is a Consultant Clinical Oncologist at the Colchester campus of East Suffolk and North Essex NHS Foundation Trust. He graduated from Barts and the London School of Medicine and trained in clinical oncology in Cambridge. He was appointed as a consultant in 2014. He specialises in the management of sarcoma, upper gastrointestinal, hepatobiliary, gynaecological and testicular cancers.

Practical Radiotherapy Planning

Fifth Edition

Stephen Morris, MRCP, FRCR
Consultant Clinical Oncologist, Guy's and
St Thomas' Cancer Centre, London

Tom Roques, MRCP, FRCR
Consultant Clinical Oncologist, Norfolk and Norwich University
Hospitals NHS Foundation Trust, Norwich

Shahreen Ahmad, MRCP, FRCR, MD (Res)
Consultant Clinical Oncologist, Guy's and St Thomas' Cancer Centre, London

Suat Loo, MRCP, FRCR
Consultant Clinical Oncologist, East Suffolk and
North Essex NHS Foundation Trust, Colchester

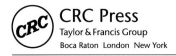

CRC Press
Taylor & Francis Group
Boca Raton London New York

CRC Press is an imprint of the
Taylor & Francis Group, an **informa** business

Fifth edition published 2024
by CRC Press
6000 Broken Sound Parkway NW, Suite 300, Boca Raton, FL 33487-2742

and by CRC Press
4 Park Square, Milton Park, Abingdon, Oxon, OX14 4RN

CRC Press is an imprint of Taylor & Francis Group, LLC

© 2024 Taylor & Francis Group, LLC

This book contains information obtained from authentic and highly regarded sources. While all reasonable efforts have been made to publish reliable data and information, neither the author[s] nor the publisher can accept any legal responsibility or liability for any errors or omissions that may be made. The publishers wish to make clear that any views or opinions expressed in this book by individual editors, authors or contributors are personal to them and do not necessarily reflect the views/opinions of the publishers. The information or guidance contained in this book is intended for use by medical, scientific or health-care professionals and is provided strictly as a supplement to the medical or other professional's own judgement, their knowledge of the patient's medical history, relevant manufacturer's instructions and the appropriate best practice guidelines. Because of the rapid advances in medical science, any information or advice on dosages, procedures or diagnoses should be independently verified. The reader is strongly urged to consult the relevant national drug formulary and the drug companies' and device or material manufacturers' printed instructions, and their websites, before administering or utilizing any of the drugs, devices or materials mentioned in this book. This book does not indicate whether a particular treatment is appropriate or suitable for a particular individual. Ultimately it is the sole responsibility of the medical professional to make his or her own professional judgements, so as to advise and treat patients appropriately. The authors and publishers have also attempted to trace the copyright holders of all material reproduced in this publication and apologize to copyright holders if permission to publish in this form has not been obtained. If any copyright material has not been acknowledged, please write and let us know so we may rectify in any future reprint.

Except as permitted under U.S. Copyright Law, no part of this book may be reprinted, reproduced, transmitted, or utilized in any form by any electronic, mechanical, or other means, now known or hereafter invented, including photocopying, microfilming, and recording, or in any information storage or retrieval system, without written permission from the publishers.

For permission to photocopy or use material electronically from this work, access www.copyright.com or contact the Copyright Clearance Center, Inc. (CCC), 222 Rosewood Drive, Danvers, MA 01923, 978-750-8400. For works that are not available on CCC, please contact mpkbookspermissions@tandf.co.uk

Trademark notice: Product or corporate names may be trademarks or registered trademarks and are used only for identification and explanation without intent to infringe.

ISBN: 9781138045989 (hbk)
ISBN: 9781138045972 (pbk)
ISBN: 9781315171562 (ebk)

DOI: 10.1201/9781315171562

Typeset in Times
by KnowledgeWorks Global Ltd.

Contents

Preface vii

1   **What You Need to Know before Planning Radiotherapy Treatment** 1

2   **Principles of Radiotherapy Planning** 7

3   **Radiobiology and Treatment Planning** 27

4   **Organs at Risk and Tolerance of Normal Tissues** 38

5   **Principles of Brachytherapy** 49

6   **Emergency and Palliative Radiotherapy** 56

7   **Skin** 65

8   **Head and Neck: General Considerations** 81

9   **Lip, Ear, Nose and Treatment of the Neck in Skin Cancer** 103

10   **Oral Cavity** 112

11   **Oropharynx Cancer and Unknown Primary Tumours of the Head and Neck** 122

12   **Hypopharynx** 136

13   **Nasopharynx** 145

14   **Larynx** 154

15   **Salivary Glands** 163

16   **Sinuses: Maxilla, Ethmoid and Nasal Cavity Tumours** 170

17   **Orbit** 179

18   **Central Nervous System** 186

19   **Thyroid and Thymoma** 205

20   **Lung** 214

21   **Mesothelioma** 234

22   **Breast** 240

23 Haematological Malignancies 260

24 Oesophagus and Stomach 283

25 Pancreas and Liver 296

26 Rectum 305

27 Anus 318

28 Prostate 328

29 Bladder 348

30 Testis 358

31 Penis 364

32 Cervix 368

33 Uterus 381

34 Vagina 393

35 Vulva 399

36 Sarcoma 405

37 Paediatric Tumours 415

38 Radiotherapy for Benign Disease 431

Index 439

Preface

The practice of radiotherapy has changed in many ways since the last edition of *Practical Radiotherapy Planning* was published in 2009. Advances in imaging have been incorporated into radiotherapy planning to improve the accuracy of volume definition. CT has advanced with new algorithms enhancing image quality and new techniques such as perfusion CT and dynamic contrast-enhanced CT improving the accuracy of tumour delineation. Diffusion-weighted MRI has been widely adopted to enhance soft tissue contrast, and apparent diffusion coefficient (ADC) maps can identify areas of increased cellularity due to tumour growth. Quantitative functional assessment with MRI has improved, so whole-body scans can be used for the accurate staging of some tumour types. Intensity-modulated radiotherapy (IMRT) has been superseded by more advanced techniques such as volumetric modulated arc therapy (VMAT). Stereotactic ablative radiotherapy (SABR) has been commissioned in most cancer centres in the UK, and proton beam therapy is now available in Manchester and London. Hypofractionation is increasingly used in breast and prostate cancers. Image-guided radiotherapy (IGRT) has become more advanced, with image-guided adaptive radiotherapy implemented for some tumour types.

There are now target volume and organ at-risk contouring guidelines and atlases for most body sites, many of which are available online. The ICRU has continued to update and publish international recommendations such as the principles of prescribing, recording and reporting photon therapy (ICRU report 62), electron beam therapy (ICRU report 71), intensity modulated photon beam therapy IMRT (ICRU report 82) and stereotactic treatments (ICRU report 91). Newer systemic treatments such as immunotherapy have changed treatment options for some cancers, and sometimes provided new indications for radiotherapy.

The previous edition of this book introduced the newly developing concepts of IMRT and IGRT. This edition explains how these new techniques have advanced and are now being used to deliver very advanced, highly accurate radiotherapy. Simpler techniques are also described where relevant to current practice. The overall aim of the book remains the same – to provide a clear description of modern radiotherapy treatment that is based on sound pathological and anatomical principles and backed by high-quality evidence.

Most radiotherapy treatment is given according to local, national and international protocols, which should always be consulted as appropriate. In a rapidly changing discipline like radiotherapy there will often be alternative protocols and techniques to those described here. We intend our text to provide guidance for radiotherapy that can be followed by practitioners anywhere in the world so they can deliver safe and effective treatment.

To improve the optimal reproduction of plans we have tried to use the following colour scheme in illustrations unless indicated otherwise:

GTV   dark blue
CTVs   cyan (light blue), magenta (purple)
PTVs   red, lime green
OARs   yellow, light yellow, light green, dark green

We are very grateful for all those in our hospitals and further afield with whom we work and collaborate; they challenge and inspire us. The current authors would like to thank the initial authors of this book – Jane Dobbs, Ann Barrett, and Dan Ash – and hope this edition continues to inspire many future versions. It would be impossible to produce a book like this one in the age of specialized practice and multidisciplinary team working without particular collaboration from expert colleagues who have helped with certain sections of the text. Special thanks to Omar Al-Salihi, Jessica Brady, Yen Chang,

Adam Dobson, Dinos Geropantas, Andrew Ho, Simon Hughes, Sarah Jefferies, Pei Lim, Asad Qureshi, Angela Swampillai, Nicky Thorp, Alison Tree, Rob Urwin and Sadaf Usman.

This small textbook cannot describe all the research which has been undertaken to develop radiotherapy schedules. We have aimed to describe evidence-based treatment protocols as used in our departments around the UK. We have included a list of key trials and information sources at the end of each chapter where more detailed information may be found. We give an introduction to the principles and practice of brachytherapy, but more detailed information can be found in dedicated brachytherapy papers and books. Commonly used abbreviations have been spelled out at first mention in the book and are included in the appendix for further reference.

We hope that trainees in clinical and radiation oncology, therapeutic radiographers, dosimetrists and physicists, all working collaboratively within their multidisciplinary teams, will continue to use our book to produce safe and appropriate plans for common tumours.

Shahreen Ahmad, Suat Loo, Stephen Morris, Tom Roques, 2023

1

What You Need to Know before Planning Radiotherapy Treatment

Introduction

Radiotherapy has been used to treat cancer for more than a hundred years. Following the discovery of X-rays by William Röntgen in 1895, X-rays were used to treat breast cancer in Chicago in 1896. The first reported cancer cured by radiotherapy was a squamous cell cancer on the nose treated in 1899. Radiotherapy is now the most important nonsurgical treatment for cancer.

Radiotherapy can only produce beneficial effects if it is delivered in an appropriate clinical context. Attempting curative radical treatment for a patient with metastatic disease or one who is likely to die soon from cardiac or lung disease is inappropriate. These decisions require a fine balance of judgement between therapeutic optimism and nihilism, and must be firmly based in good clinical history taking and examination. The clinician must then be able to synthesise all the information about the patient, tumour, investigations and previous treatment to make a decision about whether radiotherapy should be used and, if so, with curative radical or palliative intent. Comorbidities which could affect the toxicity of treatment, such as diabetes or vascular disease, must also be considered.

Sometimes the decision to offer radiotherapy may be relatively simple if the disease is common, the treatment effective and standardised, the histological features are well categorised and imaging is easy to interpret. Some breast cancers fit well into this category. In contrast, decisions may be very difficult if there is no treatment of proven benefit, the prognosis is uncertain, the patient's general performance status is poor, imaging is of limited utility or there is histological uncertainty. Clinical experience and judgement then become critically important. This expertise is built on the foundation of good history taking which enables clinicians to set a patient's disease in the context of their own ideas, concerns and expectations. Have other family members had radiotherapy with good or bad outcomes? Are they so claustrophobic that they will not go into a scanner or treatment room? Do they have other problems which would affect the feasibility of radiotherapy – arthritis which limits joint movement, shortness of breath which prevents them lying flat, pacemakers or prostheses which may affect dose delivery?

Clinicians may consider that the new era of cross-sectional and functional imaging has made examination of the patient irrelevant, but it remains the essential foundation of appropriate clinical judgements; for example, detection of a lymph node in the axilla, otherwise overlooked in imaging, or the progression of a tumour since the last scan, may change a decision taken earlier in a multidisciplinary team meeting.

Classification Systems

Many classification systems have been developed to ensure that clinicians throughout the world share a common language as they describe patients, tumours and treatment. This is essential to allow effective cancer registration and comparisons of incidence, prognosis and outcome of treatments. Many protocols for treatment are also based on such classification systems.

DOI: 10.1201/9781315171562-1

Pathological Classification

The International Classification of Disease (ICD) version 11, of the World Health Organization (WHO), was updated in 2019. It is the international standard diagnostic classification for epidemiology and health management. It is used in hospital records and on death certificates, which, in turn, are the basis for compiling mortality and morbidity statistics nationally and internationally. There is a subclassification, the International Classification of Disease for Oncology version 3 (ICD-O-3.2, updated 2019), which is used in cancer/tumour registries to code site (topography) and type (morphology) of neoplasms from the histopathology report.

Information about malignancy (malignant, benign, in situ or uncertain) and differentiation is also coded. In the UK, this information is abstracted from clinical notes by trained coders. The introduction of computerised systems suggests that clinicians will be required to develop greater awareness of this classification, at least in their own areas of expertise, especially if the information becomes essential data before income is assured. ICD 11 and ICD-O-3.2 are available online.

The morphological information for ICD-O-3.2 coding comes from the pathologist, whose expertise is essential to establish a precise diagnosis and choose appropriate treatment volumes. A pathology report will contain a description of the macroscopic appearance of the gross tumour specimen, its size, resection margins and anatomical relationships. It will describe the microscopic appearance after appropriate staining of cut sections of the tumour, including features such as areas of necrosis. Recognition of the tissue of origin and grading of the tumour will then often be possible.

There has been an explosion of new techniques in pathology, such as immunocytochemical staining, immunophenotyping and fluorescence in situ hybridisation, which may help to remove uncertainties about diagnoses following conventional histopathological examination. New molecular diagnostic tests and genetic profiling methods are increasingly being developed to identify tumour-targeted molecular profiles which inform the choice of targeted treatments. Oncologists must be in constant dialogue with their pathology colleagues to ensure that they understand the significance of results of these special investigations and know how to assess the degree of certainty of the report.

Staging

Tumour stage, histological classification and grade determine prognosis and treatment decisions. An internationally agreed staging system is essential to interpret outcomes of treatment and compare results in different treatment centres. The behaviour of tumours in different sites is determined by the anatomical situation, blood supply and lymphatic drainage, along with the histological classification and grading. Any staging system must take into account this variability. The most commonly used systems are the UICC (Union Internationale Contre le Cancer) TNM, AJCC (American Joint Committee on Cancer) and FIGO (Federation Internationale de Gynecologie et d'Obstetrique) for gynaecological malignancy. The TNM system describes the tumour extent (T), nodal involvement (N) and distant metastases (M). This defines a clinical classification (cTNM) or a pathological classification (pTNM) which incorporates information derived from an excised tumour and any draining lymph nodes that are also removed or sampled. Details of this system are given in the TNM atlas, which should be available and used wherever patients are seen or results of investigations are correlated.

T staging includes measurement of the tumour either clinically, by imaging techniques, or by macroscopic examination of an excised specimen. Correct pathological T staging can only be assured if the pathologist receives a completely excised tumour with a rim of surrounding tissue. The tumour should not be cut into or fixed except by the pathologist. Examination of the whole specimen is needed to determine the highest grade of tumour (as there is frequently inhomogeneity across the tumour), any vascular or lymphatic invasion or invasion of adjacent tissues. Spread into a body space such as the pleural or peritoneal cavity affects T staging, as it changes prognosis.

Numbers are added to indicate the extent of the disease. For example, T0 implies no primary tumour (as after spontaneous regression of a melanoma). Categories T1–4 indicate tumours of increasing size and/or involvement of lymphatic vessels or surrounding tissue. If it is impossible to ascertain the size or extent of the primary tumour, it is designated Tx.

N classification describes whether there is lymph node involvement and, if so, how many nodes are involved. Pathological staging requires adequate excision of the relevant lymph node compartment, and a minimum number of nodes which indicates that this has been achieved may be defined for each site. If there are positive nodes, the ratio of negative to positive is of prognostic significance. For example, one node positive out of four removed indicates a worse prognosis than one out of 12. The size of tumour in the nodes must be recorded, along with any extension through the capsule. Micrometastases are classified differently from tumour emboli in vessels, and this affects the N staging.

Identification and sampling of a sentinel node may give useful prognostic information about other potential node involvement and help to choose appropriate treatment strategies. In breast cancer, for example, it appears highly predictive (90 per cent) for axillary node involvement.

M category indicates presence (M1) or absence (M0) of metastases to distant sites.

For some sites, other staging systems have proved clinically more useful. These include the FIGO system for gynaecological malignancy and Dukes' classification of colonic tumours. Useful atlases of patterns of lymph node involvement have been devised for several tumor sites. These are included in subsequent chapters where relevant. Recommendations for the most appropriate imaging techniques for staging in different sites have been published.

Residual tumour after surgical excision is an important poor prognostic factor. Examination of resection margins assigns tumours to categories: R0, no residual tumour; R1, histologically detectable tumour at margins; and R2, macroscopic evidence of residual tumour. Where serum markers (S) convey important prognostic information, as in tumours of the testis, an S category has been introduced to the TNM system.

TNM categorisation is often used to group tumours subsequently into stages indicating local and metastatic extent and correlating with likely outcome.

Grading is defined by degree of differentiation: G1, resemblance to tissue of origin; G2, moderately well differentiated; G3, poorly differentiated; and G4, undifferentiated tumours; with Gx used when it is not possible to determine grading, as for example from a damaged specimen. GB signifies a borderline malignant tumour (for example in the ovary). Grading systems reduce the subjective element of these assessments.

Performance Status and PROMs

Performance status measures attempt to quantify cancer patients' general well-being. They are used to help to decide whether a patient is likely to tolerate a particular treatment such as curative radical radiotherapy or palliative chemotherapy, whether doses of treatment need to be adjusted or whether the patient's life expectancy is good enough to allow them to survive to see a benefit from treatment. The status of all patients should be recorded using one of these scores at presentation and with any change in treatment or the disease. They are also used as a measure of quality of life in clinical trials.

There are various scoring systems; the most commonly used are the Karnofsky (KPS) and WHO performance status scales for adults, and the Lansky score for children. The SF-36 is a short form (SF) survey (originally with 36 questions, now 12) which gives a profile of overall mental and physical health. It has produced statistically reliable and valid results in many reported studies. There are modifications of this questionnaire for specific tumour sites. Another commonly used scale in quality-of-life assessment is the HADS (Hospital Anxiety and Depression Scale), which is used to measure changes in mental and emotional well-being during treatment or with the progression of the disease. For palliative radiotherapy, the Chow score and TEACHH models use factors such as site of metastases, primary cancer site, previous radiotherapy and KPS to produce a score that may assist in identifying those patients most likely to benefit from treatment.

Patient-reported outcome measures (PROMs) are increasingly used in cancer patients. They are valuable to collect data on a patient's quality of life. The data is documented by patients directly without interpretation or bias from a clinician. PROMs were initially developed for use in research but are being increasingly introduced in routine clinical settings. PROMs provide more detailed and patient-centred measures than performance status alone. Patients complete questionnaires on their health and quality of life.

Patients are often involved in the designing and development of PROMs, including the time points during their cancer journey that the data is collected. The data from PROMs can be used to tailor an individual patient's care as well as being utilised by health care providers to improve patient services in general. EORTC QLQ-C30 is an example of a questionnaire with a nine multi-item scale that evaluates functional status, symptoms, and global health and quality of life.

Prognostic Factors

All possible information which may help in predicting prognosis should be collected in order to advise the patient and help make the most appropriate treatment decision.

Screen-detected cancers may have a better prognosis than tumours presenting symptomatically because diagnosis is made earlier. The UK has three screening programmes: bowel cancer, breast cancer and cervical cancer. Screening for prostate cancer is available but controversial. There is no national lung cancer screening programme, but the NHS offers a service called Targeted Lung Health Checks.

Histological tumour type, grading and staging are most influential in determining the outcome for an individual patient, and new techniques of tumour examination are yielding more information on gene function and expression, which may affect prognosis. Other factors which must also be considered include epidemiological factors such as age and sex; lifestyle factors such as smoking, alcohol and other drug use; obesity; and family history of disease. Other biological factors such as performance status, which may reflect comorbidities, must be considered.

Biochemical tumour markers may be specific enough to give prognostic information by their absolute value, as for example β subunit of human chorionic gonadotrophin (β-hCG) levels in testicular cancer. Tumour markers may be only relatively poorly correlated with tumour volume, such as carcinoembryonic antigen (CEA) in bowel cancer, but still be useful to indicate treatment response or disease progression by their rise or fall.

One of the most important prognostic factors is whether there is effective treatment for the condition. Because new treatments are being introduced all the time, prognostic predictions must also be constantly reviewed and validated in prospective controlled clinical trials. An example is Oncotype DX assay (21 gene assay) test predicting the likelihood of chemotherapy benefit in women with early breast cancer based on TailorX study.

For some tumours, predictive tools based on population data sets are available, such as 'Predict' for breast cancer, and Partin tables and the Memorial Sloane Kettering nomogram for prostate cancer.

Predictive indicators are variables determined before treatment which give information on the probability of a response to a specific treatment. Predictive indices based on multiple indicators give an individual score which may help to make decisions. These tools can only be developed by painstaking retrospective analysis and careful prospective studies, but it is likely that their use will increase steadily. They are important in determining strategies for treating different tumour subsets in guidelines and protocols.

Increasingly, specific genetic profiles are correlated with natural history of disease or outcome of treatment. Examples are the predictive value of MYCN amplification in neuroblastoma, oestrogen/HER2 receptor status and response to hormone therapy or trastuzumab, and predilection of patients with Li–Fraumeni syndrome to develop second tumours. Microarray technology will provide more genetically determined prognostic factors which will have to be taken into account in planning treatment.

Influence of Other Treatments on Radiotherapy

Surgery is most commonly used as a primary treatment for cancer. If performed before radiotherapy, it removes the gross tumour volume (GTV) so that a clinical target volume alone (CTV) is used for planning (see Chapter 2).

If it is known from the time of diagnosis that both treatments will be needed, the best sequence has to be decided. If the tumour is initially inoperable, radiotherapy first may produce tumour shrinkage which makes complete excision possible, thereby improving outcome. Radiotherapy may increase surgical complications if the interval between the two treatments is not optimal. Surgery before radiotherapy will alter normal anatomy, causing problems for planning unless pre- and postsurgical image co-registration is used.

Effective systemic therapy may produce complete resolution of the primary tumour (no residual GTV), and potentially increased acute normal tissue effects. The treatment the patient receives will be the best possible only if all these potential interactions are taken into consideration by all members of the team working together.

A true therapeutic gain from radiotherapy and chemotherapy together requires either more cell kill for the same level of normal tissue damage (which is useful in radio-resistant tumours) or the same cell kill with reduced normal tissue effects (useful for tumours cured with low-dose radiotherapy). Radiotherapy with concomitant chemotherapy is now used for many tumours. It may improve outcomes by promoting spatial cooperation in cell killing, where the chemotherapy kills metastatic cells and the radiotherapy kills those cells in the local tumour, or in-field cooperation where exploitation of differing molecular, cellular or tissue effects produces more cell kill than when the two agents are given sequentially. There has been a recent increase in the use of immunotherapy, which has significantly improved outcomes in some cancers. Radiation-induced cancer cell damage exposes tumour-specific antigens, making them visible to immune surveillance, and can also modulate the tumour microenvironment, facilitating the recruitment and infiltration of immune cells. Clinical studies are currently underway combining radiation with immunotherapy check point inhibitors.

Patients themselves may be using alternative therapies with possible effects on efficacy and complications of surgery, radiotherapy and systemic therapies. Antioxidants may interfere with free radical production, which effects radiotherapy cell kill. St John's wort, used for depression, may affect the metabolism of some drugs. Aspirin and gingko biloba may increase risk of bleeding, and phytooestrogens may affect hormonally sensitive cancers. Lifestyle factors such as smoking or eating too many vegetables during radiotherapy may influence the severity of acute treatment side effects such as mucositis or diarrhoea.

Systems for Recording Outcomes of Treatment

The most commonly used set of tumour response criteria is the Response Evaluation Criteria in Solid Tumours (RECIST). There are other response criteria used for specific tumour types. Other outcomes are recorded as the time to a specific event: time to progression for tumours with partial response (progression-free survival), time to local recurrence where there has been a complete response (relapse-free survival), time to distant metastases, time to death from any cause (overall survival) or time to second malignancy. The start and end dates for these time periods must be clearly defined and stated as, for example, date of first treatment, date of randomisation, date of imaging of relapse or date of histological proof of relapse. There is still no clear convention for defining these dates.

Quality-of-life measures are also essential for assessing treatment effects. Standardised scales such as the EORTC, QLQ-C36 and C30 have been validated and can be used for many cancer sites and in many countries.

Acute side effects can be recorded using the Common Terminology Criteria for Adverse Events (CTCAE V5.0, November 2017). This is a comprehensive system that is used in all clinical trials. Late effects are recorded either using the Radiation Therapy Oncology Group (RTOG) criteria, the European LENT-SOMA classification or other simpler schemes for individual body sites.

Clinical Anatomy

Modern radiotherapy planning requires a comprehensive knowledge of cross-sectional anatomy and the ability to visualise structures in three dimensions. Formal teaching in anatomy should be part of training, using standard atlases and various online resources, e.g. RTOG contouring atlases. We attempt to give some relevant anatomical details in the following chapters, but collaboration with a diagnostic radiologist can be essential for accurate GTV delineation. Oncologists will tend to develop expertise in their own specialist areas but are unlikely to be familiar with all the possible normal variants and anomalies which may occur.

Protocols and Guidelines

In the UK, there has been a proliferation of guidance, guidelines and protocols for the management of cancer. Some, such as Improving Outcomes Guidance (IOG) and decisions of the National Institute for Health and Clinical Excellence (NICE), have a mandatory element which ensures their adoption. The firmest base for clinical decision-making is evidence of effectiveness of treatment from well-designed prospective randomised clinical trials (RCTs). Where this is lacking, careful analysis of outcomes data can be very informative and has the advantage of wider generalisability. National and international trial protocols offer useful information for treatment planning, as they represent current consensus on best clinical practice; for example, how to scan lung cancers for treatment planning, or what quality assurance programme to use. Departments must have their own written protocols for treatment at different sites to ensure consistency and quality and to avoid errors.

Not all patients' circumstances will fit within standardised guidelines and protocols, although these should be followed whenever possible for best outcomes. However, with the rate of change in treatment in oncology, there should be a constant cycle of writing guidelines and then using, auditing, challenging and rewriting them.

INFORMATION SOURCES

Amin JB, et al. AJCC Cancer Staging Manual, 8th ed. Springer, 2017: www.cancerstaging.org.

Chow E, et al. Predictive model for survival in patients with advanced cancer. J Clin Oncol 2008;26:5863–5869.

Common Terminology Criteria for Adverse Events (CTCAE) v5.0, 2017: www.ctep.cancer.gov.

Eisenhauer EA, et al. New response evaluation criteria in solid tumors: Revised RECIST guideline (Version 1.1). Eur J Cancer 2009;45:228–247.

Krishan MS, et al. Predicting life expectancy in patients with metastatic cancer receiving palliative radiotherapy: The TEACHH model. Cancer 2014;120:134–141.

National Institute for Clinical Excellence (NICE), Guidelines: www.nice.org.uk/guidance.

Schwartz LH, et al. RECIST 1.1 – Update and clarification: From the RECIST committee. Eur J Cancer 2016 Jul;62:132–137.

World Health Organization, International Classification of Disease (ICD), v11, 2020: https://www.who.int/standards/classifications/classification-of-diseases.

World Health Organization, International Classification of Disease for Oncology, v3 (ICD-O-3.2), 2019: https://www.who.int/standards/classifications/other-classifications/international-classification-of-diseases-for-oncology.

2

Principles of Radiotherapy Planning

The practice of radiotherapy requires not only excellent clinical skills but also appropriate technical expertise. Chapter 1 considered some of the factors that contribute to making good clinical judgements; Chapter 2 outlines the specialist knowledge required to plan radiotherapy treatment.

Target Volume Definition

A common international language for describing target volumes is found in International Commission on Radiation Units (ICRU) published recommendations Report 50 (1993), 62 (1999), 71 (2004) and 83 (2010). These contain clear definitions (Figure 2.1) to enable centres to use the same criteria for delineating tumours for radiation so that their treatment results can be compared. The latest report includes definitions for Intensity Modulated Radiotherapy (IMRT).

The American Association of Physicists in Medicine Report 263 gives guidance on the naming of target volumes. These should be followed wherever possible to enable better data analysis within and between departments.

Gross Tumour Volume

Gross tumour volume (GTV) is the primary tumour or other tumour mass shown by clinical examination, at examination under anaesthetic (EUA) or by imaging. GTV is classified by staging systems such as TNM (UICC), AJCC or FIGO. Tumour size, site and shape may appear to vary depending on the imaging technique used, and an optimal imaging method for each particular tumour site must therefore also be specified. A GTV may consist of a primary tumour (GTVp) and/or a metastatic lymphadenopathy (GTVn). GTV always contains the highest tumour cell density, and is absent after complete surgical resection.

Clinical Target Volume

Clinical target volume (CTV) contains the GTV when present and/or subclinical microscopic disease that has to be eradicated to cure the tumour. The CTV definition is based on histological examination

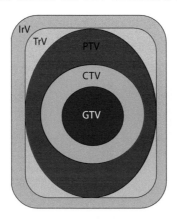

FIGURE 2.1 ICRU target volume definitions showing GTV, CTV, PTV, treated volume and irradiated volume. (Reproduced with permission from ICRU [1993] Prescribing, Recording and Reporting Photon Beam Therapy. ICRU report 50.)

DOI: 10.1201/9781315171562-2

of postmortem or surgical specimens that assesses the extent of tumour cell spread around the gross GTV, as described by Holland et al. (1985) for breast cancer. The GTV-CTV margin is also derived from biological characteristics of the tumour, local recurrence patterns and experience of the radiation oncologist. A CTV containing a primary tumour may lie in continuity with a nodal CTV to form a contiguous combined CTV (e.g. tonsillar tumour and ipsilateral cervical nodes). When a potentially involved adjacent lymph node which may require elective irradiation lies at a distance from the primary tumour, separate CTVp and CTVn are used (Figure 2.2), e.g. an anal tumour and the inguinal nodes.

Variation in CTV delineation by the clinician ('doctor's delineation error') is the greatest geometrical uncertainty in the whole treatment process. Studies comparing outlining by radiologists and oncologists have shown a significant inter-observer variability for both the GTV and/or CTV at a variety of tumour

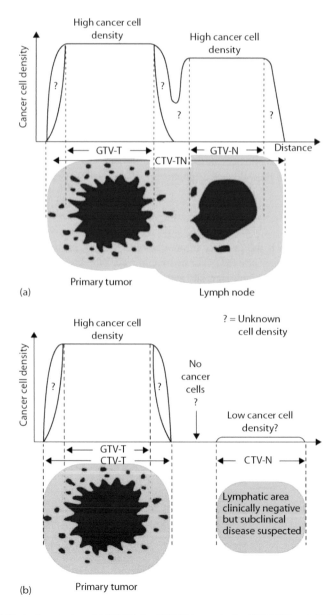

FIGURE 2.2   ICRU illustrations to show (a) GTV-T plus GTV-N in continuity (CTV-TN) and (b) CTV-T and CTV-N at a distance. (Reproduced with permission from ICRU [2004] Prescribing, Recording and Reporting Electron Beam Therapy. ICRU report 71.)

sites. This is greater than any intra-observer variation. Published results for nasopharynx, brain, lung, prostate, medulloblastoma and breast all show significant discrepancies in the volumes outlined by different clinicians. Improvements can be made with training in radiological anatomy, which enables clinicians to distinguish blood vessels from lymph nodes and to identify structures accurately on computed tomography (CT) and magnetic resonance imaging (MRI). Joint outlining by radiologists and oncologists can improve consistency and ensure accurate interpretation of imaging of the GTV. Consensus guidelines such as those for defining CTV for head and neck nodes (Gregoire et al. 2013) and pelvic nodes (Taylor et al. 2005) have improved CTV delineation greatly. Protocols for outlining GTV and CTV at all tumour sites are needed, and suggestions are made in each individual chapter.

Planning Target Volume

When the patient moves or internal organs change in size and shape during a fraction of treatment or between fractions (intra- or inter-fractionally), the position of the CTV may also move. Therefore, to ensure a homogeneous dose to the CTV throughout a fractionated course of irradiation, margins must be added around the CTV. These allow for physiological organ motion (internal margin) and variations in patient positioning and alignment of treatment beams (set-up margin), creating a geometric planning target volume. The planning target volume (PTV) is used in treatment planning to select appropriate beams to ensure that the prescribed dose is actually delivered to the CTV.

Organ Motion/Internal Margin

Variations in organ motion may be small (e.g. brain), larger and predictable (e.g. respiration or cardiac pulsation), or unpredictable (e.g. rectal and bladder filling).

When treating lung tumours, the displacement of the CTV caused by respiration can be dealt with in several ways. Most commonly, a solution based on 4D CT acquisition is used. Patients should be scanned over a few breathing cycles, using an external surrogate or fiducial marker to determine the position of the tumour and lung over different phases of the respiratory cycle. The CTV can then be edited over the phases of respiration to create an internal target volume (ITV) (ICRU 62). In addition, tumour and organ motion should be accounted for during treatment delivery with image guided radiotherapy (IGRT). IGRT techniques include active breathing control (ABC), linac-based respiratory gating and abdominal compression. See Chapter 20 for details.

Protocols for minimising effects on the CTV of variations in bladder and rectal filling are described in relevant chapters. Uncertainties from organ motion can also be reduced by using fiducial markers, and published results are available for lung, prostate and breast tumours. Radio-opaque markers are inserted and imaged at localisation using CT or MRI, and at treatment verification, using portal films, electronic portal imaging devices (EPIDs) or online cone beam CT image-guided radiotherapy (IGRT). The internal margin therefore allows for inter- and intra-fractional variations in organ position and shape which cannot be eliminated.

Set-up Variations/Set-up Margin

During a fractionated course of radiotherapy, variations in patient position and in alignment of beams will occur both intra- and inter-fractionally, and a margin for set-up error must be incorporated into the CTV-PTV margin. Errors may be systematic or random.

Systematic errors may result from incorrect data transfer from planning to dose delivery, or inaccurate placing of devices such as compensators, shields, etc. Such systematic errors can be corrected.

Random errors in set-up may be operator dependent, or result from changes in patient anatomy from day to day which are impossible to correct. Accuracy of set-up may be improved with better immobilisation, attention to staff training and/or implanted opaque fiducial markers, such as gold seeds, whose position can be determined in three dimensions at planning and checked during treatment using portal imaging or IGRT. Translational errors can thereby be reduced to as little as 1 mm, and rotational errors to 1°.

Each department should measure its own systematic and random errors for each treatment technique by comparing portal imaging and digitally reconstructed radiographs (DRRs). These measurements are then incorporated into the CTV-PTV margin using the formula devised by van Herk, where the CTV is covered for 90 per cent of the patients with the 95 per cent isodoses:

$$PTV \ margin = 2.5\Sigma + 0.74\sigma$$

where Σ = total standard deviation (SD) computed as the square root of the sum of the squared individual SD values of all systematic errors for organ motion and set up; and σ = total SD of all random errors combined quadratically in a similar way.

This provides a population-derived standard CTV-PTV margin for a particular technique in a given department and can be non-isotropic in cranio-caudal, transverse and anteroposterior (AP) directions. Accurate treatment delivery depends on reducing or eliminating systematic errors and requires a high level of awareness of all staff throughout the many different work areas from localisation through to treatment.

Other theories about how to incorporate organ motion and the uncertainty of the 'mean' position of the CTV on a snapshot CT scan used for localisation have been proposed. van Herk suggests a volume large enough to contain the mean position of the CTV in 90 per cent of cases, called the systematic target volume (STV) (van Herk et al. 2000). Collection of data on the precise CT location of tumour recurrences in relation to the original target volume is important to improve margin definition.

Treated Volume

This is the volume of tissue that is planned to receive a specified dose and is enclosed by the isodose surface corresponding to that dose level, e.g. 95 per cent. The shape, size and position of the treated volume in relation to the PTV should be recorded to evaluate and interpret local recurrences (in field versus marginal) and complications in normal tissues, which may be outside the PTV but within the treated volume.

Conformity Index

This is the ratio of PTV to the treated volume, and indicates how well the PTV is covered by the treatment while minimising dose to normal tissues.

Irradiated Volume

This is the volume of tissue that is irradiated to a dose considered significant in terms of normal tissue tolerance and is dependent on the treatment technique used. The size of the irradiated volume relative to the treated volume (and integral dose) may increase with increasing numbers of beams, but both volumes can be reduced by beam shaping and conformal therapy.

Organs at Risk

These are critical normal tissues whose radiation sensitivity may significantly influence treatment planning and/or prescribed dose. Any movements of the organs at risk (OAR) or uncertainties of set up may be accounted for with a margin similar to the principles for PTV, to create a planning organ at risk volume (PRV). The size of the margin may vary in different directions. Where a PTV and PRV are close or overlap, a clinical decision about relative risks of tumour relapse or normal tissue damage must be made. Shielding of parts of normal organs is possible with the use of multi-leaf collimation (MLC). Dose–volume histograms (DVHs) are used to calculate normal tissue dose distributions.

Immobilisation

The patient must be in a position that is comfortable and reproducible (whether supine or prone), and suitable for acquisition of images for CT scanning and treatment delivery. Immobilisation systems are widely available for every anatomical tumour site and are important in reducing systematic setup errors.

Complex stereotactic or relocatable frames (e.g. Gill–Thomas) are secured to the head by insertion into the mouth of a dental impression of the upper teeth and an occipital impression on the head frame, and are used for stereotactic radiotherapy with a reproducibility of within 1 mm or less. Thermoplastic shells are made by direct moulding of heat-softened material on the patient and can reduce movement in head and neck treatments to about 2 mm. The technician preparing the shell must have details of the tumour site to be treated, e.g. position of the patient (prone, supine, flexion or extension of neck, arm position, etc.). The shell fits over the patient and fastens to a device on the couch with pegs in at least five places.

Relocatable whole body fixation systems using vacuum-moulded bags of polystyrene beads on a stereotactic table top restrict movement to 3–4 mm, and are used to immobilise the trunk and limbs with markings on the bag instead of on the patient's skin. Where the patient has kyphosis, scoliosis or limitation of joint movement, extra limb pads or immobilisation devices may be required. Metallic prostheses, abdominal stomata and the batteries of pacemakers must be located and excluded from the radiation volume where possible. Details of immobilisation devices are discussed in each tumour site chapter.

Parameters of limb rests, thoracic or belly boards, foot rests and leg restraints, thermoplastic shells and skin tattoos should be clearly recorded to avoid transfer errors between the planning process and subsequent treatment. Gantry and couch top flexibility should be measured and couch sag avoided by using rigid radiolucent carbon fibre tables. Table tops must have fixtures for immobilisation devices and laser light systems are essential in CT simulator and treatment units (Figure 2.3). Protocols for bladder and rectal filling, respiration and other patient parameters must be documented at localisation, and reproduced daily during treatment to minimise uncertainties.

CT scans taken for localisation are only a single snapshot, and the CT scan can be repeated daily on several days to measure variation in organ motion and systematic set-up errors for an individual patient. These values can then be used to inform the CTV-PTV margin on an individual basis rather than using population-derived margin values. This is known as adaptive radiotherapy (ART). Kilovoltage (kV), cone beam CT and megavoltage (MV) imaging on treatment machines make it possible to obtain CT

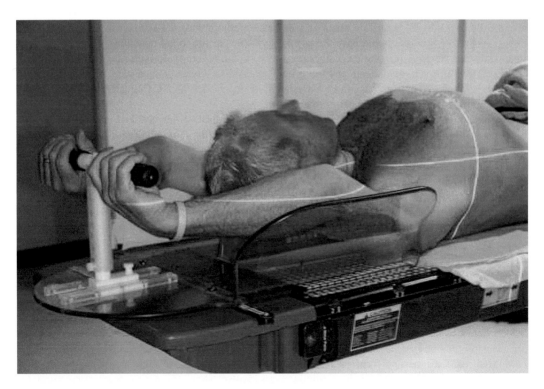

FIGURE 2.3 Patient positioned to show immobilisation on the CT scanner with arms up and laser lights used to prevent rotational setup errors.

images immediately before treatment. While resolution is not as good as with diagnostic CT, the use of fiducial markers and image registration protocols enables daily online IGRT. With this technique only intra-fractional variations and the doctor's CTV delineation error remain.

Data Acquisition

Accurate 3D data about tumours, target volumes and organs at risk are acquired in relation to external reference points under exactly the same conditions as those used for subsequent treatment. Optimal diagnostic imaging modalities are chosen for each tumour site according to protocols developed with diagnostic radiologists. Multi-slice CT, MR with dynamic scanning, 3D ultrasound, positron emission tomography (PET) and single photon emission computed tomography (SPECT) have provided a wealth of anatomical, functional and metabolic information about the GTV. MRI and PET images can be fused with CT planning scans to optimise tumour localisation.

CT Scanning

CT scanning provides detailed cross-sectional anatomy of the normal organs, as well as 3D tumour information. These images provide density data for radiation dose calculations by conversion of CT Hounsfield units into relative electron densities using calibration curves. Compton scattering is the main process of tissue interaction for megavoltage beams and is directly proportional to electron density. Hence CT provides ideal density information for dose corrections for tissue inhomogeneity, such as occurs in lung tissue. Clinical studies have shown that 30–80 per cent of patients undergoing radiotherapy benefit from the increased accuracy of target volume delineation with CT scanning compared with conventional simulation. It has been estimated that the use of CT improves overall five-year survival rates by around 3.5 per cent, with the greatest impact on small volume treatments.

CT scans taken for radiotherapy treatment planning usually differ from those taken for diagnostic use. Ideally, planning CT scans are taken on a dedicated radiotherapy CT scanner by a therapy-trained radiographer. The scanner should have the largest possible aperture to aid positioning of the patient for treatment. The standard diagnostic CT aperture is 70 cm, but 85-cm wide-bore scanners are available, which are helpful for large patients and those being treated for breast cancer, who lie with both arms elevated on an inclined plane that can be extended up to around 15°. The CT couch must be flat topped with accurate couch registration to better than 1 mm.

The patient is positioned using supporting aids and immobilisation devices, and is aligned using tattoos and midline and lateral laser lights identical to those used for subsequent radiotherapy treatment. A tattoo is made on the skin over an immobile bony landmark nearest to the centre of the target volume (e.g. pubic symphysis). It is marked with radio-opaque material such as a catheter or barium paste for visualisation on the CT image. Additional lateral tattoos are used to prevent lateral rotation of the patient and are aligned using horizontal lasers (see Figure 2.3).

Oral contrast medium is used in a small concentrated dose to outline the small bowel as an organ at risk (e.g. for pelvic intensity-modulated radiotherapy [IMRT] treatment), but care must be taken to avoid large quantities, which may cause diuresis and overfill the bladder. Intravenous contrast is given for many patients, for example in lung and mediastinal tumours to differentiate between mediastinal vascular structures, tumour and lymph nodes, and in the pelvis to enhance blood vessels for CTV delineation of lymph nodes. Structures such as the vulva, vaginal introitus, anal margin, stomata and surgical scars may be marked with radio-opaque material. Patients with locally advanced tumours should be examined in the treatment position, and tumour margins clearly marked. Protocols to reduce organ motion, for example by emptying the bladder before bladder radiotherapy and the rectum before prostate treatment, need to be in place. Patients are given information leaflets to explain the importance of, and rationale for, these procedures.

Multi-slice CT scanners perform a scan of the entire chest or abdomen in a few seconds with the patient breathing normally. Scanning for lung tumours can involve 'slow' CT scans, respiratory-correlated CT scans using a 4D technique with external surrogate or fiducial marker, abdominal compression or use of the ABC device to cope with the effect of respiratory movement.

Protocols for CT scanning are developed with radiologists to optimise tumour information, to ensure full body contour in the reconstruction circle and scanning of relevant whole organs for DVHs. DRRs are produced from CT density information and are compared with electronic portal images (EPIs). Contiguous thin CT slices are obtained at 2–5-mm intervals for the head and 3–10 mm for the body. Some tumour sites such as the brain or lung benefit from image fusion techniques to aid target volume contouring. MRI or PET-scan images are fused with the planning CT. Care must be taken that the scans are performed with corresponding setup and immobilisation to ensure accurate registration. MRI images can provide improved delineation by offering superior soft tissue contrast to allow the oncologist to contour the tumour and organs at risk with greater confidence. There is increasing interest and research in implementing MRI-only radiotherapy work flows. The registration of CT and MRI imaging is not needed, and a method for assigning electron densities to the MRI for dosimetric calculation is used. This is an area of active research including nonrigid registration of MRI to CT atlases, segmentation techniques to assign bulk electron densities and using MRI to create pseudo-CT images. Commercial solutions for MRI simulation and radiotherapy planning and delivery are emerging, and clinical trials using MRI-linear accelerator radiotherapy systems are currently underway.

Contouring

CT scans are transferred digitally to the target volume localisation console using an electronic network system, which must be compliant with DICOM 3 and DICOM RT protocols (Figure 2.4). The GTV, CTV, PTV, body contour and normal organs are outlined by a team of radiation oncologist, specialist radiologist and planning technician, with appropriate training. Where MRI is the optimal imaging modality for tumours such as those in the prostate, uterus, brain, head and neck and sarcomas, it is incorporated into target volume definition by image fusion. Treatment planning based on MR images alone is under investigation, but more commonly CT and MR images are co-registered, ideally scanning using a flat MRI couch top to aid matching. PET or PET-CT images may give additional information for head and neck tumours, lymphomas, lung and gynaecological tumours, and SPECT for brain tumours. Multimodality image fusion of all these images in the treatment planning process is ideal for accurate delineation of the target.

Departmental protocols for target volume delineation are essential for each tumour site; these should define optimal window settings, how to construct the CTV, 3D values for CTV-PTV margins, type of 3D expansion software and method of outlining for each OAR to be used. 'Doctor's delineation errors' resulting from contouring are said to be the most uncertain part of the whole planning process, and training in, and validation of, these procedures is essential. It has become standard practice in many centres to peer review all complex volume contours to improve quality assurance.

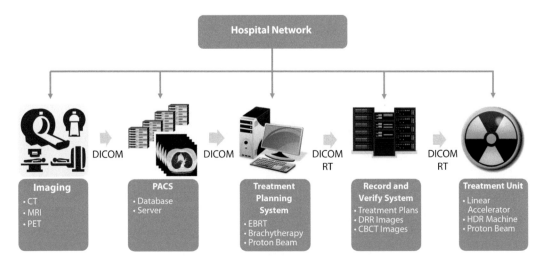

FIGURE 2.4   Network for transferring data between steps in the radiotherapy planning process. (Guys Cancer centre.)

Contouring starts with definition of the GTV on a central slice of the primary tumour, and then on each axial CT image moving superiorly and then inferiorly. Involved nodes can then be defined in the same way. Viewing the GTV on coronal and sagittal DRRs ensures consistency of definition between slices so that no artificial steps in the volume are created. A volume should not be copied or cut and pasted onto sequential slices for risk of pasting an error: it is more accurate to redraw the GTV on each slice. If there are slices where the GTV cannot be defined – for example, due to a dental artefact – the planning software will usually allow the missing contours to be interpolated from those either side.

CT Virtual Simulation

Using CT data, software generates images from a beam's eye perspective, which are equivalent to conventional simulator images. External landmarks are used to define an internal isocentre for treatment set-up. The CT simulator provides maximal tumour information along with full 3D capabilities (unlike the simulator CT facility). It is particularly useful for designing palliative treatments such as for lung and vertebral metastases, along with some breast treatments using tangential beams, which can be virtually simulated and then 3D planned. The ability to derive CT scans, and provide target volume definition, margin generation and simulation all on one workstation, provides a rapid solution.

Conventional Simulator

For palliative treatments, a simulator may still be used to define field borders following the 50 per cent isodose line of the beam, rather than a target volume. A simulator is an isocentrically mounted diagnostic X-ray machine that can reproduce all the movements of the treatment unit and has an image intensifier for screening. The patient is prepared in the treatment position exactly as described earlier for CT scanning. The machine rotates around the patient on an axis centred on a fixed point, the isocentre, which is 100 cm from the focal spot and is placed at the centre of the target volume. Digital images or radiographs are used to record the field borders chosen by reference to bony landmarks. The simulator is commonly used either for palliative single field treatments of bone metastases or to define opposing anterior and posterior fields for palliative treatment to locally advanced tumour masses.

Dose Solutions

When the PTV and normal organs have been defined in 3D, the optimal dose distribution for treating the tumour is devised. Consultation with a dosimetrist or physicist is vital to select the best parameters. For example, a treatment machine must be chosen according to percentage depth dose characteristics and buildup depth, which will vary with energy and beam size, as shown in Table 2.1. These can be used to calculate doses for treatment using single fields and to learn the construction of isodose distributions using computer modelling. Other factors to be considered in the choice of machine are the effect of penumbra on beam definition, the availability of independent or multi-leaf collimators, facilities for

TABLE 2.1

Data from Treatment Machines in Common Use, Showing Variation of D_{max} and Percentage Depth Dose (DD) with Energy

			10 x 10 cm Field[a]	
Machine	Energy (MV)	FSD (cm)	D_{max} Depth (cm)	% DD at 10 cm
Cobalt-60	1.25	100	0.5	58.7
Linear accelerator	6	100	1.5	67.5
	10	100	2.3	73
	16	100	2.8	76.8

[a] Maximum field size at 100 cm is 40×40 cm.

beam modification and portal imaging. Most dose computation is done using 3D computerised treatment planning systems which are programmed with beam data from therapy machines. These systems require careful quality control programmes. Following production of a satisfactory isodose distribution to a given target volume using 2D or 3D algorithms, the calculations are checked by a physicist, and detailed instructions for delivery are prepared by radiographers on the therapy unit.

There are different types of planning and treatment solutions of increasing complexity and special techniques described under the following headings:

- *Simple treatment* involves single or opposing beams, with or without 2D dose distributions, with compensators and simple shielding. Simple treatments include direct fields with electrons and superficial/orthovoltage photons.
- *Conformal treatment* involves target volume delineation of tumours and normal organs according to ICRU principles, with 3D dose calculations using MLC to shape beams.
- *Complex treatment* involves the use of static or dynamic IMRT, VMAT or Tomotherapy, IGRT and 3D or 4D delivery.
- *Special techniques* include stereotactic radiotherapy and protons.

Simple Treatment

Single fields may be used with borders defined by the 50 per cent isodose for bone metastases. Parallel opposing beams can be used for speed and ease of set-up for palliative treatments (e.g. lung), for target volumes of small separation (e.g. early larynx cancer) or tangential volumes (e.g. breast). Isodose distributions show that the 95 per cent isodose does not conform closely to the target volume, the distribution of dose is not homogeneous and much normal tissue is irradiated to the same dose as the tumour. Beam modification with the use of wedges alters the dose distribution to compensate for missing tissue, obliquity of body contour or a sloping target volume, and may produce a more homogeneous result.

For many tumours seated at depth, a curative radical tumour dose can only be achieved with a combination of several beams, if overdose to the skin and other superficial tissues is to be avoided. When multiple beams are chosen for a plan, variable wedges can be used to attenuate the beam and thereby avoid a high dose area at beam intersections. To achieve the same dose at the patient, the number of monitor units set will have to be increased compared with those for an open field. Computerised dose planning systems are used to construct an isodose distribution with beams of appropriate energy, size, weighting, gantry angle and wedge to give a homogeneous result over the target volume.

Inhomogeneity Corrections

Attenuation of an X-ray beam is affected by tissue density, being less in lung than bone. This variation affects both the shape of the dose distribution and the values of the isodoses. Lung tissue should therefore be localised when planning treatment for tumours of the thorax (e.g. lung, breast, oesophagus, mediastinum). The relative electron density of lung compared with water is in the range 0.2–0.3 and these values are used to correct for inhomogeneity.

When 2D conventional planning is used, correction is only valid at the planned central slice of the target volume, e.g. breast treatment planned with a simulator using central lung distance (CLD). Using CT scanning, the whole lung is localised in 3D and a pixel by pixel correction made for all tissue densities by conversion of CT numbers into relative electron densities using calibration curves. CT numbers are affected by contrast agents, but dose distributions in the chest and abdomen are not significantly changed by the quantities used in most CT scanning protocols. However, large amounts of gas in the rectum can cause organ motion of the prostate and uterus along with affecting CT densities. When complex planning is used, commercial treatment planning systems apply heterogeneity-corrected calculation algorithms classified as Type A to Type C. Type A are conventional homogenous dose calculations, Type B are convolution/superposition algorithms and the most recent Type C include fast Monte Carlo and Acuros XB algorithms.

Beam Junctions

When treatment is given to target volumes that lie adjacent to one another, consideration must be given to the nonuniformity of dose in the potential overlap regions caused by divergence of the adjacent beams. If the beams abut on the skin surface, they will overlap with excess dose at depth. If there is a gap between beams at the skin, there will be a cold area in the superficial tissues. Clinical examples of this problem include treatment of adjacent vertebrae with single posterior fields which may be separated in time, where there is a risk of overlap of dose at the underlying spinal cord, and the treatment of primary breast cancer and adjacent lymph nodes, where a single isocentric technique centred at the junction can be used (see Chapter 22).

Various techniques have been developed to minimise dose heterogeneity at beam junctions in these different clinical situations. Half-beam blocking using shielding or independent collimator jaws can be used to eliminate divergence up to the match line, but accuracy is then dependent on precise immobilisation and reliability of skin marks to reproduce the match perfectly. Couch rotation can be used to remove beam divergence when matching breast and lymph node irradiation. However, for some sites, it is still common to match beams by using a gap between beams so that the beam edges converge at a planned depth (Figure 2.5). The dose in the triangular gap (x) below the skin surface will be lower than at the point P where the beams converge because it lies outside the geometric margins of both beams. Doses at (y) are higher because they include contributions from both beams. The positioning of point P anatomically will vary according to the aim of treatment. If treatment is for medulloblastoma, a homogeneous dose is required for potential tumour cells within the spinal cord, which is therefore placed at point P, and point P is moved in a cranio-caudal direction at regular intervals to prevent any risk of overdose at junctions. Where treatment is aimed at metastases in adjacent vertebral bodies, it is important to avoid overdosage at the spinal cord, which is therefore placed in the superficial cold triangle (x) with point P anterior to it. The gap on the skin is the sum of the beam divergence of each beam. It is calculated as the distance from the edge of the beam, as defined by the 50 per cent isodose, to the point of convergence P measured perpendicular to the central axis and marked (s) spread (beam divergence) for each beam. Graphs have been drawn up expressing beam divergence as a function of the depth below the skin for different field sizes and focus skin distance (FSD). Once the gap has been calculated, it may be necessary to increase it slightly to allow for possible movement of patient or skin tattoos, to ensure that there is no overdosage. Whenever possible, a patient should be treated in the same position (supine or prone) for matching adjacent fields.

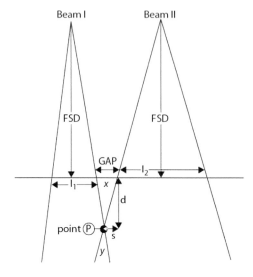

FIGURE 2.5   Technique for matching two beams I and II (length I_1 and I_2) at a point P at depth d by allowing a gap on the skin surface (x, y, s – see text).

When planning a new treatment for metastatic disease in the spine, previous treatment fields should be reconstructed from previous CT simulation data, films and records, and the patient placed in the same position to ensure there is no overlap.

Electron Therapy

Electron therapy may be used to treat superficial tumours overlying cartilage and bone (for example nose, ear, scalp and dorsum of hand), in preference to superficial or orthovoltage therapy where there is increased bone absorption due to the photoelectric effect. There is a sharp fall in dose beyond the 90 per cent isodose (4–12 MeV) and electron energy is chosen so that the target volume is encompassed by the 90–95 per cent isodose at the deep margin. Electrons at higher energies (15–25 MeV) may be used for treating cervical lymph nodes overlying spinal cord, parotid tumours and in mixed beams with photons. The effective treatment depth in centimetres is about one-third of the beam energy in MeV and the total range about half (Figure 2.6), but this is dependent on field size. Different tissue densities such as bone and air (as found in ribs overlying lung and facial bones containing air-filled sinuses) cause inhomogeneous dose distributions. Doses beyond air cavities may be higher than expected, even after density corrections, and this limits the usefulness of electrons for treatment in these clinical situations. Electron beam edges do not diverge geometrically due to lateral scatter, which is greater at low energies with the characteristic shape shown in Figure 2.7. Wider margins must be added when choosing the beam width for adequate treatment of tumours at depth. Where there is tumour infiltration of skin, the skin-sparing characteristics of electron beams below 16 MeV should be removed by adding bolus material, which can also be used to provide tissue equivalent material for an irregular contour such as the nose or ear. Beam sizes <40 × 40 mm should be avoided because of inadequate depth of penetration and loss of beam flatness.

Conformal Treatment

3D conformal radiotherapy (CFRT) links 3D CT visualisation of the tumour with the capability of the linear accelerator to shape the beams geometrically to fit the profile of the target from a beam's eye view using a multi-leaf collimator (MLC). Typical MLCs have 20–80 leaves arranged in opposing pairs which

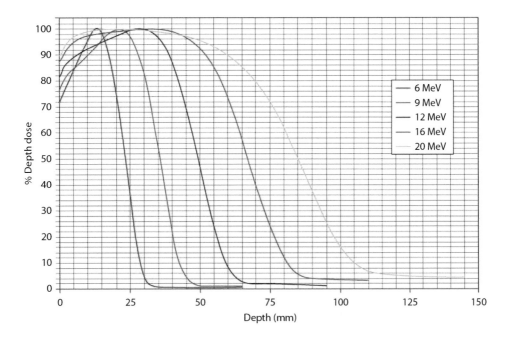

FIGURE 2.6 Percentage depth dose of varying electron energies for 10 × 10 cm applicator.

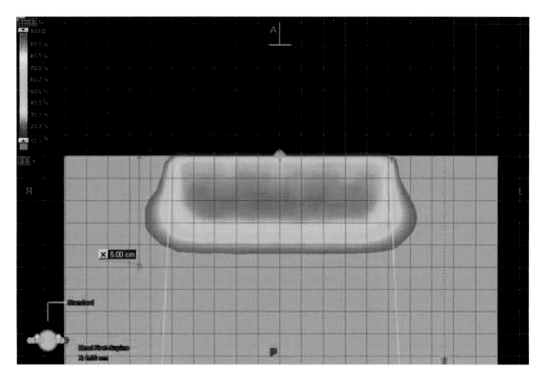

FIGURE 2.7   9 MeV electron dose distribution.

can be positioned under computer control to create an irregular beam conforming to the target shape. Along with eliminating the hazards of production and use of alloy blocks, this system allows rapid adjustment of shaping to match the beam's eye view of the PTV. This encloses the target volume as closely as possible while reducing the dose to adjacent normal tissues. The radiation oncologist and dosimetrist agree on the final PTV, which has been created using 3D growth algorithm software and departmental protocols, taking into consideration OARs. Discussions between oncologist and dosimetrist include an understanding of the tumour cell density pattern within the PTV, requirements for homogeneity of dose distribution, dose constraints to adjacent OARs, avoidance of maximum or minimum dose spots in 3D and review of a preliminary plan of likely beam arrangements. Basic CFRT may consist of coplanar and static beams with MLC or conformal blocks shaping the volume. Conformal therapy may involve the use of mixed beams combining photons and electrons for part of the treatment. Beams can be modified using bolus, wedges, compensators, MLCs and shielding blocks. Optimisation of skin dose is achieved by skin sparing using higher megavoltage energies, or by maximising skin dose with tissue equivalent bolus. Higher beam energies (10–18 MV) are preferred for pelvic treatments, to increase dose to the centre and reduce dose to skin and subcutaneous tissues. Lower energies (6–8 MV) are used for breast and head and neck treatments to avoid excess skin sparing and treat the relatively superficial target volume. For coplanar non-standard configuration of beams, DVHs may aid selection of the best plan, but they do not indicate which part of the organ is receiving a high or low dose; DVHs of the PTV, CTV and all PRVs are needed to allow subsequent correlation with clinical outcome. Selection of the final dose plan is made at the treatment-planning terminal by inspecting 3D physical dose distributions and DVHs. Good communication is important between radiographer, dosimetrist, physicist and clinician to avoid transfer errors occurring between CT, treatment planning and treatment machine.

Complex Treatment

IMRT improves the ability to conform the treatment volume to concave tumour shapes. It uses the MLC to define the beam intensity independently in different regions of each incident beam, to produce the desired uniform distribution of dose, or a deliberate non-uniform dose distribution, in the target volume. The position of the leaves of the MLC can be varied in time with a fixed or moving gantry. Step and shoot or static IMRT is where the MLC divide each radiation beam into a set of smaller segments of differing MLC shape, and the radiation is delivered while the MLC leaves are stationary, with the beam switched off between the segments.

Sliding window or dynamic IMRT is where each beam is modulated by continuously moving the MLC and the radiation is delivered while the MLC leaves are moving. An increased number of monitor units is needed to deliver an IMRT plan compared to a 3D conformal plan. The delivery time and number of monitor units needed is decreased using modern arc therapy techniques such as volumetric arc therapy (VMAT). VMAT delivers radiation while the gantry rotates using one or more arcs, varying dose rates and gantry speeds with dynamic continuous changing shape of the MLC. Other methods include tomotherapy, where there is intensity-modulated rotational delivery with a fan beam where serial or axial dose distributions are delivered slice by slice.

IMRT can be forward or inverse planned. Forward planning is a manual trial and error process where the planner places beams onto the radiotherapy planning system and then the planning system calculates the required monitor units and the dose distribution. It is only used for relatively simple cases. Inverse planning is where the oncologist defines the patient's tumour volumes and the organs at risk volumes, the planner gives an importance factor to each structure and constraints, and then an optimisation programme is run to find the treatment plan which best matches all the input criteria.

The decision about which planning technique to use is multifactorial. The factors include software differences such as dose calculation algorithms and how these relate to tumour and OAR dose to create the optimum treatment plan. Tissue differences should be considered, such as lung tissue vs solid tumour and how that affects dose distribution. Quality assurance checks are different with different techniques and may determine which technique to use along with treatment delivery time.

Plans can be produced with concave shapes, and critical structures at sites such as head and neck (eye or spinal cord) and prostate (rectum) can be avoided. Late toxicity can be reduced significantly for tumour sites such as prostate, pelvis, breast and head and neck. Dose escalation studies in prostate cancer show an improvement in biochemical relapse-free survival using IMRT with reduced late rectal toxicity. There is proof of sparing of salivary gland function with IMRT for head and neck cancer with no loss of tumour control. Late fibrotic changes in the breast can be reduced, and IMRT pelvic treatments, more conformal to the tumour lymph node drainage, have reduced bone marrow and acute bowel and bladder toxicity. However, integral dose may be greater with some IMRT solutions, with increased risk of late malignancies. IMRT dose plans with steep dose gradients may risk underdosage of tumour, if margins are close and organ motion still present.

Verification of an IMRT plan requires either measurement of the dose distribution in a phantom, or an independent monitor unit calculation with portal dosimetry. Dose delivery is verified throughout the course of treatment using radiographic film or adapted EPIDs or transit dosimetry. Accurate patient positioning, target volume delineation and reduction of organ and patient motion uncertainties, especially respiration, are critical for safe IMRT. Centres with the relevant experience and quality assurance programmes should use IMRT whenever it offers a superior dosimetric solution in terms of reduced toxicity and improved tumour control.

Special Techniques

Stereotactic Radiotherapy

Stereotactic radiotherapy is precise irradiation of image-defined lesions with a high radiation dose delivered in a small number of fractions. Stereotactic radiosurgery (SRS) is a single fraction of stereotactic-directed radiation of a limited volume in the brain or in the skull base using a rigid immobilisation frame. Stereotactic radiotherapy (SRT) is fractionated stereotactic-directed radiation of a limited volume in the brain. Stereotactic body radiotherapy (SABR) is the use of stereotactic-directed radiation therapy to structures outside the brain and skull. A principle of stereotactic radiotherapy is the use of real-time IGRT to account for tumour and organ motion.

SRS and SRT are mainly used for the treatment of small brain tumours and arteriovenous malformations. Accuracy of patient positioning to approximately 1 mm is maintained using a stereotactic frame attached to the patient's skull. Radiotherapy may be delivered as a single or multiple fractions and may be considered as an alternative to surgery. The gamma knife device uses multiple cobalt sources arranged around a half circle, which irradiate a very conformal volume by blocking selected collimator openings with different collimation helmets for different time intervals. Alternatively, a linear accelerator with specialised collimators can be used to deliver multiple arc therapy. This technique requires very careful quality assurance because of steep dose gradients and problems of electron equilibration with very small beams. It also requires close collaboration within a team of people with relevant expertise in imaging, neuroanatomy, tumour management and physics.

SABR has an established role in the treatment of non-small cell lung cancer, prostate cancer, liver metastases, hepatocellular carcinoma, re-irradiation of pelvis and spine and oligometastases. It has been introduced in the UK via the commissioning through Evaluation (CtE) programme. There are several SABR treatment delivery systems available. Cyberknife is an image-guided robotic radiosurgery system purpose built for the delivery of SRT and SABR. There are a number of modern linear accelerators with onboard imaging capabilities that meet the IGRT requirements for delivering SABR, e.g. Varian Trilogy, RapidArc, TrueBeam, Electa Synergy and Tomotherapy HiArt. These systems use rigid immobilisation specific to the body region being treated and IMRT or VMAT to achieve the best dose distribution with a steep dose fall off to minimise the dose to the organs at risk. They all include advanced IGRT solutions, including respiratory gating and other techniques using implanted fiducial markers. SABR delivers large doses per fraction (e.g. >8 Gy/#) with the aim of ablating all the tissue within the PTV.

SABR is typically prescribed to a prescription isodose of 60–80 per cent, creating considerable dose inhomogeneity within the target volume – more than recommended by ICRU 50. Radiation schedules used in SABR cannot be directly compared to those used with conventional fractionation. To compare regimens, the BED must be calculated. Normal tissue organ at risk (OAR) dose constraints are based on BED calculations and experience from clinical trials. For serial organs, constraints are described as the maximum volume of the organ that can receive a threshold dose or more, e.g. the volume of small bowel receiving a dose of 15 Gy or more should be less than 120 cc (D120 cc<15 Gy). For parallel organs, the constraints are described as a maximum percentage volume of the organ that received a threshold dose or more. E.g. the volume of lung receiving a dose of 20 Gy or more should be less than 10 per cent of the total lung volume (V20 Gy<10%).

Protons

Proton therapy is where radiation treatment is delivered by accelerated proton beams rather than X-rays. Protons are accelerated using cyclotrons, which produce protons with energies in the range of 70 to 250 MeV. The dose delivered to the tissue is maximum over the last few millimetres of the particles' range; this is called the Bragg peak. In most treatments, protons of different energies with Bragg peaks at different depths are used to encompass the target for treatment within the spread out Pristine Bragg peak (SOBP); see Figure 2.8.

In the UK there has long been a proton beam therapy centre in Clatterbridge which delivered low-energy proton beam therapy for NHS patients with eye tumours. There are now two new UK proton therapy centres, one in Manchester and the other in London.

There are indications that the benefits of protons have been established, such as some paediatric tumours, skull-based tumours and some radio-resistant tumours in difficult sites such as vertebral chondrosarcoma. Current evidence does not show an established benefit to recommend proton therapy over IMRT for most head and neck, breast, lung, gastrointestinal tract and pelvic cancers, including prostate cancer. The UK proton programme is uniquely placed to undertake randomised controlled trials of proton vs photon radiation, and trials are now being designed in a wide variety of tumour types.

There is a UK national panel of clinical experts who review individual cases referred for proton therapy. This panel decides on whether a case is suitable for proton beam therapy in line with the NHS England clinical commissioning policies and confirms if the case can be referred to one of the UK NHS centres.

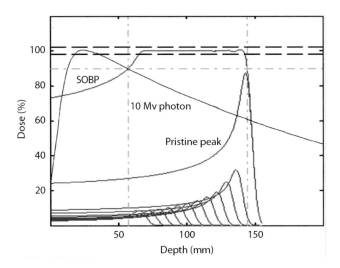

FIGURE 2.8 Depth dose of photons and protons. (From Proton beam therapy. *Br J Cancer* 2005 Oct 2017;93(8):849–854.)

Dose Fractionation

Prescription of radiotherapy treatment is the responsibility of the radiation oncologist and usually follows agreed guidelines, taking into consideration individual patient factors, such as the expected risk–benefit ratio of treatment, comorbidities and consideration of scheduling of other treatment modalities. Radiotherapy regimens vary internationally. Fractions of 2 Gy or less delivered five days a week are the standard of care in much of North America and Europe. Regimens given in this book are safe evidence-based schedules, but national and international protocols or trials should be used as appropriate.

Alternative fractionation schedules using fewer larger fractions in a shorter overall time (hypofractionation) have been developed, especially in the UK and Canada, driven initially by resource constraints, but now supported by extensive published clinical data, e.g. for breast and prostate cancer along with palliative treatments. Accelerated fractionation gives the same overall dose in a shorter time, often using smaller fraction sizes to reduce toxicity, and has been used successfully in head and neck cancer trials. Hyperfractionation regimens deliver treatment twice or three times a day using smaller fraction sizes, thereby increasing the total dose and remaining within tolerance for late toxicity (see Table 3.2, p. 34).

The linear quadratic (LQ) model of radiation-induced cell killing is currently the most useful for comparing different fractionation schedules (see Chapter 3), taking into account the effect of dose per fraction and repopulation on tumour and normal tissue late effects. Clinical outcome depends on the total dose, dose per fraction, overall treatment time, volume of tumour and normal tissues irradiated, dose specification points and quality control procedures. If treatment has to be stopped unexpectedly for operational or clinical reasons, causing an unscheduled gap in treatment, the dose fractionation schedule may need to be altered (see Chapter 3).

Dose Specification

All dose distributions are inhomogeneous, and so the dose throughout the PTV varies. The biological effect of a given dose is difficult to predict because of variations in cell density at the centre and periphery of the CTV, heterogeneity of tumour cell populations and inadequate knowledge of cellular radiosensitivity. Nevertheless, one must attempt to specify a dose which is representative of the absorbed dose in the target volume as a whole, to assess effectiveness of treatment.

To facilitate understanding and exchange of precise and accurate radiotherapy treatment data, it is important that all centres report their results using the same volume concepts and prescribing definitions.

The ICRU reports 50 and 62 recommend that the radiation dose should be reported, and hence is also best prescribed at or near the centre of the PTV, and when possible at the intersection of the beam axes (ICRU reference dose). This ICRU reference point for prescription is selected because it is clinically relevant, usually situated where there is maximum tumour cell density, easy to define, often lies on the central axis of the beam where dose can be accurately determined, and is not in a region of steep dose gradient. It is essential that this dose specification point is accompanied by a statement of the homogeneity of the irradiation as defined by at least the maximum and minimum doses to the PTV. The maximum target dose is the highest dose in the target volume which is clinically significant (to a volume greater than 15 mm³, unless in a critical tissue where special considerations apply). The minimum target dose is an important parameter because it correlates with the probability of tumour control. The ICRU report 83 evolved and adapted the previous recommendations for IMRT and the technological advances. The report recommended a dose-volume-based specification of absorbed dose employing the concept of DVHs. The minimum and maximum absorbed doses have been replaced by the near minimum D98 per cent, and near maximum D2 per cent. The report recommends that the median absorbed dose specified by the D50 per cent should be reported and is considered to correspond best with the previous ICRU reference point. See an example IMRT plan and DVH in Figure 2.9.

Superficial treatment machines, with energies ranging from 50 kV to 150 kV, and appropriate filtration, which defines percentage depth dose characteristics, are used to treat superficial skin tumours. The dose prescription point is at D_{max}, the maximum dose, which is at the skin surface. An appropriate energy

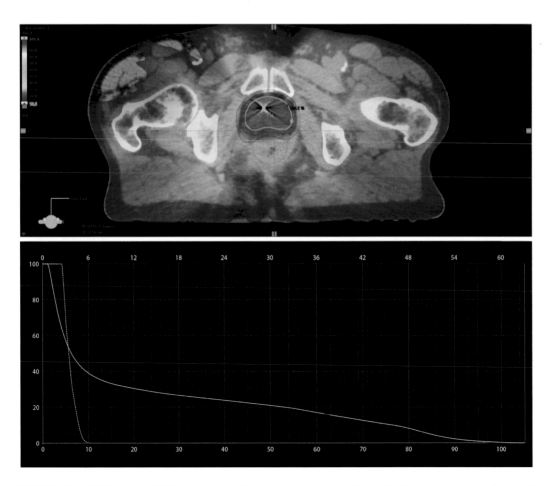

FIGURE 2.9   IMRT plan and DVH for treatment of prostate cancer (rectum brown, bladder yellow, penile bulb dotted yellow, spacer orange, CTV cyan, PTV red).

is selected from tables for different beam sizes for a given FSD to encompass the target volume both on the skin and at depth with a 90 per cent isodose.

When a single megavoltage beam is used, dose is prescribed to the ICRU point at the centre of the target volume rather than to D_{max}. For example, for bone metastases, the prescription point may be at the centre of the vertebra, e.g. 40–50 mm depth for a thoracic vertebra. Alternatively, for palliative treatments, the ICRU point may be chosen at the dose-limiting structure, such as the spinal cord, and a dose prescribed to maximum tolerance.

For co-axial opposing lateral or AP beams, the dose is specified at the midplane dose (MPD) on the central axis of the beam, as recommended by ICRU. In subsequent chapters of this book, these ICRU dose specification conventions have been followed for all dose distributions and prescriptions.

Verification and IGRT

The increased conformity of radiotherapy planning with IMRT heightens the need to ensure the accuracy of the radiation field placement and to reduce the exposure of the organs at risk. Organ motion during treatment makes it necessary to consider the fourth dimension of time. IGRT refers to imaging techniques that are used to check that the actual treatment delivered matches that which has been planned.

Both inter- and intra-fraction uncertainties may be a result of a combination of systematic and random errors. As discussed earlier, margins are added to the CTV to take account of these errors. Improving IGRT allows confident use of smaller PTV margins but must be done with care with coordination between the planning process and image guidance process with a feedback loop so that the expected accuracy of the treatment is actually delivered.

Offline IGRT correction is where images are acquired before treatment and matched to the reference image at a later time to determine the individual systematic set-up error and attempt to reduce it. When combined with the set-up data of other patients treated on the same protocol it allows definition of the standard error for the treatment in that centre. Published offline correction protocols are widely used, including the shrinking action level and no action level protocols.

Online IGRT correction is where images are acquired and any corrections are made prior to that day's treatment. Daily imaging is often used for treating sites in the abdomen, pelvis and thorax and where even small shifts are important close to critical structures.

There are several IGRT imaging methods in current use. Non-radiation-based systems include ultrasound bases systems such as BAT, SonArray and Clarity, which are used in prostate, lung and breast radiotherapy; camera-based infrared or optical tracking systems such as AlignRT; and electromagnetic tracking systems such as Calypso, which uses electromagnetic transponders. Radiation-based systems include EPIDs, Cone beam CT (kV or MV), FanBeam Kv CT (CT on rails) and FanBeam MV CT (Tomotherapy HiART II). Real-time 4D tracing for intra-fraction IGRT using fiducial markers can be done using Autobeam hold on Rapidarc machines or with 2D KV stereoscopic imaging on Cyberknife.

Variations in overall positioning of the body during treatment can be monitored using optical imaging devices, sometimes in association with markers attached to the skin. To avoid respiratory motion, treatment may be delivered while patients hold their breath using the ABC device. This demands cooperation from the patient and may be difficult in those with lung diseases. Treatment may be gated to a specific phase of the respiratory cycle, usually expiration, using optical devices or X-ray fluoroscopic measurements. CT scans obtained by imaging devices on the linear accelerator can be compared with respiration-correlated spiral CT planning images. Treatment delivery is triggered when the two images match. For other tumours, e.g. prostate or liver, internal fiducial markers may need to be placed within or in direct contact with the tumour, so that the tumour motion can be tracked by monitoring the position of the fiducials during translations, rotations and deformation. Ideally, the moving tumour outline is imaged during treatment using daily EPIs or real-time cone beam CT. Alternatively, EPIs can be taken on the first few days of treatment and used to adjust treatment volumes where necessary.

Adaptive radiotherapy (ART) involves regular changes (weekly or daily) to treatment delivery for an individual patient based on analysis of images taken offline between treatments, online immediately before treatment and in real time during treatment. Linear accelerator-mounted imaging devices and

IGRT are essential. The treatment plan delivered to the patient is changed based on observed anatomic changes caused by tumour shrinkage, internal motion, weight loss or other changes such as bladder filling, rectal emptying or stomach emptying. No one solution for ART exists. Corrective plans can be based on a predetermined set of scenarios, for example current trials in bladder cancer generate three radiotherapy plans with the most appropriate plan on the day selected depending on variations in bladder filling and position. More advanced ART techniques are being researched using deformable image registration, automatic treatment planning, deformable dose summation and real-time imaging.

Verification of the dose delivered to the patient can be measured using semiconductor silicon diodes with instant readout, or thermo-luminescent dosimetry (TLD) with delayed readout, and is usually performed on the first day of each patient's treatment. Transit dosimetry uses a transmission portal image to measure the dose delivered to the patient, which can be compared with the planned dose distribution. Equally important are the mechanical checks of MLC that are required to ensure safe delivery of treatments. These must include examination of the stability of leaf speed, accuracy of leaf position and transmission through and between leaves.

Patient Care during Treatment

Response to treatment, both in terms of tumour and acute side effects, should be monitored regularly. Weekly clinics are held, often led by a therapy radiographer or radiotherapy clinical nurse specialist, to check for early acute side effects, and to answer patients' questions and give them and their carers psychological and emotional support. Information sheets listing common and uncommon side effects for each tumour site are discussed with individual patients when they give informed consent. Protocols for scoring acute side effects, such as NCI-CTC-3 or RTOG, should be used to document acute reactions and guide appropriate investigations.

The radiation oncologist specifies imaging or blood tests that are required during treatment and is responsible for overseeing the review clinics. Patients receiving radiotherapy with concomitant or sequential chemotherapy may experience increased side effects and require special interventions. Specific instructions for dealing with different acute reactions are dealt with in each individual tumour site chapter.

Quality Assurance

A comprehensive quality assurance programme is needed to ensure that the best possible care is delivered to the patient by defining and documenting all procedures involved in radiotherapy treatments. A quality assurance policy must be formulated by a radiotherapy manager with overall responsibility for implementation, although large parts of this responsibility may be delegated to other appropriately trained and qualified members of the radiotherapy team. Internal quality assurance systems are supplemented by external accreditation visits. Individual treatment techniques may be checked before trials begin, by requiring participants to submit sample treatment plans and descriptions of treatment techniques. Phantom measurements are routinely used to give a composite check of all factors, including dose homogeneity and beam matching. Any internal or external system must be periodically reviewed with documentation of all activity according to a defined protocol. Reference values must be specified with tolerances and action to be taken if these are exceeded. A departmental procedure for investigation of deviations or errors must be in place for every part of the system.

Practical Considerations

Routine checks of the following must be included in the quality assurance protocol:

- Machine checks
- Dosimetry protocols
- Planning checks
- Patient documentation

Machine Checks

During installation and acceptance of a new unit of equipment, calibration data are obtained to provide reference against which subsequent checks are made. Inter-comparisons between different institutions or with national or international standards are useful for detecting systematic errors. Quality control should then ensure that a unit performs according to its specification and is safe for both patients and staff. It should guarantee accuracy of dose delivered, prevent major errors, minimise downtime for machines and encourage preventative machine maintenance. There should be a specific quality control protocol for each unit which outlines the test to be performed, the methods to be used to ensure consistency in the performance of each unit, parameters to be tested, frequency of measurement, staff responsibilities, reference values, tolerances, action to be taken in case of deviation and rules for documentation. Daily, weekly and extended testing of dosimetry beam alignment and safety checks are necessary. Regular checks include tests of optical, mechanical and computer hardware and software systems. Action levels are defined where correction is needed before treatment can proceed. Similar checks must be carried out for all imaging equipment and treatment planning systems. The results of daily checks must be recorded in the control room of the treatment units, and radiographers must also record any problems in machine functioning. All other checks, actions and maintenance work are recorded in a separate log book. Good cooperation is needed between all staff groups. A physicist, who coordinates all quality control activity, checks that tests are up to standard and reports any major deviations to the clinicians.

Dosimetry Protocols

These include dose monitor calibration checks, checks of beam quality and symmetry and evaluation of beam flatness. In vivo dosimetry systems such as TLDs and silicon diodes must also be regularly checked and calibrated.

Planning Checks

Treatment prescriptions are now mostly electronic, and recording of treatment delivery parameters is automatic by computer systems attached to treatment machines. Reports of activity obtained from these systems can be used for audit, and central collection of these output data may give very useful information about patterns of radiotherapy delivery. Individual weekly review of patients' treatment records should verify that treatment is being delivered as planned.

Patient Documentation

Electronic patient record systems are increasingly being used. Radiation treatment records are often kept separately from other hospital documents to ensure reliable rapid access. Records should identify the patient, give clinical history and examination findings, histological diagnosis, staging of the tumour and proposed treatment plan. There should be written treatment policies for specific tumour sites, and data should be recorded to enable subsequent evaluation of the outcome of treatment. Written consent for treatment is required. At the end of treatment, a summary detailing actual treatment parameters must be prepared, and appropriate continuing care of the patient assured.

Staffing

A quality programme as just described is essential for the safe delivery of treatment. It can only be achieved if each member of the team clearly understands the boundaries of responsibility and if there is excellent coordination of all quality control activity by a highly qualified physicist acting with the relevant professional leads responsible for overall management of the radiotherapy department. Careful training of all staff members must therefore be an integral part of any effective quality assurance system.

INFORMATION SOURCES

Choudhury A, Budgell R, Mackay R, et al. The future of image – Guided radiotherapy. Clin Oncol 2017;29(910):662–666.

Green OL, Henke LE, Hugo GD. Practical clinical workflows for online and offline adaptive radiation therapy. Sem in Rad Oncol 2019;29(3):219–227.

Grégoire V, Ang K, Budach W, et al. Delineation of the neck node levels for head and neck tumors: A 2013 update. DAHANCA, EORTC, HKNPCSG, NCIC CTG, NCRI, RTOG, TROG consensus guidelines. Radiother Oncol 2014 Jan;110(1):172–181.

Holland R, Veiling S, Mravunac M, et al. Histologic multifocality of Tis, T1-2 breast carcinomas. Implications for clinical trials of breast conserving surgery. Cancer 1985;56: 979–90.

International Commission on Radiation Units and Measurements. Prescribing, recording and reporting photon beam therapy ICRU: Report 50. ICRU, Bethesda, Maryland, USA, 1993.

International Commission on Radiation Units and Measurements. Prescribing, recording and reporting photon beam therapy (supplement to ICRU report 50): ICRU report 62. ICRU, Bethesda, Maryland, USA, 1999.

International Commission on Radiation Units and Measurements. Prescribing, recording and reporting electron beam therapy: ICRU report 71. ICRU, Bethesda, Maryland, USA, 2004.

International Commission on Radiation Units and Measurements. Prescribing, recording, and reporting proton beam therapy report 78. J ICRU 2007;7(2).

International Commission on Radiation Units and Measurements. Prescribing, recording and reporting photon beam IMRT report 83. J ICRU 2010;10(1). Report 83.

International Commission on Radiation Units and Measurements. Prescribing, recording and reporting of stereotactic treatment with small photon beams ICRU report no. 91. J ICRU 2017;14(2).

NHS England proton beam therapy policies, standard operating procedure and service specification Nov 2018: www.england.nhs.uk.

Proton Beam Therapy (eProton) web based e learning programme: www.e-lfh.org.uk.

Royal College of Radiologists. Radiotherapy Target Volume Definition and Peer Review, 2 edn – RCR Guidance. London: The Royal College of Radiologists, 2022.

Royal College of Radiologists. Radiotherapy Dose Fractionation, 3rd ed. London: The Royal College of Radiologists, 2019.

Royal College of Radiologists. The Timely Delivery of Radical Radiotherapy: Guidelines for the Management of Unscheduled Treatment Interruptions, 4th ed. London: The Royal College of Radiologists, 2019.

Royal College of Radiologists. On Target 2: Updated Guidance for Image-Guided Radiotherapy. London: The Royal College of Radiologists, 2021.

Standardizing Nomenclature in Radiation Oncology. The report of AAPM Task Group 263. American Association of Physicists in Medicine 2018: https://www.aapm.org/pubs/reports/RPT_263.pdf.

Stereotactic Ablative Radiotherapy (SABR) Commissioning through Evaluation Sep 2019: www.england.nhs.uk.

Taylor A, Rockall AG, Reznek RH, et al. Mapping pelvic lymph nodes: Guidelines for delineation in intensity-modulated radiotherapy. Int J Rad Oncol Biol Phys 2005;63:1604–1612.

Tree AC, Huddart R, Choudhury A. Magnetic Resonance-guided Radiotherapy - Can We Justify More Expensive Technology? Clin Oncol (R Coll Radiol) 2018 Nov;30(11):677–679.

van Herk M, Remeijer P, Rasch C, et al. The probability of correct target dosage: Dose-population histograms for deriving treatment margins in radiotherapy. Int J Rad Oncol Biol Phys 2000;47:1121–1135.

World Health Organization. Quality Assurance in Radiotherapy. Geneva: WHO, 1988.

3

Radiobiology and Treatment Planning

Radiation and Cell Kill

Ionising radiation interacts with molecules within the cell, resulting in damage to DNA, organelles and cellular and nuclear membranes. Radiation can cause irreparable cellular DNA damage, either directly or indirectly through the production of reactive oxygen species and other free radicals from ionisation and radiolysis of cellular water. The mechanism of DNA damage differs according to the type of radiation. Electromagnetic radiation damages DNA indirectly through the generation of free radicals, whereas heavy particles such as protons directly ionise and damage DNA. This DNA damage can be in the form of single- and double-strand breaks in the sugar-phosphate backbone of the DNA molecule or cross-links between DNA strands and chromosomal proteins. The most lethal type of radiation-induced DNA damage is double-strand breaks. Ionising radiation creates significant levels of clustered DNA damage, including complex double-strand breaks, which are difficult for cells to repair. Radiation cell damage can manifest as loss of cellular reproductive ability and cell death through induction of apoptosis. Irradiated cells however may not exhibit morphologic evidence of radiation damage until they attempt to divide. Radiation can also induce a bystander effect whereby non-irradiated cells adjacent to or located away from the irradiated tissues demonstrate similar responses to that of the directly irradiated cells through cytokine-mediated cellular toxicity and activation of various signalling pathways.

The loss of proliferative ability by all cells within a tumour is a prerequisite for tumour cure. Partial sterilisation of the tumour cell population results in tumour stasis or regression, followed by regrowth of the tumour from those cells which have retained their proliferative ability. Tumour radiosensitivity can potentially be enhanced by targeting the pathways involved in the repair of radiation-induced cluster damage and complex DNA double-strand breaks.

Cell Survival Curves

Cell culture techniques and in vitro experiments irradiating cultured tumour cells with single fractions of X-rays have been important in allowing the proliferative sterilisation of cells to be investigated quantitatively. For an irradiated cell population, the proportion of cells that still retains the ability to proliferate (relative to an unirradiated control population) is called the surviving fraction. A plot of log surviving fraction against the radiation dose gives a survival curve for the cells concerned, with an increasing dose resulting in an exponential reduction in the fraction of surviving cells. Typically, survival curves are continuously bending with both linear and quadratic components. It is characterised by an initial shoulder followed by an exponential decrease in the fraction of surviving cells at higher doses, with a slope that steepens as the dose increases (Figure 3.1). Mathematically, a continuously bending curve is best described by a linear quadratic (LQ) equation of the form:

$$SF = Exp\left(-\alpha d - \beta d^2\right) \tag{3.1}$$

where SF is the surviving fraction, d is the dose given and α and β are the parameter characteristics of the cells concerned.

DOI: 10.1201/9781315171562-3

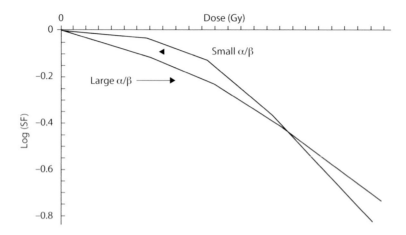

FIGURE 3.1   Two contrasting survival curves for irradiated cells, with log of the surviving fraction (SF) plotted against single radiation dose. The more steeply curving survival curve has the lower α/β ratio when fitted to the linear quadratic equation.

The α/β ratio is derived from this equation. It is a term that describes the sensitivity of tissues to radiotherapy fraction size. It gives the relative importance of the linear and quadratic dose term for those cells, and controls the slope of the survival curve. When α/β ratio is high, as is the case for many tumours such as head and neck squamous cell carcinoma or for early normal tissue reactions, the linear term predominates, so a plot of log (SF) against d is relatively straight, indicating a lower sensitivity to fraction size. When α/β ratio is low, as is the case for prostate and breast adenocarcinomas along with late toxicity reactions, the quadratic term is more important, giving a plot with greater curvature. For cells whose survival curves have a low α/β ratio, doubling the dose leads to more than doubling of the effect on log (SF). Such cells are particularly sensitive to changes in fraction size when radiation is given as a fractionated schedule.

Acute and Late Effects of Tissues

The dose-response relationship for normal tissue injury depends on the survival curve of the tissue stem cells. The timing of expression of injury is influenced by the rate of turnover of mature cells within the tissue. Epithelial and haemopoietic tissues have rapid cell turnover; thus they manifest acute effects (with a timescale of days or weeks). Late effects (with a timescale of months or years) occur in tissues and organs with slow cell turnover, such as endothelial and neuroglial tissues, and parenchymal tissues of the lung, liver and kidney. The risk of major late effects is usually dose-limiting in radiotherapy. Stem cells of late-responding tissues have more curved survival curves (low α/β ratio) than cells of acute-responding tissues (high α/β ratio). Radiobiologically, this difference is due to slow cell turnover in late-responding tissues. Consequently, late-responding tissues are particularly sensitive to changes in fraction size; larger fractions are more damaging to these tissues, whereas small fractions are well tolerated. Acute- and late-responding tissues are also affected differently by changes in the overall treatment time. Because surviving stem cells of acute-responding tissues initiate repopulation during the course of radiotherapy, the duration of radiation makes a difference to the final level of damage. Late-responding tissues do not experience repopulation during the course of radiotherapy and are thus relatively unaffected by the overall treatment time. In addition, the expression of late effects is influenced by the organisation of functional subunits within the organ. In serially arranged subunits, such as the spinal cord, damage to some subunits will lead to a change in the whole organ, whereas in organs where subunits are arranged in parallel, such as the lung, each subunit acts independently, and continuing function is possible even if some of the subunits are damaged.

The Linear Quadratic Model for Tissues

Differences between acute- and late-responding tissues and tumours must be taken into account when considering the biological consequences of replacing one treatment schedule with another. From experience, radiation oncologists developed 'rules of thumb' when altering treatment schedules, e.g. a dose reduction might be necessary if fraction size was to be increased. It is now recognised that tissues react differently to changes in treatment schedule and there is better understanding of how changes in scheduling may affect different tissues. The application of the LQ model is based on the idea that the severity of tissue damage is inversely proportional to stem cell survival, and that stem cell survival can be calculated using mathematical development of the LQ survival curve so that it can be applied to fractionated treatments. In particular, two different schedules will have equal biological effect on a tissue if each schedule produces the same level of stem cell survival. We shall not attempt to derive the mathematics of the LQ model in detail, but we will state some results which are useful in clinical practice.

Consider two different treatment schedules, namely total dose D_1 or D_2 given as fraction size d_1 or d_2. We shall assume for now that both schedules are given over the same overall duration. For a tissue whose cells have a survival curve described by the LQ parameters α and β, it can be shown that the two schedules are isoeffective for that tissue when:

$$D_1\left(\alpha/\beta+d_1\right)=D_2\left(\alpha/\beta+d_2\right) \tag{3.2}$$

Notice that the survival curve parameters appear as a ratio in this expression, which means that only the α/β ratio for a tissue needs to be known in order to apply the equation. In fact, α/β estimates have already been made for most tissues. Late-responding tissues usually have low α/β values (about 3 Gy), whereas acute-responding tissues have higher values (about 10 Gy). (This means that cells of late-responding tissues have more steeply curving survival curves). Tumours are more variable; many act like acute-responding tissues with α/β values of 10 Gy or more, but recent estimates for breast and prostate adenocarcinomas suggest lower values. In practice, Equation 3.2 is often used to compare an unfamiliar treatment schedule with a standard one. Most usefully, the unfamiliar schedule can be assessed by determining what total dose, given as 2 Gy fractions, would produce the same effect on that tissue. This is helpful for determining whether the unfamiliar schedule is 'hot' or 'cold'. For example, consider a schedule which consists of ten twice-weekly fractions of 4 Gy to a total dose of 40 Gy in five weeks. In Equation 3.2, let d_1 be 4 Gy and D_1 be 40 Gy. If we now set d_2 as 2 Gy, and calculate D_2 (for a particular choice of tissue α/β), we shall get the total dose given as 2 Gy fractions which would have the same effect on that tissue as schedule D_1, d_1. Notice, however, that the calculation depends on the assumed value of α/β. For this example, we shall repeat the calculation for acute- and late-responding tissues. For acute-responding tissues ($\alpha/\beta = 10$ Gy), we find that $D_2 = 47$ Gy, while for late-responding tissues ($\alpha/\beta = 3$ Gy), $D_2 = 56$ Gy. Therefore, the new schedule is expected to be 'hotter' in terms of its effects on late-responding tissues compared with acute-responding tissues, but it is no 'hotter' than a conventional radical regimen (e.g. 60 Gy in 2 Gy fractions).

It should be noted that the simple LQ model does not allow for differences in total treatment duration between the schedules, which are presumed to be given in the same overall time (five weeks in this case), despite their different fractionation patterns. This restriction is not so important for late-responding tissues (for which total time is a minor variable), but the results for acute-responding tissues (for which the time factor can be significant) need to be interpreted cautiously with this limitation of the model in mind.

The LQ model has been developed extensively and applied to more complex treatment schedules, including brachytherapy. The standard schedule against which an unfamiliar schedule is to be compared may not necessarily be one using 2 Gy fractions. A rather abstract standard schedule, more appealing to mathematicians than to clinicians, is a hypothetical regimen in which a very large number of small fractions are given (mathematically, an infinite number of zero-sized fractions are given, but to a finite total dose). Linear quadratic calculations performed using biologically effective dose (BED) are mathematically equivalent to those performed with the standard regimen of 2 Gy fractions, although the latter has the advantage of clinical familiarity. An important feature of the LQ model in its various forms is the recognition that cells of different tissues differ in the shape of their survival curve and therefore respond differently to changes in fraction size. Since a target volume may contain several tissue types in addition to the tumour, a change of fractionation regimen will affect these components differently. Therefore, there is no such thing as a regimen which is 'generally equivalent' to some other regimen – the regimens can only be matched (by choice of total dose) for equivalent effects on each specific tissue.

BED, formulated from the linear quadratic model, can be used to compare dose fractionation regimens.

$$\mathrm{BED} = n.d.\frac{1+d}{\alpha/\beta} - K.(T - T_k) \tag{3.3}$$

where n = total number of fractions, T = time of delivery (days), T_k = kick-off day for repopulation (days) and K = daily BED equivalent repopulation (Gy.days^{-1}).

An alternative formulation is the EQD2 or the equivalent dose in 2 Gy fractions. This permits the comparison of dose fractionation regimens to 2 Gy per fraction schedules.

$$\mathrm{EQD2} = n.d.\frac{\left(d + \dfrac{\alpha}{\beta}\right)}{\left(2 + \dfrac{\alpha}{\beta}\right)} \tag{3.4}$$

A number of online calculation tools and mobile phone apps are now available to assist these calculations.

Volume Effects

Together with the total dose and fractionation schedule, target volume is a major variable in radiotherapy. For a given fractionation regimen, higher doses can usually be given when treatment volumes are small rather than large. Most normal tissues cannot regenerate from a single surviving cell. However, tissue recovery may be assisted by immigration of unirradiated neighbouring cells, especially if the treatment volume is small. Volume is also an important determinant of normal tissue response to a given dose, firstly because larger treatment volumes provide less opportunity for tissues to draw on their 'functional reserve', and secondly because larger irradiated volumes make it more likely that a critical volume element will exceed the upper dose limit. These factors differ according to tissue structure, and vary from one treatment to another.

In general, the normal tissue complication probability (NTCP) increases with dose (for a given fractionation regimen) and with the irradiated volume. It is important to know, at least approximately, how changes in the irradiated volume at a particular site affect the tolerance dose that can safely be given. The 'tolerance dose' is defined as that dose which gives no more than 5 per cent incidence of significant side effects, based on clinical experience. A body of data has been amassed which provides some simple 'rules of thumb' concerning the trade-off between treatment volume and tolerance dose, but these need to be used cautiously. Tolerance is affected not only by volume but also by radiation sensitivity and fraction size. Tissue tolerance to the various new treatment schedules in use must be carefully studied. In some cases, radiation injury may result from an excessively high dose to a small tissue element within the treatment volume. The possibility of improved homogeneity of the dose distribution with IMRT may help to ameliorate this problem.

Radiation Dose and Tumour Cure Probability

In radical radiotherapy, the objective is complete sterilisation of all tumour cells without incurring an unacceptably high risk of serious injury to normal tissues.

Radiation kills cells randomly, which means that each tumour cell has the same probability of surviving irradiation. That probability is dependent on the given dose. Suppose that SF$_2$ is the probability of any tumour cell surviving a single dose of 2 Gy, the most commonly used fraction size. For example, if SF_2 is 0.5 for a given carcinoma, after the first 2 Gy fraction, 50 per cent of the cells survive; after the second dose, 50 per cent of those survivors still survive (i.e. 25 per cent of the original population); after the third dose, 50 per cent of those survivors still survive (i.e. 12.5 per cent of the original population), and so on. Therefore, after F fractions, the final survival probability will be $(SF_2)^F$. For a conventional treatment regimen consisting of 30 treatments of 2 Gy each, the final survival probability (in this example) would be 0.5^{30}, or 9×10^{-10}.

These relationships have some interesting clinical implications. First, there is no dose which gives zero probability of cell survival; even after a large dose there will still be some probability, possibly very small, of survival of each cell. A visible tumour will contain a large number of cells; even if each cell only has a small chance of surviving, there is still a chance that at least one cell will survive and regenerate the tumour. We therefore need to know the relationship between a given dose and the probability that the entire cell population will be sterilised with not a single cell surviving – the basic requirement for tumour cure. This can be computed using the theory of Poisson statistics. We can then calculate the number of treatments required to achieve some value of cure probability, such as 90 per cent (remember that 100 per cent cure probability cannot be achieved by any finite dose).

We can repeat the calculation for tumours of different sizes (different cell population numbers), not just for our example of $SF_2 = 0.5$, but also for other values of SF_2 representing more sensitive or less sensitive tumour types. Figure 3.2 shows these relationships. Although we have used a rather simple model for these calculations, we can observe some features which turn up in more complex and realistic models.

First, note that the relationship between tumour cell number and number of treatments required is logarithmic, i.e. a large change in cell number corresponds to a rather modest change in the number of treatments and hence the total dose required. For example, the number of treatments required for a tumour of 10^4 cells is half the number required for 10^8 cells. It is because of this logarithmic relationship that quite high total doses are required for regions containing only microscopic spread. Within regions of microscopic spread, it is likely that the tumour cell density will gradually decrease with increasing distance from the visible tumour edge. This suggests that the radiotherapy dose should similarly decrease with distance,

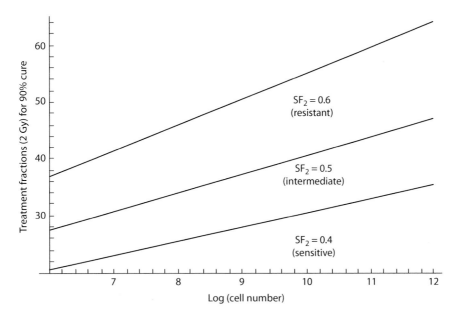

FIGURE 3.2 Shows the calculated number of 2 Gy fractions required to achieve 90 per cent cure probability, as a function of tumour cell population number, for differing values of cellular intrinsic radiosensitivity (expressed as the surviving fraction following a single 2 Gy treatment, SF_2). Moderate variation in SF_2, as seen between cells of different tumour types, leads to large differences in the number of 2 Gy treatment fractions required to achieve 90 per cent cure probability. In some cases, the predicted number of fractions required is larger than could be safely given.

roughly in proportion to log cell density. Although the cell density distribution may not be known, it is possible that a tapering dose distribution, as occurs in a conventional plan with a peripheral dose gradient, or with IMRT and deliberate dose modulation within the volume, could be advantageous. A second feature of the model is that a small change in SF_2 has quite a profound effect on the total dose required (compare the three curves shown in Figure 3.2). Small variations in the intrinsic radiosensitivity of tumour cells could result in a tumour being easily curable, or completely incurable, by a radiotherapy regimen.

Another feature of the dose–cure relationship is the steepness of the increase in tumour cure probability with total dose, illustrated in Figure 3.3. In this figure, the solid curves show the dose–cure relationship for a series of tumours with slightly different parameters; they can be seen to increase steeply with total dose in all cases. This implies that relatively small differences in total dose could result in significant differences in cure probability for each tumour. However, these steep relationships are not seen in the dose–cure relationships following treatment of groups of tumours with differing parameters, such as that seen in clinical studies with patient groups. The broken line in Figure 3.3 shows the much swallower gradient that is typically observed in such studies. The shallow gradient of the curve for tumour groups is the result of a series of steep curves for individual tumours with differing radiosensitivities. This has significance when we consider the importance of moderate changes in the total dose when treating individual patients. The importance of a dose increment in treating an individual tumour depends on how close the treatment regimen is to achieving cure. For a large or resistant tumour such as sarcoma with cure probability close to zero, a modest dose increment will make little difference. Conversely, for a small or highly sensitive tumour such as seminoma with cure probability close to 100 per cent, a small dose increment again makes little difference. However, if the treatment regimen achieves a cure probability of close to 50 per cent such as with some head and neck tumours, the dose-response curve will be as steep as that calculated from the Poisson model. This means that for any individual patient there is some likelihood that a large change in tumour control probability can result from a small change in the delivered dose. Even where the average dose-response curve for patient groups is known to be shallow, a minority of patients may still benefit substantially from small changes in the given dose. It is these patients for whom the choice of treatment plan may be critical.

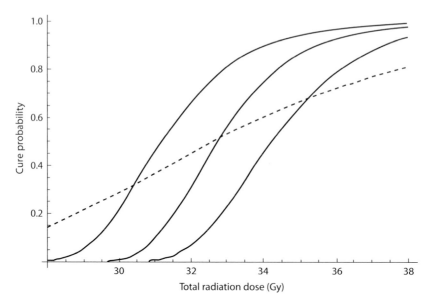

FIGURE 3.3   The solid lines in this figure show the expected relationship between total radiation dose and cure probability for individual tumours with differing radiosensitivity and cell number. The curves are sigmoid in shape, located at different positions on the dose axis, and each is quite steep. The broken line shows the much shallower dose response usually seen in clinical studies when proportion cured is plotted against dose for groups of tumours. The shallower response is thought to be due to tumour heterogeneity in each dose group.

TABLE 3.1

Radiobiological Factors Controlling Response to Fractionated Radiotherapy (the 'Five Rs') and Their Clinical Relevance

Radiobiological Factor	Mechanism of Effect on Response	Clinical Relevance
Radiosensitivity	Intrinsic radiosensitivity differs between cells of tumours and normal tissue types, and strongly determines final surviving fraction.	Can account for variable response of tumours to radiation. Curative dose is proportional to the log of cell number (subclinical disease needs smaller dose).
Repair	Cells differ in their capacity to repair DNA damage, particularly after small doses of radiation. The repair process can take at least six hours to complete.	Repair is maximal when late-responding tissues are given small fractions of radiation. Hyperfractionation may be advantageous. Treatments need to be well separated in order to avoid compromising repair.
Repopulation	Surviving cells in many tumours and acute-responding (but not in late-responding) normal tissues proliferate more rapidly once treatment is in progress.	Shortened treatment times (accelerated therapy) may be advantageous for some tumours. Acute (but not late) effects will be increased. Gaps should be avoided.
Reoxygenation	Hypoxic cells, which occur especially in tumours, are relatively resistant to radiation. Hypoxic surviving cells reoxygenate and become more radiosensitive as treatment proceeds.	Very short treatment times may lead to resistance due to persistence of hypoxic cells. Treatment of anaemia may optimise tumour response.
Redistribution	Cells in certain phases of the proliferative cycle (e.g. late S) are relatively resistant to radiation and survive preferentially. With time between fractions, cells redistribute themselves over all phases of the proliferative cycle.	Closely spaced treatment fractions may lead to resistance due to persistence of cells in the less sensitive phases of proliferation.

Tumour Radiobiology

The so-called five Rs of radiobiology are the main factors controlling tumour response to fractionated radiotherapy (Table 3.1). Currently, the most important of these factors are thought to be the intrinsic radiosensitivity of cells and the kinetics of repopulation of surviving tumour cells.

Intrinsic radiosensitivity varies between different tumour cell lines in culture, with cell lines derived from clinically resistant tumour types having a tendency towards higher SF_2 values. Although tumours are diverse, the radiobiological properties of most tumours are similar to those of acute-responding tissues with a high α/β ratio, moderate sensitivity to changes in fraction size and some dependence on total treatment time. It is now widely believed that many tumours repopulate rapidly during the latter part of a course of radiotherapy, and that any factor which prolongs the treatment duration could lead to significantly reduced tumour cure probability.

Avoidance of Gaps during Treatment

The occurrence of rapid repopulation in irradiated tumours, sometimes with doubling times as short as three or four days, has important implications for treatment interruption. Unscheduled gaps occur not infrequently in radiotherapy schedules due to patient intercurrent illness, non-attendance or machine breakdown. Gaps are important, as they may lead to prolongation of the overall treatment time, allowing opportunities for rapid repopulation of surviving tumour cells towards the end of the radiotherapy schedule. Although prolongation will often spare acute normal tissue reactions, the risk of late effects is not reduced. It has been shown for squamous cell carcinomas of the head and neck that the probability of cure may reduce by 1–2 per cent with each day of treatment prolongation. If gaps occur, the best management strategy is 'post-gap acceleration' with the use of twice-daily treatments separated by more than six hours or weekend treatments to enable 'catching up' so that treatment is completed within the intended period. This does not require any changes to fraction size or total dose. However, these approaches are not always feasible in practice. Avoidance of treatment gaps should be an important consideration for all radiotherapy departments.

Treatment Scheduling

Conventionally, radiotherapy schedules have consisted of multiple fractions of 2 Gy delivered for five days a week over several weeks. The total dose is usually limited by anticipated risk of injury to late-responding tissues, although there are situations where acute responses such as mucosal reactions are the main concern. Treatment schedules with this structure take advantage of differences in the survival curves of cells between late-responding tissues (with low α/β ratio and fraction size sensitivity) and typical tumours (with higher α/β ratio). This means that late-responding tissues are spared to a greater extent than most tumours through the use of small fraction sizes. Late responses are not strongly influenced by overall treatment time. It would thus be desirable to make the overall treatment time as short as possible in order to minimise the opportunities for tumour repopulation. However, this must be balanced against the potential adverse effect of reduced treatment time on acute-responding tissues.

When designing rational radiotherapy treatment schedules, one has to take into consideration the tumour control probability (TCP) and normal tissue complication probability (NTCP). TCP is the likelihood of achieving local control. In radical radiotherapy, the tumour BED must be sufficient to achieve a clinically acceptable TCP. The therapeutic ratio describes the ratio of TCP:NTCP. Dose fractionation schedules should aim to maximise the therapeutic ratio. This can be attained by altering the total radiation dose, fraction size and total duration of the treatment schedule.

There is now considerable experience with different schedules of treatment (for details, see Table 3.2). All these changes in scheduling may bring important gains in tumour control. However, tumours are

TABLE 3.2

Effects of Alterations in Radiotherapy Scheduling on Tumour and Normal Tissues

Fractionation Scheme	Rationale	Mode of Delivery	Effect on Tumour	Effect on Acute-Responding Tissues	Effect on Late-Responding Tissues
Hyperfractionation	Tumours resemble acute-responding tissues with high α/β ratio.	Multiple daily fractions of less than 1.8 Gy using an increased number of fractions to give an increased total dose.	Increased tumour cell kill.	Increased.	Decreased or same.
Accelerated	Accelerated repopulation in tumours. Time factor for late effects relatively unimportant.	Reduced overall treatment time. Same fraction size, six-hour interval between treatments if used with hyperfractionation. Six or seven treatments a week for daily fractions.	Increased tumour cell kill.	Increased.	Minimal increase.
Accelerated hyperfractionation (CHART)	Combines the advantages of hyperfractionation and acceleration.	Benefit of this approach either with reduced total dose or shorter overall treatment time.	Increased tumour cell kill.	Increased.	Decreased or same.
Hypofractionation	May help to overcome radio-resistance. Possible for some tumour sites where normal tissue reactions are not dose limiting. Reduced overall treatment time.	Fraction size greater than 2 Gy. Decreased number of fractions. Suitable for small-volume, high-precision treatments.	Same or increased cell kill.	Same or increased.	Increased if total dose is unchanged. Decreased if total dose is reduced.

extremely heterogeneous with regard to cell survival parameters and growth kinetics, along with other properties. It is unlikely that any one schedule is ideal for all tumours, even those of a single pathological type. Treatment schedules for individual patients should be selected based on the radiobiological and kinetic parameters of the tumour.

Treatment Plan, Schedules and 'Double Trouble'

The design of physical treatment plans usually proceeds without regard to the treatment schedule. However, there may be interplay between dose distributions and treatment schedules, giving an altered biological effect sometimes known as 'double trouble'. Consider a treatment plan in which the spread of dose within the target volume is 10 per cent; if the intended treatment is 30 fractions of 2 Gy to give a total dose of 60 Gy, the spread of dose will be 57 Gy to 63 Gy. However, the low- and high-point doses will not have been delivered as 2 Gy per fraction (the dose variation of 10 per cent affects each dose fraction, so the fraction size will range from 1.9 Gy to 2.1 Gy). A treatment schedule of 30×2.1 Gy = 63 Gy will be what is 'seen' by cells located close to the high-dose point, and this 63 Gy dose is more damaging to late-responding tissues with low α/β ratio, than 63 Gy given as 2 Gy fractions (which is what is implied when only the physical total dose is cited). Therefore, the spread of radiobiological damage within the target volume has two components, namely that due to variation in total dose, and that due to variation in fraction size by which that total dose is given. This 'double trouble' effect is most marked for late-responding tissues, for large treatment volumes with considerable dose variation and for intended treatment schedules where the prescribed fraction size is large.

Two ways of accounting for 'double trouble' can be envisaged. First, IMRT makes it possible to ensure homogeneity of dose distribution across a treatment volume and this approach is now being used extensively, as it has been shown, for example, to reduce late normal tissue effects of fibrosis following treatment for breast cancer. Second, radiobiological dose plans can be constructed with the physical dose replaced by some radiobiological equivalent that includes the effect of variation in fraction size. For example, the physical dose at each point in the dose matrix could be replaced by a dose calculated using the LQ model to show the same effect on late-responding tissues as 2 Gy fractions. Isodose curves can be constructed using the 'radiobiological dose' and compared with conventional isodose plots using the physical dose. Algorithms have been developed which can be incorporated into commercial treatment planning systems to compute radiobiological treatment plans. In addition, LQ-transformed DVHs (which incorporate the biological effects of variations in fraction size within the volume) can be computed and the biologically equivalent dose to the hottest and coldest parts of the volume calculated.

Integrating the Five Rs of Radiobiology into the Hallmarks of Cancer

In a landmark publication in 2000, Hanahan and Weinberg described six hallmarks of cancer: sustained proliferative signalling, evasion of growth suppressors, resistance to cell death, induction of angiogenesis, acquisition of unlimited replicative capacity and activation of invasive and metastatic phenotypes. Two new emerging hallmarks have also been identified: evading immune destruction and reprogramming energy metabolism. These hallmarks of cancer provide insights into the underlying mechanisms of the five Rs of radiobiology and radiation response. They present potential routes to novel therapeutic strategies in the field of radiation oncology.

Sustained Proliferative Signalling

Sustained proliferative signalling facilitates tumour repopulation. Targeting this hallmark of cancer may enhance radiation sensitivity. Sustained proliferation and genomic instability enabled by a mutation in one aspect of the DNA damage response may lead to dependency on another DNA damage response pathway. Blockade of this pathway, in combination with radiation, may result in enhanced cell death.

An example of the clinical exploitation of this 'synthetic lethality' is the use of poly(ADP-ribose) polymerase (PARP) inhibitors in tumours harbouring BRCA mutations. These tumours have defective homologous recombination repair; thus they rely on base excision repair to maintain their genomic integrity. By inhibiting DNA repair functions, PARP inhibitors enhance radiation-induced cell death. Several early-phase studies are currently underway to assess the safety, tolerability and efficacy of PARP inhibitors in combination with radiotherapy.

Evasion of Growth Suppressors

In human cancer, there is loss or impaired function of tumour suppressor genes, enabling cancer cells to ignore signals such as transforming growth factor beta (TGF-β) that would normally stop cell proliferation. Cancer cells can also secrete TGF-β in an autocrine fashion. This may in turn trigger epithelial-mesenchymal transition through which cancer cells gain the ability to invade and metastasise. In addition, radiation can induce release of TGF-β, and this can contribute to normal tissue effects such as fibrosis, micro-thrombus formation and tissue ischaemia. Thus, TGF-β has multiple roles in human cancer. It is a tumour suppressor in normal cells and early cancers. However, as tumours develop and progress, the protective effects of TGF-β are lost and it switches to promote tumour progression, invasion and metastasis. Blockade of TGF-β signalling therefore has the potential to simultaneously enhance radiation-induced cell kill, improve normal tissue sparing and prevent radiation-induced epithelial-mesenchymal transition of tumour cells.

Resistance to Cell Death

Radiation can lead to cancer cell death in a number of ways. These include immediate apoptosis when cancer cells self-destruct with little impact on the surrounding tissues; mitotic catastrophe in which cancer cells with unrepaired DNA damage undergo one or more mitoses before apoptotic death; necrosis, which is a form of programmed cell death; and autophagy in response to stress induced by radiation.

Cancer cells can acquire the ability to circumvent various regulators of cell death and senescence. For example, mutation of p53 can prevent apoptosis secondary to radiation-induced DNA damage. Loss of p53 also results in cell cycle redistribution following radiotherapy, where cancer cells utilise the G2/M checkpoint to allow time for the repair of potentially lethal DNA damage. Inhibitors targeting checkpoint kinase 1, which regulate the G2/M checkpoint, have the potential to render p53 defective cells more sensitive to radiation-induced apoptosis. A number of checkpoint kinase 1 inhibitors are currently in clinical development.

Induction of Angiogenesis

Many tumours sustain a hypoxic environment. Hypoxia makes tumour cells significantly less sensitive to radiation, which can in turn lead to treatment failure. So far, attempts to combine radiotherapy with modulators of tumour hypoxia have achieved limited success. Enhancing the concentration of inspired oxygen may improve clinical outcomes in patients with laryngeal and bladder cancer. Nimorazole, an oxygen mimetic, induces formation of free radicals and sensitises hypoxic tumour cells to the cytotoxic effects of ionising radiation. However, its availability is limited. Drugs, such as tirapazamine, which are selectively toxic to hypoxic cells have produced disappointing clinical results. The addition of bevacizumab, a VEGF-blocking antibody, to preoperative chemoradiation in rectal cancer led to increased toxicity with no improvement in the rate of pathological complete response.

Acquisition of Unlimited Replicative Capacity

Telomere shortening and loss of telomerase are associated with sensitivity to radiation. Telomerase is expressed by most cancer cells. Radiation may in itself also enhance telomerase expression in cancer cells, and this may in turn lead to tumour repopulation during treatment.

Evading Immune Destruction

Cancer cells can evade immune destruction. They can reduce immune reactivity within the tumour microenvironment, suppressing the cytolytic ability of infiltrating T cells and forming blood vessels which are less permissive to extravasation by T cells and natural killer cells. Radiation can overcome the immunosuppression observed within the tumour microenvironment. It can generate and release novel tumour-associated antigens and increase the infiltration of lymphocytes into tumour. Radiotherapy may thus make tumours more immunogenic. The combination of hypofractionated radiotherapy and ipilimumab, a monoclonal antibody against immune checkpoint inhibitor CTLA-4, can potentially trigger anticancer immunity, leading to an 'abscopal effect' where there is regression of disease outside the irradiated volume.

Reprogramming Energy Metabolism

Glycolysis is favoured over oxidative phosphorylation as a source of energy by cancer cells, even in the presence of oxygen. The subsequent intracellular buildup of lactate, glutathione and pyruvate results in more effective scavenging of radiation-induced reactive oxygen species, thus reducing the number of double-strand DNA breaks induced by radiation. Targeting such tumour metabolism through the use of metformin has been shown to improve the rate of pathological complete response following chemoradiation in rectal cancer.

Future Directions

Continued research efforts to enhance our understanding of the mechanisms of tumour and normal tissue response to radiation can result in an improvement in the therapeutic ratio of radiotherapy. Predictive biomarkers will also need to be identified to enable rational selection of treatments to combine with radiotherapy. The next quantum leap in progress in radiotherapy will require radiation oncologists to engage themselves in the biological basis of cancer and its response to radiation.

INFORMATION SOURCES

Brand DH, Yarnold JR. The linear-quadratic model and implications for fractionation. Clin Oncol 2019;31:673–677.

Good JS, Harrington KJ. The hallmarks of cancer and the radiation oncologist: Updating the 5Rs of radiobiology. Clin Oncol 2013;25:569–577.

Hanahan D, Weinberg RA. The hallmarks of cancer. Cell 2000;100:57–70.

Hanahan D, Weinberg RA. Hallmarks of cancer: The next generation. Cell 2011;144:646–674.

Joiner M, van der Kogel A (ed). Basic Clinical Radiobiology, 4th ed. London: Hodder Arnold, 2009.

The Royal College of Radiologists (2019) The timely delivery of radical radiotherapy: guidelines for the management of unscheduled treatment interruptions, Fourth edition.

4

Organs at Risk and Tolerance of Normal Tissues

Therapeutic Ratio

Radiation is potentially harmful to all normal tissues. Every country will have a legal framework to protect patients from unnecessary radiation exposure such as the Ionising Radiation (Medical Exposures) Regulations in the UK. The fundamental principle of radiation protection is to make all exposures as low as reasonably achievable (ALARA). So whilst normal tissue radiation exposure is impossible to avoid in radiotherapy, and relatively safe dose limits have been established for different tissues, it is always important to keep in mind that there are no absolute limits of radiation dose that are completely safe.

When considering how to achieve the best outcome from radiotherapy in the treatment of tumours, it is critical to understand the concept of therapeutic ratio. Cure is always achieved at some cost in terms of normal tissue damage. There must be a balance between trying to ensure that all tumour cells receive a lethal dose of radiation and that acute and late effects are tolerable. The total dose, dose per fraction, treated volume and concomitant drugs will all affect this balance, as will individual factors for each patient such as age, comorbidity and intrinsic tissue radiosensitivity.

In some clinical situations, the frequency or severity of late effects drives a reduction in radiotherapy dose. For example, concern about the high incidence of second malignancies after radiotherapy for Hodgkin lymphoma has led to chemotherapy being used in preference. In some paediatric tumours with high cure rates (Wilms', germ cell tumours), research has focused on lowering radiotherapy dose to see if late effects can be reduced without compromising cure. There is considerable interest in de-intensifying the dose and target volume of radiotherapy treatment for HPV-positive oropharyngeal cancer to reduce dysphagia and other late effects of treatment.

More commonly, a desire to increase radiotherapy dose to improve cure rates may be limited by the response of normal tissues to radiation. Although the optimal balance of cure and side effects may have been reached for one radiotherapy technique, further dose escalation may be possible with more precise treatment delivery or better patient support. The dose that can be safely delivered in prostate cancer has increased with the use of IMRT and with a better understanding of how to control for prostate, bladder and bowel motion. Improvements in patient support, such as dietetic advice and feeding tubes to support nutrition for patients undergoing head and neck radiotherapy, may make acute effects more tolerable. A better understanding of the mechanisms of late effects is helping to produce a less nihilistic approach to their management. There are specialist teams now providing a multidisciplinary therapeutic approach to the management of late effects of radiotherapy, particularly in the pelvis.

Any change to a treatment regimen, such as the use of IMRT, an increase in dose or addition of chemotherapy or biological agents, will change the therapeutic ratio. The challenge for the radiation oncologist is to ensure that this change improves the ratio and that an increase in dose is not counteracted by an increase in unmanageable acute or serious late effects. TCP (tumour control probability) and NTCP (normal tissue complication probability) are models used to predict the effects of such changes. However, to know whether a new treatment has really produced better outcomes overall, and to inform and improve the reliability of these modelling estimates, good clinical data must be collected, not only for outcome measures relating to tumour control but also for acute and late normal tissue damage.

Figure 4.1 illustrates how a change in delivered dose may affect TCP and NTCP. With dose A, the chance of cure is low but there is no risk of complications to the normal tissue. Dose B gives a much higher chance of cure but with a small risk of complications. Dose C gives an excellent chance of cure

DOI: 10.1201/9781315171562-4

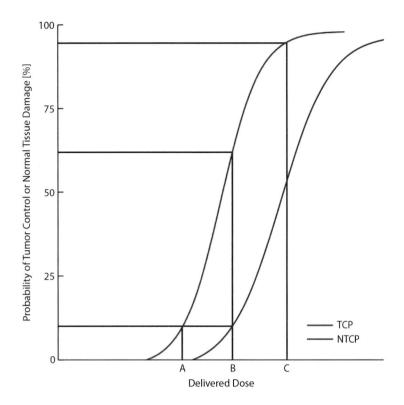

FIGURE 4.1 Graphical depiction of therapeutic ratio.

but with about a 50 per cent chance of complications. The actual dose chosen for the patient will depend on the organ in question and the severity of the complication that is being considered. A change to the treatment regimen which moves the blue NTCP curve to the right, such as the addition of concomitant drugs, will improve the therapeutic ratio.

Modern radiotherapy techniques such as IMRT and arc therapy mean that homogeneous dose distributions within the target volumes are much more easily achieved than with older techniques. As more beam angles are used in a single plan, more of the surrounding tissues receive some radiation dose. Consequently, there is more flexibility in deciding which volume of adjacent tissues will be collaterally irradiated and to what dose. An understanding of the 3D dose-volume effects of radiation on normal tissues is therefore key.

Early and Late Effects of Radiation

Normal tissue effects can be specified in relation to the probability of them occurring, their severity and their timing. Radiation injury may be expressed soon after treatment (early effects) or after six months and up to many years later (late effects). Subsequent treatment, as for example with anthracyclines, may reveal latent, previously asymptomatic, damage. Expression of damage depends on genetic susceptibility. It has been estimated that 20 per cent of the observed variation in normal tissue sensitivity to radiation is random and 80 per cent deterministic, including that due to genetic variations. Several conditions are known to predispose to abnormal radiation sensitivity, including ataxia telangiectasia, Fanconi's anaemia and Bloom's syndrome.

As the understanding of genetic variation has increased with the ability to sequence whole genomes more quickly and cheaply, a new science of radiogenomics is evolving. It tries to identify genomic markers of normal tissue sensitivity to radiation with the goal of being able to test for predictive markers of radiation sensitivity and to personalise radiotherapy treatment. If the risk of late effects in an individual is low, then the dose could be increased to give a higher chance of cure. If the risk is particularly high, other treatments might be preferable to radiotherapy.

Underlying all normal tissue damage, there is a mechanism of dysregulated repair of the radiation injury. Fibroblastic proliferation and extracellular matrix deposition are influenced by oxidative stress, the release of cytokines such as TGF-ß and by the immune response, and may lead to endothelial proliferation and subsequent fibrosis. This is common in soft tissues such as skin, breast, bowel, lung, kidney and liver. Alternatively, cell death may lead to atrophy or necrosis of tissues as may occur with bone, nerves or brain.

Late damage will also depend on the functional organisation of the irradiated tissue. In an organ where the cells are arranged in serial such as at the spinal cord, a high dose to one part of the organ can stop function completely and cause paralysis, whereas a lower dose to a larger volume may have no effect on function. Where there is a more parallel arrangement of functioning subunits such as in the liver, a moderate dose to the whole organ is potentially more harmful than a high dose to a small part of it.

Organs at Risk

The International Commission on Radiation Units (ICRU) defines OAR (organs at risk) as those normal tissues which lie adjacent to tumours and may therefore be included within treated volumes, with a risk that the radiation may impair their normal functioning. Preparation of a treatment plan involves outlining in three dimensions not only the tumour and its potential extensions but also any OAR.

OAR should be outlined according to protocols so that dose can be correlated accurately with end effect and comparisons made between institutions. For example, in lung cancer, the OAR volume for the normal lung is variously defined as the whole of both lungs, lungs with GTV subtracted or lungs with PTV subtracted. Contouring atlases have been produced to help reduce variation in contouring OARs, and the Global Harmonisation Group published consensus guidelines in 2020. The volume of OAR can be expanded in three dimensions to take account of organ movement and of systematic and random errors in treatment delivery. This will create a planning organ at risk volume (PRV) in the same way that a CTV is expanded to form a PTV. It is important to name OARs consistently using internationally agreed nomenclature. The use of a common language will make it much easier to compare treatment plans between radiotherapy centres.

There is a risk that the increasing awareness of organ motion and treatment delivery errors will lead to larger PTVs and larger PRVs, which may overlap when a dose solution is chosen. While it may be theoretically correct to generate a PRV for each organ so that with each fraction the true location of that organ will be within the PRV, in practice, dose limits for organs at risk are usually applied to the OAR as defined on the planning images. One exception is the spinal cord, where a more conservative approach is often taken because of the potential severity of late effects (paralysis). The cord itself can be contoured and a 3–5 mm margin added isotropically to produce a PRV. Alternatively, the spinal canal is contoured as the organ at risk, which effectively adds a margin to the OAR. This approach also makes it possible to make comparisons with data derived from 2D planning where the spinal canal was considered to represent the cord.

For some tumours, the PTV can be treated with a plan where accepted tolerance doses to normal tissues are not exceeded. But sometimes the clinician may need to make a value judgement about the relative risks of possible normal tissue damage and loss of tumour control. It is important to consider the type and severity of the effect, the possible consequences of a local tumour recurrence and how an individual patient may tolerate radiotherapy. For example, late damage to the spinal cord resulting in paralysis may be catastrophic, whereas an oesophageal stricture or a cataract may be treatable. It may be acceptable to irradiate one kidney to high dose if the contralateral one is functioning normally, but not in the presence of hypertensive nephropathy. In postoperative radiotherapy for a tumour close to the optic nerve, using a lower dose of radiation to try to keep within accepted tolerance may increase the risk of blindness from a local recurrence. In trying to prevent blindness, the risk of not giving an adequate dose to the PTV may be greater than the risk of normal tissue damage. In the same patient, the acceptable dose to the ipsilateral and contralateral optic nerves may therefore be different. Ascertaining the patient's perspective through careful discussion and listening is key to helping to inform these complex decisions in individual cases.

Tolerance Doses

There are very few prospective dose escalation studies of radiation, analogous to phase 1 studies of new drugs, to help determine the maximum tolerated dose of radiotherapy. The tables of tolerance doses which are used in clinical practice are often extrapolated from laboratory or animal studies, or at best relate to radiotherapy given many years ago with techniques and technology which have been superseded by 3D planning and treatment delivery. In addition, the fraction size, dose rate, volume treated, concomitant therapy, comorbidity and length of life will all affect the probability of late effects occurring in an individual. A tolerance dose needs to be interpreted in this context. Moreover, tolerance doses will change over time as 3D dose distributions are correlated with late effects in the modern era. Nevertheless, it is possible to give guidance as to the chance that a given dose will produce a given side effect and to define reasonable safe limits to use when devising a plan.

Correlating the risk of side effects with 2D dose distributions led to the production of TD5/5 tables. These provide an estimate of the dose which gives a 5 per cent probability of a given late effect five years after treatment. Similarly, a TD50/5 is the dose giving a 50 per cent risk of a particular effect at five years. From these point estimates, models to predict probability of normal tissue complications were developed, such as the Lyman-probit and the Kallman-relative seriality models.

While point doses or absolute dose thresholds such as TD5/5 may be useful for some serial organs such as the spinal cord, where exceeding a dose threshold at any point can compromise whole organ function, they are less useful in organs composed of parallel subunits. The advent of 3D planning has made it possible to describe the dose given to a volume of tissue and to correlate it with acute and late effects. This description is usually in the form of a cumulative dose-volume histogram or DVH.

A DVH is a plot of dose of radiation on the x-axis and per cent volume of the structure of interest on the y-axis. The DVH curve can be used to ensure that dose to critical structures in a plan is within acceptable limits and to compare different plans (Figure 4.2). DVHs assume that the function

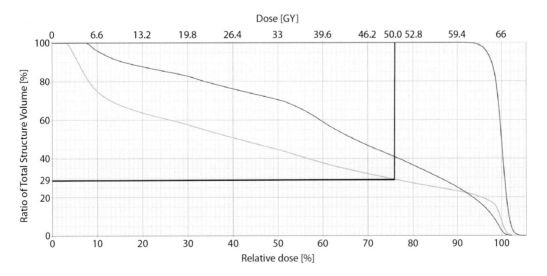

FIGURE 4.2 Sample DVHs for radiotherapy to the prostate bed. The PTV is shown in red, rectum in blue and bladder in green. The black lines show that the volume of the bladder receiving 50 Gy is just under 30 per cent of the total organ volume. This is less than the tolerance dose in Table 4.1 below.

of that structure is uniform, whereas in reality different parts of the same organ may have different functions. A 3D planning system can calculate the dose in each pixel of the organ outlined and sum these to produce a DVH. This can be used to calculate the percentage of the volume of an organ receiving a dose of x Gy (Vx), or to see the minimum dose received by y per cent or y cc of the organ (Dy). Alternatively, the mean, maximum doses, etc. can be calculated. DVHs can also be used to ensure that a PTV receives a uniform dose. A plan should ideally produce a steep curve showing that the dose within the PTV varies from no more than 95 per cent to 107 per cent of that prescribed in accordance with ICRU report 50; DVHs for multiple volumes can be plotted on the same axes. (See Figure 4.2.)

If DVHs are obtained from a series of patients in whom acute or late effects are recorded, points on the DVH can be correlated with the probability of these effects occurring. In 2010, the QUANTEC initiative published a series of papers summarising the published evidence for safe or acceptable dose limits for normal structures. It must be remembered that these limits essentially still simplify a 3D dose distribution into a single parameter, albeit the parameter that is best correlated with effect measured in a series of patients. It is therefore important to view and record the whole DVH for a volume rather than just one dose point.

DVH calculations do not take into account all the biological variables which may determine a treatment outcome, and the concept of BED has been developed by Withers and colleagues (see Wilson 2007), based on the LQ model (see Chapter 3) to allow comparison of equivalent doses delivered to a particular structure for other dose fractionation schedules. The formula for BED is:

$$\text{BED} = \left\{ n * d \left[1 + d / \left(\alpha / \beta \right) \right] \right\} - \left[\left(0.693 * T \right) / \left(\alpha * Tp \right) \right] \tag{4.1}$$

where n = number of treatments, d = dose per fraction, T = treatment time and α/β = 3 Gy (for late effects). Tp (potential doubling time) and α (linear component of cell killing) are taken from published data for each tumour.

Equivalent uniform dose (EUD) is another method of summarising and reporting inhomogeneous dose distributions, which assumes that any two dose distributions are equivalent if they cause the same radiobiological effect.

Individual Organ Tolerances

Using QUANTEC and subsequent evidence, departments and clinical trial protocols have developed tables of dose–volume limits which plans should try to achieve. These are used as constraints in the IMRT planning process to optimise the plan, or as targets that can be assessed when the plan is being evaluated. The limits for an organ often vary slightly between departments and protocols or between tumour sites for the same organ. The QUANTEC papers provide a detailed summary of the complexities of deciding what a safe dose is for each organ, but later we suggest dose thresholds and dose–volume constraints for commonly irradiated organs. They assume radiation is prescribed at a standard fractionation of 1.8–2 Gy per fraction. Site-specific chapters discuss critical organ tolerance doses in more depth where relevant.

Spinal Cord

- Spinal cord – D_{max} <50 Gy; D_{max} <48 Gy if concomitant chemotherapy used

Because a possible consequence of late radiation damage is irreversible paralysis, treatments have been appropriately cautious, so there are few real-world examples of severe radiation myelitis on which to base estimates of spinal cord tolerance. Conversely, radiation oncologists are appropriately conservative in the limits accepted. QUANTEC estimates doses of 50 Gy and 60 Gy to the whole cord at one level result in a 0.2 per cent and 6 per cent risk of any myelopathy (defined as G2 or greater myelitis on CTCAE v5). With IMRT, it is usually only part of a cross section of the cord which receives a dose close to 50 Gy, and the dose per fraction received by the cord is usually lower than that prescribed to the PTV. A spinal cord PRV is usually defined rather than just contouring the cord itself. The spinal cord should either be defined with a 5-mm margin to produce a PRV or the spinal canal contoured as a PRV.

Dose to any part of the cord should be less than 50 Gy. When concomitant chemotherapy is used, a D_{max} of 48 Gy is recommended whilst allowing a small part (<1 cm^3) to receive up to 50 Gy. If more than a 15-cm length of cord is treated, the dose to any part of the cord should be less than 44 Gy. Milder myelopathy symptoms, such as Lhermitte's syndrome, can still occur at lower doses.

When palliative radiotherapy is repeated – for example, for spinal cord compression or when the prognosis is short – a higher dose may be used if withholding treatment is more likely to give a poor outcome than exceeding a theoretical dose limit.

Brain, Brainstem and Peripheral Nerves

- Brain – D_{max} <60 Gy for non-CNS tumours
- Brainstem – D_{max} <54 Gy (allow <59 Gy for 1–10 cc)
- Peripheral nerves e.g. brachial plexus – D_{max} < 60 Gy

QUANTEC suggest a 5 per cent risk of symptomatic radiation necrosis of the brain at five years if 72 Gy is delivered. The use of tolerance doses is more applicable to head and neck cancers where the PTV is close to neural tissue. If the brain is not part of the target volume, dose to any part should not exceed 60 Gy, as a 5 per cent risk of brain necrosis is too high to accept in this patient group.

For primary brain tumours, high doses of radiation rarely exceed 60 Gy and are usually employed only where there is a high risk of local recurrence with consequent brain injury, or when prognosis is poor. The dose to the remaining normal brain should be kept as low as possible and hot spots should be avoided.

The cognitive effects of radiotherapy to the normal brain in adults are not well evaluated, but there is increasing evidence that even low doses such as those in palliative whole brain radiotherapy can produce measurable, symptomatic effects.

The brainstem is traditionally regarded as more radiosensitive than the cerebrum and, like the spinal cord, radiation-induced damage could have very severe consequences, so acceptable dose levels are necessarily conservative.

Damage to peripheral nerves with modern radiotherapy dose distributions is very rare and there is no QUANTEC recommendation for peripheral nerves. When part of the nervous system such as the brachial plexus is considered to be an OAR, dose should be limited to <60 Gy.

Optic Nerves and Orbital Tissues

- Optic nerve – D_{max} <55 Gy. Consider accepting <60 Gy if the PTV is very close to one optic nerve.
- Optic chiasm – D_{max} <55 Gy
- Lacrimal gland – D_{max} <40 Gy
- Lens – D_{max} <10 Gy
- Retina – aim for dose to whole retina <45 Gy; D_{max} <50 Gy

Tolerance doses to optic structures are usually considered when the PTV is very close to those structures. Underdosing the PTV and increasing the risk of local recurrence may threaten sight more than potentially overdosing the optic pathway. It can be hard to assess radiation toxicity and ascribe damage to one part of the optic system as many subsections may have received a potentially harmful radiation dose (e.g. retina and optic nerve). Optic nerves and chiasm are best contoured on MRI images fused with the planning CT. Care should be taken not to have gaps in the optic nerve contour, for example at the orbital apex. QUANTEC report optic neuropathy as very rare for D_{max} <55 Gy; 3–7 per cent for D_{max} 55–60 Gy but then increasing more quickly with higher dose.

The lens is very sensitive to radiation, with doses as low as 6 Gy in 2 Gy/fraction causing cataracts. Usually the dose/fraction received in a fractionated plan is substantially less than this and cataracts can be monitored and successfully treated with relative ease. A D_{max} of <10 Gy is recommended but may be exceeded to ensure optimal PTV coverage with consent of the patient.

Radiation can cause lacrimal gland damage at relatively low doses and this can be very uncomfortable for the patient and cause subsequent damage to the cornea. A D_{max} of <40 Gy is recommended.

Mucosa

Acute radiation-induced mucositis can produce pain, nausea and diarrhoea and can affect nutrition and therefore recovery from treatment. In general, the volume of normal mucosa irradiated should be minimised, but to reduce severe acute toxicity the following are suggested.

- Small bowel – V15 <120 cc when contouring individual loops of bowel; V45 <195 cc when contouring the entire peritoneal cavity as a space for small bowel to move within
- Stomach – D_{max} < 45 Gy
- Oesophagus – limit length within treated volume as much as possible

Late radiation damage to the rectum with prostate cancer radiotherapy, including diarrhoea and incontinence, can have a major effect on quality of life. Several dose limits are usually stipulated (see Table 4.1 and Chapter 28).

Lung

There are several controversies in assessing radiation-induced pneumonitis. Breathlessness may be multifactorial, tumour shrinkage may improve lung function, and obscure radiation damage and toxicity scoring scales often relate to steroid use so more frequent prescribers may record more damage. In addition, a range of parameters are reported to correlate with late radiation fibrosis.

We recommend subtracting the GTV from the whole lung volume and then aiming for V20 <35 per cent and mean lung dose <18 Gy. In patients at higher risk of symptomatic pneumonitis we recommend V20 <25 per cent. Such patients have two or more co-existing risk factors: (i) significant lung volume loss such as previous pneumonectomy, atelectasis, effusion; (ii) concomitant chemotherapy; (iii) poor respiratory function and/or moderate to severe COPD and/or restrictive lung disease.

Testes and Ovaries

For the testis, 0.2 Gy can cause transient brief oligospermia; 2–3 Gy can lower sperm counts for two to three years. Doses of more than 6 Gy cause permanent sterility, and doses of more than 20 Gy affect hormone production.

For the ovaries, menses are suppressed at 1.5 Gy, and 6–15 Gy causes permanent ovarian failure. Increasing age lowers the threshold for these effects.

We recommend doses to ovaries and testes be kept as low as possible in order to preserve fertility when this is relevant.

OAR Tolerance Table

No radiation dose is absolutely safe, and the chosen dose constraints for an individual patient may differ from those listed in Table 4.1 for reasons explained in the text. The doses in Table 4.1 should therefore be regarded as a safe guide when radiotherapy is prescribed at 2 Gy per fraction. Please see individual tumour chapters for more detailed discussion of OAR doses.

TABLE 4.1

OAR Dose Constraints

Organ	Constraint	Optimal	Mandatory
Nervous system			
Brain	D_{max}	<60 Gy	
Brainstem	D_{max} whole organ		54 Gy (60 Gy if PRV used)
	D(1–10 cc)		<59 Gy
Peripheral nerves	D_{max}	<60 Gy	
Spinal cord	D_{max} to PRV (cord +5 mm or spinal canal)		<50 Gy (48 Gy if concomitant chemotherapy)
Head and neck			
Cochlea	Mean dose	<45 Gy	
Lacrimal gland	D_{max}		<40 Gy
Larynx	Mean dose	<45 Gy, <35 Gy where feasible	
Lens	D_{max}	<10 Gy	
Optic nerve and chiasm	D_{max}		<55 Gy <60 Gy if PTV very close to one optic nerve
Parotid gland	Mean dose	<24 Gy	
Pharyngeal constrictors	Mean dose	<50 Gy	
Retina	D_{max}	<50 Gy	
Submandibular gland	Mean dose	<39 Gy	
Thorax			
Heart	Mean dose	<25 Gy	<30 Gy
	V30 Gy	<45%	
	V40 Gy	<30%	
Lung (whole lung volume minus GTV)	V20 Gy	<35% (<25% if risk factors – see text)	
	Mean lung dose	<18 Gy	
Oesophagus (e.g. in lung cancer treatment)	Length within treated volume	<8 cm	<12 cm
Abdomen and pelvis			
Bladder	V50 Gy	<50%	
	V60 Gy	<25%	<50%
Femoral heads	V50 Gy	<5%	<50%
Kidney (each)	V20 Gy	<25%	<30%
Kidney (both)	V20 Gy	<30%	<35%
Liver	V30 Gy		<30%
	Mean	<28 Gy	<30 Gy
Ovary	D_{max}	<1.5 Gy	<15 Gy
Penile bulb	V50 Gy	<50%	
	V60 Gy	<10%	
Rectum	V30 Gy	<70%	<80%
	V40 Gy	<51%	<65%
	V50 Gy	<38%	<50%
	V60 Gy	<27%	<35%
	V70 Gy	<15%	<20%
Small bowel	D_{max} (0.1 cc)	<58 Gy	<60 Gy
	V50 Gy	<10 cc	
	V15 Gy	<120 cc	
Spleen	Mean dose	<10 Gy	
Testis	D_{max}	<2 Gy	<6 Gy

Second Malignancies

Any radiation dose increases the risk of second malignancy, so no safe dose limits can be given. In principle, the irradiated volume should be kept as small as possible. Techniques such as IMRT which use multiple beams may increase the volume of normal tissue irradiated and theoretically increase the risk of second malignancy. It will take decades before data on the incidence of second malignancies is obtained, so the possible increase can only be estimated from biological modelling. Clinical experience with radiotherapy for Hodgkin lymphoma, where the absolute incidence of second malignancies after mantle radiotherapy is 30 per cent at 30 years, shows the importance of long-term follow-up and data collection in the assessment of late effects, particularly when a new treatment technique is introduced.

Cardiac Devices

The risk of pacemaker or implantable cardioverter defibrillator (ICD) malfunction with radiotherapy increases with higher doses and should be assessed in the context of whether the patient is dependent on pacing or not. Close liaison with the pacemaker technicians and cardiologists is important. The dose to a cardiac device should be kept below 2 Gy if possible. Appropriate monitoring should be carried out during and after radiotherapy.

Special Situations

Hypofractionation

The tolerance doses described earlier assume radiotherapy is being delivered to that organ at 1.8–2 Gy per fraction, but hypofractionation is also often used particularly to treat small target volumes. The ultimate example of this is stereotactic radiotherapy. The UK SABR consortium has published guidance on optimal and mandatory critical organ tolerance doses that should be achieved with different fractionation schedules. As an example, the mandatory spinal cord PRV tolerance of 50 Gy in 2 Gy fractions becomes 14 Gy for a single fraction, 20.3 Gy for 3 fractions and 25.3 Gy for 5 fractions. These hypofractionated tolerance doses can be estimated using the linear quadratic equation, but such estimations should be used cautiously as there is often less evidence for the tolerance of tissues to new hypofractionated schedules than with standard fractionation that has been used for decades.

It is useful to be able to convert the preceding tolerance doses to other dose fractionation schedules. To do this, the equivalent dose equation described in Chapter 3 is used.

$$D_1(\alpha/\beta+d_1) = D_2(\alpha/\beta+d_2) \tag{4.2}$$

For example – what should cord tolerance be for 55 Gy in 20 fractions (2.75 Gy/fraction)? Assuming cord $\alpha/\beta = 3$, the parameters D_1 (50 Gy), d_1 (2 Gy) and d_2 (2.75 Gy) are known and D_2 can therefore be calculated by rearranging Equation 4.2:

$$D_2 = \frac{D_1(\alpha/\beta+d_1)}{(\alpha/\beta+d_2)} \text{ so } D_2 = 50(3+2)/(3+2.75) \tag{4.3}$$

So at 2.75 Gy per fraction, the equivalent cord tolerance is 43.5 Gy. This will be an overestimate, as the actual dose per fraction to the cord PRV over 20 fractions will be slightly less than 2.75 Gy.

Comorbidities

Autoimmune connective tissue diseases, such as systemic lupus erythematosus, scleroderma or rheumatoid arthritis, have long been considered an absolute or relative contraindication to radiotherapy because of concerns about an increased risk of acute or late effects. The evidence for these concerns is poor and limited to small retrospective studies, often using old radiation techniques, many of which show no increase in toxicity. As with any radiation treatment, care should be taken to minimise dose to adjacent normal structures by accurate contouring and careful planning, and the possible short- and long-term side effects should be carefully explained to patients. There is no good evidence that tolerance doses should be modified in connective tissue disease.

Inflammatory bowel disease (IBD) is usually felt to be a contraindication to pelvic radiotherapy because radiotherapy is thought to be a risk factor for flare up of IBD. The evidence for this is not strong. We recommend careful discussion with the patient and a gastroenterologist before considering pelvic radiotherapy in patients with IBD, but with proactive management of IBD and the acute side effects of treatment, radiotherapy can be used in some patients. As chemotherapy can cause flare-ups, concomitant chemotherapy with radiation should be avoided if possible.

Highly active antiretroviral therapy (HAART) has transformed the treatment of HIV infection. People with HIV have a similar increase in cancer incidence to those immunosuppressed because of a solid organ transplant. If they have a CD4 count of more than 200 cells per microlitre, are on HAART and have a good performance status then there is no good evidence that radiation tolerance doses are different to the general population.

Measurement of Late Effects

Local control and survival are usually relatively easy to assess with clinical examination, imaging and population databases. In contrast, estimation of the frequency and severity of late effects is often haphazard and incomplete and will depend on the sensitivity of the test used for their detection. Over time treatments change frequently, making it difficult to evaluate the role of each component of treatment to the outcome.

Adverse outcomes of treatment are often poorly documented by physicians and data are usually only collected retrospectively. Pressurised doctors prioritise care of the patient before recording outcomes, and there is no simple internationally standardised measure of late effects. Most scales involve grading of late effects from the physician's perspective and have been shown to underestimate late effects from the patient's point of view.

Existing scales include the RTOG/EORTC, the French/Italian scheme for gynaecological cancer, LENT-SOMA (late effects of normal tissues – subjective, objective, measured and analytic) and the NCI-CTC (common toxicity criteria) v5 – the National Cancer Institute of USA terminology criteria for adverse events recording with a severity scale for each item. This is used widely for clinical trials but is rather complex for day-to-day clinic use.

Most endpoints in these scales are clinical. Modern imaging modalities will be more sensitive at detecting abnormalities than are ascertained by clinical signs and symptoms or laboratory markers. Currently, imaging is rarely used for the documentation of late effects of radiation, unless subclinical damage progresses to a clinical problem, there is some early preventative intervention possible or the patient is being treated within a trial of a new modality.

Patient reported outcome measures (PROMS) are standardised, validated questionnaires that are completed by patients to measure their perceptions of their own functional status. Scales such as EORTC QLQ-C30 and Functional Assessment of Cancer Therapy G (FACT G) have generic cancer sections to which tumour-specific modules can be added. Studies of simpler scales for routine use by physicians or for self-reporting by patients are in progress.

Treatment of Late Effects

Until recently, little attempt has been made to modify any radiation-associated damage. Restricting aggravating factors to damage by stopping smoking, maintaining good control of blood pressure and blood sugar levels, and avoiding use of fibrogenic drugs such as bleomycin may help. Unfortunately, there is still a lack of phase 3 data to support the many drugs that have been proposed as ways to treat late effects when they begin to occur or to support the use of hyperbaric oxygen in established osteora-dionecrosis. At the end of their radiotherapy treatment, patients should be informed of possible late side effects and of who to report them to. Multidisciplinary late effects clinics are being set up with the hope that new treatments for radiation damage, better psychological support and the treatment of co-existing pathologies will improve quality of life. Preventing late effects by improving the therapeutic ratio when radiation is delivered and the promise of radiogenomics to individualise treatment are likely to be the best ways to reduce late radiation morbidity.

INFORMATION SOURCES

Alongi F, Giaj-Levra N, Sciascia S et al. Radiotherapy in patients with HIV: Current issues and review of the literature. Lancet Oncol 2017;18(7):e379–e393.

Annede P, Seisen T, Klotz C, et al. Inflammatory bowel diseases activity in patients undergoing pelvic radiation therapy. J Gastrointest Oncol 2017;8(1):173–179. doi:10.21037/jgo.2017.01.13.

Diez P, Hanna GG, Aitken KL et al. UK 2022 consensus on normal tissue dose-volume constraints for oligo-metastatic, primary lung and hepatocellular carcinoma stereotactic ablative radiotherapy. Clin Oncol 2022;34(5):288–300.

Emani B, Lyman J, Brown A et al. Tolerance of normal tissue to irradiation. Int J Radiat Oncol Biol Phys 1991;21:109–122.

Faithfull S, Lemanska A, Chen T. Patient-reported outcome measures in radiotherapy: Clinical advances and research opportunities in measurement for survivorship. Clin Oncol 2015;11:679–685.

Giaj-Levra N, Sciascia S, Fiorentino A et al. Radiotherapy in patients with connective tissue diseases. Lancet Oncol 2016;17:e109–117.

Hurkmans CW, Knegjens JL, Oei BS et al. Management of radiation oncology patients with a pacemaker or ICD: A new comprehensive practical guideline in the Netherlands. Radiat Oncol 2012;7:198–209.

Lawrie TA, Green JT, Beresford M et al. Interventions to reduce acute and late adverse gastrointestinal effects of pelvic radiotherapy for primary pelvic cancers. Cochrane Database Syst Rev 2018 Jan 23;1:CD012529.

Mir R, Kelly SM, Xiao Y et al. Organ at risk delineation for radiation therapy clinical trials: Global Harmonisation Group consensus guidelines. Radiother Oncol 2020;150:30–39.

QUANTEC - quantitative analyses of normal tissue effects in the clinic. Int J Radiat Oncol Biol Phys 2010;76(3):S1–S160.

Rosenstein BS. Radiogenomics: Identification of genomic predictors for radiation toxicity. Semin Radiat Oncol 2017;27:300–309.

Scoccianti S, Detti B, Gadda D et al. Organs at risk in the brain and their dose-constraints in adults and in children: A radiation oncologist's guide for delineation in everyday practice. Radiother Oncol 2015;114:230–238.

The Radiotherapy Board (made up of the Society and College of Radiographers, Institute of Physics and Engineering in Medicine and The Royal College of Radiologists). Management of Cancer Patients Receiving Radiotherapy With a Cardiac Implanted Electronic Device: A Clinical Guideline. London: The Royal College of Radiologists, 2015.

The Radiotherapy Board (made up of the Society and College of Radiographers, Institute of Physics and Engineering in Medicine and The Royal College of Radiologists). Ionising Radiation (Medical Exposure) Regulations: Implications for Clinical Practice in Radiotherapy. London: The Royal College of Radiologists, 2020.

Wilson G. Cell kinetics. Clin Oncol 2007;19:370–384.

5

Principles of Brachytherapy

Introduction

Brachy is from the Greek word for 'short' so brachytherapy (also known as sealed source radiotherapy), roughly translated, means short-distance therapy. Traditional brachytherapy is where a radioactive material is inserted directly into or next to a tumour and concentrates the dose there. The dose falls off very rapidly according to the inverse square law, and surrounding normal tissues receive substantially lower doses than the tumour. When 65 Gy are delivered at 0.5 cm from the source, the dose at 2 cm is only 4.06 Gy. Electronic brachytherapy is a relatively new technique using miniaturised, low-power X-ray sources operating between 50 and 100 kV.

Along with its physical advantages, there are also biological advantages. Low dose rate (LDR) brachytherapy is a type of extreme hyperfractionation and is therefore relatively sparing to normal tissues. The dose rate may be low but it is delivered continuously, which shortens overall treatment time and reduces the opportunity for tumour repopulation during treatment. Conversely, high dose rate (HDR) brachytherapy must be fractionated to avoid normal tissue morbidity. Three dose rate bands are defined: LDR (1 Gy/h), medium dose rate (MDR) (1 to 12 Gy/h) and HDR (12 Gy/h). It is important to remember that if the dose rate is increased, a dose reduction is needed to give a biologically isoeffective dose. When changing from low to medium dose rate (e.g. changing from LDR intracavitary brachytherapy to MDR), a dose correction of approximately minus 15 per cent is needed. Other advantages of brachytherapy include accurate localisation and immobilisation of the tumour, which removes the problems of organ movement and set-up errors seen with external beam radiotherapy (EBRT).

The disadvantages of brachytherapy are the operative nature of the procedures often needed to access the tumour, the requirement for skilled personnel and the radiation protection measures needed to protect patient, staff and general public.

Brachytherapy is considered whenever possible for accessible localised tumours of relatively small volume. It is contraindicated where tumour infiltrates bone, where the margins of the tumour or target volume are not clearly identifiable and where there is active infection in the tissues. Brachytherapy is used as a radical single modality treatment or in combination with EBRT to deliver a boost dose. It can be used after surgical excision to irradiate a tumour bed. Isotopes used for brachytherapy are shown in Table 5.1.

Delivery Systems

With interstitial brachytherapy, sources are inserted directly into tissue. Iridium-192 wire is ideal and can be cut to any length and curved as required. It is used as hair pins to treat cancer of the anterior tongue, or looped to treat base-of-tongue tumours. Prostate cancer brachytherapy with iodine-125 or palladium-103 seeds is also classed as interstitial therapy.

Intracavitary brachytherapy places applicators inside a body cavity such as the uterine canal or vagina. These applicators can then be afterloaded with radioactive sources. Caesium-137 is the isotope of choice for low dose rate treatments, and small iridium-192 sources for HDR afterloading systems. Surface applicator brachytherapy can be used for very superficial lesions less than 1 mm thick, such as strontium-90 eye plaque therapy after resection of pterygium.

DOI: 10.1201/9781315171562-5

TABLE 5.1

Isotopes for Brachytherapy

Source	Form	Dose Rate	Emissions	Half-Life
Radium-226	Tubes, needles	LDR	2.45 MV gamma	1620 years
Caesium-137	Tubes, needles	LDR	0.662 MV gamma	30 years
	Afterloading pellets			
Cobalt-60	Tubes	HDR	1.17, 1.33 MV gamma	5 years
	Afterloading pellets			
Iridium-192	Wires	LDR	0.38 MV gamma	74 days
	Afterloading pellets	HDR		
Iodine-125	Seeds	LDR	27.4, 31.4, 35.5 kV	60 days
Palladium-103	Seeds	LDR	21 kV	17 days
Strontium-90	Eye plaques	HDR	2.27 MeV beta	28.8 years

Mould brachytherapy uses sealed sources held in a fixed arrangement and distance from the surface by a custom-made mould. It is usually used to treat superficial lesions of skin, mouth or vagina. Intraluminal brachytherapy places applicators loaded with radioactive sources in a lumen such as the bronchus or oesophagus.

For tumour sites where it would be difficult to remove the sources, or where very low dose rate is preferred, a permanent implant can be performed with sources such as iodine-125 seeds for prostate cancer. High dose rate intracavitary afterloading systems place sources temporarily using flexible catheters. Temporary interstitial HDR prostate implants are also possible.

To reduce radiation dose to staff, techniques of afterloading have been developed which involve the initial implantation of nonradioactive applicators, catheters or carriers into the patient. The radioactive sources can then be 'manually afterloaded' by the operator into the applicators, or 'remotely afterloaded' by a machine under computer control. Remote afterloading reduces the doses to staff, patients and visitors to a minimum and, with appropriately shielded rooms, can be used for LDR continuous, and HDR fractionated, treatments.

There are several types of electronic brachytherapy (EB) systems available, e.g. Intrabeam (Zeiss), Papillon (Ariane) and Esteya (Electa). It is mainly being used to treat non-melanomatous skin cancers and partial breast irradiation. There is early data showing promising results, but prospective long-term data is needed, and there is a lack of data comparing EB to traditional radiotherapy techniques. There are also no consensus dosimetry data available, and further trials are needed to investigate potential differences in RBE. An Randomised Controlled Trial (RCT) of EB for Intra operative radiotherapy (IORT) in breast cancer has shown a higher rate of recurrence than other standard techniques. Current guidelines do not recommend EB outside of prospective clinical trials. Research into designing miniaturised X-ray tunes closer to the dimension of an Ir-192 wire may allow future research into interstitial electronic brachytherapy.

Clinical Use

Table 5.2 shows some of the common sites treated with brachytherapy techniques.

Dosimetry

The spatial configuration of brachytherapy sources in a target volume is chosen to achieve as homogeneous a dose as possible. The dose distribution is inherently inhomogeneous with high doses around each source, which can cause necrosis, and low doses between sources, which can result in recurrence. An established set of rules for implantation must be followed to achieve good dose distributions. Several systems have been used to calculate and describe the dose distributions of brachytherapy implants. The

TABLE 5.2

Brachytherapy Treatments

Site	Indications	Technique	Source and Dose Rate
Anterior Tongue	Small T1/T2	Hair pins	Iridium 192 LDR
Buccal Mucosa	Small T1/T2	Plastic tube	Iridium 192 LDR
Base of Tongue	Boost after EBRT	Loop	Iridium 192 LDR
Lip	Small T1/T2 Boost after EBRT	Needle	Iridium 192 LDR
Nasopharynx	Boost after EBRT Re-treatment	Moulds NPC applicators	Iridium 192 LDR or HDR
Recurrent Disease in Neck	Re-treatment	Plastic tube	Iridium 192 LDR or HDR
Uterine Tumours	Postoperative Palliative	Vaginal applicator Tube and ovoids	HDR or LDR
Cervical Tumours	Boost after EBRT	Tube and ovoids	HDR or LDR
Vagina	Small stage 1 Boost after EBRT Palliative	Perineal template	HDR or LDR
Vulva	Boost after EBRT Palliative	Perineal template	HDR or LDR
Anal	Small T1 Boost after EBRT Palliative	Perineal implant through template	HDR or LDR
Breast	Boost after EBRT Palliative	Plastic tubes Needles Bridge template	HDR or LDR
Prostate	Low risk disease Boost to EBRT	Permanent seeds Perineal template	LDR I-125 or Pd 103 HDR or LDR
Skin	NMSC with complex curved surfaces	3D-printed mould therapy Freiburg flap applicator	HDR HDR

Manchester system is widely used for gynaecological implants. The GEC-ESTRO/ICRU group has published recommendations on target volume concepts and plan evaluation using DVHs (see Chapter 32). The Paris system was specifically designed for use with iridium wire afterloading techniques. Both these systems use traditional dose formalism for manual calculations with reference to precalculated data such as Paterson–Parker tables for needle implants, and the cross-line graphs or escargot curves for iridium wire. These systems have been adapted for computer calculations which follow the TG43 formalism, published in 1995 by the American Association of Physicists in Medicine (AAPM) Task Group 43. The sources must be distributed according to the particular dosimetry system used and the method of dose specification and prescription adhered to. Previously, it was always important to plan in advance the number and distribution of radioactive sources. With modern implant and dosimetry techniques, it is now possible to perform dynamic intraoperative dosimetry, e.g. for prostate seed implants, which reduces the amount of preplanning needed and avoids repositioning errors. An estimate of the volume to be implanted and the number of sources still needs to be made and the sources must be distributed according to the system used.

The Manchester System for Interstitial Implants

The Manchester system was based on the use of radium sources with dose tables that gave the amount of radium and time needed (mg h tables) to give 1000 roentgens (1000 cGy) to the treated surface. The Paterson–Parker rules provide sets of distribution rules for planar or volume implants. For a simple planar rectangular implant, the sources must be parallel and the distance between sources should not exceed 10 mm. The end of rows of parallel needles is crossed by needles at right angles with two-thirds of the sources at the periphery and one-third in the central area. If an end is not crossed, 10 per cent is deducted from the area when reading from the mg h tables.

The Paris System for Iridium Wire Implants and Afterloading Techniques

The Paris system was developed for iridium-192 wire implants and can also be used to calculate doses for computer-based HDR systems. The distribution rules for iridium-192 implants are as follows:

- Active sources should be parallel and straight.
- The lines should be equidistant.
- The line or plane on which the midpoint of the sources lies (central plane) should be at right angles to the axis of the sources.
- The linear activity should be uniform along the length of each line, and identical for all lines.
- The separation of sources may be varied from one implant to another. A minimum of 8 mm separation is acceptable for the smallest volumes, rising to 20 mm for the largest.
- For volume implants, the distribution of sources in cross section (central plane) should be either in equilateral triangles or in squares.
- Because it is not usual to cross the ends of the sources, the average length of active wire must be longer than the target volume by 25–30 per cent, depending on the number and separation of sources used.

A Paris implant can be a single plane with regularly spaced wires, a circular arrangement of needles/catheters or a multiple plane arrangement to treat thicker tumours. The multiple plane arrangement can be triangular, rectangular or square. The dose calculation is then based on the distribution of sources in the central plane, that is, the plane which is at right angles to the axis of the midpoint of the sources. An example of a rectangular implant is when hairpins are used to treat anterior tongue tumours. Here the central plane should be halfway down the legs of the hairpin, ignoring the cross piece. Computer systems can now allow rotation of the implant in 3D to visualise the implant and central plane.

The calculation then uses the basal dose rate, which is the dose in the middle of the implanted volume where the dose rate is lowest. The basal dose rate at a point is the summation of dose rate contributions from each source according to the distance of the source from the point. In the case of a large implant, there may be several basal dose rate points, and a mean basal dose rate is taken for the implant as a whole (Figure 5.1).

Once the basal dose rate at the centre of the implant is known, the reference dose is taken as 85 per cent of the basal dose rate. This is then used to calculate the duration of the implant, and the 85 per cent isodose defines the treated volume. The time needed for the implant is derived by dividing the prescribed

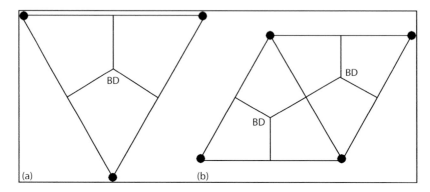

FIGURE 5.1   Basal dose (BD) rate point for two different volume implants arranged in (a) one and (b) two equilateral triangles.

TABLE 5.3

Calculation for Breast Implant

Two-plane implant to deliver 25 Gy
Superficial plane = 5-cm wires × 2
Deep plane = 7-cm wires × 3
Separation between sources = 18 mm
Activity of wire (midway through treatment) = air kerma rate 0.5 μGy/h/mm at 1 m (0.1193 mG/mm)

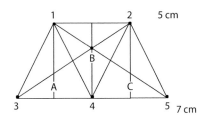

Wire	A		B		C	
	Distance (mm)	Dose Rate (Gy/h)	Distance (mm)	Dose Rate (Gy/h)	Distance (mm)	Dose Rate (Gy/h)
1	10.4	0.1245	10.4	0.1245	20.8	0.0465
2	20.8	0.0465	10.4	0.1245	10.4	0.1245
3	10.4	0.1340	20.8	0.0555	27.5	0.0365
4	10.4	0.1340	10.4	0.1340	10.4	0.1340
5	27.5	0.0365	20.8	0.0555	10.4	0.1340
Total		0.4755		0.4940		0.4755

$$\text{Mean basal dose rate} = \frac{0.4755 + 0.4940 + 0.4755 \text{ Gy/h}}{3}$$

$$= 0.4817 \text{ Gy/h}$$

$$\text{Reference dose rate } (85\%) = 0.4817 \times 0.85$$

$$= 0.4095 \text{ Gy/h}$$

$$\text{Treatment time} = \frac{25.00}{0.4095}$$

$$= 61.05 \text{ h}$$

$$= 2 \text{ days } 13 \text{ h}$$

dose by the reference dose rate and takes into account the activity of the wire used and radioactive decay during the implant. An example is shown in Table 5.3.

It is important to know the relationship between volume treated and length and separation of sources used when performing an implant. The following apply to implants according to the Paris system:

- The length of the treated volume is approximately 70 per cent of the length of the active sources (Figure 5.2).
- The thickness of the treated volume in a single-plane implant is approximately 50 per cent of the separation between the sources.
- The treatment margin around a volume implant performed in triangles is 30–40 per cent of the distance between the sides of the triangle.
- The ratio of treated volume to source length or separation increases as more sources are used.

With the increased use of computer programmes for dose calculation, there is a tendency to prescribe to computer-derived isodoses. The isodose for prescription is chosen where the dose gradient is very steep, and there

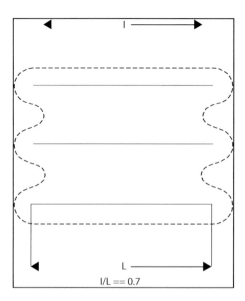

FIGURE 5.2   Relationship between treated volume (I) and length of active sources (L).

may be wide variation between the dose at the periphery and that at the centre of the target volume. A considerable proportion of the implanted volume may therefore receive a higher dose than that at the periphery. For safe treatment, it is advised that the central dose should be no more than 20 per cent higher than the peripheral dose.

Dose Reporting

The ICRU report 38 (1985) gives guidance on reporting absorbed doses and volumes for intracavitary brachytherapy. It recommends that a combination of total reference air kerma, description of the reference volume and absorbed dose at reference points be used to specify intracavitary applications for cervix carcinoma.

The ICRU report 58 (1997) recommends that the following information should be reported following an interstitial implant:

- Description of volumes:
  - Gross tumour volume
  - Clinical tumour volume
  - Treated volume
- Description of sources and techniques:
  - Description of time pattern
  - Total reference air kerma (TRAK) (the sum of the products of the reference air kerma rate and irradiation time for each source)
- Description of doses:
  - Prescribed dose
  - Mean central dose in the central plane (equivalent to basal dose in the Paris system)
  - Peripheral dose (equivalent to the reference dose in the Paris system)
- Description of high and low dose volumes

The ICRU GEC-ESTRO report 89 (2013) gives guidance on reporting brachytherapy for cancer of the cervix, with a key element being the 4D adaptive target concept at certain time points during treatment, and recommends reporting dose and volume parameters to contours and reference points.

A highly skilled and trained team is essential to perform brachytherapy implants safely. Everyone in the team should be trained in the principles of radiation safety so that the patient, staff and public are not at risk of unnecessary irradiation. Protective measures should be in place to keep dose levels as low as reasonably practicable (ALARP).

Legislation Pertaining to Brachytherapy

The following legislation governs the use of sealed brachytherapy sources in hospitals in the UK:

- Ionising Radiations Regulations 2017, Statutory Instrument 2017 No. 1075, London: HMSO
- Ionising Radiation (Medical Exposure) Regulations 2017, Statutory Instrument 2017 No. 1322, London: HMSO
- Ionising Radiation (Medical Exposure) Regulations (Amendment) 2018, Statutory Instrument 2018 No. 121, London: HMSO
- The Environmental Permitting (England and Wales) Regulations 2016, Statutory Instrument 2016 No. 1154, London: HMSO
- The Carriage of Dangerous Goods (Amendment) Regulations 2019, Statutory Instrument 2019 No. 598, London: HMSO
- High Activity Sealed Sources (HASS) and Orphan Source Regulations 2005, Statutory Instrument 2005 No. 2686. London: HMSO
- Health and Safety at Work etc. Act 1974

The Ionising Radiation Medical Exposure Regulations (IR[ME]R) requires employers and practitioners to hold a licence for the administration of radioactive substances for a specified purpose at any given medical radiological installation.

- Each employer is required to hold a licence for each administration at each medical radiological installation for the purpose of the administration of radioactive substances to humans.
- Every practitioner is required to hold a licence in order to justify the administration of radioactive substances to humans.

ARSAC (Administration of Radioactive Substances Advisory Committee) provides advice on the issue of licences to the relevant licencing authority. Applications are processed by Public Health England (PHE). The purpose for which each radioactive substance specified in a licence may be administered is defined as research, diagnosis or treatment. The majority of licences are issued for five years.

INFORMATION SOURCES

Gerbaulet A, Pötter R, Mazeron J-J, et al. The GEC ESTRO Handbook of Brachytherapy. Brussels: ESTRO, 2002.

Gyn GEC-ESTRO/ICRU Report 89. Prescribing, recording and reporting brachytherapy for cancer of the cervix. J ICRU 2013;13(1–2).

Hoskin P, Coyle C. Radiotherapy in Practice. Oxford: Oxford University Press, 2005.

International Commission on Radiation Units and Measurements. Dose and Volume Specification for Reporting Intracavitary Therapy in Gynecology, ICRU Report 38. Bethesda, Maryland, USA, 1985.

International Commission on Radiation Units and Measurements. Dose and Volume Specification for Reporting Interstitial Therapy, ICRU Report 58. Bethesda, Maryland, USA, 1997.

Report of American Association of Physicists in Medicine Radiation Therapy Committee Task Group 43. Med Phys 22 1995:209–235. www.oxfordjournals.org/jicru/backissues/reports.html. Reports 50, 62 and 71.

Tom MC, Hepel JT, Patel R, et al. The American brachytherapy society consensus statement for electronic brachytherapy. Brachytherapy 2019;18(3):292–298.

6

Emergency and Palliative Radiotherapy

Indications for Radiotherapy

Emergency radiotherapy, which should be given within 24 hours of diagnosis, is only indicated for selected patients with spinal cord compression. Urgent palliative radiotherapy, used to treat various other symptoms from primary disease or metastases, should be given as soon as possible. The set-up and planning are kept as simple as possible for palliative treatments, but they have to be individualised for each patient. Palliation requires as much skill as radical treatment. Accurate definition of the tumour causing the symptom is important, and side effects of treatment must be minimised to ensure overall benefit to the patient.

Stereotactic ablative radiotherapy (SABR) has an established role in the treatment of oligometastases with improvement in disease-free survival. The oligometastatic phenotype is being increasingly identified with the use of sensitive modern imaging such as MRI and PET CT. More complex specialist planning techniques are used as described in Chapter 2. An experienced multidisciplinary team is essential for the delivery of SABR.

Spinal Cord Compression

This is a medical emergency. The spinal cord is compressed most commonly by metastatic tumour involving the vertebrae, or less commonly by a benign cause such as a vertebral fracture, abscess or ruptured intervertebral disc. The spinal cord ends at approximately L1, and compression below this level causes cauda equina syndrome.

Metastatic spinal cord compression (MSCC) occurs in approximately 5 per cent of patients with cancer, most commonly with primary tumours of the lung, prostate, breast, kidney and thyroid, and with lymphoma and multiple myeloma.

The most important determinant of outcome is the severity of neurological damage at the time treatment is initiated, which is why treatment must be considered as an emergency. Of patients without significant neurological deficit, 80 per cent remain ambulant or regain the ability to walk, whereas only 50 per cent of those with even a mild transverse myelopathy and 5 per cent of those with paraplegia do so. The prognosis is dependent on the type and extent of the primary malignancy. Untreated patients with MSCC often die within a month. With treatment, the median overall survival ranges from 3 to 16 months.

Clinical Features

A high index of suspicion is needed to detect cases early while neurological function is still intact. Common features of MSCC in the thoracic area are back pain (typically radicular), sensory disturbance in the lower limbs, bladder or bowel dysfunction and leg weakness. The neurological signs are of bilateral upper motor neuron lesions in the legs and a sensory level. Cervical cord involvement may be suspected if there are signs and symptoms in the arms. In the lumbar spine area, compression may be of the cauda equina, causing nerve root pain in the back and legs, urinary disturbance, signs of a lower motor neuron lesion in the

DOI: 10.1201/9781315171562-6

legs and patchy asymmetrical sensory loss. Nerve root irritation may be shown by limitation of straight leg raising. Onset of symptoms may be insidious, or occasionally paraplegia may develop rapidly with few preceding symptoms. Any delay in diagnosis and treatment will impact on functional outcome. Complete, sudden paraplegia is usually associated with vascular damage and is commonly irreversible.

Investigations

A patient with suspected MSCC needs an emergency MRI scan of the whole spine, which is the most informative and least invasive technique. There are frequently multiple levels involved, and clinical signs can appear to be out of keeping with the vertebral level involved (Figure 6.1).

A diagnosis of malignancy may already be known. If not, a good history and general examination should be undertaken to search for a primary tumour. Investigations such as a chest X-ray, CT chest/abdo/pelvis, tumour marker estimations, biopsy or fine needle aspiration and cytology should be performed.

Treatment

At presentation, all patients suspected to have MSCC should be given high dose steroids (e.g. dexamethasone 16 mg daily).

Sequencing of Multimodality Treatment

When planning treatment, the overall picture of the patient's health status, neurological function, site and histology of the primary, sites of metastases, prognosis and further treatment options, performance status and previous treatments, especially with radiotherapy, need to be taken into account. In patients who are not known to have malignancy, surgical decompression should be the first consideration; or if malignancy is highly suspected and the patient is not fit for surgery, an image guided vertebral biopsy can be performed.

A neurosurgeon should urgently assess all patients who are fit for surgery, reviewing clinical features and MRI to assess whether there is a place for multimodality treatment. Immediate consultation is made

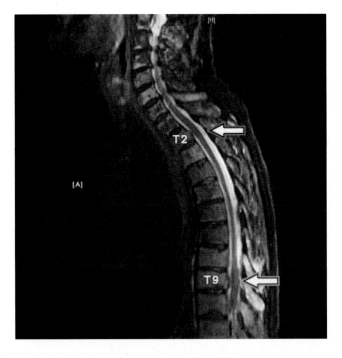

FIGURE 6.1 MRI of spine showing spinal cord compression at T2 and T9.

possible with remote image viewing. Surgery for MSCC usually involves decompression and stabilisation of the spine. The indications for surgery are:

- Unknown primary tumour
- Unstable spine or vertebral displacement
- Relapse following spinal radiotherapy
- Neurological symptoms which progress during radiotherapy
- Relatively radio-resistant tumour
- Paralysis of rapid onset

There is evidence that some patients have a better functional outcome if treated with emergency spinal decompressive surgery followed by postoperative radiotherapy than with radiotherapy alone.

In patients with very chemo-sensitive tumours such as lymphoma or small cell carcinoma of the lung, chemotherapy can be started urgently before radiotherapy.

If surgery or chemotherapy are not appropriate, Radiotherapy is given immediately to prevent further neurological damage, to improve function and for pain relief.

Clinical and Radiological Anatomy

A full neurological examination should include search for motor impairment, sensory levels and local pain and tenderness. These symptoms and signs should be correlated with MRI appearances in consultation with a radiologist. Metastases may be lytic or sclerotic, and collapse, compression, laterally or posteriorly, and any paravertebral soft tissue mass should be noted. The sensory level detected in a skin dermatome arises from compression of the corresponding cord segment, which lies at a higher level than the vertebral body of the same number, e.g. a sensory level at T10 on the skin arises from compression of its cord segment at the level of the T8 vertebra.

Data Acquisition

The patient is planned and treated ideally in the prone position using a direct posterior beam to avoid increased skin dose from treatment through the couch top. However, the supine position using an undercouch beam may be easier and more comfortable for the patient. Treatment should be planned using a CT scanner for virtual simulation or a simulator. Information from clinical examination and the MR scan is used to design the target volume.

Reference tattoos are placed at the isocentre and bilaterally.

Target Volume Definition

The GTV includes vertebral and soft tissue tumour as seen on CT planning scan and diagnostic MRI. The CTV includes the spinal canal, the width of the vertebra and one vertebra above and below the MSCC, if the planning is based on MRI, or two vertebrae above and below if based on X-ray or CT, to allow for uncertainty about the extent of microscopic disease. The CTV to PTV margin is 1 cm.

In patients who have had surgery, the CTV will also include any metal that has been used to stabilise the spine.

Dose Solutions

Simple single beam or conformal techniques can be used (Figure 6.2). To treat the PTV adequately at depth, a direct 6 MV photon beam may be used. For lumbosacral lesions, a better dose distribution may be obtained with opposing beams. If treatment is delivered with a cobalt-60 source, an extra margin for the penumbra should be added according to departmental protocol. The field edge defined at the simulator to cover the PTV represents the 50 per cent isodose.

The dose prescription point is the depth of the anterior spinal canal. This can be assessed from axial imaging and is usually at 5–7 cm in the cervical and thoracic region, and at 7–8 cm in the lumbar region.

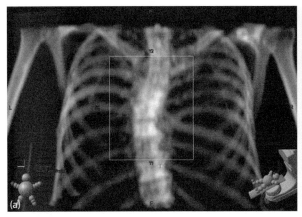 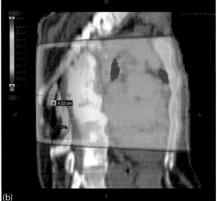

FIGURE 6.2 Virtual simulation for treatment of spinal cord compression showing (a) posterior beam arrangement, and (b) sagittal dose distribution from 6 MV beam (depth to anterior spinal canal 4.52 cm).

Occasionally, spinal cord compression is caused by a primary tumour such as a plasmacytoma, and radical radiotherapy can produce permanent local control or even cure. In this situation, a planned homogeneous dose distribution using IMRT or with wedged posterior oblique beams with or without a direct posterior beam (Figure 6.3) can be used.

Dose Fractionation

Palliative Radiotherapy

In patients with a good prognosis, when radiotherapy is the first definitive treatment or post operatively the following schedules are used:

- 20 Gy in 5 daily fractions of 4 Gy given in one week
- 30 Gy in 10 daily fractions of 3 Gy given in two weeks

For the palliation of pain in patients with a poor prognosis, poor performance status of established paraplegia for 24 hours a single dose of 8Gy may be used.

The SCORE-2 randomised controlled trial showed that short course 20 Gy in 5 fractions was not significantly inferior to 30 Gy in 10 fractions in patients with poor to intermediate expected survival.

The SCORAD randomised controlled trial showed that a single fraction of 8 Gy versus 20 Gy in 5 fractions did not meet the criteria for noninferiority, but the lower bound of the CI overlap with the noninferiority margin was very close. The trial showed that patients with metastases in the distal spine or cauda equina may have less toxicity with 20 Gy in 5 fractions.

Curative Radiotherapy

Solitary plasmacytoma: 45 Gy in 25 daily fractions of 1.8 Gy given in five weeks. Lymphoma: 30–36 Gy in 15–18 daily fractions given in three to three and a half weeks.

Treatment Delivery and Patient Care

An experienced multidisciplinary team should care for a patient during treatment. A patient with an unstable spine or undergoing surgery needs specialist nursing and physiotherapy. Those undergoing radiotherapy need specialist input from experienced radiographers, nurses and physiotherapists to help them to rehabilitate and regain neurological function. Ongoing oncological management needs to be

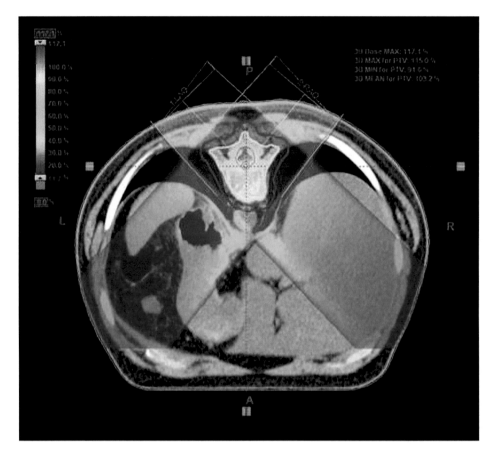

FIGURE 6.3   CT plan (with dose color wash) to treat tumour of vertebral body using 6 MV posterior oblique wedged beams.

planned, and the palliative care team should be involved for symptom control and support. Doses of dexamethasone should be reduced gradually after completion of radiotherapy.

Superior Vena Cava Obstruction

Indications for Radiotherapy

Over 90 per cent of cases of superior vena cava obstruction (SVCO) have a malignant cause. Although uncommon in patients with lung cancer, the commonest cause of SVCO is nevertheless small cell and non-small cell lung cancer. Other malignant causes are lymphoma and metastasis from mesothelioma, thymoma or any tumour that spreads to the mediastinal lymph nodes.

The obstruction arises from compression of the SVC by tumour at the right main or upper lobe bronchus or by large volume mediastinal lymphadenopathy. Symptoms may be severe when the obstruction is below the entry of the azygous vein. The clinical features are neck swelling and distended veins over the chest. There may be swelling of one or both arms, shortness of breath, hoarse voice and headaches. The diagnosis is made on contrast-enhanced spiral or multi-slice CT scans, which can accurately identify the site of occlusion or stenosis and the presence of intravascular thrombus. Impending SVCO may also be diagnosed on CT scans.

SVCO is no longer considered a radiotherapy emergency, as outcome is not related to the duration of symptoms. Urgent action may be needed to prevent SVCO leading to airway obstruction from laryngeal or bronchial oedema, or coma from cerebral oedema.

Confirmation of histology is important and can be obtained by biopsy of the primary tumour at bronchoscopy or mediastinoscopy, by percutaneous CT-guided biopsy or by biopsy of an involved cervical lymph node. Tumour markers such as alpha-fetoprotein (AFP) and ß-hCG for germ cell tumours, lactic dehydrogenase for lymphoma and prostate-specific antigen (PSA) for prostate cancer may be helpful.

Sequencing of Multimodality Treatment

Steroids such as high-dose dexamethasone are traditionally given as part of SVCO management. Their use should be of short duration.

SVC stenting has been shown to be the most effective treatment, with rapid relief of symptoms, and should be considered first wherever available or for patients who fail to respond to chemotherapy or radiotherapy. Patients with a locally advanced cancer may still be amenable to radical treatment with chemotherapy and radiotherapy once the acute SVCO has been managed with a stent.

Chemotherapy should be considered in chemo-sensitive tumours such as small cell lung cancer, lymphoma, leukaemia and germ cell tumours. Radiotherapy should be considered in non-small cell lung cancer and other less chemo-sensitive tumours and when SVC stenting is not available.

Data Acquisition

Ideally, patients should be treated supine with 3D conformal CT planning, virtual CT simulation or simulator planning. The CT scans are taken with 3–5 mm slices from the lower neck to the diaphragm. As SVC stenting is the initial treatment for patients with respiratory compromise, they should be able to lie flat, and a treatment volume can be determined in order to deliver the best treatment for their cancer.

Target Volume Definition

The GTV is defined on the contrast-enhanced CT scans, including any mediastinal mass and the site of SVCO (Figure 6.4).

The CTV is chosen according to tumour type and patterns of spread. The CTV-PTV margin is 1–2 cm. The margin is modified to spare normal lung tissue if possible.

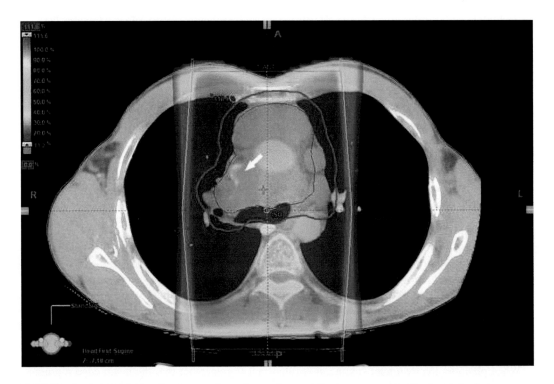

FIGURE 6.4 Axial CT slice showing anterior and posterior opposing beams created with virtual simulation to treat SVCO (arrowed).

Dose Solutions

3D conformal planning can be used to treat the PTV and spare as much normal lung and spinal cord as possible. Conventionally, treatment is given with anterior and posterior beams with MLC or lead shielding.

Dose Fractionation

- 20 Gy in 5 daily fractions of 4 Gy given in one week
- 30 Gy in 10 daily fractions of 3 Gy given in two weeks

Bone Metastases

Indications for Radiotherapy

Pain from bone metastases which persists in spite of analgesia can be successfully treated by radiotherapy with good relief in 80 per cent of cases. The most common tumours to metastasise to bone are prostate, breast and lung cancers, but bone metastases may occur from any primary tumour site. Assessment of metastatic bone pain may require a full evaluation of the sites of metastases by isotope bone scanning or MRI to determine whether local or systemic therapy is appropriate. If the cortex of the bone is eroded and there is risk of fracture, or if the bone has already fractured, surgical stabilisation should be performed followed by postoperative radiotherapy. Isotope therapy of diffuse prostatic cancer bone metastases may be considered.

Data Acquisition

Immobilisation is individualised to the patient and the site of the bone metastases to be treated. Most sites can be treated with the patient supine, except vertebral lesions, which are ideally treated with the patient prone. This is especially relevant for cancers with a long natural history where a possible need for re-treatment makes skin sparing desirable, particularly over the sacrum. Ankle stocks and headrests can be used to aid immobilisation. Lesions in the upper cervical spine are best treated with the patient supine, immobilised in a thermoplastic shell so that opposing lateral beams can be used to avoid irradiating the oral cavity and pharynx. Patients who are to be treated with electron or orthovoltage applicators can be immobilised supine, prone or on their sides.

The area to be treated is planned using a virtual CT or conventional simulation with reference to diagnostic X-rays, bone scans, CT, MRI and sites of symptoms.

Target Volume Definition

The origin of the pain must be carefully ascertained to ensure the correct site is treated. For example, knee pain may radiate from the hip, femur or spine, and rib pain may radiate from the vertebral body. The volume chosen must balance symptom relief with sparing of normal tissues to minimise side effects (e.g. avoiding the small bowel with pelvic treatments).

Where possible, the whole structure should be treated, e.g. a whole vertebra, so that it is easier to match adjacent fields that may be required with subsequent treatments. It is usual to include one or two vertebrae above and below the site of involvement.

When treating a bone postoperatively, the entire prosthesis or intramedullary nail should be covered with a margin of normal bone. This is the area most at risk of residual tumour. In patients with multiple painful bone metastases, wide field half-body volumes can be treated. Treatment portals are marked on the patient with reference tattoos as a permanent record. Photographs, DRRs or simulator films should be taken as a record and for reference for future treatment planning.

When planning the treatment volume, it is important to remember that the beam edge represents the 50 per cent isodose, and a margin must be added to ensure the target volume is covered by the 90–95 per cent isodose.

Dose Solutions

The majority of treatments are given with a single direct photon beam, for example to the spine, or as opposing anterior and posterior beams, e.g. pelvis. Sites such as the ribs can be treated with direct electron or orthovoltage beams. For sites close to organs at risk or for re-treatment, more conformal or complex techniques can be used. A single fraction of 8 Gy has been shown overall to be equivalent to higher doses. For large volumes, situations where long-term survival is expected or where long segments of spinal cord are included, a fractionated course of treatment may reduce acute and late morbidity.

Anterior and posterior opposing beams are used for half-body radiotherapy. A lower dose is used for upper half-body radiotherapy to keep lung dose within tolerance. The prescription point for a single beam, e.g. spine, should be the depth of the vertebral body taken from imaging, and is usually between 5 cm and 7 cm in the cervical and thoracic region and 7–8 cm in the lumbar region. The prescription point for opposing anterior and posterior beams is the MPD. The prescription point for electron therapy is 100 per cent on the central axis, and the energy is chosen to cover the target volume at depth by the 90 per cent isodose.

Orthovoltage beams are prescribed to D_{max} at 100 per cent. A 250–500 kV beam will give an 80 per cent isodose at a depth of 3–3.5 cm, with a relative increase in the dose to bone compared with megavoltage and electron beams.

Dose Fractionation

- 8 Gy single fraction
- 20 Gy in 5 daily fractions of 4 Gy given in one week
- 30 Gy in 10 daily fractions of 3 Gy given in two weeks

Half body Radiotherapy

- Lower 8 Gy single fraction
- Upper 6 Gy single fraction

Haemorrhage

Bleeding from advanced tumours of the breast, bladder, bronchus, oesophagus and other sites can be effectively palliated with radiotherapy. Simple arrangements such as opposing anterior and posterior beams for treatment of the bronchus or bladder, or small tangential beams for breast tumours, can be used. The field size is chosen clinically as the smallest needed to palliate the bleeding effectively with the fewest side effects, and so may not include the whole tumour.

The following dose fractionations can be used:

- Single 8 Gy fraction
- 20 Gy in 5 daily fractions given in one week
- 30 Gy in 5 fractions given in six weeks (6 Gy once weekly) can be used for patient convenience where higher doses are needed

SABR for Oligometastases

The aim of SABR in patients with oligometastases is to achieve local control at the limited number of metastatic sites, improve disease-free survival, delay systemic therapy, improve quality of life and, hopefully, improve overall survival. To identify patients with truly oligometastatic disease, staging should be carried out with PET CT and/or whole-body MRI. Brain imaging should be performed to exclude occult brain metastases in disease subtypes such as NSCLC with a high propensity for cerebral metastases. The maximum number of sites and size considered for SABR are two sites of spinal metastatic disease, one to three sites and <5 cm for liver metastases, <6 cm for adrenal metastases, up to three sites and <5 cm for lung metastases and one to three sites for lymph node metastases. SABR may be used for re-irradiation,

TABLE 6.1

SABR Oligometastatic Treatment Dose and Fractionation Recommendations

Metastasis Site	Total Dose (Gy)	No. of Fractions	Dose Fraction (Gy)	Frequency
Lung	54	3	18	Alt daily
	55	5	11	Alt daily
	60	8	7.5	Alt daily
Adrenal	30–36	3	10–12	Daily or alt daily
Liver	45	3	15	Alt daily
	50–60	5	10–12	Daily or alt daily
Spine	24–27	3	8–9	Alt daily
Bone	30–40	3	10–13.3	Alt daily
Lymph node	30–40	3	10–13.3	Alt daily
Re-irradiation	Up to 30 Gy depending on previous dose	5	Up to 6	Daily or alt daily

for example in the spine with full MDT assessment and careful calculation of the remaining spinal cord tolerance. The following are the eligibility criteria for oligometastatic disease treated within the UK Commissioning Through Evaluation (CTE) programme.

- Metastatic carcinoma with either a histologically or cytologically proven primary site or a male patient with a PSA >50 and clinical evidence of prostate cancer
- One to three sites of metastatic disease (defined after appropriate imaging) which can be treated with stereotactic radiotherapy to a radical radiation dose
- A maximum of two sites of spinal metastatic disease
- Maximum size of any single metastasis 6 cm (5 cm for lung or liver metastases)
- Disease-free interval greater than six months; unless synchronous liver metastases from colorectal primary (see liver metastases section)
- Not more than three oligometastatic sites treated in total per patient
- Expected life expectancy greater than six months
- Performance status less than or equal to two
- All patients to be discussed at stereotactic MDT with presence of, or prior discussion with, a disease site-specific oncologist

Doses and recommendations are given in Table 6.1.

INFORMATION SOURCES

Hoskin PJ, Hopkins K, Misra V, et al. Effect of single-fraction vs multifraction radiotherapy on ambulatory status among patients with spinal canal compression from metastatic cancer: The SCORAD randomized clinical trial. JAMA 2019;322(21):2084–2094. doi:10.1001/jama.2019.17913

NICE. Metastatic Spinal Cord Compression. Guideline 75, 2008: www.nice.org.uk/guidance/index (Accessed December 4, 2008).

Patchell RA, Tibbs PA, Regine WF, et al. Direct decompressive surgical resection in the treatment of spinal cord compression caused by metastatic cancer. A randomized trial. Lancet 2005 Aug 20–26;336:643–648.

Rades D, Šegedin B, Conde-Moreno AJ, et al. Radiotherapy with 4 Gy × 5 versus 3 Gy × 10 for metastatic epidural spinal cord compression: Final results of the SCORE-2 trial (ARO 2009/01). J Clin Oncol 2016;34(6):597–602. doi:10.1200/JCO.2015.64.0862

Rowell NP, Gleeson FV. Steroids, radiotherapy, chemotherapy and stents for superior vena caval obstruction in carcinoma of the bronchus: A systematic review. Clin Oncol 2002;14:338–351.

Sze WM, Shelley MD, Held I, et al. Palliation of metastatic bone pain: Single fraction versus multifraction radiotherapy – A systematic review of randomized trials. Clin Oncol 2003;15:345–352.

UK SABR consortium guidance: www.sabr.org.uk.

7

Skin

Each cell type in the skin can give rise to a different type of cancer. It is convenient to classify skin tumours into non-melanoma skin cancers (NMSC) and malignant melanoma (MM). Secondary deposits from other cancers can also present in the skin. This chapter covers the role of radiotherapy for NMSC (basal and squamous cell carcinomas), MM and other rare tumours such as primary cutaneous lymphoma, Kaposi sarcoma, angiosarcoma and Merkel cell tumours.

Non-Melanoma Skin Cancer

Basal Cell Carcinoma

Indications for Radiotherapy

Radiotherapy cures more than 90 per cent of primary or recurrent basal cell carcinoma (BCC), with reported five-year recurrence rates of 7.4 per cent.

BCCs are defined as low and high risk:

- Low-risk BCCs are generally small (<2 cm) and well defined in a noncritical site with nonaggressive histology. Only 5 per cent of well-defined BCCs <2 cm show subclinical spread beyond 5 mm.
- High-risk BCCs are generally large (>2 cm); indistinct or morphoeic; in a critical site (eyes, ears, lips, nose and nasolabial folds); and show aggressive histology such as morphoeic, infiltrative, micronodular or perineural spread.

In many cases, BCCs can be managed equally effectively by surgery or radiotherapy. Indications for radiotherapy include:

- Large superficial lesions where a better cosmetic result can be obtained with radiotherapy.
- Large lesions where surgery would cause major loss of function, such as paralysis, numbness, dribbling or ectropion.
- Extensive lesions where surgery may require nasectomy, ear amputation or eye enucleation.
- Older patients where long-term skin atrophy caused by RT may not be relevant.
- Multiple superficial lesions where surgery would be onerous for the patient.
- Patients who are unfit for, or refuse, surgery.
- Selected tumours of the eyelids and canthi of the eyes.
- Selected tumours on the nose, ears and lips. Larger lesions overlying cartilage are best treated with electron rather than superficial radiotherapy.
- Large lesions on the cheek, which often respond with minimum scarring.
- Recurrent lesions after surgery, or with incomplete excision or perineural invasion.

Relative contraindications include:

- Patients under 45 years: there is potential for deterioration of the cosmetic outcome over time (more than five to ten years) and risk of second malignancy.

DOI: 10.1201/9781315171562-7

- Large lesions involving cartilage, bone, tendons or joints: the risk of radionecrosis is high, and cure rates are lower.
- Lesions where there is uncertainty over the histology.
- Lesions that recur after radiotherapy.
- Hair-bearing skin such as scalp, eyebrow and eyelashes: risk of permanent epilation.
- Lesions around the upper eyelid: risk of lacrimal gland dryness and upper lid conjunctival keratinisation.
- Inner canthus lesions: risk of nasolacrimal duct stenosis.
- Lesions on the lower leg, back and dorsum of the hand: poor healing and radiation sequelae, particularly telangiectasia, pigmentation, ulceration, and atrophic scarring.

These relative contraindications need to be reviewed in each individual case, as alternative treatments may produce even more problems.

Mohs micrographic surgery can be used in selected patients with BCCs in critical sites such as the eyelids, ears, lips, nose and nasolabial folds; morphoeic or infiltrative histological subtype; and patients with recurrent BCC, especially after radiotherapy.

Incompletely excised high-risk BCCs may be treated by re-excision or by postoperative radiotherapy.

Not all BCCs require treatment. Aggressive treatment may not be appropriate for patients of advanced age or poor general health, especially for asymptomatic low-risk lesions that are unlikely to cause significant morbidity. In these cases, expectant or palliative treatment may be preferable.

Assessment of Primary Disease

A biopsy is essential to obtain a histological diagnosis. The six clinicopathological subtypes of BCC are nodular, pigmented, cystic, morphoeic, superficial and linear. BCC rarely metastasises, and a staging workup is not necessary.

The primary tumour should be examined under a bright light. By palpation and using a magnifying glass, the edges and depth of the tumour are defined. Dermoscopy is now a key tool for the diagnosis of BCC and enables discrimination from other skin tumours. Edges of morphoeic lesions are difficult to define due to their wide area of spread. Deep penetration may occur at the inner canthus where a tumour may infiltrate along the medial border of the orbit and also at the nasolabial fold, ala nasi, tragus and post-auricular areas. Imaging with MRI may be useful to define extensive lesions.

Data Acquisition

The majority of skin radiotherapy is based on clinical definition of the treatment volumes and the use of single superficial X-ray or electron beams. In very advanced cases with deep infiltration, a CT planned photon or electron treatment may be needed.

Immobilisation

The patient is positioned supine, prone or semi-prone so that the tumour to be treated can be accessed by the superficial X-ray machine or electron applicators. Head rests, pillows, sandbags and other supports are used to aid immobilisation as necessary. If the patient requires a plan to treat an extensive tumour, immobilisation will be similar to that for a head and neck cancer using a Perspex shell.

Target Volume Definition

The gross tumour volume (GTV) is defined clinically as described earlier and marked on the skin.

A peripheral and deep margin is added to the GTV to create the CTV depending on the clinico-pathological type of BCC, the site and size of the lesion being treated and the organs at risk. A further margin for set-up error is added to create the PTV. The field size is chosen to ensure the PTV receives 95 per cent of prescribed dose and will vary between superficial and electron beam radiotherapy. This margin needs to be increased when electron therapy is used to allow for the shape of the isodoses. This will depend on the size of the lesion and the energy of the electron beam. For a 6 MeV electron beam treating a 5-cm circle, an extra 1 cm should be added to the margins above to define the field size with an electron applicator.

Low risk well-defined BCC:

$$\text{Superficial / Orthovoltage Field size} = \text{GTV} + 5 - 8 \ \text{mm}$$

$$\text{Electrons Field Size} = \text{GTV} + 15 - 18 \ \text{mm}$$

High risk, large >3 cm, poorly defined or morphoeic BCC:

$$\text{Superficial / Orthovoltage Field size} = \text{GTV} + 10 - 15 \ \text{mm}$$

$$\text{Electrons Field Size} = \text{GTV} + 20 - 25 \ \text{mm}$$

Shielding

Superficial Radiotherapy Lead shielding is used to define the treatment field and protect surrounding structures. The superficial machine applicators are applied directly to the skin or standard lead cut-outs may be used. Irregular lesions need individualised lead cut-outs, which on the face can be made into lead masks (Figure 7.1a). The thickness of lead depends on the energy of the beam used: 1.5 mm is adequate for 90–150 KV.

When treating lesions of the eyelids, a lead shield must be used to protect the eye. Internal lead contact lenses are available in various sizes and shapes (Figure 7.2a). They are inserted after instillation of local anaesthetic eye drops. The eye must be protected following treatment until the local anaesthetic wears off and the corneal reflex returns. Alternatively, a spade-shaped eye shield may be used under the lower or upper eyelid (Figure 7.2b). An intranasal shield is used to protect the mucosa and cartilage of the nasal septum. The gums can be protected with an internal lead shield when lesions on the skin above the upper lip are treated, but it is important to ensure the shield does not alter the shape of the area, causing stand-off.

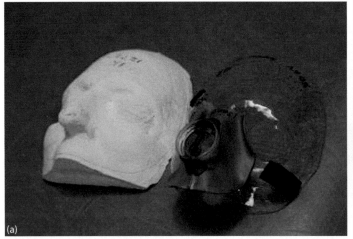
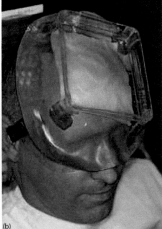

FIGURE 7.1 Lead mask with area cut out for treatment of (a) BCC of nose for superficial radiotherapy and (b) squamous cell carcinoma of the scalp with wax bolus for electron treatment.

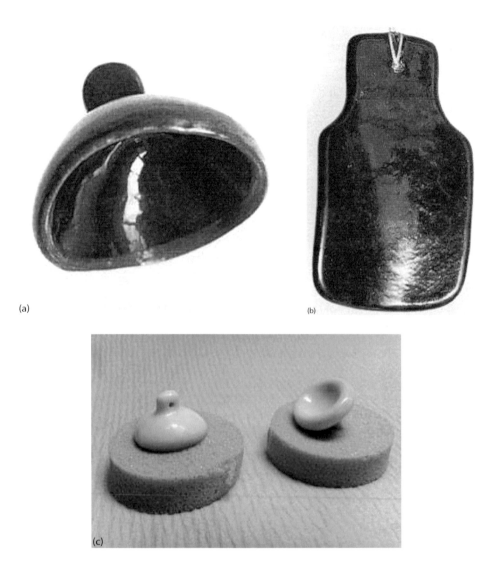

FIGURE 7.2   (a) Internal lead eye shield; (b) spade-shaped eye shield and (c) electron eye shield.

Electron Beam Radiotherapy   Electron beams may be defined by an electron end plate cut-out inserted into the electron applicator or by shaped lead placed on the skin. Four millimetres of lead is adequate for electrons up to 10 MeV. The lead shields for electrons need to be lined with wax or plastic on the inner surface to absorb secondary electrons. Internal eye contact lenses have been designed for use with electron beam therapy around the eye and are made of 3–4-mm lead with 2–3-mm silicon lining, depending on the electron energy used (Figure 7.2c).

Dose Solutions

Superficial/Orthovoltage Radiotherapy

Most lesions are treated with superficial (40–100 kV) or orthovoltage (100 kV–300 kV) energies with appropriate filtration which defines the beam characteristics. Percentage depth doses for different field diameters and energies are obtained from tables drawn up for each therapy unit,

TABLE 7.1

Percentage Depth Dose Table for 140 kV (8.0 mm Al HVL)

	Equivalent Field Diameter (cm)								
	20 cm SSD					30 cm SSD			
	E	F	G	H	I	K	L	J	M
Depth (cm)	4.0	4.5	5.0	6.0	8.0	9.9 (8x10)	11.2 (10x10)	12.5	13.3 (10x15)
0.0	100.0	100	100	100	100	100	100	100	100
0.5	91.0	91.5	92.0	92.5	94.0	96.0	96.2	96.5	96.7
1.0	82.5	83.5	84.5	86.0	87.5	91.5	92.0	92.5	92.8
2.0	66.0	67.3	68.5	71.0	75.0	82.4	83.5	84.5	85.1
3.0	52.5	54.0	55.5	58.0	62.5	72.9	74.1	75.3	76.0
4.0	41.5	42.8	44.0	46.5	51.0	61.9	63.4	65.0	66.0
5.0	32.0	33.0	34.0	36.5	40.5	51.4	52.9	54.5	55.5
6.0	24.5	25.5	26.5	28.5	32.5	41.9	43.3	44.9	45.8
7.0	19.5	20.5	21.5	23.0	26.5	35.4	36.7	38.1	38.9
8.0	16.0	16.8	17.5	19.0	22.0	29.9	31.1	32.3	33.0
9.0	12.5	13.3	14.0	15.5	18.0	24.9	26.1	27.3	28.0
10.0	10.0	10.8	11.5	12.5	14.5	20.4	21.6	22.8	23.5

and an appropriate energy is selected to encompass the target volume within the 90 per cent iso-dose (Table 7.1).

Because of curving body contours, it may not be possible to appose the applicator of the machine to the lead mask, which will result in positive or negative stand-off (Figure 7.3). An allowance for this stand-off must be made according to the inverse square law. Tables for superficial X-ray therapy units are available which give multiplication factors to correct for different amounts of both positive and negative stand-off (Table 7.2).

Example Calculation for Superficial Radiotherapy

Modern orthovoltage machines use treatment monitor units (MU) to calculate the applied dose needed per field to give the prescribed dose at the skin surface.

$$\text{Treatment MU} = \frac{\text{Applied dose per field}\left(\text{cGy}\right)}{\text{OF}_{\text{S,d}} \times \text{SOF} \times \left(\text{BSF}_{\text{c}} / \text{BSF}_{\text{A}}\right)}$$

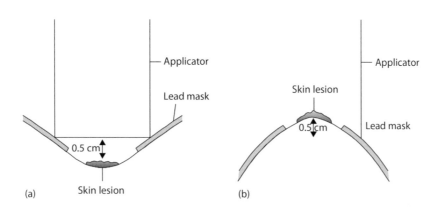

FIGURE 7.3 (a) Positive stand-off of 0.5 cm between lesion and applicator and (b) negative stand-off of 0.5 cm.

TABLE 7.2

Backscatter Factors Table (the Equivalent Diameters of Rectangular Applicators Are in Parentheses)

	Open Ended Applicator						30cm FSD			
								J	K	L	M
Filter	Energy (kV)	9 cm	10 cm	11 cm	12 cm	13 cm	12.5 cm	8x10 cm (9.9 cm)	10x10 cm (11.2 cm)	10x15 cm (13.3 cm)
1	45	1.159	1.165	1.166	1.168	1.170	1.169	1.164	1.167	1.170
2	70	1.231	1.240	1.245	1.250	1.256	1.253	1.239	1.246	1.257
3	125	1.314	1.328	1.338	1.348	1.358	1.353	1.327	1.340	1.361
4	140	1.343	1.365	1.377	1.390	1.404	1.397	1.362	1.380	1.408
5	220	1.235	1.255	1.267	1.280	1.292	1.286	1.253	1.270	1.296

Treatment MU = Monitor units required to deliver prescribed dose at prescribed depth

Prescribed dose = Dose prescribed at depth d in cGy

$OF_{S,d}$ = Output factor at depth d and for equivalent diameter S at the prescribed energy

SOF = Stand-off/incorrection factor for the prescribed SSD

BSF_C = Backscatter factor for the lead cut-out equivalent diameter at the prescribed energy

BSF_A = Backscatter factor for the applicator equivalent diameter at the prescribed energy

BSF_c/BSF_A = Cut-out correction factor (less than 1.00 if there is a cut-out)

Calculate the Treatment MU for a prescription of 300 cGy at the skin surface using 140 kVp, a 12.5-cm applicator (30-cm SSD), 10-cm equivalent diameter cut-out and stand-off of -1.5 cm.

Prescription depth = 0 cm

$OF_{S,d}$ = 0.475 (Table 7.3)

SOF = 1.11 (Table 7.4)

BSF_{10} = 1.365 (Table 7.2)

$BSF_{12.5}$ = 1.397 (Table 7.2)

$$\text{Treatment MU} = \frac{300}{0.475 \times 1.11 \times (1.365 / 1.397)} = 582\text{MU}$$

TABLE 7.3

Applicator Output Factors Table (the Equivalent Diameters of Rectangular Applicators Are in Parentheses)

		20 cm FSD					30 cm FSD			
		E	F	G	H	I	J	K	L	M
Filter	Energy (kV)	4 cm	4.5 cm	5 cm	6 cm	8 cm	12.5 cm	8x10 cm (9.9 cm)	10x10 cm (11.2 cm)	10x15 cm (13.3 cm)
1	45	0.951	0.957	0.967	0.965	1.00	0.445	0.441	0.443	0.446
2	70	0.933	0.944	0.958	0.982		0.459	0.451	0.455	0.461
3	125	0.907	0.923	0.933	0.959		0.467	0.454	0.459	0.470
4	140	0.890	0.905	0.929	0.954		0.475	0.463	0.469	0.484
5	220						3.119	3.015	3.072	3.175

TABLE 7.4

Stand-off/Incorrection Factors

Stand Off Distance (cm)	Applicator SSD (cm)		
	20	**30**	**50**
-2.0	1.23	1.15	1.09
-1.5	1.17	1.11	1.06
-1.0	1.11	1.07	1.04
-0.5	1.05	1.03	1.02
0.0	1.00	1.00	1.00
0.5	0.95	0.97	0.98
1.0	0.91	0.94	0.96
1.5	0.87	0.91	0.94
2.0	0.83	0.88	0.92

Electron Beam Therapy

Beam sizes of less than 4-cm diameter should not be used because the advantage of beam flatness is lost. The physical characteristics of electron beams are shown in Figure 2.6. The energy of the electron beam is chosen so that the deep surface of the target volume is encompassed by the 90 per cent isodose with a sharp fall in dose beyond. This spares the underlying tissues. The effective treatment depth expressed in centimetres is about one-third of the beam energy in MeV but depends on the beam size and depth dose data for any particular machine. Bolus is placed on the skin surface to increase dose to 100 per cent and to compensate for irregular surfaces (Figure 7.1b). This reduces the depth of the 90 per cent isodose which must be taken into account when choosing the electron energy. A correction for any stand-off between the applicator and skin surface can be made using the inverse square law and effective SSD. Tables for varying electron energy and applicator size should be used. In complex cases, CT planning of electrons is possible with modern planning solutions such as the Eclipse electron Monte Carlo Algorithm (see Figure 7.4), and patient specific bolus can be created using 3D-printing technology.

Dose Fractionation

The daily dose and fractionation scheme depend on the site and size of the lesion, and the age and performance status of the patient. The convenience of shorter regimens must be balanced against risks of normal tissue damage. When treating areas of the skin that may be near to critical structures, the normal tissue constraints as defined by Emani et al and Quantec (see Chapter 4). should be adhered to. Special considerations are the lacrimal gland and lens when treating near and around the eye, the spinal cord when treating near the spine, the small bowel when treating the pelvis, testis and fertility when treating the perineal area and of course permanent hair loss on any hair-bearing skin.

For superficial radiotherapy, the dose is specified at D_{max} and for electrons at 100 per cent on the central axis, ensuring a minimum dose of 90–95 per cent to the whole target volume.

Many different regimens have been shown to be effective and are in widespread use.

Curative Radiotherapy

- Lesions <3-cm diameter
  (Superficial radiotherapy [SRT] 80–140 kV)
  - 45 Gy in 9 fractions over 22 days (alternate weekdays)
  - 37.8 Gy in 6 fractions over 15 days (alternate weekdays)
  - 32.4 Gy in 3 fractions over 15 days (once a week)
  - 18 Gy in a single fraction

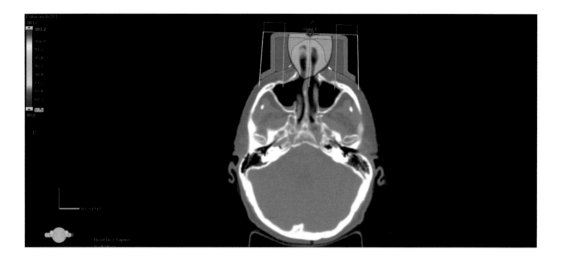

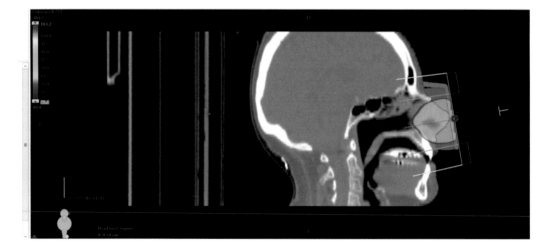

FIGURE 7.4   Eclipse electron plan treating a cutaneous lymphoma on the nose.

- Lesions >3-cm diameter or nose/pinna/poorly vascularised skin
  (SRT or electron beam* radiotherapy)
  - 45 Gy in 9 fractions over 22 days (alternate weekdays)
  - 50 Gy in 20 daily fractions over four weeks
- Lesions >5-cm diameter
  (Electron beam* or megavoltage radiotherapy)
  - 50 Gy in 20 daily fractions over four weeks
  - 60 Gy in 30 daily fractions over six weeks

Treatment Delivery and Patient Care

The patient lies on the treatment couch with lead mask, cut-out and other shielding such as internal eye shields in place. Any bolus required is applied and the treatment applicator positioned over the target

---

* Consider increasing dose by 10 per cent to account for the reduced relative biological dose of electrons.

volume. Skin marks, tattoos, if appropriate, and photographs of the planned treatment position are used to ensure the correct set-up each day.

Scabs over lesions may need to be removed before treatment to ensure adequate depth dose. Skin should be kept dry, and shaving and the application of makeup and chemicals to the area should be avoided. Erythema usually develops in the first week of treatment followed by an exudative reaction. Acute erythema is treated with aqueous cream or soft paraffin. If the skin becomes broken, paraffin gauze or hydrogel is applied with a dry dressing. Vaseline can be used inside the nostril to help prevent scabbing and nose bleeds. If the dose to the lacrimal gland is kept below 35 Gy, the risk of the late complication of dry eye may be minimised.

Long-term side effects include atrophy, hyper- and hypopigmentation, telangiectasia and alopecia. Nonhealing skin ulceration, persistent pain and secondary skin cancers are more serious late side effects. Patients should be advised to avoid exposure to cold winds and sun, to use ultraviolet sun barrier cream and to wear a hat.

Squamous Cell Carcinoma

Cutaneous squamous cell carcinoma (SCC) is the second most common skin cancer after BCC. Treatments are highly effective and can achieve cure rates of 90 per cent. In the head and neck area, 20 per cent of NMSC are cutaneous SCC, but this rises to 43 per cent in sites such as the pinna. The common pre-malignant lesion is actinic keratosis.

Primary cutaneous SCC may grow slowly or rapidly. They may metastasise initially to regional lymph nodes, and later to viscera, with an overall mortality of 3 per cent. Cutaneous SCCs of the head and neck can spread haematogenously to the CNS, or via the perineural space.

Overall, lesions recur locally in 25 per cent. Risk factors for local or nodal recurrence include site (lip and ear SCCs have a higher recurrence rate and are discussed in Chapter 9), size (tumours >2 cm diameter), depth of invasion (>4 mm), cellular differentiation, perineural involvement, host immune status and previous treatment. Tumours arising in non-sun-exposed sites, and areas of previous radiation, thermal injury, scarring, or chronic ulceration, have higher risk of recurrence and metastases. Poorly differentiated and anaplastic SCCs metastasise more frequently than well-differentiated SCCs. Those on the mid face and lip are especially prone to neural involvement. Careful follow-up of patients with these high-risk features is essential.

Indications for Radiotherapy

Treatment of SCC is similar to that described for BCC. However, more radical surgery with larger margins is required because of the greater metastatic potential. Patients with high-risk SCC presenting with involved lymph nodes should be reviewed by a multidisciplinary oncology team including a dermatologist, pathologist, plastic or maxillofacial surgeon, oncologist and clinical nurse specialist.

Radiotherapy is generally reserved for patients over 45 years old because of the theoretical risk of inducing further malignancies. It is not suitable for tumours invading underlying cartilage where the risk of radiochondritis is high and cure rates are lower. There is a relative contraindication to treating SCCs in cardiac or renal transplant patients, as they may be particularly susceptible to further cutaneous malignancies. The five-year cure rate for NMSC with radiotherapy is as high as 90 per cent, and the cosmetic results are good or acceptable in 84 per cent of cases. The early and late complication rates are low.

There is limited evidence for the role of adjuvant radiotherapy for cutaneous SCC. Single centre retrospective studies have reported that for head and neck SCC with high-risk features, e.g. lesions over 2 cm with perineural invasion, adjuvant radiotherapy may reduce the risk of local recurrence. This has to be weighed against the risk of toxicity. Adjuvant radiotherapy following therapeutic lymphadenectomy can be considered in high-risk cases, e.g. lymph node >3 cm, multiple involved lymph nodes, extracapsular spread. Radiotherapy may also be used palliatively for patients with lymph node metastases.

Afterloading brachytherapy can be used for SCCs on the dorsum of the hand, lower limb or curved surfaces such as the scalp. A mould of the area to be treated is made and catheters distributed over the area to be treated following the Manchester or Paris rules for an interstitial implant. Modern brachytherapy computer planning systems use powerful inverse planning optimisation and automated volume-based planning.

Methods of assessment and target volume definition are similar to those described for BCC. However a larger margin of 10–20 mm is added to the GTV to create the PTV according to risk factors. Dose fractionation regimens are similar to those described for BCC, but for larger lesions, longer dose fractionation schedules are preferred.

Dose Fractionation

Curative Radiotherapy

- Lesions <5-cm diameter (see also dose fractionation regimens for BCC)
  - 45 Gy in 9 fractions over 21 days treating on alternate weekdays
  - 54 Gy in 20 fractions over four weeks
- Lesions >5-cm diameter (Electron beam* or megavoltage radiotherapy)
  - 54 Gy in 20 daily fractions over four weeks
  - 66 Gy in 33 daily fractions over six and a half weeks

Postoperative Radiotherapy

Electron beam* or megavoltage radiotherapy

- Skin: (*note limited evidence)
- 50 Gy in 20 daily fractions over four weeks
- 60 Gy in 30 daily fractions over six weeks
- Lymph node regions:
- 50–60 Gy in 25–30 fractions over five to six weeks
- 66 Gy in 33 fractions over six and a half weeks (in high-risk head and neck region)

HDR Brachytherapy

- 45 Gy in 10 fractions over two weeks.
- A more prolonged fractionation may be advisable in the lower limb.

Palliative Radiotherapy

- 8 Gy in a single fraction
- 20 Gy in 5 daily fractions over one week
- 36 Gy in 6 fractions weekly over six weeks
- 27 Gy in 6 fractions twice a week over three weeks

Malignant Melanoma

The primary treatment of melanoma is surgery. Radiotherapy has a primary role in treating in situ lentigo maligna, an adjuvant role for postoperative lymph node areas and a palliative role for skin, nodal and visceral metastases. In vitro studies have shown a wide shoulder to the cell survival curve for melanoma cell lines, suggesting a possible advantage for hypofractionation. This has to be balanced against the risk of increased normal tissue reactions with larger fractions.

Lentigo maligna is the superficial in situ phase that progresses to lentigo maligna melanoma in 30–40 per cent of cases. It is typically a large, flat, pigmented area most commonly on the face. The treatment

---

* Increase dose by 10 per cent to account for reduced relative biological dose of electrons.

is surgical excision or radiotherapy. Radiotherapy is very effective with a recurrence rate of 7 per cent, and is a good option for older patients. The lesions may be treated with superficial or electron beam radiotherapy as described for NMSC. The margins need to be carefully defined, as there is often a large area of subclinical disease requiring a margin of up to 20 mm from GTV to PTV. The dose used is the same as for NMSC described earlier.

Adjuvant radiotherapy has been shown in an RCT to reduce the risk of local recurrence from 36 per cent to 21 per cent following lymph node dissection in patients with high-risk features, but does not improve survival. The high-risk features are number of nodes involved (one parotid, two cervical or axillary, three inguinal), size of involved nodes (≥ 3 cm cervical, ≥ 4 cm axilla or inguinal), presence of extracapsular extension, matted nodes, free tumour in the surrounding tissues or lympho-vascular invasion. There is a high risk of lymphoedema when treating the axillae or groins and 20 per cent of patients develop grade 3 skin or subcutaneous tissue toxicity. The NICE guidelines advise against adjuvant radiotherapy accept in patients with stage IIIB or IIIC melanoma where the risk of local recurrence is estimated to outweigh the risk toxicity. Radiotherapy is planned to the nodal sites following the principles of involved field radiotherapy discussed in Chapter 23 for lymphoma. IMRT planning is now used to spare as much normal tissue as possible and reduce the risk of toxicity.

Radiotherapy may be used palliatively to relieve pain and bleeding from skin metastases, in transit metastases, nodal, bone and visceral metastases. Solitary metastases may benefit from treatment with stereotactic ablative radiotherapy (SABR).

Brain metastases can be palliated in patients with a good performance status. The recursive partitioning analysis (RPA) classification is helpful is selecting patients for treatment.

- RPA class 1: age <65, Karnovsky PS >70, controlled primary, no extra cranial metastases
- RPA class 2: all others
- RPA class 3: Karnovsky PS <70

Patients in RPA class 1 may benefit from surgical excision and postoperative whole-brain radiotherapy, or SABR. Patients in RPA class 3 and those with meningeal involvement have such a poor survival that they are best managed with palliative care only. Patients in RPA class 2 may benefit from palliative whole-brain radiotherapy.

Dose Fractionation

Lentigo Maligna

- Curative radiotherapy
  - 45 Gy in 10 fractions over two weeks

Malignant Melanoma

- Adjuvant radiotherapy after lymph node dissection
  - 48 Gy in 20 fractions over four weeks
  - 50 to 60 Gy in 25 to 30 fractions over five to six weeks
- Palliative radiotherapy
  - 8 Gy in a single fraction
  - 20 Gy in 5 fractions over oneweek
  - 36 Gy in 6 fractions weekly over six weeks
- Whole-brain radiotherapy
  - 12 Gy in 2 daily fractions given on consecutive days
  - 20 Gy in 5 fractions over one week

Cutaneous Lymphoma

Primary cutaneous lymphomas are rare, with an incidence of 0.4 per 100,000, but most are low grade with long survival and therefore the prevalence is much higher. Two-thirds are T cell in origin, the majority of which are mycosis fungoides (MF). The WHO EORTC (2018) classification is now used, and specialist multidisciplinary teams should manage these patients.

Primary Cutaneous T Cell Lymphoma

Radiotherapy is a very effective single agent for the treatment of MF. It is used in every stage to treat patches and plaques, tumours and lymph nodes. Mycosis fungoides is extremely sensitive to radiotherapy and low doses can be used, allowing adjacent areas to be treated, and recurrences can be re-treated safely.

In early stage IA–IIB MF, radiotherapy is used with skin-directed therapy such as PUVA to treat patches and plaques, which are planned for treatment in a similar way to NMSC as described earlier. The margins from GTV to field edge depend on the area being treated and are usually 5–10 mm.

In stage IIB–IVB MF, radiotherapy can be used alone or with systemic therapies to treat skin patches, plaques and tumours, nodal and visceral metastases. Mucosal involvement of the nasopharynx or pharynx responds well to radiotherapy, which is fractionated to reduce normal tissue toxicity.

Total Skin Electron Beam Therapy (TSEB)

TSEB can be used to treat the whole skin in any stage of MF. It is used in stage IB disease that is becoming resistant to skin-directed treatment such as PUVA, in stage IIB disease to debulk tumours, in stage III disease to treat erythroderma, and palliatively in stage IV disease where patients are of good performance status or as conditioning for a reduced intensity allograft stem cell transplant in selected patients with advanced disease. The current standard is the modified Stanford technique (Figure 7.5) using a conventional linear accelerator in high-dose-rate electron mode to deliver matched dual fields at a distance of 3.5–4.5 m. A Perspex screen is placed close to the patient to degrade the beam to meet the EORTC consensus of dose maximum at 1 mm depth, 80 per cent isodose at 9-mm depth and 20 per cent isodose at <20 mm. The patient is treated standing and rotates through the six positions shown to maximise unfolding of the skin. On days 1 and 5, TLD measurements are taken from various sites on the skin to map dosimetry accurately. Areas of low dose and inherently shielded areas such as the scalp and soles of the feet are treated separately. Using modern techniques, the whole-body photon contamination dose is less than 2.3 per cent (<0.7 Gy). Acute adverse effects of TSEB are usually minor with attention to care of the patient's skin. They include fatigue, temporary alopecia, nail loss, leg swelling and blisters, minor nose bleeds, reduced sweating, minor parotitis, gynecomastia and skin infection which is rare but must be treated aggressively. Late effects include skin atrophy, hypothyroidism, nail and finger changes, sun sensitivity and infertility in men. Combined with the risk from PUVA, TSEB adds to the patient's risk of other cutaneous malignancies. Low-dose TSEB schedules are now more commonly used and have been shown to have a lower complete response rate but very high, very good partial response rate, much less toxicity and a similar median response duration to the high-dose schedules.

There are other non-MF cutaneous T cell lymphomas that can be effectively treated with radiotherapy using similar doses to MF.

Dose Fractionation

Patch and plaque:	• 8 Gy in 2 fractions over two to four days
Tumour:	• 12 Gy in 3 fractions over three to five days
Mucosal disease:	• 20 Gy in 10 daily fractions over two weeks
Lymph nodes:	• 30 Gy in 15 daily fractions over three weeks
TSEB:	• High-dose 30 Gy in 20 fractions over five weeks
	• Low-dose 12 Gy in 8 fractions over two weeks

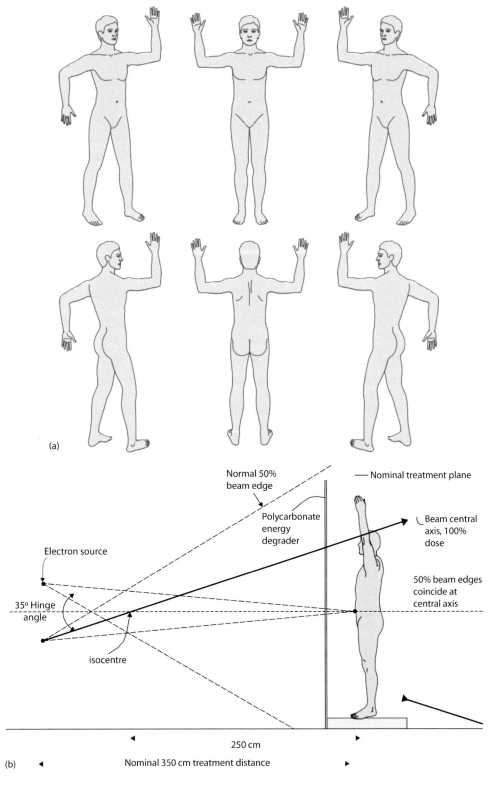

(a)

(b)

Normal 50% beam edge

Nominal treatment plane

Polycarbonate energy degrader

Beam central axis, 100% dose

Electron source

50% beam edges coincide at central axis

35° Hinge angle

isocentre

250 cm

Nominal 350 cm treatment distance

FIGURE 7.5 TSEBT technique used at Guy's and St. Thomas' Hospital modified from the Stanford technique: (a) six standing positions and (b) dual field arrangement. (Courtesy of Dr P. Rudd.)

Primary Cutaneous B Cell Lymphoma

Primary cutaneous B cell lymphomas (PCBCL) are a heterogeneous group that present in the skin without evidence of extra-cutaneous disease at diagnosis. The EORTC WHO (2018) classification describes two indolent types, i.e. primary cutaneous marginal zone lymphoma (PCMZL) and primary cutaneous follicle centre lymphoma (PCFCL), and the more aggressive primary cutaneous diffuse large B cell lymphoma leg type (PCLBCL LT). The indolent PCMZL and PCFCL are treated with radiotherapy alone, with an excellent five-year disease-specific survival of over 95 per cent. The more aggressive PCLBCL LT has a five-year disease-specific survival of 50 per cent and is best treated with CHOP-R chemotherapy followed by involved field radiotherapy to the primary skin lesions and regional lymph nodes.

If radiotherapy planning margins are inadequate, the relapse rate is much higher. It is currently recommended that margins of 20 to 30 mm are added to the GTV to form the treatment field when planning superficial radiotherapy, and margins of 30 to 50 mm are added to the GTV when planning electron beam radiotherapy. Lymph node regions are treated in the same way as nodal lymphoma.

Dose Fractionation

PCMZL & PCFCL:
- 24 Gy in 12 daily fractions over one and a half weeks
- 15 Gy in 5 daily fractions of 3 Gy given in one week
- 8 Gy in 2 daily fractions over two days for small lesions

PCLBCL LT:
- 30 Gy in 15 daily fractions over three weeks

Kaposi Sarcoma

Radiotherapy can be used in all the forms of Kaposi sarcoma (KS): classical, equatorial Africa endemic, secondary to iatrogenic immunosuppression and HIV/AIDS related. It is very useful for treatment of localised lesions and for the palliation of pain, bleeding and oedema. Nodular localised disease can be treated with superficial or electron therapy with a 5–10 mm margin. More widespread lower-limb skin involvement can be treated by covering the limb in bolus to deliver opposing photon beams, or by surface mould HDR brachytherapy. Mucosal lesions (such as the mouth and conjunctiva) are best treated with fractionated courses to avoid the severe mucosal reactions to radiotherapy seen in patients with HIV. Modern, highly active antiretroviral therapy (HAART) is very effective in HIV/AIDS-related Kaposi sarcoma and some lesions respond very quickly without the need for radiotherapy.

Dose Fractionation

Skin:
- Single lesions/small fields:
  - 8 Gy in a single fraction
  - 15 Gy in 3 fractions over one week
- Multiple lesions/large fields:
  - 24 Gy in 12 fractions over two and a half weeks
  - 30 Gy in 10–15 fractions over two to three weeks

Mucosal:
- 20 Gy in 10 daily fractions over two weeks

Cutaneous Angiosarcoma

Cutaneous angiosarcoma of the scalp and face is a rare condition that primarily affects elderly patients. The tumours have ill-defined margins, are often multifocal and the scalp and face location makes complete resection difficult. It is biologically aggressive with a high risk of metastases. Combined modality treatment with surgery and radiotherapy improves the five-year survival from 16 per cent to 46 per cent.

The primary treatment is surgical excision if possible. In cases with involved or close margins, postoperative adjuvant radiotherapy is advised. For inoperable disease, high-dose palliative electron therapy with large margins around the tumour produces local control and palliation. There is no standard chemotherapy approach and patients should be referred to experienced sarcoma units. Lesions on the scalp need to be treated with wide margins and often require several electron fields with moving match lines to avoid overdose when matching fields. Lesions involving the face require large electron fields with electron eye shielding.

Dose Fractionation

Adjuvant: • 50Gy in 25 fractions over five weeks

Palliative: • 44Gy in 11 fractions of 4 Gy over three and a half weeks
Or
• 60Gy in 30 daily fractions over six weeks

Merkel Cell Carcinoma

Merkel cell carcinoma (MCC) is a rare primary dermal tumour that is known to have a high local recurrence rate, frequent nodal involvement and high risk of metastases. It most commonly occurs on the head and neck and extremities. The overall three-year survival has improved to 70 per cent with a multidisciplinary approach. Wide local excision (WLE) of the primary tumour with a 2–3-cm margin is the initial treatment. There is only one RCT of adjuvant radiotherapy, which was carried out in patients with stage 1 (T1 tumour ≤2 cm N0 M0), which showed no improvement in survival but did show a reduction in regional recurrence. Observation is the standard after complete excision in stage 1 cancers. The evidence for adjuvant therapy for higher stage cases is lacking and is based on retrospective reviews and pooled data reviews. When the margins are involved or the tumour is larger than 2 cm in diameter, postoperative adjuvant radiotherapy to the tumour bed and scar using electrons with a 5-cm margin where possible may be considered. In particularly high-risk cases where there are positive margins or residual disease present after surgery, postoperative chemoradiotherapy protocols may be considered. But it is important that the toxicity of treatment is considered. In patients unfit for surgery, or where the tumour is inoperable, radiotherapy alone or combined with chemotherapy can be used as the primary treatment.

The regional lymph nodes should be managed by sentinel node biopsy followed by a completion lymph node dissection (CLND). For patients with extensive lymph node disease, adjuvant radiotherapy following the CLND may be considered. This is planned in the same way as regional lymph nodes for lymphoma. The in-transit lymphatics are not treated unless the primary is close to the nodal region. Locally advanced and metastatic Merkel cell tumours can be treated with standard palliative radiotherapy doses, palliative chemotherapy or immunotherapy.

Dose Fractionation

- Curative radical radiotherapy:
  - 60 Gy in 30 daily fractions over six weeks
- Curative radical radiotherapy with concomitant chemotherapy:
  - 50 Gy in 25 daily fractions over five weeks
- Postoperative adjuvant radiotherapy:
  - Adjuvant tumour bed:
    - 56 Gy in 28 daily fractions over five and a half weeks
    - 50 Gy in 20 daily fractions over four weeks
    - 45 Gy in 15 daily fractions over three weeks
  - Adjuvant lymph nodes:
    - 50 Gy in 25 daily fractions over five weeks
- Postoperative adjuvant radiotherapy with concomitant chemotherapy:
  - Tumour bed +/- lymph nodes:
    - 50 Gy in 25 fractions over five weeks

INFORMATION SOURCES

Bichakjian CK, Olencki T, Aasi SZ, et al. Merkel cell carcinoma, version 1.2018, NCCN clinical practice guidelines in oncology. J Natl Compr Canc Netw 2018 Jun;16(6):742–774.

British Association of Dermatology. Clinical guidelines for the management of Basal Cell Carcinoma, Squamous Cell Carcinoma, Melanoma and Primary cutaneous lymphoma: www.bad.org.uk.

DermIS. Dermatology Information System 1991: www.dermis.net.

Holden CA, Spittle MF, Jones EW. Angiosarcoma of the face and scalp, prognosis and treatment. Cancer 1987;59:1046–1057.

Schlienger P, Brunin F, Desjardins L, et al. External radiotherapy for carcinoma of the eyelid. Report of 850 cases treated. Int J Radiat Oncol Biol Phys 1996;34(2):277–287.

Specht L, Dabaja B, Illidge T, et al. international lymphoma radiation oncology group. Modern radiation therapy for primary cutaneous lymphomas: Field and dose guidelines from the international lymphoma radiation oncology group. Int J Radiat Oncol Biol Phys 2015 May 1;92(1):32–39.

Willemze R, Cerroni L, Kempf W, et al. The 2018 update of the WHO-EORTC classification for primary cutaneous lymphomas. Blood 2019 Apr 18;133(16):1703–1714.

8

Head and Neck: General Considerations

Conformal volume-based radiotherapy of head and neck cancers requires knowledge of anatomy and patterns of spread of disease which are often specific to each tumour site. This chapter explains the common principles of treatment of these tumours.

Initial Patient Assessment

Head and neck tumours and their treatments can cause complex anatomical and functional deficits. A thorough initial assessment of tumour and patient factors, including function, comorbidity and personal preference, is essential to choose the optimal treatment. The ideal forum for this assessment is a multidisciplinary clinic where surgeon and oncologist assess the patient together with input from a clinical nurse specialist, dietician, speech and language therapist and restorative dentist.

The extent of the primary tumour should be clearly recorded in the patient record with the aid of diagrams and photographs. This can be especially useful if postoperative radiotherapy is later recommended. Both sides of the neck should be examined, and any palpable lymph nodes recorded with a measurement of their size and position.

Assessments by a dietician and a speech and language therapist are important to document initial functional problems and to plan support through radiotherapy and surgery. A dental assessment should be performed before any radiotherapy that may cause salivary gland dysfunction or where the mandible is in the treatment volume. At-risk teeth should be removed prior to radiotherapy planning.

Smoking and alcohol abuse are two principal causes of head and neck tumours, and their role in cardiovascular and respiratory diseases means patients often have comorbidities. A formal frailty assessment is useful in elderly patients or those with other significant illnesses.

Cross-sectional imaging to document local tumour extent and assess nodes is recommended in all but very early vocal cord tumours. A chest CT or PET-CT should be performed in patients with locally advanced disease to look for metastases or a synchronous primary cancer. Histological confirmation should be obtained by fine needle aspiration or core biopsy of lymph nodes or by incisional biopsy of the primary tumour or nodes. Tissue samples should be reviewed by a specialist head and neck pathologist.

Indications for Radiotherapy Including Sequencing with Surgery

Although the primary site and involved or at-risk cervical lymph nodes are usually treated with the same modality, it is useful to consider the indications for radiotherapy for the primary site and nodes separately.

Primary Tumour – Curative Treatment

If a tumour is technically resectable with clear margins, local control rates with nonsurgical therapy can never exceed those with surgery. However, it is important to consider not only tumour control but also long-term function – particularly swallowing and speech. A radiotherapy-based approach can provide equivalent local control rates but better long-term function, as long as there is careful follow-up, so that salvage surgery can be considered if tumours recur. Improvements in radiotherapy with more conformal treatments and the addition of concomitant chemotherapy mean that radiotherapy is the treatment of choice for many patients with head and neck cancer. The indications for primary radiotherapy as opposed to primary surgery are considered in site-specific chapters. For stage I–II cancers, single modality treatment should be used where possible. Combinations of surgery, radiotherapy and chemotherapy are usually required for advanced-stage disease.

Primary Tumour – Adjuvant Treatment

After a curative resection, the surgeon, pathologist and oncologist should meet to discuss the role and extent of adjuvant radiotherapy. For each patient, the most likely sites of residual disease or recurrence can be specifically targeted. The clearest indication for adjuvant radiotherapy is where resection margins are positive and further surgery is not possible. It should also be considered when factors predicting local recurrence after surgery are present, including locally advanced tumours (usually T 3/4), close resection margins (<3–5 mm), high tumour grade and perineural or vascular invasion. A clinicopathological discussion is especially important when a laser excision has been carried out: the piecemeal excision of a tumour and frozen section analysis of radial margins will preclude measurement of margins of excision, which is the most useful indicator of the need for adjuvant radiotherapy. Adjuvant radiotherapy approximately halves the risk of local recurrence but has little measurable effect on survival for most tumour subtypes.

Cervical Nodes – Prophylactic Treatment

Historical series of neck dissections or observational follow-up provide the best evidence for estimating the risk of recurrence in clinically negative neck nodes. If the risk is greater than 15–20 percent the relevant nodal levels should be removed surgically or irradiated prophylactically. Modern imaging techniques are more likely to discover involved nodes and stage patients N+ so patients may be upstaged when compared with historical controls. The AJCC TNM (8th edition, 2018) staging for head and neck nodes – excluding nasopharyngeal, HPV-positive oropharyngeal and thyroid cancer – is shown in Table 8.1.

Selecting the appropriate nodal levels depends on a thorough knowledge of lymph node drainage pathways of the head and neck along with data from previous series of patients found to have nodal metastases when clinically N0.

The choice of surgery or radiotherapy to treat the N0 neck is usually determined by the treatment of the primary tumour.

Cervical Nodes – Curative Treatment

When staging indicates lymph node involvement, the neck is treated with a neck dissection, radiotherapy or a combination of the two.

Surgery followed by radiotherapy has the advantages of quickly obtaining local control of disease (useful if there is a rapidly growing mass or skin involvement) and providing definitive staging information. But radiotherapy volumes are more difficult to define with certainty and precision postoperatively than in the unoperated neck, and there is good evidence that radiation (usually combined with systemic therapy) can control neck disease, particularly when involved nodes are smaller than 3 cm at diagnosis. If the primary tumour is to be treated with radiotherapy an initial neck dissection is only recommended if the neck nodes are fungating. A selective neck dissection can be considered three months after radiation if there is evidence of residual nodal disease. There is increasing data that PET-CT is most useful in providing this evidence, supported by fine needle aspiration or biopsy of any borderline nodes.

In a selective neck dissection the surgeon will remove the affected nodes and at-risk nodal levels but not the internal jugular vein, accessory nerve or sternocleidomastoid muscle in order to reduce morbidity. If the node is invading or is one or more of these structures they can be removed in a modified radical or radical neck dissection. A neck dissection provides definitive information on extracapsular nodal spread and can help inform prognosis and the need for adjuvant treatment. Surgical and CT-based descriptions of lymph node levels are similar though not identical.

TABLE 8.1

Nodal Staging for Head and Neck Cancer – Excluding Nasopharyngeal, HPV-Positive Oropharyngeal and Thyroid Cancer

Clinical		Pathological	
cNx	Regional lymph nodes cannot be assessed	**pNx**	Regional lymph nodes cannot be assessed
cN0	No regional lymph node metastasis	**pN0**	No regional lymph node metastasis
cN1	Metastasis in a single ipsilateral lymph node, 3 cm or smaller in greatest dimension with no extranodal extension	**pN1**	Metastasis in a single ipsilateral lymph node, 3 cm or smaller in greatest dimension with no extranodal extension
cN2a	Metastasis in a single ipsilateral lymph node, larger than 3 cm but not larger than 6 cm in greatest dimension with no extranodal extension	**pN2a**	Metastasis in a single ipsilateral lymph node, 3 cm or smaller in greatest dimension with extranodal extension, or Metastasis in a single ipsilateral lymph node, larger than 3 cm but not larger than 6 cm in greatest dimension with no extranodal extension
cN2b	Metastasis in multiple ipsilateral lymph nodes, none larger than 6 cm in greatest dimension with no extranodal extension	**pN2b**	Metastasis in multiple ipsilateral lymph nodes, none larger than 6 cm in greatest dimension with no extranodal extension
cN2c	Metastasis in bilateral or contralateral lymph nodes, none larger than 6 cm in greatest dimension with no extranodal extension	**pN2c**	Metastasis in bilateral or contralateral lymph nodes, none larger than 6 cm in greatest dimension with no extranodal extension
cN3a	Metastasis in a lymph node larger than 6 cm in greatest dimension with no extranodal extension	**pN3a**	Metastasis in a lymph node larger than 6 cm in greatest dimension with no extranodal extension
cN3b	Metastasis in any lymph node(s) with clinically overt extranodal extension	**pN3b**	Metastasis in a single ipsilateral lymph node, larger than 3 cm in greatest dimension with extranodal extension, or Metastasis in multiple ipsilateral, bilateral or contralateral lymph nodes with any extranodal extension, or Metastasis in a single contralateral node of any size with extranodal extension

Source: Adapted from AJCC TNM (8th edn, 2018).

Cervical Nodes – Adjuvant Treatment

If an initial neck dissection is carried out, adjuvant radiotherapy is recommended if there is macroscopic residual disease (e.g. nodes dissected off the carotid artery), microscopic extracapsular nodal spread or if two or more nodes contain tumour. Adjuvant radiotherapy should also be considered if a single involved node is >3 cm in greatest dimension.

Palliative Treatment

It is often challenging to select patients for a palliative approach when they present with locally advanced disease that is theoretically curable with surgery and or radiation. When the chance of cure is low or potential cure would entail significant morbidity – for example when a total glossectomy or laryngo-pharyngectomy is proposed – or when comorbidity precludes optimal curative approaches, palliative radiotherapy may provide control of local symptoms such as pain and airways obstruction. Palliative radiotherapy to the primary site can also be useful when metastases are present at diagnosis, or in locally recurrent disease to ameliorate fungating tumour or reduce bleeding.

Dose Fractionation

For many years, daily 2 Gy fractions, five days a week, was the standard of care in curative radiotherapy for head and neck cancer with the target volume and fields becoming smaller during the course of treatment to deliver different doses to different parts of the volume. A dose of 70 Gy in 35 fractions has

TABLE 8.2

Comparison of Different Dose Levels with Different Curative IMRT/VMAT Dose
Fractionation Schedules for Head and Neck Cancer

Prescribed Dose	PTV_HIGH	PTV_MID	PTV_LOW
70 Gy in 35 fractions	70 Gy (95%)	63 Gy (85.5%)	56 Gy (76%)
65 Gy in 30 fractions	65 Gy (95%)	60 Gy (87.7%)	54 Gy (78.9%)
55 Gy in 20 fractions	55 Gy (95%)	50 Gy (86.4%)	46 Gy (79.4%)
68 Gy in 34 fractions (DAHANCA)	68 Gy (95%)	62 Gy (86.6%)	56 Gy (78.2%)

Note: Percentage Total Dose for 95 Percent Isodose Coverage in Brackets

been the international standard for treatment of the primary site and involved nodes with 60 Gy to treat uninvolved nodal regions at particular high risk of disease. The prophylactic dose to uninvolved lower risk nodal levels is 44–50 Gy. In adjuvant radiotherapy, 60 Gy has been the standard dose with 66 Gy to small, defined volumes if there are positive resection margins or extranodal spread.

With simultaneous integrated boost techniques using IMRT now a standard, different tumour volumes receive different radiation doses each day. This has required a recalculation of doses based on knowledge of radiobiology. In the UK, a schedule of 30 fractions over six weeks has been widely adopted with doses of 65, 60 and 54 Gy prescribed to high-, intermediate- and low-risk target volumes. If 35 fractions are used, 70, 63 and 56 Gy are prescribed. More hypofractionated protocols are sometimes used for smaller treatment volumes but with the risk of more late effects. See Table 8.2 for a comparison of fractionation schedules.

There is now good evidence that improved local control and cure rates can be achieved for stage III–IV disease by combining chemotherapy drugs with radiation or by employing altered fractionation schedules. The choice depends on the ability of the patient to tolerate combination treatment and the resources available, but for locally advanced (T3/4 or N+) head and neck cancer in patients able to tolerate more toxic therapy, one of these methods should be used.

Each of these approaches not only improves local control but also increases acute and/or late side effects, suggesting that they make dose escalation possible rather than improving the therapeutic ratio. Careful collection of data on side effects is as important as local control rates in assessing outcomes.

Refining target volumes in the context of increasingly conformal radiotherapy will, on the other hand, improve the therapeutic ratio. Better imaging techniques and clinical expertise lead to more accurate selection and definition of target volumes, and improvements in treatment delivery such as IMRT lead to more conformal dose solutions. This allows the same dose to be delivered to the tumour with reduced side effects, or may make dose escalation possible without increasing side effects.

Altered Fractionation Radiotherapy

Accelerated radiation schedules shorten the overall treatment time to reduce tumour repopulation during a course of radiotherapy and theoretically increase local control or cure. In a moderately accelerated schedule, overall treatment time is reduced by about a week whilst keeping the total dose similar. Examples of moderately accelerated techniques include using six fractions per week (DAHANCA) or a concomitant boost schedule where the smaller second-phase volume is treated at the same time as the larger prophylactic volume rather than after it (Figure 8.1). There should be a gap of at least six hours between fractions given on the same day to allow normal tissues to repair sublethal damage. In a very accelerated schedule, the overall time is reduced by at least 50 percent with a reduction in total dose. The GORTEC group has used a very accelerated regimen of twice daily 2 Gy fractions throughout a course of treatment and shown that 62–64 Gy over 32–33 days produces better local control and equivalent survival to 70 Gy in 35 daily fractions, but with more acute toxicity.

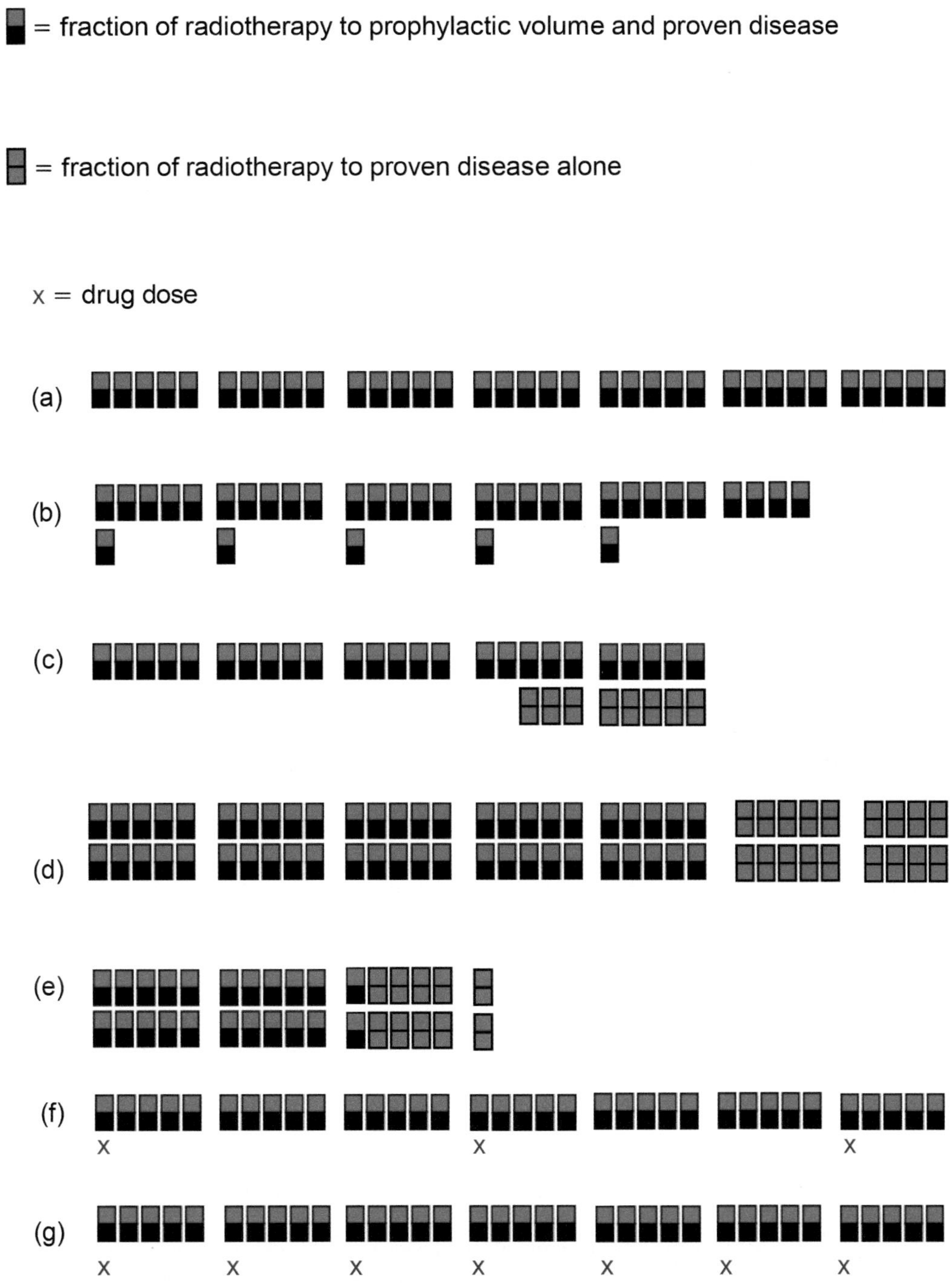

■ = fraction of radiotherapy to prophylactic volume and proven disease

▨ = fraction of radiotherapy to proven disease alone

x = drug dose

FIGURE 8.1 Schematic examples of fractionation and radiochemotherapy schedules for head and neck cancer. (a) Conventional 2 Gy/fraction. (b) Accelerated DAHANCA – 6 fractions/week. (c) Concomitant boost. (d) Hyperfractionation (1.2 Gy/fraction). (e) GORTEC very accelerated regimen (2 Gy/fraction). (f) Radiochemotherapy with 3 weekly cisplatin. (g) Radiochemotherapy with weekly cisplatin or cetuximab.

Hyperfractionation uses a higher total dose given in two daily fractions with the same overall treatment time. An example is the RTOG 9003 schedule of 1.2 Gy given twice daily to a total dose of 81.6 Gy in 68 fractions. Some altered fractionation regimens are both accelerated and hyperfractionated. The CHART protocol used 54 Gy in 36 fractions of 1.5 Gy over 12 days and has been shown to produce equivalent local control to 66 Gy in 33 daily fractions. The benefit of hyperfractionation needs to outweigh the total dose reduction necessary to make acute side effects tolerable.

Individual trials have shown that altered fractionation schedules can improve locoregional control and overall survival compared to standard fractionation, but meta-analysis has shown that altered fractionation only improves five-year overall survival by 3.1 percent. The improvement was seen with hyperfractionated schedules (absolute survival benefit 8 percent) but not accelerated regimens. Acute effects are increased so careful support through radiotherapy is necessary.

Hypofractionation

There is evidence that more hypofractionated regimens can produce local control and survival rates comparable with the regimens described earlier, but there are few RCT data to support this. Examples are 50 Gy in 16 fractions, 55 Gy in 20 fractions and 60 Gy in 25 fractions. A shorter overall treatment time will reduce the risk of tumour repopulation at the cost of a theoretical increase in late effects due to the higher dose per fraction. The small volumes in early laryngeal cancer make this less of a concern, and 55 Gy in 20 fractions is used for T1/2 N0 laryngeal tumours in many centres.

Palliative

When the goal of treatment is to improve symptoms and quality of life, a short course of radiotherapy with minimal side effects is ideal. Several regimens have been advocated, including 20 Gy in 5 daily fractions, 30 Gy in 10 fractions over two weeks, and 24 Gy in 3 fractions over three weeks. Such regimens improve symptoms in between 50 and 70 percent of patients, and responses typically last for some months but sometimes much longer.

Radiotherapy with Chemotherapy

Concomitant Radiotherapy and Chemotherapy

Chemotherapy given during a course of conventionally fractionated radiation improves survival compared with radiation alone. A meta-analysis confirms an absolute improvement in five-year survival of 6.5 percent, with various chemotherapy regimens in the curative setting. Cisplatin-based chemotherapy is particularly effective. Carboplatin is substituted in renal impairment or if cisplatin is not tolerated. Concomitant chemotherapy increases the acute side effects of radiation – particularly the intensity and duration of mucositis. Late effects are also increased compared to radiotherapy alone, but the magnitude of this increase is difficult to quantify, particularly when using modern radiotherapy techniques.

Cisplatin-based chemotherapy is most commonly used with a three-weekly dose of 100 mg/m^2 (two to three doses) or a weekly dose of 30–40 mg/m^2. Regimens including 5-fluorouracil are sometimes used but may increase mucositis. There are theoretical and practical advantages to a weekly schedule: the chemotherapy is present for more fractions, there are fewer side effects, and it is easier to omit chemotherapy if acute toxicity is a problem. There is more trial data supporting three-weekly regimens and total doses of $\geq$ 200 mg/m^2, but the largest single trial of these approaches contained mainly patients having adjuvant treatment for oral cavity cancer, so extrapolating to other subsites is difficult. The chemotherapy is usually given early in the week and before that day's fraction of radiotherapy, but there is no evidence that the timing of chemotherapy is critical.

No individual RCTs have shown superiority of radiation and concomitant chemotherapy over altered fractionation, but a meta-analysis favours combined modality treatment.

Concomitant Radiotherapy with Cetuximab

Cetuximab is a humanized monoclonal antibody against the epidermal growth factor receptor (EGFR), which is overexpressed in many head and neck cancers. An RCT adding cetuximab to conventional radiotherapy showed improvements in overall survival and local control but two trials have found cetuximab-radiotherapy to be inferior to cisplatin-radiotherapy. Cetuximab should only be considered in the rare situation that concomitant chemotherapy is contraindicated and altered fractionation radiotherapy is not possible. Mucositis is not increased but cetuximab does cause an acneiform rash which can be severe.

Concomitant Radiotherapy and Hypoxic Sensitizers

Hypoxic cell sensitizers attempt to mimic the effects of oxygen in fixing radiation-induced DNA damage in tissues thereby increasing cell kill. Many trials of hypoxic cell sensitizers have patient numbers but a meta-analysis has suggested a 3 percent overall survival benefit when compared to radiotherapy alone.

Immunotherapy

Current clinical trials are evaluating the addition of immunotherapy to radiotherapy alone or radiotherapy and concomitant chemotherapy.

Altered Fractionation with Concomitant Chemotherapy

Attempts to combine these approaches have led to unacceptable rates of toxicity and no evidence of a survival benefit. This approach is not recommended outside a clinical trial.

Induction Chemotherapy

The excellent (50–70 percent) response rate of head and neck cancers to cisplatin-based chemotherapy (cisplatin and 5-fluorouracil +/- docetaxel) makes the idea of induction chemotherapy, given before radiation, attractive, but the evidence shows only a nonsignificant 2 percent improvement in overall survival. Chemotherapy can be started quickly, can reduce the volume of disease and improve symptoms and, theoretically, may reduce the rate of distant metastases.

The side effects of induction chemotherapy mean that a proportion of patients will be less well equipped to deal with the toxicity of subsequent radiochemotherapy. There is also a concern that increasing the overall duration of anticancer therapy may lead to tumour repopulation and may negate any benefit of smaller treatment volumes. Radiochemotherapy must not be compromised by induction chemotherapy. Induction chemotherapy is therefore not recommended outside a clinical trial unless there is an urgent need for rapid response in symptomatic, locally advanced diseases (e.g. sinonasal tumours threatening vision) or as part of a larynx-preservation protocol in hypopharynx cancer, or in nasopharyngeal cancer (see Chapters 12 and 13).

Other Radiotherapy Modalities

Protons

Although there are theoretical advantages to protons in head and neck cancer, particularly in tumours close to the skull base, there is no phase 3 evidence to support their routine use. A phase 3 trial of protons in oropharyngeal cancer was opened in the UK in 2020.

Brachytherapy

Brachytherapy can be used as definitive treatment for small tumours of the lip, oral tongue, floor of mouth and buccal mucosa, when expertise is available. Treatment with intraluminal catheters can increase dose to the primary site in nasopharyngeal cancer. Interstitial brachytherapy can be used to aid local control in the neck where there is extracapsular spread.

Re-irradiation

Potentially curative re-irradiation can be given in highly selected patients with unresectable local recurrence after previous radiotherapy or for an adjacent unresectable second primary tumour. The disease-free interval should be at least two years, and the volume as small as possible. Elective nodes should not be irradiated. The patient should have excellent performance status, no serious late effects from previous treatment and be fully aware of the increased risk of potentially serious late effects. IMRT or VMAT should normally be used to conform dose more closely to target volumes and to minimize the volume treated to a high dose.

3D Data Acquisition

Immobilization

The proximity of tumour to critical normal tissues in head and neck cancer with relatively limited intra-fractional motion of organs means that good immobilization will enable smaller treatment margins and reduce side effects.

Modern thermoplastic materials provide an equally effective immobilization mask compared to a Perspex shell constructed from a plaster cast of the patient. The mask is usually constructed with the patient supine with their head on a customized headrest and as flat as possible to maintain the spinal cord parallel to the couch top, in a so-called neutral position. Some patients, particularly those with excessive secretions, need to have their head more elevated. The shell should be fixed to the couch top in at least five places to reduce movement (Figure 8.2). A mouth bite can be used to push the hard palate away from the treated volume in oral cavity tumours, or to depress the tongue when sinonasal tissues are treated. Grip bars at the side of the couch may help to pull the shoulders inferiorly. Once anterior and lateral reference marks have been made on the shell, selected parts can sometimes be cut out to reduce skin dose in regions where full dose to the skin is not required. An anterior midline tattoo below the inferior extent of the shell is useful to improve shoulder alignment.

Immobilization masks can induce anxiety in patients prone to claustrophobia. The skill of the radiographers and technicians and cutting out the shell can help alleviate this, but some patients need benzodiazepines or hypnotherapy to relax them in order to construct a mask that will be tolerable and practical.

Each department should assess the random and systematic errors of their immobilization system to help determine the margin to be added from the CTV to the PTV. A margin of 3 mm should be achievable with high-quality immobilization.

CT Scanning

CT slices should be 2–3 mm thick to aid accurate target volume definition and to produce good quality DRRs for verification. Intravenous contrast will highlight the internal jugular vein, and tumour enhancement can help to define both the primary site and involved lymph nodes more accurately.

Co-registration of diagnostic (usually MRI) and planning CT scans can help to define both tumour volumes and critical normal tissues (e.g. optic chiasm, lacrimal glands), particularly in sinonasal and oropharyngeal tumours or those involving the skull base (Figure 8.3). Care should be taken unless the MRI and CT are acquired with the patient in the same position, and registration must be carefully assessed to ensure adequate accuracy. The final volumes should always be contoured on the planning CT images. PET-CT should not be used to delineate the edge of a GTV due to lack of spatial resolution.

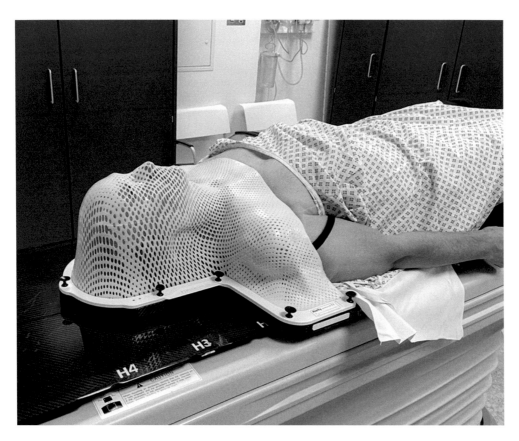

FIGURE 8.2 A thermoplastic shell fixed to the couch in nine places to reduce movement.

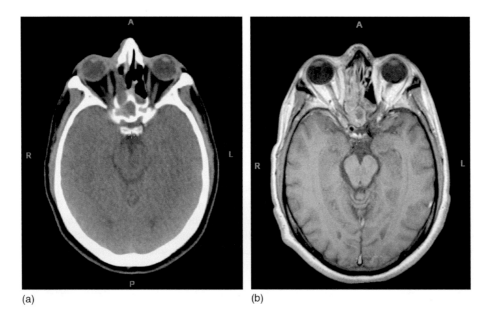

(a)　　　　　　　　　　　　　　　　　　(b)

FIGURE 8.3 Adjuvant radiotherapy of an ethmoid tumour. (a) Planning CT. (b) Fused MRI–CT of the same axial slice to help to define volumes and critical normal structures. Note ethmoid opacities seen on CT are shown to be postoperative secretions on MRI.

Target Volume Definition

General principles for target volume definition which can be applied throughout the head and neck are defined here. For curative radiotherapy, three dose levels are usually defined: CTV_HIGH, CTV_MID and CTV_LOW.

GTV

The GTV is defined as the primary tumour (GTVp) and any involved neck nodes thought to contain tumour – lateral neck lymph nodes over 10 mm in short axis dimension, retropharyngeal nodes over 5 mm or smaller nodes with necrotic centres or rounded contours (GTVn). If induction chemotherapy has been used, the post-chemotherapy GTV is contoured, but the pre-chemotherapy extent of tumour should be included in the CTV_HIGH.

The diagnostic images and records and photographs of initial evaluation in clinic or at examination under anaesthesia (EUA) are critical to assess the extent of the primary tumour and the exact site of involved lymph nodes. Discussion with the surgeon performing the endoscopic assessment and with an experienced radiologist will enable GTV to be defined as accurately as possible. Radiological expertise can be particularly useful when assessing sagittal or coronal planes, as oncologists work mainly in the axial plane. A planning CT scan performed at an interval from the diagnostic one or after surgery should be carefully reviewed for evidence of unexpected new sites of disease. We recommend reviewing the planning system settings with a radiologist and defining optimal settings for each region of the body, always using these settings when defining volumes.

Starting on a central slice of the primary tumour, the GTV is defined on each axial CT image, moving superiorly and then inferiorly. Involved nodes can then be defined in the same way. Viewing the GTV on coronal and sagittal plane reconstructions ensures consistency of definition between slices so that no artificial steps in the volume are created. A volume should not be cut and pasted onto sequential slices for risk of pasting an error: it is more accurate to redraw the GTV on each slice. If there are slices where the GTV cannot be defined – for example due to dental artefact – the planning software will allow the missing contours to be interpolated from those either side.

Some guidelines recommend a larger margin around nodes with radiological evidence of extracapsular spread (ECS). Such nodes should be defined as GTVnes, separate to GTVn with no ECS, as it will make CTV definition easier.

Primary Tumour CTVs (CTVp)

We recommend the '5+5' technique to produce high and intermediate dose CTVs as long as the GTV can be clearly defined based on clinical and imaging findings.

The GTVp is grown by an isotropic margin of 10 mm to produce the CTV_MID. The CTV_MID is then edited slice by slice – again starting in the centre of the volume – to subtract air and adjacent structures such as bone or muscles with fascial barriers which are definitely not involved. An isotropic expansion will not understand complex head and neck anatomy so care should be taken to edit the CTV_MID from opposed mucosal surfaces where there is no method for direct tumour spread (e.g. soft palate, tongue). The CTV_MID should be edited to include any adjacent structures felt to be at higher risk of involvement – for example the medial pterygoid muscle in a tumour close to the muscle when the patient has trismus. It is often easier to edit the CTV_MID from air, then bone, then other structures in sequence.

The high-dose CTV is produced by using a 5 mm isotropic expansion margin from GTVp. The intersect of this 5 mm expansion and the edited CTV_MID is the CTV_HIGH. (Defining the CTV_MID before the CTV_HIGH is slightly faster than the other way round, as only one volume needs editing from bone, air and adjacent structures.) If there is significant uncertainty about the GTV, a single CTV with a 10 mm margin from GTV can be used (Figure 8.4).

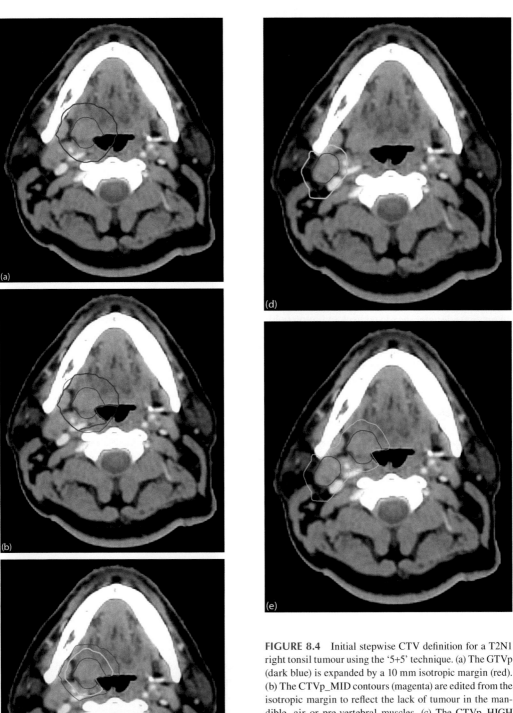

FIGURE 8.4 Initial stepwise CTV definition for a T2N1 right tonsil tumour using the '5+5' technique. (a) The GTVp (dark blue) is expanded by a 10 mm isotropic margin (red). (b) The CTVp_MID contours (magenta) are edited from the isotropic margin to reflect the lack of tumour in the mandible, air or pre-vertebral muscles. (c) The CTVp_HIGH (cyan) is formed by a 5 mm isotropic margin around the GTV and intersecting this volume with CTVp_MID. (d) Note also the involved right level II lymph node. This is contoured as GTVn (dark blue), is expanded by 5 mm and edited to form the GTVn_HIGH (cyan). (e) The sum of the two cyan volumes is the final CTV_HIGH encompassing both primary tumour and involved node with a 5 mm edited margin.

Postoperative Primary Tumour CTV

It is more difficult to specify guidance for CTV definition postoperatively, as the anatomy is distorted by the resection and by any reconstructive myocutaneous flaps. A discussion between surgeon, pathologist and oncologist is important to define the exact anatomical sites at risk of residual disease. Radio-opaque clips used to mark close or involved margins can be helpful, but should not be confused with vascular ligation clips which may be distant to the original tumour. It is not known whether the whole operative field should be included in the CTV, but a more individualized, selective approach seems reasonable in many cases. It is sometimes useful to define the site of the preoperative GTV on the planning CT to orientate the possible sites of microscopic disease, but this is less helpful when the anatomy is very different following a major resection. It can also be helpful to contour a reconstructive flap on the planning CT as the edges of the flap are the margins of resection. If there is visible residual disease, a GTV can be defined and expanded to form the CTV as shown earlier. The CTV should aim to cover the initial anatomical sites of tumour with a 5–10 mm margin.

If there is perineural invasion of large nerves, consideration should be given to specifically contouring the course of that nerve up to the base of skull and including the nerve within the CTV. Contouring atlases showing the course of different nerves are available.

Cervical Lymph Node CTV (CTVn)

In previous decades, head and neck radiation fields included all lymph nodes on both sides of the neck for all but small or well-lateralized tumours. Surgical evidence that a selective approach to neck dissection is as effective as more radical operations, and the ability to create and treat relevant smaller nodal volumes with radiotherapy, have changed this approach.

Defining nodal CTVs requires both selection of appropriate nodal levels and delineation of those levels on the CT data set. Selection is covered in individual tumour chapters, as it will necessarily differ for each site and stage of disease. Often, three nodal CTVs are selected.

The high-risk volume (CTVn_HIGH) contains involved nodes with a 5 mm margin, edited from bone and air. Sometimes multiple small nodes are included in GTVn, in which case a smaller margin (e.g. 3 mm) may be more appropriate. Where there is obvious ECS, a 10 mm margin is used to account for spread into adjacent tissues, particularly adjacent muscle. Muscle fascia provides a barrier to tumour invasion, but once breached, tumour can spread longitudinally along muscle fibres. It is not known whether part or all of an involved muscle should be included in the CTV. We recommend including 10 mm into the muscle on axial slices and 10 mm superior and inferior to the GTVn (Figure 8.5).

The CTV_MID contains the whole levels, including GTVn or levels close to the primary site, which are at particularly high risk of disease. CTV_LOW contains other levels thought to be at risk of microscopic disease.

Lymph Node Level Delineation

There are published guidelines for delineation of nodal CTVs in the node-negative, node-positive and postoperative neck. It is very useful to have the relevant guideline available on an adjacent computer screen when defining nodal CTVs. The consensus guidelines for the node-negative neck are available as an online atlas and specify CT anatomy of nodal levels in the neck. The retropharyngeal (VIIa) and retrostyloid (VIIb) nodes, levels Ia, Ib and II–V, are defined according to CT-based anatomical criteria which correspond closely to the surgical definitions of nodal levels (Table 8.3; Figure 8.6).

The nodal volumes in the positive neck are adjusted from the guidelines for the node-negative neck to take account of the risk of extracapsular spread, usually into adjacent muscles. Nodal size is related to the risk of extracapsular spread, with 25 percent of 10 mm nodes and 80 percent of 30 mm nodes having breached the capsule.

It should be remembered that the division into nodal levels is on anatomical and not functional grounds. When an involved node is at or close to a nodal level boundary, the CTV_MID should extend at least 10–20 mm into both nodal levels, though many protocols advise including the whole of both adjacent levels.

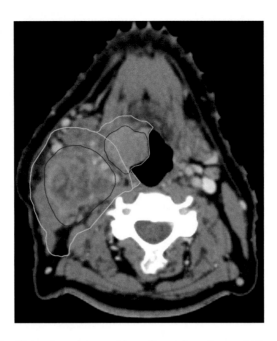

FIGURE 8.5 Level II node with extracapsular spread into adjacent fat and sternocleidomastoid muscle. GTV-N (dark blue) is therefore expanded by 10 mm to form the nodal component of CTV_HIGH (cyan) which is extended to include the whole sternocleidomastoid muscle. GTV_P (red) is expanded by 5 mm.

TABLE 8.3

CT-based Anatomical Guidelines for the Delineation of Nodal Volumes in the N0 Neck

	Anatomical Boundaries					
Level	**Cranial**	**Caudal**	**Anterior**	**Posterior**	**Lateral**	**Medial**
Ib	Cranial edge of submandibular gland	Plane through caudal edge of hyoid bone and caudal edge of mandible	Symphysis menti	Posterior edge of submandibular gland	Inner side of mandible, platysma	Lateral edge of anterior belly of digastric muscle
II	Caudal edge of lateral process of C1	Caudal edge of body of hyoid bone	Posterior edge of submandibular gland	Posterior edge of sternocleidomastoid muscle	Deep surface of sternocleidomastoid muscle	Medial edge of internal carotid artery/paraspinal muscles
III	Caudal edge of body of hyoid bone	Caudal edge of cricoid cartilage	Anterior edge of sternocleidomastoid muscle	Posterior edge of sternocleidomastoid muscle	Deep surface of sternocleidomastoid muscle	Medial edge of internal carotid artery/paraspinal muscles
IVa	Caudal edge of cricoid cartilage	2-cm cranial to sternoclavicular joint	Anterior edge of sternocleidomastoid muscle	Posterior edge of sternocleidomastoid muscle	Deep surface of sternocleidomastoid muscle	Medial edge of internal carotid artery/paraspinal muscles/lateral edge of thyroid gland
V	Cranial edge of body of hyoid bone	CT slice including the transverse cervical vessels	Posterior edge of sternocleidomastoid muscle	Anterior border of trapezius muscle	Platysma muscle, skin	Paraspinal muscles

Source: Adapted from Gregoire (2014).

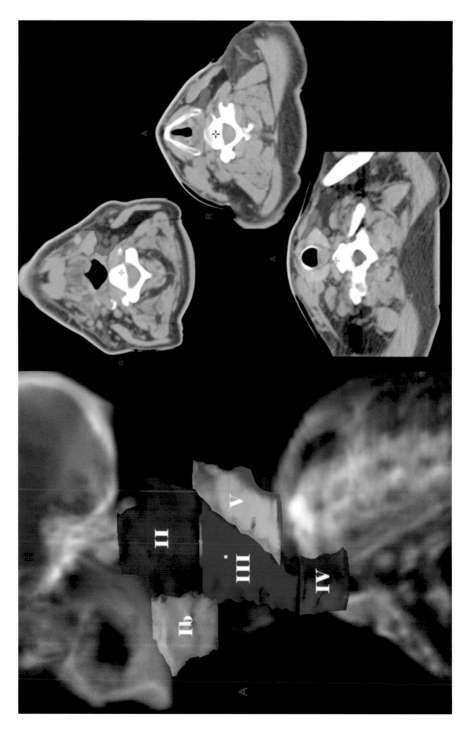

FIGURE 8.6   Lateral DRR and corresponding axial planning CT slices to illustrate cervical lymph node levels Ib–V.

When a matched anterior neck field is used to treat the uninvolved low neck, nodal volumes need not be defined on all slices. If there are involved nodes in the low neck, nodal GTV and CTV should be contoured to ensure adequate coverage (see more on this later in the chapter).

For postoperative neck irradiation, all nodal levels where there was tumour should be treated, particularly when there was extracapsular spread. Where nodes abutted muscles or other structures not removed at operation, those structures should be included in the CTV. It is not clear whether there is also an advantage to postoperative irradiation of dissected nodal levels that did not contain tumour.

PTV

Each CTV is grown isotropically to create a PTV. By recording and analysing systematic and random errors in a series of patients, CTV-PTV margins for each centre can be defined, with the assumption that there is no intra-fractional organ motion in the head and neck. Such margins are usually 3–5 mm.

Nodal PTVs often come close to the skin surface. To artificially create a skin-sparing effect with IMRT, the PTVs are edited so as to be a minimum of 5 mm from the body contour. The only exception is when an involved node is within 5 mm of the skin surface.

OAR and PRV

OAR are outlined on serial axial CT slices in a similar fashion to the GTV. Ideally, the tumour volumes should be hidden or turned off so that they do not distract from OAR definition. Depending on the location of the PTV, OAR contours may include the spinal cord, parotid and submandibular salivary glands, pharyngeal constrictor muscles, optic nerves and chiasm, lacrimal glands and lenses. With more information on how DVHs relate to side effects, contouring of other structures may be useful in the future. Global Harmonization Group consensus guidelines should be used to define and label OARs consistently.

Owing to the catastrophic effect of late spinal cord, brainstem or optic chiasm damage, PRVs for these structures are usually defined either by adding an isotropic 3–5 mm margin. For the spinal cord, the bony spinal canal is sometimes used as a surrogate for the cord PRV.

Dose Solutions

Dose solutions for tumour subtypes will be covered in the relevant chapters, but general principles are covered here.

Complex

IMRT or VMAT are particularly useful for head and neck tumours, given the concave PTVs and their proximity to critical structures. IMRT offers parotid sparing in oropharyngeal and some nasopharyngeal cancers to reduce the risk of xerostomia, avoids the risk of underdosing or overdosing at photon–electron junctions and provides a more uniform dose distribution. For most head and neck subsites, five or seven equispaced IMRT beams or one to two arc treatments provide the most conformal coverage.

In practice, the five IMRT beam angles are selected with beam sizes chosen to cover the PTV. The computer software uses an iterative process to try to meet the constraints applied to the target volumes. The operator guides the computer by defining the constraints and weighting them according to their importance. The target constraints and weights are gradually changed until spinal cord and brainstem are within tolerance, the PTVs are adequately covered and, if possible, the mean contralateral parotid dose (or combined superficial parotid mean dose) is less than 24 Gy.

When bilateral neck nodes are being treated with IMRT it is hard to spare the midline structures of the lower aerodigestive tract to less than 40 Gy. If the lower neck nodes are being treated to a low dose, an IMRT plan can therefore be used to treat the primary site and upper part of the neck, matched to an anterior neck field for the lower neck. The borders of this anterior field are defined so as to cover the nodal levels on an AP DRR. This technique will theoretically underdose the lower neck nodes but provides good local control and avoids dose to midline structures like the hypopharynx and larynx.

In the future, careful mapping of recurrent disease and improved knowledge of the relationship between toxicity and critical organ doses should allow volume definition to be refined so that increased dose can be given to the tumour with tolerable side effects – thereby improving cure. This will be enhanced by the ability to paint dose to areas of highest risk of recurrence as identified by functional imaging or radiogenomics.

Tissue Equivalent Bolus

When volumes are defined as described earlier, the nodal PTV often comes close to the skin surface. Unless there is felt to be a risk of tumour in the epidermis or dermis, it is preferable to accept a slight underdosing of this part of the volume rather than use tissue equivalent bolus which will increase skin reactions significantly.

Plan Review

When assessing a plan with the dosimetry and physics teams, the physician should first make sure that the tolerance of the spinal cord, brainstem or optic nerves are not exceeded. Then coverage of each PTV is assessed to ensure that the PTV is enclosed by the 95 percent isodose (see Table 8.2). Any organs at risk that have been defined are then assessed, such as the salivary glands. The maximum dose for the plan and on each slice should be assessed to ensure it is <107 percent and is within the high dose PTV where possible. Finally, lower isodoses should be reviewed to ensure that other normal tissues such as the uninvolved oral cavity are not irradiated to a higher dose than is desirable.

Conventional/Conformal

Opposed Laterals and an Anterior Neck Field

The standard conventional beam arrangement of opposing lateral beams or a unilateral plan to treat the primary site and involved nodes is matched to an anterior neck beam. With this arrangement, recurrences in the low neck are uncommon, but if nodal volumes are delineated as described earlier, a 6-MV anterior photon beam will not provide adequate coverage of level III and IV nodal volumes (Figure 8.7). In most patients, the risk of recurrence in the low neck is low, and we recommend continuing with an anterior beam. The lateral border is 1 cm lateral to the intersection of the first rib and clavicle on a posteroanterior radiograph, and the inferior border is at the inferior head of the clavicle. If the target volume is unilateral, the medial border is 1 cm from midline to avoid the cord, pharynx and larynx. If it is bilateral, 2-cm midline shielding is added. MLC shielding is used inferior to the clavicle to spare the apex of the lung (Figure 8.8).

When the low neck is included in the high-risk volume (e.g. involved level IV nodes or in the high-risk postoperative neck), the nodal CTV should be formally delineated. Either anteroposterior opposing photon beams can be used (which will increase dose to the posterior neck) or an anterior beam with dose prescribed at 3-cm depth is used to improve coverage at the expense of a hot-spot underneath the skin surface.

Matching Techniques

The common practice of using an anterior beam to treat the low neck nodes necessitates matching at the junction with superior fields. The problems are the divergent edges of the photon beams in different planes and the beam penumbra.

The most elegant solution – which deals with both problems – is to use a single isocentre technique. Both the anterior neck beam and the plan superior to it use only half the beam (the other half shielded by an asymmetric jaw) so that they match at the isocentre without penumbra or beam divergence.

Another technique is to calculate angles required so that both beam edges diverge perpendicular to the match plane. This will result in slight overlap at depth as the width of the penumbra increases. Simpler solutions are to match the beams at the 50 percent (light beam) isodose or to leave a gap of 5–10 mm

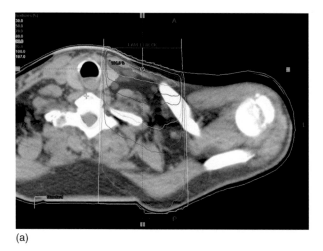

(a)

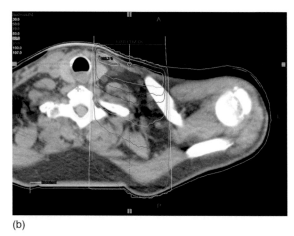

(b)

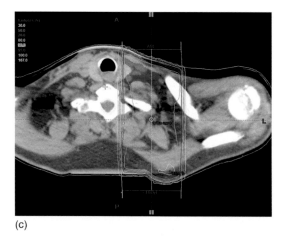

(c)

FIGURE 8.7 Possible beam arrangements for prophylactic treatment of low neck (level IV) nodes. Beam edges are chosen as described in the text. (a) Anterior beam prescribed to D_{max}. (b) Anterior beam prescribed to 3 cm. (c) Anterior and posterior opposing beams.

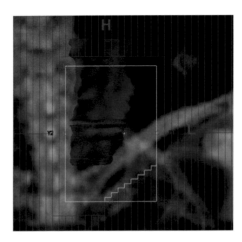

FIGURE 8.8 Standard borders of an anterior neck beam to treat the low neck prophylactically. The superior border is determined by the inferior extent of the high dose planning target volume. Sites of normal level III (blue) and IV (pink) nodal volumes are shown for illustration.

on the skin surface. Both will produce a perfect match at one depth but underdose anterior to this and overdose posteriorly where the divergent beams overlap.

The level at which the anterior beam is matched depends on the PTV. Ideally it should be below the high dose PTV or in between nodal CTVs as matches overlying the PTV risk underdosing disease at the match plane. If this is unavoidable the junction can be moved by 1 cm halfway through the course of treatment to blur this match.

Electron Therapy

If IMRT is not available, electron beams of 9–12 MeV may be used to treat posterior nodes overlying the spinal cord, especially if the prescribed dose would exceed spinal cord tolerance, i.e. if 50 Gy in 25 fractions is chosen as the prophylactic dose rather than 44 Gy in 22 fractions. The lateral 'bowing' of electron isodoses at depth means perfect matching with the photon beam is not possible, so a compromise of matching the 50 percent photon surface isodose with the 50 percent electron surface isodose is usually chosen. This is achieved by matching the edges of the two light beams on the surface of the shell. With CT algorithms for electron beams, it is possible to view electron isodoses on a three-dimensional plan so that underdosing at areas of high risk (e.g. involved nodes) can be avoided if possible.

Treatment Delivery and Verification

Gaps in Treatment Delivery

Squamous cell cancers of the head and neck are particularly sensitive to prolongation of a course of treatment, so gaps in therapy should be avoided whenever possible. If an unintended gap occurs, hyperfractionation is used, avoiding days when chemotherapy is also given.

Verification and Image Guidance

High-quality imaging during treatment is important in head and neck tumours because of the steep dose gradients provided by IMRT and the close proximity of PTVs to OARs. Volumetric imaging with cone beam CT is superior to orthogonal films, and kV CBCT is preferred to MV CBCT as it allows assessment of target volumes.

Daily kV CBCTs with online correction provide the most accurate information, but this approach is resource intensive. It is particularly helpful when contours are expected to change significantly during radiotherapy because of weight loss or tumour shrinkage, or when PTVs and OARs are very close such as at the base of skull. Routine use of daily CBCTs in a department should facilitate a reduction in CTV-PTV margins. Another common protocol is imaging on days 1–3 with an offline correction for systematic errors followed by weekly imaging to check for trends over the course of treatment.

Inter-Fraction Motion

During a course of head and neck radiotherapy, tumour shrinkage or unintentional weight loss can occur, leading to two problems.

First, immobilization may become less effective, introducing error into treatment delivery. The mould room technician may be able to adjust the immobilization shell, for example with shims underneath the head rest. Second, a reduction in tissue volume due to tumour shrinkage or weight loss (usually manifest as a gap between the shell and the skin) may compromise target volume coverage or risk increased dose to critical normal structures. Daily CBCT with online correction can mitigate this.

It can be helpful, and often reassuring, to repeat a planning CT and recalculate the treatment plan on the new CT dataset to assess the dosimetric effect of a change in body contour. Occasionally weight loss or tumour shrinkage can necessitate replanning midway through a course of radiotherapy, but with proactive nutritional support this should rarely be needed.

Patient Care before and during Radiotherapy

The severity of acute side effects of head and neck radiotherapy mandates meticulous assessment and support before, during and after radiotherapy. This is particularly important where dose escalation with altered fractionation and/or concomitant drugs are used. Those most at risk of nutritional problems are men living alone without support, and this should be taken into account when supporting them through treatment or even when deciding on dose-escalation approaches. Psychological support from the multidisciplinary on-treatment team can be as important as mitigating the physical side effects.

Dental Assessment

Before radiotherapy commences, a thorough dental assessment should be carried out and an orthopantomogram (OPG) performed to look for signs of decay in teeth likely to be within the treated volume. Any teeth at risk of decay should be removed to avoid the potential for radionecrosis and chronic infection that can occur when dental work is carried out in a previously irradiated mandible or in patients with xerostomia. Patients should be given advice about maintaining good oral hygiene.

Smoking

Continued smoking increases the severity of mucositis, and patients still smoking should be offered formal cessation advice.

Haemoglobin

There is evidence that low haemoglobin predicts poor outcomes in head and neck cancer. There is less good evidence that maintaining haemoglobin above 12 g/dL with transfusions improves survival. In fact, the use of weekly darbepoetin during radiotherapy has been shown to make outcomes worse. Anaemia may therefore be a marker of poor prognosis rather than a correctable influence of survival.

Weight Loss

The common acute side effects of mucositis, pain, altered taste and altered saliva all contribute to a reduction in calorie intake during radiotherapy. Patients with pre-existing swallowing problems (e.g. tongue base or hypopharyngeal tumours or significant oral or pharyngeal pain) are at particular risk of losing weight, but we recommend that all head and neck patients are assessed by a specialist dietician before radiotherapy. Losing more than 10 percent weight during treatment is associated with delayed recovery and increased complications, along with making immobilization more uncertain. When a patient is felt to be at risk of losing more than 10 percent of their weight during treatment, a prophylactic enteral feeding tube is recommended.

During treatment, patients should be seen weekly by a dietician as part of a multidisciplinary assessment team (with a specialist radiographer, nurse specialist or doctor and a speech and language therapist) and weighed each week. Soft and high calorie diets and high-energy protein-based supplement drinks can be useful to maintain oral intake when it is limited by pain or dysphagia.

Speech and language therapy can be valuable during treatment to maintain effective swallowing, to assess aspiration risk and to advise on vocal care. When swallowing stops completely, rehabilitation after treatment is more difficult and therefore only patients with risk of aspiration should be denied oral intake.

When part of the eyes is in the treated volume (e.g. sinonasal tumours), patients should be seen regularly throughout treatment by an ophthalmologist for advice on preventing corneal damage with lubricating drops and to treat corneal abrasions or infections promptly.

As mucosal reactions peak up to two weeks after therapy, particularly with accelerated fractionation or hypofractionation, careful weekly assessment should continue until acute effects are subsiding.

Pain and Mucositis

Mucositis and the consequent pain are the principal side effects for most patients having head and neck radiotherapy. Benzydamine hydrochloride (Difflam) is the only substance shown to delay the onset of mucositis in an RCT and should be used four to eight times a day from the start of treatment, diluted with water if necessary. No other topical mouthwashes are of proven value and alcohol-based washes should be avoided. Topical anaesthetic agents such as lidocaine (Xylocaine) can be helpful if used before eating, but they have a short duration of action. Candida infections are common and should be treated with fluconazole, or nystatin if less severe.

Pain should be managed proactively with systemic analgesia to avoid a reduction in oral intake as much as possible. Many patients having significant portions of their oral cavity or pharynx irradiated require opioids or anti-neuropathic agents such as gabapentin or pregabalin. Transdermal opiate patches can be especially effective when oral intake is difficult.

Systemic steroids can occasionally be useful if pharyngeal or laryngeal oedema is severe, but they should be avoided if the patient has a gastrotomy tube, as they can precipitate a cutaneous fistula at the site of the tube.

Saliva and Taste

The combination of dysphagia and the buildup of thick, sticky saliva is a major problem during treatment. Good oral hygiene is important, while a humid atmosphere helps keep secretions moist and easier to swallow. Nausea caused by secretions stimulating the soft palate is best managed with 5-hydroxytryptamine antagonists. Taste is commonly affected by radiotherapy, but the mechanisms of dysgeusia are complex and poorly understood.

Skin

Skin reactions can be minimized by applying aqueous cream topically four times daily to treated areas. Tight collars should be avoided, and men should avoid wet shaving.

Key Trials

Bauml JM, Vinnakota R, Anna Park YH, et al. Cisplatin every 3 weeks versus weekly with definitive concurrent radiotherapy for squamous cell carcinoma of the head and neck. J Natl Cancer Inst 2019;111:490–497.

Beitler JJ, Zhang Q, Fu KK, et al. Final results of local-regional control and late toxicity of RTOG 9003: A randomized trial of altered fractionation radiation for locally advanced head and neck cancer. Int J Radiat Oncol Biol Phys 2014;89(1):13–20.

Bernier J, Domenge C, Ozsahin M, et al. Postoperative irradiation with or without concomitant chemotherapy for locally advanced head and neck cancer. N Engl J Med 2004;350:1945–1952.

Bourhis J, Sire C, Graff P, et al. Concomitant chemoradiotherapy versus acceleration of radiotherapy with or without concomitant chemo- therapy in locally advanced head and neck carcinoma (GORTEC 99-02): An open-label phase 3 randomised trial. Lancet Oncol 2012;13:145–153.

Cooper JS, Zhang Q, Pajak TF, et al. Long-term follow-up of the RTOG 9501/intergroup phase III trial: Postoperative concurrent radiation therapy and chemotherapy in high-risk squamous cell carcinoma of the head and neck. Int J Radiat Oncol Biol Phys 2012;84:1198–205.

Gillison ML, Trotti AM, Harris J, et al. Radiotherapy plus cetuximab or cisplatin in human papillomavirus-positive oropharyngeal cancer (NRG oncology RTOG 1016): A randomised, multicentre, noninferiority trial. Lancet 2019;393:40–50.

Mehanna H, Robinson M, Hartley A, et al. Radiotherapy plus cisplatin or cetuximab in low-risk human papillomavirus- positive oropharyngeal cancer (De-ESCALaTE HPV): An open-label randomized controlled phase 3 trial. Lancet 2019;393:51–60.

Mehanna H, Wong WL, McConkey CC, et al. PET-CT surveillance versus neck dissection in advanced head and neck cancer. N Engl J Med 2016;374:1444–1454.

Nguyen-Tan PF, Zhang Q, Ang KK, et al. Randomized phase III trial to test accelerated versus standard fractionation in combination with concurrent cisplatin for head and neck carcinomas in the radiation therapy oncology group 0129 trial: Long-term report of efficacy and toxicity. J Clin Oncol 2014;32:3858–3866.

Noronha V, Joshi A, Patil VM, et al. Once-a-week versus once-every-3-weeks cisplatin chemoradiation for locally advanced head and neck cancer: A phase III randomized noninferiority trial. J Clin Oncol 2018;36:1064–1072.

Nutting CM, Morden JP, Harrington KJ, et al. Parotid-sparing intensity modulated versus conventional radiotherapy in head and neck cancer (PARSPORT): A phase 3 multicentre randomised controlled trial. Lancet Oncol 2011;12:127–136.

Overgaard J, Hansen HS, Sprecht L, et al. Five compared with six fractions per week of conventional radiotherapy of squamous-cell carcinoma of head and neck: DAHNACA 6&7 randomised controlled trial. Lancet 2003;362:933–940.

INFORMATION SOURCES

Ang KK, Harris J, Wheeler R, et al. Human papillomavirus and survival of patients with oropharyngeal cancer. N Engl J Med 2010;363:24–35.

Biau J, Dunet V, Lapeyre M, et al. Practical clinical guidelines for contouring the trigeminal nerve (V) and its branches in head and neck cancers Radiother Oncol 2019;131:192–201.

Biau J, Lapeyre M, Troussier I, et al. Selection of lymph node target volumes for definitive head and neck radiation therapy: A 2019 update. Radiother Oncol 2019;134:1–9.

Blanchard P, Bourhis J, Lacas B, et al. Meta-analysis of chemotherapy in head and neck cancer, induction project, collaborative group. Taxane-cisplatin-fluorouracil as induction chemotherapy in locally advanced head and neck cancers: An individual patient data meta-analysis of the meta-analysis of chemotherapy in head and neck cancer group. J Clin Oncol 2013;31:2854–2860.

Blanchard P, Landais C, Petit C, et al. Meta-analysis of chemotherapy in head and neck cancer (MACH-NC): An update on 100 randomized trials and 19,248 patients, on behalf of MACH-NC group. Ann Oncol 2016;27:328–350.

Budach W, Bölke E, Kammers K, et al. Induction chemotherapy followed by concurrent radio-chemotherapy versus concurrent radio - chemotherapy alone as treatment of locally advanced squamous cell carcinoma of the head and neck (HNSCC): A meta-analysis of randomized trials. Radiother Oncol 2016;118:238–243.

Chow LQM. Head and neck cancer. N Engl J Med 2020;382:60–72.

Evans M, Beasley M. Target delineation for postoperative treatment of head and neck cancer Oral Onocol 2018;86:288–295.

Grégoire V, Eisbruch A, Hamoir M, et al. Proposal for the delineation of the nodal CTV in the node-positive and the post-operative neck. Radiother Oncol 2006;79:15–20.

Grégoire V, Ang K, Budach W, et al. Delineation of the neck node levels for head and neck tumors: A 2013 update. DAHANCA, EORTC, HKNPCSG, NCIC CTG, NCRI, RTOG, TROG consensus guidelines. Radiother Oncol 2014;110:172–181.

Grégoire V, Evans M, Le QT, et al. Delineation of the primary tumour clinical target volumes (CTV-P) in laryngeal, hypopharyngeal, oropharyngeal and oral cavity squamous cell carcinoma: AIRO, CACA, DAHANCA, EORTC, GEORCC, GORTEC, HKNPCSG, HNCIG, IAG-KHT, LPRHHT, NCIC CTG, NCRI, NRG oncology, PHNS, SBRT, SOMERA, SRO, SSHNO, TROG consensus guidelines. Radiother Oncol 2018;126:3–24.

Hansen CR, Johansen J, Samsoe E, et al. Consequences of introducing geometric GTV to CTV margin expansion in DAHANCA contouring guidelines for head and neck radiotherapy. Radiother Oncol 2018;126:43–47.

Ko HC, Gupta V, Mourad WF, et al. A contouring guide for head and neck cancers with perineural invasion. Pract Radiat Oncol 2014;4:247–258.

Lacas B, Bourhis J, Overgaard J, et al. Role of radiotherapy fractionation in head and neck cancers (MARCH): An updated meta-analysis. Lancet Oncol 2017;18:1221–1237.

Le Guevelou J, Bastit V, Marcy PY, et al. Flap delineation guidelines in postoperative head and neck radiation therapy for head and neck cancers Radiother Oncol 2020;151:256–265.

Lengele B, Hamoir M, Scalliet P, et al. Anatomical bases for the radiological delineation of lymph node areas. Major collecting trunks, head and neck. Radiother Oncol 2007;85:146–155.

Machiels J-P, René Leemans C, Golusinski W, et al. Squamous cell carcinoma of the oral cavity, larynx, oropharynx and hypopharynx: EHNS-ESMO-ESTRO clinical practice guidelines for diagnosis, treatment and follow-up. Ann Onc 2020;31:1462–1475.

NICE Guideline NG36. Cancer of the upper aerodigestive tract: Assessment and management in people aged 16 and over, 2016.

Overgaard J. Hypoxic modification of radiotherapy in squamous cell carcinoma of the head and neck–A systematic review and meta-analysis. Radiother Oncol 2011;100:22–32.

Paleri V, Roland N. Head and neck cancer: United Kingdom National multidisciplinary guidelines. J Laryngol Otol 2016;130:S2.

The Royal College of Radiologists. Head and Neck Cancer. RCR Consensus Statements. London: The Royal College of Radiologists, 2022

9

Lip, Ear, Nose and Treatment of the Neck in Skin Cancer

This chapter describes radiotherapy for squamous cell cancers of the lip, external ear canal and middle ear, and nasal vestibule, along with management of the neck in skin cancers of the head and neck. Superficial skin tumours of the nose and pinna are considered in Chapter 7.

Lip

Indications for Radiotherapy

Most lip cancers arise on the vermillion border of the lower lip – the junction between the skin and the lip itself – and are diagnosed at an early stage because they are visible. They are usually superficial squamous cell tumours linked to long-term sun exposure and smoking but are also more common with long-term immunosuppression. Commissure tumours have higher rates of local recurrence than lower lip cancers. Surgery, EBRT and brachytherapy all give local control rates of 90 percent or higher at five years. The choice of treatment depends on the expertise available, the likely cosmetic and functional outcomes and patient choice. Radiotherapy is particularly appropriate when the commissure of the lip is involved (as function may not be as good after surgery), and for larger tumours where more extensive resection and reconstruction would be required, which may result in a smaller oral aperture affecting speaking and eating.

If excision margins are positive or close (<3 mm), adjuvant radiotherapy should be considered if it would result in better function and cosmesis than a further excision. In elderly patients with significant comorbidity it may be appropriate to observe clinically rather than treat with adjuvant radiotherapy, even if margins are close. Involved neck nodes are usually managed with a neck dissection and postoperative radiotherapy if required (see more on that later in the chapter).

Sequencing of Multimodality Therapy

When adjuvant radiotherapy is indicated, it should ideally commence within six weeks of surgery, but a longer gap may be required to allow adequate recovery from a major resection.

Clinical and Radiological Anatomy

Most lip cancers are superficial and have a low risk of lymph node spread. Cross-sectional imaging is only recommended for T2 tumours and above. CT or MRI can assess local extent and bone invasion and the relevant neck node levels. The lymphatic drainage of the lower lip is to ipsilateral level Ib and then level II nodes. The midline portion drains to level Ia and then to bilateral levels Ib and II, but there can be direct drainage to level III. The upper lip drains to level Ib, sometimes via the buccal nodes, which lie under the superficial muscle layer of the face (Figure 9.1).

Assessment of Primary Disease

Careful clinical examination with a strong light and magnifying lens is essential to define the extent of the tumour. Palpation is used to assess thickness.

DOI: 10.1201/9781315171562-9

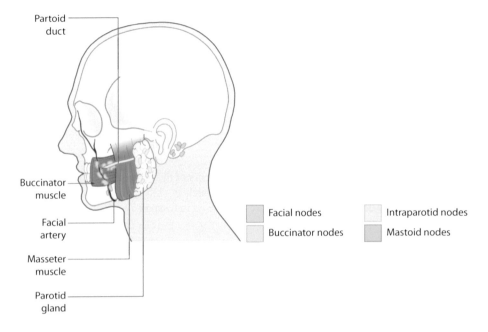

FIGURE 9.1   Superficial lymph nodes of the head and neck.

Target Volume Definition

As superficial photons or electrons are usually used, target volumes are defined on the patient rather than on a planning CT. For small (<2-cm diameter) well-defined tumours, a 3–5 mm margin can be added to the GTV to produce a CTV with a further 5 mm CTV to PTV margin. In practice, the PTV is usually drawn directly on the surface of the skin and lip with a fine marker pen using a strong light, magnifying lens and a ruler to measure the margin from the visible GTV. Larger tumours or those with indistinct edges need a larger GTV-CTV margin of 5–10 mm.

When adjuvant radiotherapy is used, a 5 mm margin from the resection edge is used to define the CTV.

Dose Solutions

The PTV should be covered by the 90 percent isodose of the electron or superficial X-ray beam. Once the PTV has been defined and marked as just described, isodose charts are used to select the required energy to give 90 percent coverage from the surface to the deep margin. Tissue equivalent bolus is used as required either to increase the surface dose or to reduce unwanted deep penetration. The applicator size can then be calculated. If electrons are used, the 90 percent isodose in the lateral plane is 3–5 mm inside the edge of the applicator, which represents the 50 percent dose. Electrons bow inwards at depth at higher energies, so if a high energy is chosen the applicator size will need to be correspondingly larger to avoid underdosing the deep lateral margin.

A 3–4 mm-thick lead mask is then constructed with a cut-out area over the target volume. An intraoral lead shield is used to protect the gums and teeth from the exit beam. It has wax on the anterior surface to absorb secondary electrons.

Dose Fractionation

- 55 Gy in 20 fractions over four weeks
- Consider 66 Gy in 33 fractions over six and a half weeks for larger volumes

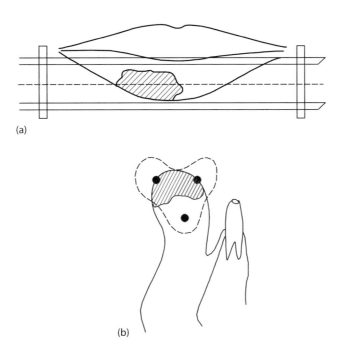

(a)

(b)

FIGURE 9.2 Three-source implant for carcinoma of the lip. (a) Anterior view; (b) sagittal view showing arrangement of sources in an equilateral triangle.

Verification

Verification is by daily inspection of the set-up compared with photographs taken at planning.

Treatment Delivery and Patient Care

Mucositis of the outer and inner lip occurs from the third week of treatment. White soft paraffin is used to keep the lips moisturized, and systemic analgesics should be prescribed if necessary. Sun exposure and smoking should be avoided.

Other Points

Brachytherapy for Lip Squamous Cell Cancer

Where technical expertise exists, brachytherapy can produce excellent local control rates, cosmesis and function. The target volume is defined as just described. Rigid needles are implanted horizontally along the axis of the lip, using either a single plane for superficial lesions, or three or more sources distributed in an equilateral triangle or square in the cross-sectional plane for deeper tumours. A plastic template can be used to provide stability. Sources are usually 10 mm apart and 5–8 cm long, which inevitably means treating most of the lip, making this a useful technique in more extensive tumours or those with indistinct margins (Figure 9.2).

Ear

Indications for Radiotherapy

Cancers of the external auditory canal and middle ear are rare. There is no agreed staging system but most tumours present when locally advanced with bone erosion or cranial nerve palsies. Surgery should be carried out by a lateral skull base team with expertise in temporal bone resections. Local invasion and the complexity of a temporal bone resection mean that close or positive resection margins are common. For these patients, surgery and postoperative radiotherapy are recommended and can produce five-year survival rates of 40–60 percent. Early tumours confined to the external ear canal without soft tissue or bone involvement can be treated with either primary radiotherapy or surgery.

Sequencing of Multimodality Therapy

When adjuvant radiotherapy is indicated, it should ideally commence within six weeks of surgery, but a longer gap may be required to allow adequate recovery from a major resection.

Clinical and Radiological Anatomy

The external ear canal is a 25 mm-long tube with an outer cartilaginous portion and an inner bony segment lined with mucosa. The middle ear contains the ossicles and semicircular canals and communicates posteriorly with the mastoid air cells.

Ulceration and submucosal spread in the ear canal is best assessed by otoscopy. Medially, tumour can spread into the temporal bone (causing VII nerve palsy), around the internal carotid artery and through the Eustachian tube into the nasopharynx. Anterior extension into the temporomandibular joint, parotid gland and masticator space can cause trismus. Posterior spread occurs into the mastoid air cells and thence to the posterior cranial fossa. Superiorly, tumour can invade into the middle cranial fossa and inferiorly into the jugular foramen, causing IX, X and XI cranial nerve palsies, or into the cervical vertebrae.

Lymph node spread at presentation is uncommon. Tumour can spread to the parotid nodes (sometimes divided into the preauricular, subparotid and superficial and deep intraparotid). The posterior part of the external canal drains to the mastoid nodes. Further spread to level II can occur. If tumour reaches the nasopharynx, it can spread to the retropharyngeal nodes.

Assessment of Primary Disease

A combination of clinical examination to look for cranial nerve palsies, MRI for soft tissue extent and CT to evaluate bone destruction is most useful to assess local spread.

Data Acquisition

Immobilization

The patient is immobilized lying supine in a custom-made thermoplastic shell with the neck extended to move the orbit superiorly out of the treatment plane.

CT Scanning

CT slices are obtained from the skull base to the hyoid bone. Slices should be no more than 3 mm thick, and intravenous contrast should be used to highlight vessels at the base of skull, which will help define the medial extent of the CTV. Fusion of diagnostic MR and CT planning images can be particularly helpful to define skull base anatomy.

Target Volume Definition

Discussion with the surgeon and pathologist is critical to establish the sites at highest risk of recurrence after a temporal bone resection. It can be helpful to delineate the original site of disease on the post-op planning CT and to mark any sites where resection margins were involved or close.

For adjuvant treatment, the CTV is contoured on each axial CT slice with the aid of the corresponding slices on preoperative imaging and the operation details, aiming to encompass all resection margins and to have a 10 mm margin from the resection edge at high-risk sites. This 10 mm margin should be individualized depending on natural tumour barriers and possible routes of spread. Recurrences at the skull base are not usually treatable with surgery and cause significant pain and cranial nerve morbidity, so the lateral base of skull and cranial foramina should be included in the CTV. Though the risk of involvement is low, adjacent parotid, mastoid and high level II nodes are included in the CTV, as they tend to be superficial to the resection margins and can be treated without a significant increase in morbidity. A CTV_Boost can be defined if there is macroscopic residual disease or resection margins are positive at a clearly defined site. CTV_Boost should be the residual GTV or site of positive resection with a 5 mm margin.

The CTV is expanded isotropically to form the PTV by a margin determined for each department by the observed random and systematic errors – usually 3–5 mm.

The brainstem, spinal cord and adjacent temporal lobe should be contoured as organs at risk. The CTV and PTV should be defined without reference to the organs at risk and vice versa. The PTV may end up overlapping a critical structure but the dosimetrist and oncologist can then evaluate the beam arrangements and MLC shielding to optimize the treatment plan. If the CTV or PTV is edited away from an organ at risk to protect that organ, the opportunity to deliver dose to the whole target by an innovative treatment plan may be lost and the good coverage of the PTV will be falsely reassuring. It is better to accept a compromise in dose to the PTV when the plan is produced, than to guess where this compromise needs to be made at the volume definition stage.

For early external ear canal tumours confined to the mucosa and treated with primary radiotherapy, the GTV as defined by clinical examination is outlined on a planning CT. A 5 mm isotropic margin is added to produce a CTV_HIGH. The GTV is then expanded by 10 mm to produce the CTV_MID, which is edited to include the adjacent temporal bone. If there is concern about accuracy of GTV delineation, a single target volume can be defined and treated to the prescribed dose.

Dose Solutions

The proximity of the PTV to brain, brainstem and optic structures means IMRT or VMAT is preferable. Up to five ipsilateral beams are usually employed with individualized beam angles to avoid entering through normal tissues or exiting through critical structures as much as possible. As the PTV is often close to the temporal lobe or brainstem, the risk of late radiation damage must be weighed against the risk of tumour recurrence, and the decision about the possible risks of late effects and possible benefits of giving more dose to high-risk sites should be discussed with the patient.

If a compromise is needed, it may be better to use two phases of treatment rather than underdose part of the PTV throughout the whole course. The whole PTV can be treated in a phase 1 volume (usually for 20–25 fractions), with a smaller phase 2 shaped prioritizing the sparing of critical structures at the expense of coverage of some of the PTV. A summed plan is created from the two phases to allow evaluation of DVHs. The number of fractions for each phase can be varied so that the best compromise can be achieved for individual patients. It may also be necessary to reduce the total dose to protect OARs (Figure 9.3).

Dose Fractionation

Adjuvant

- 60 Gy in 30 fractions over six weeks
- Consider 65 Gy in 30 fractions over six weeks if resection margin involved

Curative

- 65 Gy in 30 fractions over six weeks
- 55 Gy in 20 fractions over four weeks for small volumes

Verification

See Chapter 8.

Treatment Delivery and Patient Care

After a temporal bone resection, patients often have considerable morbidity with cranial nerve palsies affecting swallowing and speech, and a feeding gastrostomy tube may be in place. A dietician and speech and language therapist should assess patients each week along with other members of the radiation therapy

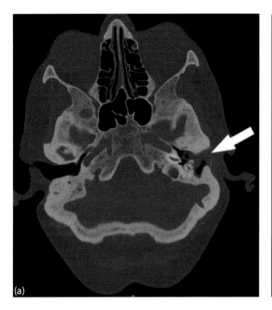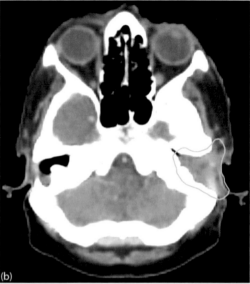

FIGURE 9.3   Cancer of the middle ear invading the lateral base of skull. (a) Temporal bone diagnostic CT showing tumour (arrowed) invading mastoid and lateral skull base; (b) planning CT scan showing CTV.

team. Although the local acute effects of radiotherapy are limited to skin erythema and localized mucositis, lethargy and anorexia can be debilitating when radiotherapy follows such major surgery. The shell can be cut out over the treated volume to reduce skin reaction if the PTV is not close to the skin surface.

Nose

Indications for Radiotherapy

Cancers of the nasal vestibule behave like skin tumours, are usually diagnosed when small and have a 90 percent local control rate with radiotherapy or surgery. Radiation gives better cosmesis except for very small lesions as surgery often necessitates a partial or total rhinectomy. Larger tumours or those with bone involvement have a low chance of cure by radiation alone. Resection may be followed by adjuvant radiotherapy.

Sequencing of Multimodality Therapy

When adjuvant radiotherapy is indicated, it should ideally commence within six weeks of surgery, but a longer gap may be required to allow adequate recovery from a major resection.

Clinical and Radiological Anatomy

The nasal vestibule is the entrance to the nasal cavity, lined by squamous epithelium. Tumours of the proximal nasal cavity lined by respiratory epithelium are covered in Chapter 16. The columella is the midline, medial wall of the vestibule and tumours arising here can spread submucosally onto the upper lip or posteriorly along the roof of the hard palate. Cross-sectional imaging with MR or CT is important to define their extent.

Lymph node spread is uncommon at diagnosis but the vestibule drains to levels Ia and Ib or to the buccinator node overlying the buccinator muscle and then to level II.

Assessment of Primary Disease

Careful clinical examination with a strong light and magnifying lens is essential to define the extent of the tumour. Palpation is used to assess thickness.

Data Acquisition

Immobilization

The patient is immobilized in a thermoplastic shell. Wax nostril plugs are recommended to help produce a more homogeneous dose distribution, if the patient is able to tolerate them.

CT Scanning

Slices 3 mm thick are obtained from the inferior orbit to the hyoid bone to include level I nodes. Intravenous contrast may help to visualize the tumour if it enhances.

Target Volume Definition

The GTV is outlined on the planning CT scan with the help of clinical examination and diagnostic imaging. The GTV is expanded by 5 mm isotropically to form the CTV. This is then expanded posteriorly to include the soft tissue up to the bone of the hard palate. The CTV is edited from adjacent air cavities and the wax nasal plugs if used. A 10 mm margin can be considered inferiorly at the lower lip where there may be submucosal spread. The CTV-PTV margin is determined by local audit but is usually 3–5 mm.

Dose Solutions

Two lateral oblique photon beams provide the most conformal coverage plan for the PTV, sometimes with a third anterior beam. Non-coplanar beams as used for ethmoid tumours can also be employed. The angle of the beams is chosen to ensure adequate dose to any posterior extension along the roof of the hard palate. Wax is applied on the external surface of the nose and upper lip as needed to increase the surface dose. The epithelial surface thus becomes encased in wax internally and externally to allow the hollow vestibule to be treated as a block, producing a more homogeneous dose distribution (Figure 9.4). The beams can be modulated with IMRT to produce a more homogeneous dose distribution.

Electrons can also be used for superficial lesions, but the contour of the nose, small field sizes and underlying cartilage make conformal photons the preferred solution.

Dose Fractionation

- 55 Gy in 20 fractions given in four weeks
- Longer fractionation is not usually necessary given the small volumes treated

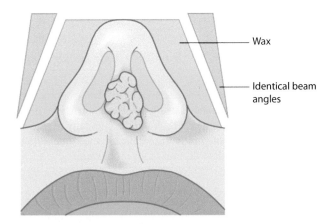

FIGURE 9.4 Beam arrangement for conformal treatment of nasal columella tumour. Note beams are angled posteriorly to cover possible tumour extension along the roof of the hard palate.

Verification

Portal images are compared with DRRs as for other head and neck tumours with in vivo dosimetry on the first day of treatment.

Treatment Delivery and Patient Care

The inside of the nasal cavity can become especially sore and topical local anaesthetic or steroid creams along with systemic analgesics are often needed to enable the patient to tolerate insertion of the wax plugs throughout treatment.

Neck Nodes from Skin Cancers

Indications for Radiotherapy

Squamous cell skin cancers of the head and neck may recur in the regional lymph nodes, with a median interval to recurrence of 12 months. Treatment at this time is usually surgical with postoperative radiotherapy indicated unless a neck dissection only reveals a solitary intraparotid or level II–V node without extracapsular spread. If comorbidity or patient choice precludes surgery, then radiation alone can be used, but the chance of cure with radiation alone is small.

It is possible to identify head and neck skin tumours at higher risk of having occult metastases with size, depth of invasion, high grade and perineural or vascular invasion all increasing the risk. Tumours on or near the external ear are at higher risk of spread to the intraparotid nodes. There is, however, no consensus on the role of prophylactic nodal radiotherapy (or neck dissection) in these tumours.

Sequencing of Multimodality Therapy

Ideally, radiotherapy should commence within six weeks of surgery, as long as there is adequate healing. There is randomized controlled trial evidence showing no benefit of adding concomitant carboplatin chemotherapy to adjuvant radiotherapy.

Clinical and Radiological Anatomy

The most common sites for skin cancers (ear, temple, forehead, anterior scalp and cheek) drain to the intraparotid nodes and thence to level II and on to levels Ib and III–V. Many patients therefore present with a parotid mass. In 25 percent of patients, a primary skin tumour is not identified and a mucosal head and neck tumour should be excluded by clinical examination and PET imaging. The pattern of lymph node spread (intraparotid nodes), immunohistochemistry and the presence of sun-damaged skin may point to the skin as the likely primary source.

Assessment of Nodal Disease

The intraparotid nodes and levels Ib–V should be assessed by clinical examination and imaging. MRI is preferred to CT for imaging the parotid. Surgery usually involves a superficial parotidectomy if there are intraparotid nodes, and a neck dissection of levels Ib–Va in the clinically negative lower neck.

Discussion with the surgeon and pathologist is important to determine which nodal levels require radiotherapy because of microscopic residual disease or for prophylaxis.

Target Volume Definition

It can be helpful to define the original site of involved nodes on the planning CT if they were visible on pre-op imaging. The CTV_HIGH encompasses the involved nodal levels ensuring at least a 10 mm

TABLE 9.1

Examples of CTV_HIGH and CTV_LOW for adjuvant radiotherapy when treating lymph nodes from squamous cell skin cancers in the head and neck depending on clinical and pathological findings

Clinically Involved Nodes	Surgery and Pathology	CTV_HIGH	CTV_LOW
Intraparotid only	Superficial parotidectomy alone	Parotid bed	Levels Ib, II, III
Intraparotid only	Superficial parotidectomy and level Ib–III neck dissection; involved intraparotid node only	Parotid bed	Not defined
Intraparotid only	Superficial parotidectomy and level Ib–III neck dissection; involved intraparotid node and level II	Parotid bed and level II	Levels Ib, III, IVa and V
Intraparotid and neck	Superficial parotidectomy and level Ib–V dissection; involved intraparotid node and level Ib–V nodes[a]	Parotid bed and levels Ib–V	Not defined

Note:

[a] Consider omitting lateral neck irradiation if only one lateral neck node involved without extranodal extension.

margin longitudinally from the original involved nodes. Dissected nodal levels that were node negative are included if the risk of recurrence there is high – for example if many nodes are involved in adjacent levels – or if it is hard to know exactly where the involved nodes were. A CTV_LOW can be defined to treat undissected nodal levels adjacent to those containing involved nodes, e.g. levels 1b, IVa/b, Vc depending on the extent of the neck dissection. (See Table 9.1.)

Dose Solutions

IMRT or VMAT is preferred to provide a more homogeneous dose distribution given the change in neck contour in the length of the volume. Three to five ipsilateral beams are used with beam angles chosen to avoid entry through normal tissue or exit through critical structures where possible.

Dose Fractionation

- 60 Gy in 30 daily fractions given in six weeks
- PTV_HIGH receives 60 Gy in 30 fractions
- PTV_LOW receives 54 Gy in 30 fractions

Treatment Delivery and Patient Care

See Chapter 8.

Verification

See Chapter 8.

Key Trials

Porceddu SV, Bressel M, Poulsen MG, et al. Postoperative concurrent chemoradiotherapy versus postoperative radiotherapy in high-risk cutaneous squamous cell carcinoma of the head and neck: The randomized phase III TROG 05.01 trial. J Clin Oncol 2018;36:1275–1283.

INFORMATION SOURCES

Porceddu SV, Daniels C, Yom SS, et al. Head and neck cancer international group (HNCIG) consensus guidelines for the delivery of postoperative radiation therapy in complex cutaneous squamous cell carcinoma of the head and neck (cSCCHN) Int J Radiation Oncol Biol Phys 2020;107(4):641–651.

10

Oral Cavity

The oral cavity comprises the anterior two-thirds of the tongue, the floor of mouth, buccal mucosa, hard palate and gingivae (Figure 10.1). Tumours of the lip are discussed in Chapter 9.

Indications for Radiotherapy

Curative Radiotherapy for Local Disease

Most T1 and T2 tumours of the oral cavity are treated with surgical excision as long as clear margins and good functional outcome can reasonably be expected. Radiotherapy can only provide equivalent local control rates to surgery if some or the entire radiation dose is given by brachytherapy. Five-year local control rates for T1 and T2 tumours are 75–95 percent and 50–85 percent, respectively. However, brachytherapy is often technically impossible (tumour is close to bone) or the necessary expertise is unavailable. There is no proven role for radiotherapy for carcinoma in situ of the oral cavity.

Primary EBRT is therefore only recommended if surgery is not technically possible with clear margins and good expected functional outcome, for example in the case of a second primary tumour close to a previous resection site, or if there are reasons precluding a general anaesthetic.

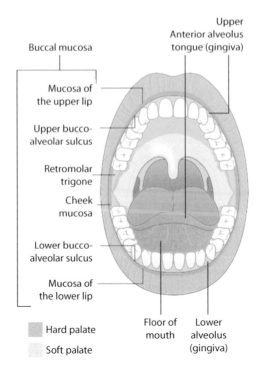

FIGURE 10.1 Subsites of the oral cavity.

DOI: 10.1201/9781315171562-10

Adjuvant Radiotherapy for Local Disease

For larger T2 (>3 cm), T3 and T4 tumours, local control is best achieved by surgery and adjuvant radiotherapy.

Adjuvant local radiotherapy is also indicated where a smaller primary tumour is excised with positive margins and the preferred option of further excision is not possible. Where a small primary tumour has been excised with close (usually considered to be <5 mm) margins, a discussion with the surgeon is important to assess the risk of microscopic residual disease. The measured margin must be considered in the context of other pathological risk factors such as perineurial invasion and tumour grade, adjacent structures (whether the margin is adjacent to bone) and how easy it may be to detect local recurrence early. Single modality treatment should be the goal for early oral cavity cancer as the best way to maintain function and reduce complications such as osteoradionecrosis. In addition, second primary oral cancers are relatively common, and once part of the oral cavity has been irradiated, further surgery or radiation may be difficult.

Primary Radiotherapy to the cN0 Neck

Treatment of the clinically and radiologically node-negative neck should be considered in all patients with oral cavity tumours. Several factors increase the risk of occult nodal metastases, including greater depth of primary tumour invasion, larger primary tumour and site (tongue and floor of mouth tumours are at higher risk owing to richer lymphatic drainage). No treatment of the neck should only be considered in people with a very low risk of occult nodal disease – for example when an excision of an area of carcinoma in situ shows a very small focus of early invasive cancer. At-risk nodal levels can be treated by a selective neck dissection or radiotherapy.

When surgery is the initial treatment for the primary cancer, a selective level I–IV neck dissection is usually performed if access to the neck is required for insertion of a reconstructive flap. If neck access is not required, a sentinel node biopsy can also be used to better assess nodal risk, proceeding to a neck dissection if positive. Radiotherapy to the N0 neck is used if radiation is used to treat the primary site or, in rare situations, when histological features of the primary tumour indicate a higher risk of occult metastases than was thought preoperatively (for example when an excision biopsy shows an unexpected cancer). If brachytherapy alone is used to treat the primary it is usually followed by radiation or surgery to the N0 neck.

Tumours of the floor of mouth or midline tongue or hard palate are at risk of bilateral neck metastases, so both sides of the neck should be treated unless the tumour is more than 10 mm from midline.

Adjuvant Radiotherapy to the Neck

When tumour is found in lymph nodes from a neck dissection, adjuvant radiotherapy to that neck is recommended unless there is only pN1 disease. When a patient has had an ipsilateral neck dissection that is pN2–3, the contralateral undissected neck is also at risk with a 12–33 percent recurrence rate, so both sides of the neck should be irradiated.

If adjuvant radiotherapy to the primary site is recommended for a pT3/4 N0 tumour, the bilateral neck should also be included in the treatment volume, as the risk of neck recurrence is likely to be >15 percent, even after a pN0 neck dissection.

Recovery from resection and reconstruction of an oral cavity cancer is a major challenge for many patients, especially if they have comorbidities. There is always a balance to be struck between irradiating more of the primary site and bilateral neck to reduce recurrence risk and irradiating less to reduce likely acute and long-term toxicity. For many patients, careful assessment with the multidisciplinary team, taking into account patient preferences and their support networks, is key to making the best decision.

Palliative Radiotherapy

Surgery may be inappropriate for locally advanced cancer if clear resection margins are not possible, if the expected functional outcome after surgery is not acceptable to the patient or if comorbidity precludes surgery. In these cases, radiotherapy alone can provide effective palliation. High doses can provide a small chance of long-term cure, especially if combined with concomitant chemotherapy, but at the cost of significant toxicity.

Sequencing of Multimodality Therapy

Where EBRT is followed by brachytherapy, the overall treatment time should be kept as short as possible to avoid tumour repopulation. A one-week gap is recommended.

If adjuvant radiotherapy is indicated, it should ideally commence within six weeks after surgery but after adequate wound healing has occurred. If radiotherapy is delayed to more than three months after surgery because of surgical complications, the potential risks of EBRT may outweigh the benefits.

Concomitant chemotherapy with adjuvant radiotherapy improves local control and disease-free survival when there is a high risk of local recurrence, especially if excision margins are positive or there is extracapsular nodal spread.

Clinical and Radiological Anatomy

Anterior tongue tumours usually present as ulcers, which can spread radially or invade deeply into the tongue muscles or grow as an exophytic mass. Adjacent field change and carcinoma in situ is relatively common. The T staging of oral cavity tumours has changed in UICC TNMv8 to include reference to tumour depth (Table 10.1).

The lateral tongue drains to ipsilateral level Ib nodes. The level Ib nodes have efferent lymphatic connections to level II and thence to levels III and IV, but there are also direct lymphatic connections from the tongue and floor of mouth to level II and level III and occasionally to level IV. This explains the relatively high incidence of skip metastases in oral cavity tumours (10–15 percent) (Figure 10.2).

Lymphatics from the floor of mouth and the tip of the tongue drain to level Ia nodes and thence to bilateral Ib nodes, but there can again be direct spread to level III nodes. Floor of mouth tumours are often infiltrative and invade the mandible anteriorly, tongue posteriorly and deep muscles of the floor inferiorly. They commonly present late so surgery and radiotherapy are often both required for local control. Oral tongue and floor of mouth tumours can spread to contralateral neck nodes, especially if they involve or are close to midline.

Primary tumours of buccal mucosa can invade deep structures including the mandible and cheek and spread initially to ipsilateral level Ib nodes or to level IX (facial) nodes. Retromolar trigone cancers can grow inferiorly into the mandible and posteriorly to invade the pterygoid muscles causing trismus.

TABLE 10.1

Tumour Staging for Oral Cavity Cancer

Tx	Primary tumour cannot be assessed
Tis	Carcinoma in situ
T1	Tumour ≤2 cm with depth of invasion (DOI)[a] ≤5 mm
T2	Tumour ≤2 cm with DOI[a] >5 mm and ≤10 mm or tumour >2 cm and ≤4 cm with DOI[a] ≤10 mm
T3	Tumour > 2 cm and ≤4 cm with DOI[a] >10 mm or tumour >4 cm with DOI[a] ≤10 mm or any tumour
T4a	Moderately advanced disease
	Tumour >4 cm with DOI[a] >10 mm or tumour invades adjacent structures only (e.g. through cortical bone of the mandible or maxilla or involves the maxillary sinus or skin of the face)
T4b	Very advanced disease
	Tumour invades masticator space, pterygoid plates or skull base or encases the internal carotid artery

Source: Adapted from UICC TNM (8th edn, 2018).
Note:
[a]   DOI is depth of invasion and not tumour thickness.

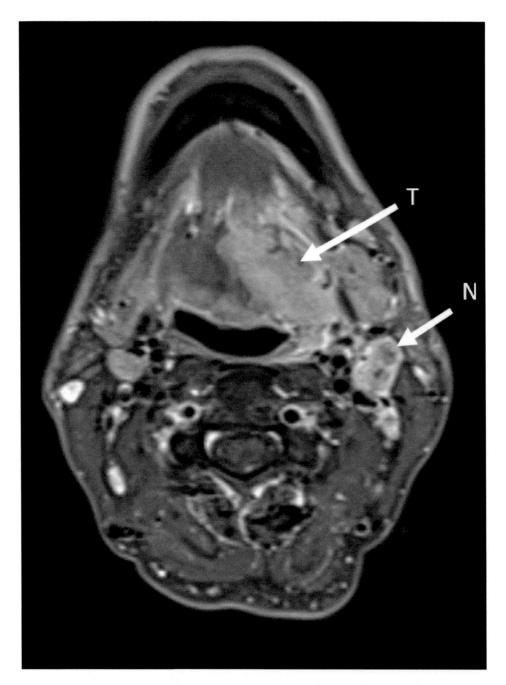

FIGURE 10.2 Primary floor of mouth tumour and lymphadenopathy. Axial T1-weighted contrast-enhanced MRI with tumour (T) and level II node (N) (both arrowed).

The mucosa of the upper and lower alveolus (gingivae) and hard palate is fixed to the underlying periosteum so invasion of the adjacent bone occurs relatively early, making these tumours less suitable for primary radiotherapy. Superficial erosion of bone/tooth socket alone by a gingival primary is not sufficient to classify a tumour as T4.

Hard palate tumours may originate from minor salivary glands and spread via nerves towards the skull base. They spread first to ipsilateral level Ib nodes. Midline tumours of the hard palate can spread bilaterally to level Ib. Hard palate tumours invading the soft palate posteriorly can also spread to level II or retropharyngeal nodes which should be specifically evaluated by cross-sectional imaging.

Assessment of Primary Disease

The oncologist and maxillofacial surgeon should assess primary disease by careful examination using bimanual palpation to assess tumour thickness when possible, as this predicts for occult metastases. EUA should be considered for more extensive tumours to assess local invasion before planning curative treatment.

MRI gives the most accurate information to assess local invasion, but a CT scan can also be useful, especially to assess bone. An OPG can also help assess invasion of the mandible. Superficial mucosal tumours can be difficult to see on cross-sectional imaging. Either MRI or CT can be used to stage neck nodes.

Data Acquisition

Immobilization

Patients should lie supine with a straight spine, immobilized in a thermoplastic shell. A custom-made mouth bite may help to push the tongue inferiorly when irradiating the hard palate or upper alveolus or to separate the roof of the mouth from the inferior oral cavity when irradiating the tongue. Mouth bites can distort the anatomy and make volumes on CT more difficult to define accurately. Some patients find them difficult to tolerate and they may precipitate swallowing and thus cause movement of critical structures.

CT Scanning

CT slices are obtained from the base of skull to the arch of the aorta with the patient immobilized in the treatment position. Slices should be no more than 3 mm thick to improve volume definition and quality of the DRR. Intravenous iodinated contrast should be used unless it is contraindicated.

Target Volume Definition

When defining volumes, it is important to have all relevant information available, including clinical assessments, EUA reports, operation notes, histology results and diagnostic imaging.

Curative Radiotherapy

The primary GTV is outlined on a planning computer with window settings adjusted to show soft tissues. It can be helpful to fuse diagnostic MRI images to better define the tumour but the quality of image fusion should be carefully assessed and the final contours should be defined on the planning CT.

The GTV is expanded isotropically by 5 mm to form the CTVp_HIGH. This is edited to take account of local patterns of tumour spread and natural tissue barriers, for example bone can be spared if not clinically involved. The medial pterygoid muscle should be included in the CTVp_HIGH if there is local invasion of part of the muscle, for example from a retromolar trigone tumour. The GTV is then expanded by 10 mm to create the CTVp_MID, which is also edited to take account of possible routes of local spread and natural tissue barriers.

Involved lymph nodes on imaging are contoured as GTVn and expanded by 5 mm to form CTVn_HIGH. A 10 mm expansion can be used if there is obvious extracapsular nodal extension. The CTVn_MID is defined to include involved nodal levels or those at particularly high risk of occult nodal disease, such as those close to a primary site or in between involved nodal levels. The CTVn_LOW is defined as in Table 10.2.

TABLE 10.2

Recommendations for the Selection of Low-Risk Nodal Levels (CTV_LOW) for Oral Cavity Tumours – Anterior Two-Thirds of the Tongue, Floor of Mouth, Buccal Mucosa, Hard Palate and Gingivae

Nodal Status (TNM8)	Ipsilateral Neck	Contralateral Neck – Consider in Patients unless N0-1 and Well-Lateralized Primary
N0-1	Ia, Ib, II, III, IVa IX for buccal mucosa tumours	Ia, Ib, II, III, IVa
N2a-2b or N3	Ia, Ib, II, III, IVa, Va,b IVb if level IVa is involved IX for buccal mucosa tumours VIIb if upper level II is involved	Ia, Ib, II, III, IVa
N2c	According to N stage on each side of the neck	According to N stage on each side of the neck

Adjuvant Radiotherapy – Primary

The CTV_HIGH is defined using the planning CT scan after discussion with the surgeon and pathologist to define the sites at risk of microscopic residual disease. Postoperative oral cavity CTVs can be difficult to define because oral mucosa is not well defined on CT, dental artefact can obscure the oral anatomy and reconstructive soft tissue flaps can be confused with normal anatomical structures. The intention is to cover the original site of primary disease with a 5–10 mm margin.

It can be helpful to contour the location of the original primary disease and sometimes to fuse pre-op images with the planning CT to help define this, though the anatomical changes that will have occurred after surgery mean that care should be taken with this approach. If there has been a reconstructive free flap, it can be helpful to contour the flap as a guide to where the resection site is, expanding this contour by 5–10 mm and editing from air (Figure 10.3).

The CTV-PTV margin should be individualized in each department according to measured random and systematic set-up errors. There should be minimal organ or tumour movement in a head and neck shell with the exception of small tumours of the oral tongue. For these, a separate internal margin may need to be added. Overall CTV-PTV margins should be 3–5 mm in each direction.

Adjuvant Radiotherapy – Neck

Pathologically involved nodal levels should be contoured as part of CTV_HIGH. Levels that were dissected but with no involved nodes, or undissected adjacent or contralateral levels, can be defined in CTV_LOW according to Table 10.2. It is always challenging to define neck levels precisely in the dissected neck, so it is often more pragmatic to treat all dissected levels of an involved neck within the high dose volume.

Prophylactic Radiotherapy – Undissected cN0 Neck, No Primary Site RT

At-risk nodal levels are defined according to patterns of lymphatic drainage from the primary site in Table 10.2. 50 Gy in 25 fractions is an adequate dose.

Palliative Radiotherapy

Whilst GTV, CTV and PTV can be defined as for curative treatment, it is usually appropriate to use smaller margins to minimize normal tissue toxicity (particularly mucositis). For example, a 5 mm margin is used from GTV to CTV and uninvolved neck levels are omitted.

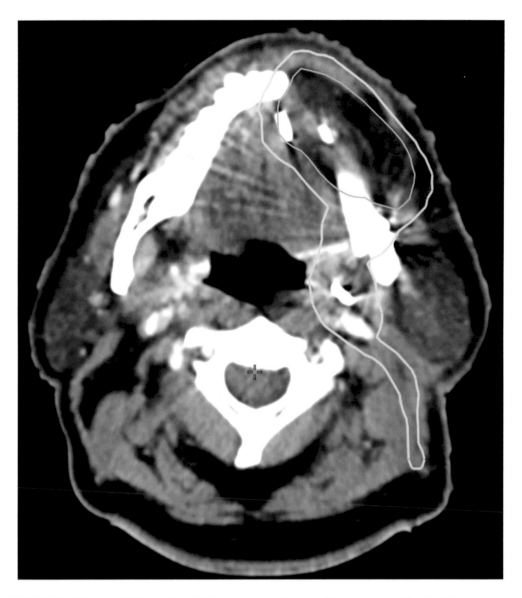

FIGURE 10.3 Adjuvant radiotherapy for pT4aN3b squamous cell cancer of the lower gum with a fibula free flap reconstruction (light green). Closest excision margin is 4 mm. CTV_HIGH (cyan) is the free flap with a 5 mm isotropic margin and level Ib and II nodal regions.

Dose Solutions

Complex

IMRT or VMAT have the potential to deliver the most conformal radiotherapy to complex target volumes with greater sparing of normal tissues, but if the target volume is ipsilateral, the added advantage of IMRT over conformal solutions is likely to be relatively small.

Beam numbers and angles are chosen depending on the location of tumour volumes. For midline tumours when bilateral nodal volumes are irradiated, five or seven equispaced IMRT beams or one to two arcs are used similar to an oropharyngeal cancer plan. For a more ipsilateral volume, three to five beams avoiding entry in the contralateral neck, or a single arc, will facilitate sparing of the contralateral mucosa and salivary glands.

Conformal

When only one side of the neck is treated, an arrangement of three coplanar beams can usually provide good PTV coverage while sparing the contralateral mucosa and parotid gland. At least one of the beams must have no exit dose through the spinal cord for this organ to remain within tolerance. In practice, this means the angle of the posterior oblique beam is chosen to provide best coverage of the PTV while avoiding the cord. A matched anterior neck beam can be used to treat low neck nodes (see Chapter 8).

For palliative doses, a midline PTV can be treated with lateral opposed beams with MLC shielding to spare normal tissues. Wedges can be used to compensate for the change in neck contour and produce a more even dose distribution.

Conventional

Where resources are not available for conformal planning, conventional techniques may be unavoidable. For tumours involving the midline or where bilateral neck nodes require radiotherapy, opposed lateral fields can be used, but this does not allow sparing of any adjacent mucosa in the treated volume. If the high dose volume extends posteriorly to the spinal cord, a two-phase technique is used with large lateral fields for phase 1 and smaller lateral fields matched to posterior electron fields for phase 2. A matched anterior neck field treats lower neck nodes with midline shielding to reduce dose to the larynx, pharynx and spinal cord.

Where treatment is unilateral, anterior and posterior oblique wedged fields are chosen, with a lateral field sometimes used to improve homogeneity medially in the target volume. An ipsilateral anterior neck field is matched to treat inferior neck nodes if required.

Dose Fractionation

Curative Treatment

- EBRT with brachytherapy
  - EBRT 50 Gy in 25 daily fractions given in five weeks
  - LDR brachytherapy boost 30 Gy to the reference isodose over three days
- LDR brachytherapy alone
  - 65 Gy to the reference isodose over seven days.
- EBRT alone
  - 70 Gy in 35 daily fractions given in seven weeks +/− concomitant cisplatin
    - PTV_HIGH receives 70 Gy in 35 fractions
    - PTV_MID receives 63 Gy in 35 fractions
    - PTV_LOW receives 56 Gy in 35 fractions
  - 65 Gy in 30 daily fractions given in six weeks +/− concomitant cisplatin
    - PTV_HIGH receives 65 Gy in 30 fractions
    - PTV_MID receives 60 Gy in 30 fractions
    - PTV_LOW receives 54 Gy in 30 fractions

Adjuvant Treatment

- 60 Gy in 30 daily fractions given in six weeks +/− concomitant cisplatin
  - PTV_HIGH receives 60 Gy in 30 fractions
  - PTV_LOW receives 54 Gy in 30 fractions

Palliative Treatment

- 30 Gy in 10 fractions of 3 Gy given in two weeks
- 20 Gy in 5 daily fractions of 4 Gy given in one week

Treatment Delivery and Patient Care

See Chapter 8. Excellent oral hygiene is particularly important when part of the oral cavity is being irradiated. Mucositis of the lip can be treated with steroid-based paste preparations if there is no concurrent infection. Fungal infections are common and can recur during a course of radiotherapy. The oral cavity should be carefully inspected at least once a week and antifungal agents used as necessary.

Verification

See Chapter 8.

Brachytherapy

Brachytherapy offers excellent conformal radiotherapy to small tumours of the tongue and buccal mucosa that are well demarcated, not close to bone and accessible for implantation. These tumours are usually treated by surgery, and the decision to treat with brachytherapy instead is often based on the expertise available. The disadvantages of brachytherapy include the risk of bleeding and infection, the radiation risk to staff and the patient isolation required.

Anterior tongue tumours or small floor-of-mouth cancers not too close to the mandible are usually treated with iridium-192 hairpins after metal gutters have been inserted. With the patient anaesthetized, the GTV is marked with ink. The depth of tumour infiltration on MRI corresponds accurately with surgical invasion and can be used to assess depth. The CTV is the GTV with a 10 mm margin. There is no margin added to form a PTV, as there is no daily set-up error or organ motion relative to the radiation. The gutters are inserted 12–15 mm apart according to Paris rules to ensure adequate CTV coverage, and their position verified by orthogonal radiographs before the iridium is inserted (Figure 10.4).

Small buccal mucosa tumours can be treated with a single plane implant using iridium-192 placed in flexible plastic tubes. After the CTV has been defined, hollow needles are placed to provide adequate

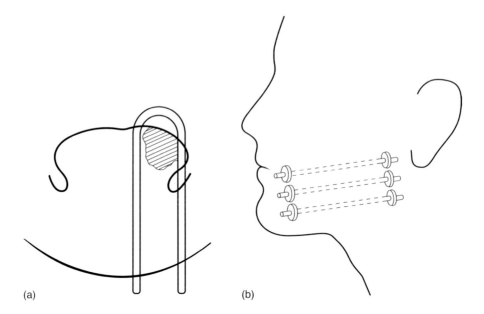

(a)   (b)

FIGURE 10.4 Source arrangements for brachytherapy of oral cavity tumours. (a) Iridium-192 hairpins for anterior tongue or floor of mouth. (b) Iridium-192 single plane implant for buccal mucosa.

CTV dose, and a guidewire is introduced over which the plastic tubes are placed. Steroids may be required if trauma during the procedure causes enough swelling to compromise the airway. The skin should be cleaned regularly with an antiseptic agent. Analgesia is provided with opiates and nonsteroidal anti-inflammatory drugs. The implant is reviewed daily.

Equivalent pulse dose rate or high dose rate schedules are sometimes used.

Key Trials

There are no phase III trials evaluating the role of radiotherapy in oral cavity cancers alone, although these patients are often included in studies of head and neck cancer in general (see key trials in Chapter 8).

D'Cruz AK, Vaish R, Kapre N, et al. Elective versus therapeutic neck dissection in node-negative oral cancer. N Engl J Med 2015;373:521–529.

Hutchison IL, Ridout F, Cheung SMY, et al. Nationwide randomised trial evaluating elective neck dissection for early stage oral cancer (SEND study) with meta-analysis and concurrent real-world cohort. Br J Cancer 2019;121:827–836.

INFORMATION SOURCES

See Chapter 8.

Chegini S, Schilling C, Walgama ES, et al. Neck failure following pathologically node-negative neck dissection (pN0) in oral squamous cell carcinoma: A systematic review and meta-analysis. Br J Oral Maxillofac Surg 2021. doi: https://doi.org/10.1016/j.bjoms.2021.04.002

Ganly I, Goldstein D, Carlson DL, et al. Long-term regional control and survival in patients with "low-risk," early stage oral tongue cancer managed by partial glossectomy and neck dissection without postoperative radiation: The importance of tumor thickness. Cancer 2013;119:1168–1176.

Kovács G, Martinez-Monge R, Budrukkar A, et al. GEC-ESTRO ACROP recommendations for head & neck brachytherapy in squamous cell carcinomas: 1st update – Improvement by cross sectional imaging based treatment planning and stepping source technology. Radiother Oncol 2017;122:248–254.

Mazeron JJ, Ardiet JM, Haie-Méder C, et al. GEC-ESTRO recommendations for brachytherapy for head and neck squamous cell carcinomas. Radiother Oncol 2009;91:150–156.

Shlomo A, Koyfman MD, Ismaila N, et al. Management of the neck in squamous cell carcinoma of the oral cavity and oropharynx: ASCO clinical practice guideline summary. J Oncol Pract 2019;15:273–278.

11

Oropharynx Cancer and Unknown Primary Tumours of the Head and Neck

Indications for Radiotherapy

Oropharyngeal squamous cell cancer is now recognized as at least two different sets of diseases. Those linked to exposure to HPV (HPV-positive) have an excellent prognosis when treated with radiotherapy with or without concomitant chemotherapy or with surgery followed by postoperative radiation with or without concomitant chemotherapy depending on pathological results. People with HPV-positive tumours tend to be younger and to have fewer comorbidities and may therefore be better able to cope with side effects. There is also an increase in HPV-positive tumours in the elderly. Clinical trials are focused on de-intensifying treatment strategies to maintain cure rates and reduce acute and late side effects. HPV-positive tumours are often diagnosed with immunohistochemical tests to show over-expression of p16, a tumour suppressor protein, and are therefore referred to as p16-positive.

Oropharyngeal cancers linked to tobacco and alcohol exposure (usually HPV-negative and p16-negative) still have a relatively poor prognosis. Clinical trials are focussed on escalating treatment by adding in more modalities or increasing radiation dose. At the moment, there is no randomized clinical trial evidence to recommend treating HPV-positive or HPV-negative tumours differently with respect to radiotherapy dose or target volume delineation, though many de-intensification trials are currently recruiting. The recommendations here thus refer to HPV-positive and HPV-negative disease unless otherwise stated.

Kian Ang et al.'s seminal paper describes three prognostic groups for oropharyngeal cancer depending mainly on HPV status and smoking history. This recognizes the fact that some people are smokers with HPV-positive disease and that other factors such as T stage also influence prognosis. Estimating prognosis at presentation may help inform treatment decisions.

Two approaches can be recommended for curative treatment of oropharyngeal squamous cell cancers: primary radiotherapy +/− chemotherapy, or surgery +/− postoperative radiation with or without concomitant chemotherapy. There are no randomized controlled trials comparing these two approaches, although there is indirect evidence suggesting cure rates are similar. The choice depends on likely functional outcomes, particularly with respect to swallowing and speech, local medical expertise, the patient's ability to tolerate treatment and individual patient choice. Treatment of the primary site and the neck can be considered separately, though one modality is usually used as the initial treatment to all sites of disease.

Oropharyngeal tumours usually have lymphadenopathy at presentation but distant metastases are uncommon. The presence of extracapsular nodal disease does not appear to be as important in HPV-positive disease. The TNM v8 staging system reflects the different prognoses of HPV-negative and HPV-positive disease. The staging for HPV-positive disease has changed considerably from previous versions. Care must be taken when assessing clinical trials or other published data which use TNM7 or older systems and applying such protocols to cancers staged using TNM v8. (See Tables 11.1–11.3. For HPV-negative N staging, see Table 8.1.)

DOI: 10.1201/9781315171562-11

TABLE 11.1

T Staging for HPV-Positive/p16-Postive Oropharyngeal Cancer

T0	No primary identified
T1	Tumour 2 cm or smaller in greatest dimension
T2	Tumour larger than 2 cm but not larger than 4 cm in greatest dimension
T3	Tumour larger than 4 cm in greatest dimension or extension to lingual surface of epiglottis
T4	Moderately advanced local disease
	Tumour invades the larynx, extrinsic muscle of the tongue, medial pterygoid, hard palate, or mandible or beyond

TABLE 11.2

T Staging for HPV-Negative/p16-Negative Oropharyngeal Cancer

Tx	Primary tumour cannot be assessed
Tis	Carcinoma in situ
T1	Tumour 2 cm or smaller in greatest dimension
T2	Tumour larger than 2 cm but not larger than 4c m in greatest dimension
T3	Tumour larger than 4 cm in greatest dimension or extension to lingual surface of epiglottis
T4a	Moderately advanced local disease
	Tumour invades the larynx, extrinsic muscle of the tongue, medial pterygoid, hard palate, or mandible
T4b	Very advanced local disease
	Tumour invades lateral pterygoid muscle, pterygoid plates, lateral nasopharynx, or skull base or encases carotid artery

TABLE 11.3

N Staging for HPV-Positive/p16-Postive Oropharyngeal Cancer

Clinical		**Pathological**	
cNx	Regional lymph nodes cannot be assessed	**pNx**	Regional lymph nodes cannot be assessed
cN0	No regional lymph node metastasis	**pN0**	No regional lymph node metastasis
cN1	One or more ipsilateral lymph nodes, none larger than 6 cm	**pN1**	Metastasis in four or fewer lymph nodes
cN2	Contralateral or bilateral lymph nodes, none larger than 6 cm	**pN2**	Metastasis in more than four lymph nodes
cN3	Lymph node(s) larger than 6 cm		

The acute and potential late side effects of oropharyngeal radiotherapy are considerable, so assessing physiological reserve, support for patients during treatment and patient preferences is important before deciding on a treatment for each individual.

For information about the additional benefits of concomitant chemotherapy, see Chapter 8.

Radiation to the Primary Tumour

Radiation to the primary site is often the preferred treatment in oropharyngeal cancer because of the difficulty in obtaining adequate surgical margins while maintaining good swallowing and speech. Transoral robotic surgery (TORS) advances allow better preservation of function than older surgical techniques – if it is available. Target volumes can be defined with greater precision if there has been no surgery prior to radiation, so surgery should only be considered if an R0 resection is expected. The use of concurrent chemotherapy or altered fractionation regimens may improve local control and survival compared with standard radiotherapy in locally advanced disease. Cure rates vary from 90 percent for early HPV-positive tonsil cancer to 40–50 percent for larger HPV-negative primary tumours with nodal involvement.

If surgery is used to treat the primary site, adjuvant radiation is recommended if surgical margins are positive, and should be considered if the margins are close or if there is vascular or perineural invasion.

Radiation to the N0 Neck or One Involved Node <3 cm

The node-negative neck or one with a single node with no obvious extracapsular spread can be managed with either radiation or surgery alone depending on the modality used to treat the primary site. If there is no clinical evidence of nodal involvement (N0), prophylactic treatment of the neck is recommended if the risk of occult metastases is greater than 10–20 percent. Because the oropharynx has a rich lymphatic network, this is usually the case. In well-lateralized tumours of the soft palate or tonsil, only the ipsilateral nodes need treatment. The risk of contralateral nodal involvement is higher in T3/4 tumours or any tumour involving the tongue base or the soft palate within 10 mm of midline. Prophylactic radiation to the contralateral neck is recommended in these circumstances.

Radiation to the Neck – Multiple or Contralateral Neck Nodes

Curative radiotherapy to involved neck nodes is recommended when treatment of the primary site is with radiotherapy. If the risk of nodal metastases at uninvolved nodal levels in the ipsilateral or contralateral neck is greater than 10–20 percent, a prophylactic dose is given to these sites. Residual neck disease after radiation requires a neck dissection. This is usually best established with a PET-CT scan three months after radiotherapy and with a biopsy to confirm residual disease.

If surgery is used as initial therapy to the primary, a neck dissection is often performed. Adjuvant radiotherapy is then recommended in the case of multiple involved nodes or if there is extracapsular nodal spread. It should be considered if a single node >3 cm is found.

Palliative Radiotherapy

Palliative radiotherapy may improve pain, dysphagia and speech in the presence of metastases, or if tumour size or patient frailty or comorbidity preclude a curative approach.

Unknown Primary Tumour Sites in the Head and Neck

Patients presenting with level II/III neck nodes without a clear primary site often have an occult primary tumour in the tonsil, base of tongue, pyriform fossa or nasopharynx. Pathology of the involved nodes obtained by biopsy or excision can suggest a likely primary site, as can careful examination of the pharynx. In particular, HPV-positive nodes are very likely to have come from a primary site in the oropharynx and are usually managed in a similar way to HPV-positive oropharyngeal cancers, even if a primary site cannot be found (T0 oropharynx cancer). EBV-positive nodes suggest a nasopharyngeal primary tumour.

Investigation should include a PET-CT scan and directed biopsies of possible primary sites (Figure 11.1). If there is no primary site visible on clinical examination or imaging, an EUA with bilateral tonsillectomies and a tongue base mucosectomy or deep biopsies of the base of tongue should be performed. For HPV-negative nodes, biopsies of the nasopharynx and pyriform fossae should also be obtained. After thorough radiological and clinical assessment, a primary site is usually discovered. If none is found, a possible skin cancer primary should be carefully evaluated in these patients.

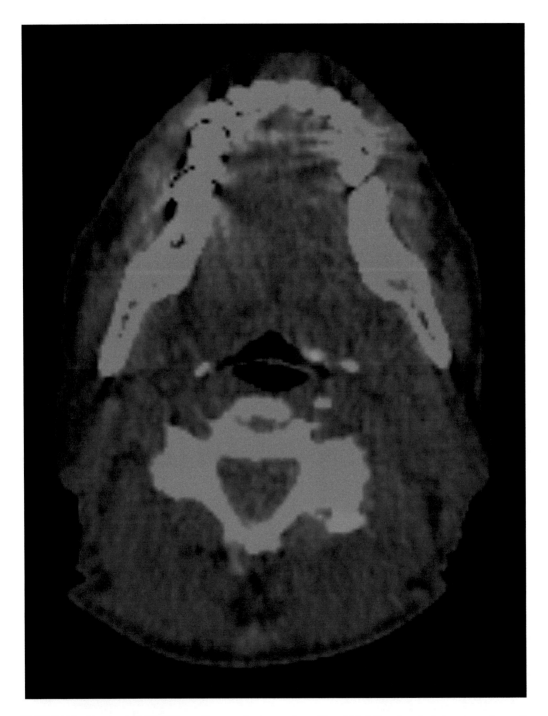

FIGURE 11.1   Fused axial PET-CT image from a patient presenting with multiple left neck nodes but no clear primary site on examination. Uptake in the right base of tongue suggests the primary site, subsequently confirmed on biopsy.

Sequencing of Multimodality Therapy

If adjuvant radiotherapy is indicated, it should ideally commence within six weeks after surgery but after adequate wound healing has occurred. If radiotherapy is delayed to more than three months after surgery because of surgical complications, the potential risks of EBRT may outweigh the benefits.

Clinical and Radiological Anatomy

The oropharynx is the posterior continuation of the oral cavity. Superiorly it joins the nasopharynx at the level of the hard palate and inferiorly it meets the hypopharynx at the level of the hyoid bone. An appreciation of the complex anatomy and physiology of this area is vital in order to understand the mechanisms for local invasion and lymph node spread (Figure 11.2).

The commonest site of oropharyngeal tumours is the lateral wall, which is made up of the tonsils, tonsillar fossae and palatoglossal and palatopharyngeal arches. Tonsil cancers tend to be infiltrative and can spread inferiorly to the tongue base or superiorly to the soft palate. The rich lymphatic drainage of the tonsils means spread to ipsilateral lymph nodes is common at presentation. The tonsil is a frequent site for occult primaries to be detected in patients presenting with enlarged neck nodes. Tonsillar tumours extending onto the tongue base have a greater risk of bilateral nodal spread.

The base of tongue extends from the circumvallate papillae anteriorly to the vallecula (glossoepiglottic fossa) inferiorly. It is covered with lymphoid tissue comprising the lingual tonsils, and it has a rich lymphatic drainage to both sides of the neck. Tumours involving the tongue base are therefore treated with bilateral neck irradiation. The infiltrative nature of most base-of-tongue tumours in a site critical for swallowing means that patients should be assessed before therapy for evidence of aspiration and a prophylactic feeding tube should be strongly considered.

HPV-positive tumours usually arise in the basal cell layer of the crypts of lymphoid tissue in the tonsils or lingual tonsils whereas HPV-negative tumours can occur at any oropharyngeal subsite. This basal cell layer is rich in intraepithelial capillaries, which may explain the higher rate of lymph node spread in HPV-positive tumours.

Tumours of the soft palate and uvula and of the posterior wall are less common. Lateral soft palate tumours spread to ipsilateral lymph nodes, while more medial tumours or those arising in the posterior wall have a higher chance of bilateral nodal involvement. The lack of submucosal tissue on the posterior pharyngeal wall means radiation to these tumours often results in a shallow ulcer which takes many months to heal, can be very painful and can be confused with residual tumour.

Level II nodes are the usual first site of spread. Disease then spreads inferiorly to levels III and IV or superiorly to upper level II and retrostyloid or retropharyngeal nodes. Level V involvement is relatively uncommon unless adjacent nodal levels are involved. The pattern of nodal spread may be less predictable in patients who have had a previous neck dissection.

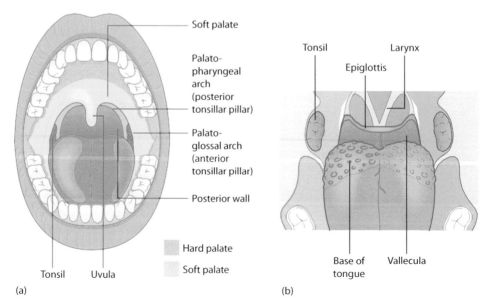

FIGURE 11.2 Anatomy of the oropharynx. (a) Anterior view; (b) superior view looking down from the nasopharynx. The vallecula (glossoepiglottic fossae) lie between the base of tongue and the epiglottis.

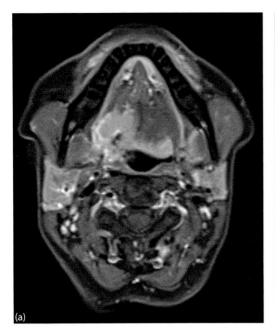 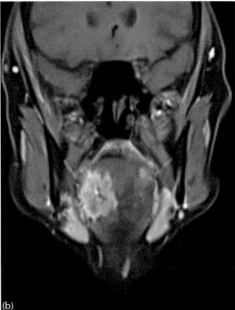

FIGURE 11.3 Axial (a) and coronal (b) T1+ contrast MRI image of a right base of tongue tumor invading the extrinsic tongue muscles anteriorly.

Assessment of Primary Disease

The oropharynx, oral cavity and larynx should be carefully examined by the radiation oncologist and ENT surgeon together to assess the exact mucosal sites of disease and invasion of adjacent sites and structures. Tonsil and soft palate tumours can be seen by inspection through the oral cavity. The tongue base and lingual tonsils are best assessed by flexible nasendoscopy combined with careful bimanual palpation. EUA may be helpful to define the extent of tumour and to obtain histology.

Cross-sectional imaging is essential to define extent of the primary tumour and MRI is preferable to CT in oropharyngeal tumours (Figure 11.3). However, MRI and CT are equally accurate at assessing neck disease. Cross-sectional imaging should include the whole neck from the skull base to the superior mediastinum to assess retropharyngeal nodes and levels I–V. A node ≥ 10 mm in short axis is considered pathological, but nodes larger than 5 mm should be regarded as suspicious if in a location typical for nodal metastases and if they have suspicious imaging characteristics such as being rounded or lacking a normal fatty hilum. Ultrasound and fine needle aspiration cytology may be useful to confirm or refute metastases in different nodal levels.

Data Acquisition

Immobilization

The patient lies supine with the spine as straight as possible and no mouth bite, but any dentures should be left in place. A thermoplastic shell with at least five fixation points is constructed to ensure immobilization (see Chapter 8).

CT Scanning

CT images – ideally with intravenous contrast – are acquired with 2–3 mm-thick slices from the skull base superiorly to the top of the aortic arch inferiorly. Many oropharyngeal tumours are more easily defined with MRI than CT, so co-registered images may help GTV definition.

Target Volume Definition

Curative Treatment

The diagnostic images and records and photographs of initial evaluation (in clinic or at EUA) are critical to assess the extent of the primary tumour and the exact site of involved lymph nodes. The GTV is defined as the primary tumour and any lymph nodes greater than 10 mm in short axis dimension or smaller nodes with necrotic centres or rounded contours thought to contain tumour. There is no good evidence correlating CT data with pathological specimens from which to derive a GTV-CTV margin, so the margins used are based on surgical data and studies of patterns of local failure after radiotherapy.

Either two or three CTV and PTV dose levels can be contoured. We recommend three dose levels as per internationally agreed guidelines.

CTV_HIGH is the GTV with a 5 mm margin for local invasion at both the primary and nodal sites. At the primary site, the CTV can be edited from uninvolved bone and from air but should not be edited from adjacent soft tissues. At the nodal sites, the CTV should conform to the tissue planes containing lymph node regions except where there is possible extracapsular spread, for example into adjacent muscles.

CTV_MID includes structures or subsites close to the primary tumour where there is possible involvement. This is best constructed by expanding the GTV isotropically by 10 mm. This volume is then edited to exclude uninvolved air and bone and to exclude soft tissues where there are natural barriers to tumour spread – for example conforming to the contour of muscle/fat boundaries such as platysma and the prevertebral fascia. It is then extended to consider possible local routes of spread – for example including the whole ipsilateral parapharyngeal space in a tonsil cancer or the tongue base in a tonsil cancer with base of tongue invasion. CTV_MID includes nodal levels at high risk of involvement – for example those levels containing involved nodes or directly draining the primary site. It should include at least 10 mm of the adjacent sternocleidomastoid muscle if there is possible extracapsular nodal spread into the muscle.

It is usually easier to define the tumour and nodal GTVs and CTVs separately before summing them together in one volume, as this allows the oncologist to concentrate on volume definition for one area at a time.

CTV_LOW includes those nodal levels thought to be at risk of occult nodal spread based on pattern of GTV disease. A suggested algorithm for deciding on low-dose nodal CTV levels is shown in Table 11.4 (also see Figure 11.4).

If there is considerable uncertainty about defining the GTV, for example if there is significant dental artefact on the planning CT or if the edge of the GTV is hard to define on diagnostic imaging, two dose levels may be used. Two dose levels are recommended if IMRT is not being used. In this case CTV_HIGH is the GTV with a 10 mm expansion edited as just described and including involved nodes with a small margin and sometimes involved whole nodal levels. CTV_LOW is those nodal levels thought to be at risk of occult nodal spread based on pattern of GTV disease.

TABLE 11.4

Nodal Levels to Be Included in CTV_LOW for Oropharynx Cancer

Nodal Status (TNM8)	Ipsilateral Neck	Contralateral Neck
N0 or one involved node <3 cm with no ECS	II, III, IVa, RP Ib if level II is involved, or the primary involves the anterior tonsillar pillar or oral cavity	No treatment if well-lateralized primary (see text) Otherwise – II, III, IVa Consider omitting high level II nodes (see text) RP if posterior pharyngeal wall involved
Multiple nodes or one node >3 cm	Ib, II, III, IVa, Va,b, RP, RS	Consider no treatment if well-lateralized primary and < 3 nodes. Otherwise – II, III, IVa Consider omitting high level II nodes (see text) RP if posterior pharyngeal wall involved
Bilateral nodes	According to N stage on each side of the neck	According to N stage on each side of the neck

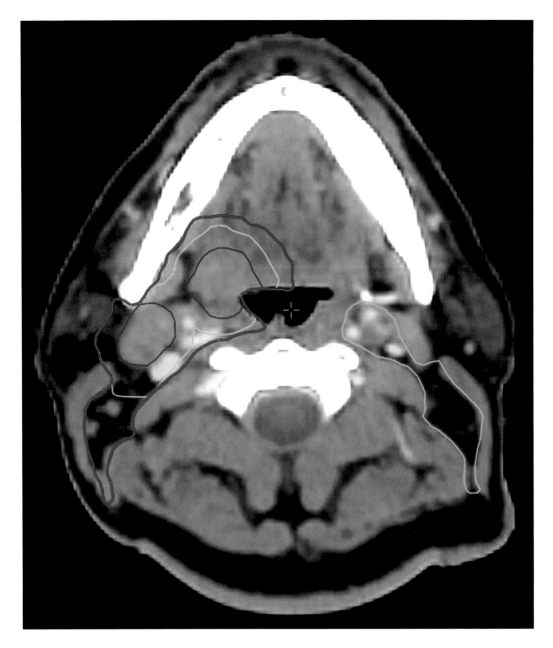

FIGURE 11.4   CTVs and GTVs for T2N1 tonsil cancer – GTV (dark blue), CTV_HIGH (cyan), CTV_MID (magenta) and CTV_LOW (green). The same patient is shown in Figure 8.4.

The CTVs are grown to PTVs by applying a margin which can be determined by the local assessment of random and systematic errors, assuming that tumour movement in head and neck cancer is negligible. This is usually 3–5 mm.

CTV for Adjuvant Radiotherapy

In addition to imaging and clinical information, discussion with the surgeon and pathologist is important in determining the sites at greatest risk of recurrent disease. CTV_HIGH is the operative tumour bed with an appropriate margin paying particular attention to sites where excision margins are positive or close. There is no GTV, but we recommend projecting the original sites of GTV onto the planning CT, for example contouring the tonsillar fossa after a tonsillectomy, and expanding by 10 mm to guide CTV definition. If radiation to the nodes is indicated, the CTV_HIGH includes the nodal levels where there were positive lymph nodes and the adjacent structures at sites of extracapsular spread. A CTV_LOW is only defined if there are nodal levels that were not operated on but have a greater than 20 percent chance of containing occult metastases (see Table 11.4).

CTV for Unknown Primary

Any macroscopically enlarged nodes are contoured as GTV. The CTV_HIGH is the involved nodes with a 5 mm margin edited to conform to the tissue planes containing lymph node regions except where there is possible extracapsular spread, for example into adjacent muscles.

The CTV_MID is the nodal levels containing tumour with at least a 10 mm margin superiorly and inferiorly and is usually the ipsilateral level II and upper level III nodes. It should include at least 10 mm of the adjacent sternocleidomastoid muscle if there is possible extracapsular nodal spread into the muscle. There are two approaches to contouring the rest of the CTV.

One approach is not to treat the possible primary sites and only include the ipsilateral levels Ib–IVa, retrostyloid and retropharyngeal nodes in the CTV_LOW. This is less toxic, as much of the oral cavity and pharyngeal mucosa can be spared but, if the primary site later becomes apparent or a second primary cancer develops, it will be very difficult to treat with radiation so close to the original CTV.

Alternatively, the most likely primary site can be deduced from the pattern of nodal spread and pathological information. An HPV-positive cancer is best thought of as a T0 oropharynx tumour. With unilateral nodes, the ipsilateral tonsil and base of tongue are the most likely sites. These are included in CTV_MID. The contralateral tonsil and base of tongue can be included within CTV_LOW or omitted. If there are bilateral nodes in an HPV-positive cancer, both tonsils and the whole base of tongue are included in CTV_MID. (See Figure 11.5.)

In an HPV-negative tumour, the whole base of tongue, both tonsils and pyriform fossa (and nasopharynx in some parts of the world) are considered to be possible primary sites. These sites are contoured as CTV_MID along with their first echelon draining lymph nodes if not already part of CTV_MID. The CTV_LOW will include levels Ib–IVa, retropharyngeal and retrostyloid nodes on the involved side and levels II–IVa contralaterally. We recommend this approach unless comorbidity and performance status suggest such that larger treatment volumes will be poorly tolerated.

Ipsilateral Radiotherapy for Tonsil Cancer

Avoiding treatment to the uninvolved contralateral neck in tonsil cancer will reduce acute and long-term side effects but might increase the risk of contralateral neck recurrence. Larger tumours, those close to midline, and with multiple involved nodes have a higher risk of contralateral node recurrence. The evidence that HPV status and ECS change the risk is less conclusive.

We recommend unilateral radiotherapy in T1–2 squamous cell carcinomas of the tonsil if the GTVp is at least from midline, invades 10 mm or less into the superficial mucosa of the base of tongue or the soft palate and does not involve the posterior pharyngeal wall and if there is no more than one involved node. That node should measure <3 cm with no obvious ECS. In similar tonsil primaries with one to three involved nodes, none more than 6 cm and with no ECS, either a unilateral or bilateral approach is an option.

Reducing the Contralateral Neck CTV

When nodal contouring was introduced, the contralateral RP nodes and all level II nodes were usually included in the CTV_LOW. The more superior the CTV_LOW extends, the harder it is to spare the

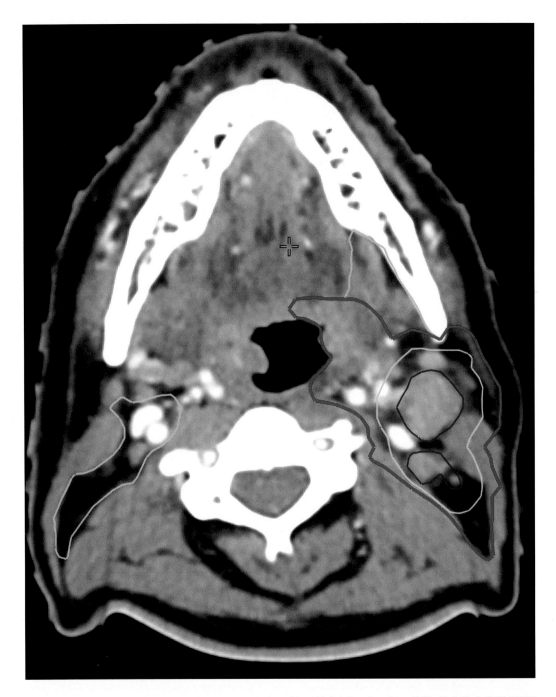

FIGURE 11.5 CTVs for T0N1 oropharynx cancer presenting with multiple left neck nodes – GTVn (dark blue), CTV_HIGH (cyan), CTV_MID (magenta) and CTV_LOW (green). Note inclusion of ipsilateral tonsil and base of tongue in CTV_MID.

parotid gland and superior constrictor muscles. The contralateral RP neck nodes in the uninvolved neck should not be treated unless the ipsilateral RP nodes are involved or the primary involves the posterior pharyngeal wall. There is also increasing evidence that it is also safe to omit the higher-level II nodes in this situation, so that the superior border of level II is defined where the posterior belly of digastric crosses the posterior aspect of the internal jugular vein (Figure 11.6).

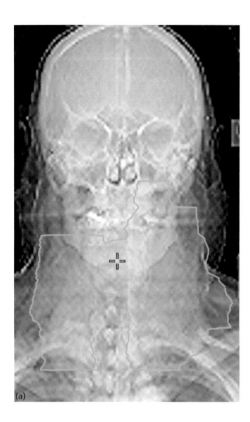

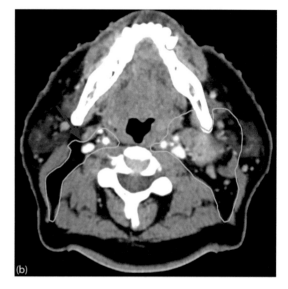

FIGURE 11.6 Sparing of high level II nodes. (a) Coronal projection of CTV_LOW showing volume extends less superiorly in the node-negative right neck than in the left neck. (b) Axial slice showing superior border of right level II is defined where the posterior belly of digastric crosses the posterior aspect of the internal jugular vein (arrow).

Dose Solutions

Complex – IMRT or Arc Therapy

IMRT is the ideal treatment for oropharyngeal cancer requiring bilateral neck irradiation as it allows parotid sparing to reduce the risk of xerostomia, obviates the need for matched electron fields and enables different PTVs to be treated to different doses within the same plan. If bilateral level II nodes contain tumour, the need to include the retrostyloid nodes in the higher-dose treated volumes may preclude parotid sparing (Figures 11.7 and 11.8).

Target volumes are defined as described earlier. Nodal PTVs often come close to the skin surface. To artificially create a skin-sparing effect with IMRT, the nodal volumes are edited so as to be a minimum of 5 mm from the body contour. The only exception is when an involved node is within 5 mm of the skin surface.

The spinal cord is outlined with a 5 mm isocentric margin as a PRV. Both parotid glands are contoured: they can be difficult to define on a planning CT, particularly when there is dental artifact, though the diagnostic MRI may be helpful. When the CTV_HIGH or CTV_MID is bilateral, the superficial parotid lobes should be defined separately and summed as one volume. The brainstem is also contoured as an OAR. There is increasing evidence that the dose to the pharyngeal constrictor muscles may relate to the risk of long-term dysphagia. They can be spared inferior to the midline PTV and can either be contoured or can be included as part of an avoidance volume, including the larynx, hypopharynx and trachea, which can help to reduce dose to these midline structures. The contralateral submandibular salivary gland can sometimes be spared.

When the high-dose PTV extends inferiorly below the inferior cricoid cartilage, the whole neck is treated in one plan, usually with a seven-beam arrangement of equispaced IMRT beams or with two arcs. If the more inferior nodes only require a prophylactic dose, they can be treated with a matched anterior neck beam as for conformal treatment, in which case the superior part of the volume can usually be treated with five equispaced IMRT beams. This has the advantage of more complete sparing of midline normal tissues in the lower neck but at the expense of worse dosimetric coverage of the inferior low-dose CTV.

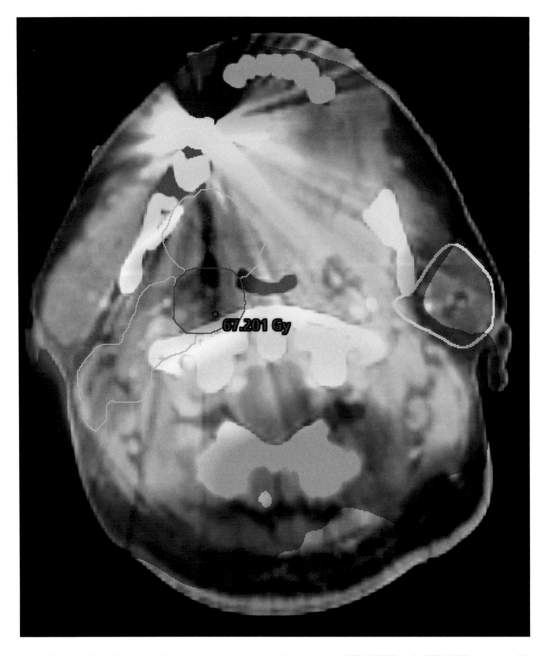

FIGURE 11.7 VMAT plan for R tonsil cancer treating the bilateral neck. PTV_HIGH (red), PTV_MID (green) and L parotid (yellow). Colour wash of 20 Gy dose is shown to illustrate sparing of the L parotid.

If the contralateral neck is not in the PTV, a single arc or four to five unilateral IMRT beams can produce a conformal dose distribution and minimize dose to contralateral or uninvolved midline structures.

Conformal without IMRT

Phase 1 aims to treat the PTV_LOW to a dose thought sufficient to eradicate microscopic disease in lymph nodes. Unilateral PTVs are treated with a plan using two or three beams unilaterally to provide dose to the PTV according to ICRU62. The angle of the posterior oblique beam is chosen so as to avoid

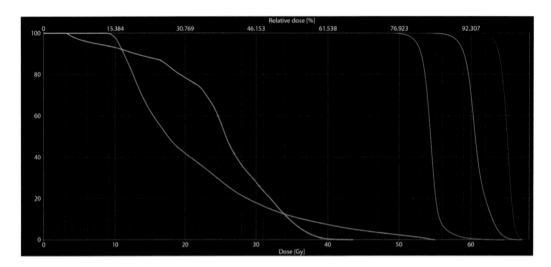

FIGURE 11.8   DVHs for PTV_HIGH (red), PTV_MID (green), PTV_LOW (blue), contralateral parotid (yellow) and spinal cord PRV (white) for a T2N1 HPV-positive tonsil cancer treated with VMAT (same patient as seen in Figures 11.4 and 11.7).

the spinal cord PRV, which can sometimes mean accepting reduced dose to the most posterior part of the nodal CTV. This is matched to an ipsilateral low neck beam.

Those PTVs extending to the contralateral side are usually treated with opposing lateral beams with AP wedges and sometimes superior–inferior wedges to compensate for changes in contour. A three-beam arrangement can sometimes be used to try to spare the contralateral parotid gland. Usually the planned superior volume is matched isocentrically to a lower anterior neck beam, with midline shielding to treat more inferior nodes without irradiating midline structures.

Phase 2 aims to treat the PTV_HIGH to a curative dose and the beam arrangements are similar to those in phase 1 but with more shielding if possible. If the PTV_HIGH extends posteriorly to the posterior level II or level V nodes, a matched posterior electron beam (9 MeV or 12 MeV) may be needed. The plans for phase 1 and phase 2 should be reviewed together to ensure PTVs are adequately covered according to ICRU62 and critical structures are not overdosed. Acute side effects will be reduced if the dose to the oral cavity and pharynx outside the PTV is minimized.

Dose Fractionation

Curative

- 70 Gy in 35 daily fractions given in seven weeks +/– concomitant cisplatin
  - PTV_HIGH receives 70 Gy in 35 fractions
  - PTV_MID receives 63 Gy in 35 fractions
  - PTV_LOW receives 56 Gy in 35 fractions
- 65 Gy in 30 daily fractions given in six weeks +/– concomitant cisplatin
  - PTV_HIGH receives 65 Gy in 30 fractions
  - PTV_MID receives 60 Gy in 30 fractions
  - PTV_LOW receives 54 Gy in 30 fractions

Adjuvant

- 60 Gy in 30 daily fractions given in six weeks +/– concomitant cisplatin
  - PTV_HIGH receives 60 Gy in 30 fractions
  - PTV_LOW receives 54 Gy in 30 fractions

- Conformal without IMRT
  - 70 Gy in 35 fractions over seven weeks to PTV_HIGH
  - 44 Gy in 22 fractions over four and a half weeks to PTV_LOW

Palliative

- 30 Gy in 10 fractions over two weeks
- 20 Gy in 5 fractions over one week

Verification

See Chapter 8.

Treatment Delivery and Patient Care

Patients are treated daily on weekdays. Any gap in treatment must be corrected – ideally by treating twice in one day. There must be at least a six-hour gap between fractions on any day when a patient receives two doses.

Weekly assessment by a doctor, nurse specialist or radiographer and by a dietician is important. Regular advice by a speech and language therapist can help maintain safe, functional swallowing and assess risk of aspiration. Most patients are at high risk of weight loss and should be considered for a gastric feeding tube inserted for prophylaxis before radiotherapy. Further details are given in Chapter 8.

> **Key Trials**
>
> See Chapter 8–most phase III trials in head and neck cancer contain a majority of patients with oropharyngeal cancers.
>
> Nichols AC, Theurer J, Prisman E, et al. Radiotherapy versus transoral robotic surgery and neck dissection for oropharyngeal squamous cell carcinoma (ORATOR): An open-label, phase 2, randomised trial. Lancet Oncol 2019;20:1349–1359.
>
> Owadally W, Hurt C, Timmins H, et al. PATHOS: A phase II/III trial of risk-stratified, reduced intensity adjuvant treatment in patients undergoing transoral surgery for Human papillomavirus (HPV) positive oropharyngeal cancer. BMC Cancer 2015;15:602.

INFORMATION SOURCES

Ang KK, Harris J, Wheeler R, et al. Human papillomavirus and survival of patients with oropharyngeal cancer. N Engl J Med 2010;363:24–35.

Huang SH, Waldron J, Bratman SV, et al. Re-evaluation of ipsilateral radiation for T1-T2N0-N2b tonsil carcinoma at the princess Margaret Hospital in the human papillomavirus era, 25 years later. Int J Radiat Oncol Biol Phys 2017;98:159–169.

O'Sullivan B, Huang SH, Su J, et al. Development and validation of a staging system for HPV-related oropharyngeal cancer by the international collaboration on oropharyngeal cancer network for staging (ICON-S): A multicentre cohort study. Lancet Oncol 2016;17:440–451.

Sher DJ, Adelstein DJ, Bajaj GK, et al. Radiation therapy for oropharyngeal squamous cell carcinoma: Executive summary of an ASTRO evidence-based clinical practice guideline. Pract Radiat Oncol 2017;7:246–253.

Spencer CR, Gay HA, Haughey BH, et al. Eliminating radiotherapy to the contralateral retropharyngeal and high level II lymph nodes in head and neck squamous cell carcinoma is safe and improves quality of life. Cancer 2014;120:3994–4002.

Tsai CJ, Galloway TJ, Margalit DN, et al. Ipsilateral radiation for squamous cell carcinoma of the tonsil: American Radium society appropriate use criteria executive summary. Head & Neck 2020;43:1–15.

12

Hypopharynx

Indications for Radiotherapy

Curative Treatment for T1/T2 N0 Tumours

Early-stage hypopharyngeal tumours are rare but can be treated with curative intent by surgery or radiotherapy. The choice depends on patient preference and local expertise, but it can be difficult to achieve clear resection margins without compromising vocal and swallowing function. There are no RCTs comparing these approaches.

Pyriform fossa tumours have the best prognosis – radiotherapy can achieve local control in 90 percent of T1 tumours and 80 percent of T2 tumours with a five-year overall survival of 50–65 percent. Involvement of the apex of the pyriform fossa (which may imply occult invasion of cartilage) predicts a lower chance of cure. Postcricoid carcinomas have a 20–50 percent cure rate with radiotherapy, which is equivalent to that in surgical series. There are fewer data available for posterior wall tumours but cure rates are similar to those for postcricoid cancer.

Curative Treatment for T3/T4 or N+ Tumors

Most hypopharyngeal cancers are locally advanced at presentation. Many patients have significant smoking and alcohol exposure and cardiac, respiratory and other comorbidities which make suitability for major surgery or for concomitant or neoadjuvant chemotherapy challenging. Treatment choice depends on the site and stage of disease and patient preference acknowledging the balance between possible cure, treatment morbidity and likely functional outcomes. Noncurative approaches (supportive and palliative care with palliative dose radiotherapy) should always be discussed as an option.

Curative surgery usually involves a laryngopharyngectomy and bilateral neck dissections with postoperative radiotherapy, with or without concomitant chemotherapy, usually recommended. Radiotherapy with concomitant or neoadjuvant chemotherapy has the advantage of potentially preserving pharyngeal and laryngeal function. It should be considered if baseline voice and swallow is good and the patient is not aspirating. There are phase III data to support an organ preserving approach for advanced pyriform fossa cancer. Large volume primary disease, particularly with cartilage destruction, is best treated with surgery and postoperative radiotherapy.

Curative dose radiotherapy alone is less effective but can be a good option for people not well enough for chemotherapy and not wanting to consider major surgery.

Adjuvant Radiotherapy

Adjuvant radiotherapy to the site of primary tumour is recommended for all resected T3/T4 tumours and for T1/T2 tumours with positive or close resection margins (usually <5 mm or where there is surgical concern). Adjuvant radiotherapy to the involved neck is recommended in pN2/3 disease.

Palliative Treatment

Locally advanced hypopharyngeal cancers – particularly those originating in the postcricoid and posterior pharyngeal wall – have a low chance of cure with any approach. Patients' wishes, advanced age and comorbidity mean that palliative treatment should be discussed with all patients with locally advanced disease. Palliative radiotherapy may improve pharyngeal pain and obstructive symptoms and help to

DOI: 10.1201/9781315171562-12

control neck disease but hardly ever improves complete dysphagia. Supportive care alone is an option for patients with incurable disease, complete dysphagia and few other symptoms.

Sequencing of Multimodality Therapy

If primary surgery is used and adjuvant radiotherapy is indicated, radiation should begin within six weeks of surgery or when adequate healing has taken place. Concomitant cisplatin chemotherapy should be considered, especially when resection margins are positive or there is extracapsular nodal spread.

If induction chemotherapy is used, radiotherapy should ideally begin three to four weeks after the start of the last chemotherapy cycle.

Clinical and Radiological Anatomy

The pyriform fossae are mucosa-lined spaces on either side of the larynx (Figure 12.1). Each is shaped like an inverted pyramid with the apex between the cricoid cartilage medially and the thyroid cartilage laterally at the level of the cervical oesophagus. The posterior pharyngeal wall is the posterior mucosa in between the pyriform fossae extending from the level of the hyoid bone to the inferior border of the cricoid cartilage. The postcricoid mucosa is the anterior surface of the hypopharynx from the arytenoid cartilages to the inferior border of the cricoid. It is continuous posterolaterally with the inferior portion of the posterior pharyngeal wall (Figure 12.2).

Tumours can spread mucosally to involve adjacent mucosal sites – other subsites of the hypopharynx, the supraglottic larynx or tongue base. It can be difficult to tell whether a tumour has arisen from the supraglottic larynx or pyriform fossa if both are involved. If other sites are invaded, lymph node target volumes should include levels draining these sites. Because the hypopharyngeal mucosa is thin, tumours readily spread into the adjacent sites – medially from the pyriform fossae to the paraglottic space (and then into the larynx), laterally into the soft tissues of the neck, or posteriorly into the prevertebral fascia. They can also invade the arytenoid, thyroid and cricoid cartilages. Postcricoid tumours can spread into the cervical oesophagus.

Lymph node spread is common at presentation and occult disease is found in up to 60 percent of patients with no lymphadenopathy. The pyriform fossae drain to ipsilateral levels II and III nodes initially, and other sites to levels II, III and IV, usually bilaterally. If the apex of the pyriform fossa or the post cricoid region is involved, level VIb is at risk. Tumours involving the posterior pharyngeal wall can also spread directly to the retropharyngeal nodes. If levels II–IV are involved, tumour can spread to level Ib or V or to retropharyngeal nodes.

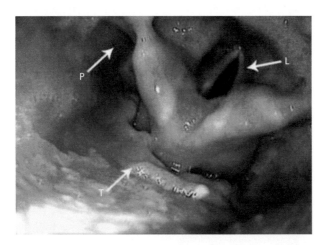

FIGURE 12.1 Transnasal oesophagoscopic view of the hypopharynx. Note the pyriform fossa (P) and larynx (L). There is a tumour of the posterior pharyngeal wall (T).

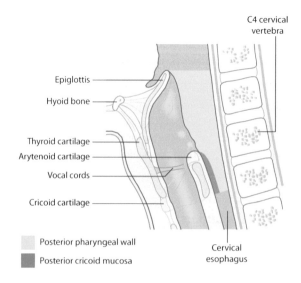

FIGURE 12.2   Midline sagittal anatomy of the hypopharynx.

Assessment of Primary Disease

Most pyriform fossa cancers are visible at nasendoscopy during which vocal cord function is assessed. Vocal cord paralysis is a poor prognostic sign. Tumours are more visible if the fossae are distended by the patient performing a Valsalva manoeuvre with the nostrils pinched. Transnasal oesophagoscopy allows other hypopharyngeal sites to be assessed and biopsies to be taken if necessary. Palpable lymphadenopathy should be recorded and fine needle aspiration or core biopsy of lymphadenopathy is often an easier way to confirm the diagnosis histologically than a biopsy of the primary site.

EUA allows assessment of mucosal extent and deep fixation of the tumour and can be performed if surgery is considered. The EUA should include laryngoscopy, oesophagoscopy and bronchoscopy to assess involvement of adjacent organs.

Cross-sectional imaging with either CT or MRI is performed (Figure 12.3). Both are equally good at demonstrating lymphadenopathy, though MRI may provide slightly better imaging of the primary

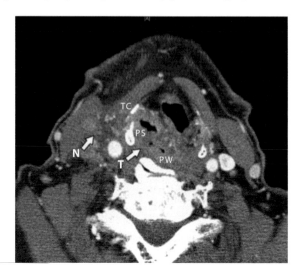

FIGURE 12.3   Diagnostic CT scan of a right pyriform fossa tumour (T) growing into the paraglottic space (PS), through the thyroid cartilage (TC) and invading onto the posterior pharyngeal wall (PW). (Note the adjacent involved lymph Node [N].)

TABLE 12.1

Tumour Staging for Hypopharyngeal Cancer

Tx	**Primary tumour cannot be assessed**
Tis	Carcinoma in situ
T1	Tumour 2 cm or smaller in greatest dimension
T2	Tumour larger than 2 cm but not larger than 4 cm in greatest dimension
T3	Tumour larger than 4 cm in greatest dimension or extension to lingual surface of epiglottis
T4a	Moderately advanced local disease
	Tumour invades the larynx, extrinsic muscle of the tongue, medial pterygoid, hard palate or mandible
T4b	Very advanced local disease
	Tumour invades lateral pterygoid muscle, pterygoid plates, lateral nasopharynx, or skull base or encases carotid artery

Source: Adapted from UICC TNM (8th edn, 2018).

tumour. CT is preferable for more inferior tumours that may have spread to the superior mediastinal nodes as it allows easy imaging of the head, neck and thorax contiguously. T staging is shown in Table 12.1.

Data Acquisition

Immobilization

Patients lie supine on a headrest to keep the spine straight, with a custom-made thermoplastic shell fixed to the couch top in at least five places to reduce movement. The treated volume will usually extend inferior to the level of the shoulders, which should be as low as possible to facilitate beam entry. No mouth bite is required.

CT Scanning

With the patient immobilized, CT images are obtained from the skull base to the carina. Slices should be no more than 3 mm thick. Intravenous contrast should be used to help define both the primary tumour and the nodal levels.

Target Volume Definition

Curative Radiotherapy T1/T2 N0

The GTV is defined using endoscopy, EUA reports and diagrams, and diagnostic imaging. It may be helpful to fuse diagnostic MRI images with the planning CT scan. There is a lack of good evidence on which to base GTV-CTV margins at the primary site, but submucosal spread is common and can extend at least 10 mm from the GTV. We recommend the GTV is expanded isotropically by 5 mm to form the CTV_HIGH, which is then edited from air and uninvolved cartilage or bone.

The CTV_MID includes the adjacent mucosa at risk of microscopic spread and is most consistently defined by expanding the GTV by 10 mm isotropically and editing it to ensure at-risk regions are included. Tumours may spread into the ipsilateral parapharyngeal space, pre-epiglottic space and the other subsites of the hypopharynx or adjacent supraglottic larynx. For early-stage disease there is no need to extend the CTV_MID outside the laryngeal cartilages, though the cartilage adjacent to the GTV can be included. Submucosal extension has been described, so consideration can be given to extending the GTV-CTV_MID margin to 15 mm longitudinally. The CTV_MID is then edited from air.

The CTV_LOW is the at-risk nodal levels. For lateral T1 pyriform fossa tumours this will only include ipsilateral levels II–IVa. For other tumours bilateral nodes are included.

Curative Radiotherapy T3/T4 or N+

As for T1/T2 disease, the CTV_HIGH is the GTV expanded isotropically by 5 mm and edited from adjacent air spaces. The CTV_MID is best defined by expanding the GTV by 10 mm (or 15 mm longitudinally) and then including tissue thought to be at risk of microscopic spread.

Anterolaterally, the CTV_MID should include at least the pre- and paraglottic fat spaces and the whole adjacent cartilages. If the GTV invades the cartilage then the strap muscle external to the cartilage is included. If there is tumour invading the strap muscle, then the adjacent subcutaneous tissue and thyroid gland are included. Posteriorly, the CTV_MID includes the pharyngeal constrictor muscle up to the prevertebral fascia. The prevertebral muscles should also be included if the GTV extends to the prevertebral fascia. Medially, the CTV_MID usually includes the hemilarynx with some extension contralaterally to keep a 10 mm mucosal margin from GTV. Superiorly, the CTV_MID may extend into the valleculae or base of tongue and inferiorly into the cervical oesophagus.

Involved nodes are contoured as GTVn and expanded by 5 mm to be included in CTV_HIGH. The nodal CTV_MID includes the nodal levels that are involved or thought to be at highest risk of nodal spread. We recommend including at least a 20 mm longitudinal margin from the GTVn. If imaging suggests extracapsular spread into adjacent muscle, the CTV_MID should extend into the muscle with at least a 10 mm margin from the GTVn. For a T3/T4 N0 tumour the adjacent N0 nodal regions (usually bilateral levels III and IVa) can be included in CTV_MID, as the risk of occult nodal spread will be high. (See Figure 12.4.)

The CTV_LOW is the uninvolved at-risk nodes on both sides of the neck as per Table 12.2.

Patients in this group may occasionally have been treated with and responded to neoadjuvant chemotherapy. CTVs should therefore be based on the initial pattern of disease as well as on the residual tumour

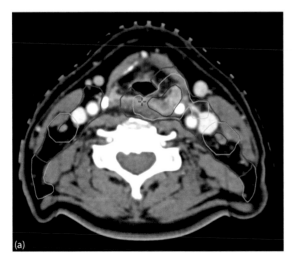

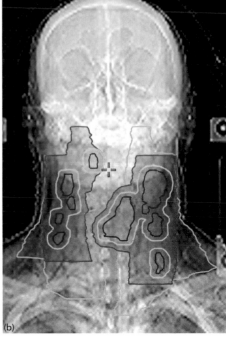

FIGURE 12.4 Target volumes for a T2N2c left piriform fossa tumour – GTV (dark blue), CTV_HIGH (cyan), CTV_MID (magenta), CTV_LOW (green). (a) Sample axial slice; (b) coronal projection.

TABLE 12.2

Recommendations for the Selection of Low Risk Nodal Levels (CTV_LOW) for Hypopharyngeal Tumours

Nodal Status (TNM8)	Ipsilateral Neck	Contralateral Neck
N0	II, III, Iva VIIa for posterior pharyngeal wall tumours VIb if pyriform apex or post-cricoid region are involved	II, III, IVa VIIa for posterior pharyngeal wall tumours VIb if post-cricoid region is involved
N1, N2a-b or N3	Ib, II, III, IVa, Va,b, VIIa IVb if level IVa is involved VIb if pyriform apex or post-cricoid region are involved VIIb if upper level II is involved	II, III, IVa VIIa for posterior pharyngeal wall tumours VIb if post-cricoid region is involved
N2c	According to N stage on each side of the neck	According to N stage on each side of the neck

seen on the planning CT. The GTVp should be defined on the planning CT based on the residual tumour volume but should include any parts of the hypopharynx or larynx that were involved at diagnosis. In the same way, any nodes that were involved at diagnosis are contoured as GTV even if they are not enlarged after chemotherapy.

CTV for Adjuvant Radiotherapy

After careful discussion with the surgeon and pathologist, the CTVp_HIGH is defined as sites of possible residual microscopic disease. After a pharyngolaryngectomy, the anatomy visible on the planning CT will be very different from that on the initial diagnostic images. It can be helpful to mark the original superior-inferior extent of the tumour on the planning CT. Asking the surgeon to review the planning CT to help define the sites they are most concerned may harbour microscopic residual disease can be very helpful.

The CTV_HIGH should include the margins of resection with at least a 10 mm margin and sites of any dissected nodal levels where there was tumour. Particular care should be given to covering the site of the pharyngolaryngeal membrane where tumours can escape between the laryngeal cartilages and the anterolateral neck soft tissues if cartilage invasion was present. When the patient has had a laryngectomy, the stoma should be included in the CTV_HIGH if subglottic extension was present, if an emergency tracheostomy was required before surgery or if the surgeon is particularly concerned about the risk of parastomal recurrence.

Pathologically involved nodal levels are included in the CTV_HIGH, though they are often hard to define precisely after major surgery. A nodal level that is pN0 after a neck dissection does not necessarily need adjuvant radiotherapy as well. In practice, the CTV_HIGH often extends into the resected nodal region so that at least the medial part of levels III and IVa are irradiated even if pN0. CTV_LOW should be contoured to ensure that all the nodal levels defined in Table 12.2 have been treated either surgically or with radiotherapy. (See Figure 12.5.)

CTV for Palliative Radiotherapy

The goal of palliative radiotherapy is to treat all symptomatic disease with minimal toxicity. The GTV is defined from clinical information and imaging and should be expanded by 5 mm to produce the CTV.

Planning Target Volume

CTVs are expanded isotropically to form PTVs by a margin depending on the measured random and systematic errors in the department – usually 3–5 mm.

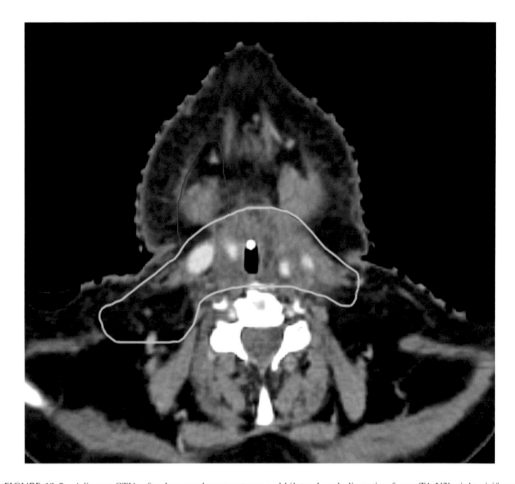

FIGURE 12.5   Adjuvant CTVs after laryngopharyngectomy and bilateral neck dissection for a pT4aN2b right piriform fossa tumour. Multiple right level II and III neck nodes were involved, including in the posterior part of level III. CTV_HIGH (cyan) includes the primary tumour bed and involved nodal levels including R level V given the number of right neck nodes involved close to this level; CTV_LOW (magenta) includes R Ib.

Dose Solutions

Complex

IMRT or VMAT will provide better PTV coverage for hypopharyngeal tumours than other techniques because of the extension of volumes longitudinally, the need to treat different volumes to different doses and the proximity of critical organs to the PTVs.

A seven-beam coplanar IMRT technique using equispaced beams is usually needed to achieve coverage though five beams are sometimes adequate. One-two arc VMAT can also be used. Spinal cord (with a 5 mm isotropic margin), parotid glands and brainstem are contoured as organs at risk. It may also be possible to spare more oral or pharyngeal mucosa outside the PTV and other structures such as the submandibular salivary glands and pharyngeal constrictor muscles if they are contoured.

Conformal

The usual conformal plan for many hypopharyngeal tumours uses opposing lateral photon beams shaped to the PTV with MLCs. Wedges in both the AP and superoinferior planes may be needed to compensate for changes in the contour of the neck.

If the high dose PTV extends posterior to the plane of the spinal cord, a two-phase technique will be needed. Opposing lateral beams in phase 1 will include the spinal cord. A second phase using smaller lateral photon beams with posterior border anterior to the spinal cord is then matched to electron beams to the posterior neck. The electron energy is chosen to keep within spinal cord tolerance but cover PTV if possible. Alternatively, the opposing photon beams can be angled to treat the PTV while avoiding the cord.

The PTV usually extends inferiorly to below the level of the shoulders. The inferior part of the volume can be treated with a matched anterior photon beam with midline shielding. The match plane should ideally be inferior to the lower border of the high dose volume to avoid matching through sites of macroscopic or high-risk microscopic disease. An alternative is to angle the opposing lateral beams caudally by 10–30°. Superoinferior wedges compensate for the change in contour of the neck but it can still be difficult to produce a homogeneous dose distribution for adequate dose to the inferior part of the volume. An anterior neck beam can help to achieve this.

If the volume extends both posterior to the cord and inferior to the shoulders, there is no conformal option other than to use opposing photon and posterior electron beams and a matched anterior neck beam. If the match plane is through a high-risk site, it should be moved once during the course of treatment to reduce the risk of under- or overdosing at the junction.

If the volume is unilateral (e.g. lateral T1 N0 pyriform fossa), a unilateral beam arrangement will provide a more conformal dose distribution while sparing contralateral pharyngeal mucosa and salivary glands. A plan with three beams can be used with beam angles chosen to avoid the spinal cord with the posterolateral beam and to minimize dose to the uninvolved mucosa.

Conventional

Patients having palliative radiotherapy can be treated conventionally with lateral opposing beams chosen by virtual simulation. If the volume extends inferior to the shoulders or for any curative treatment, a conformal CT-based plan is recommended.

Dose Fractionation

Curative

70 Gy in 35 daily fractions given in seven weeks +/− concomitant cisplatin

- PTV_HIGH receives 70 Gy in 35 fractions
- PTV_MID receives 63 Gy in 35 fractions
- PTV_LOW receives 56 Gy in 35 fractions

65 Gy in 30 daily fractions given in six weeks +/− concomitant cisplatin

- PTV_HIGH receives 65 Gy in 30 fractions
- PTV_MID receives 60 Gy in 30 fractions
- PTV_LOW receives 54 Gy in 30 fractions

Adjuvant Treatment

60 Gy in 30 daily fractions given in six weeks +/− concomitant cisplatin.

- PTV_HIGH receives 60 Gy in 30 fractions
- PTV_LOW receives 54 Gy in 30 fractions

Palliative Treatment

- 30 Gy in 10 fractions of 3 Gy given in two weeks
- 20 Gy in 5 fractions of 4 Gy given in one week

Treatment Delivery and Patient Care

Weekly assessment by doctor, specialist nurse or radiographer and dietician is important. Regular speech and language therapist advice can help maintain safe, functional swallowing and is important to help laryngectomees care for their stoma during radiotherapy. Most patients are at high risk of weight loss and should be considered for a gastric feeding tube inserted prophylactically before radiotherapy. Further details are given in Chapter 8.

Verification

See Chapter 8.

Key Trials	See Chapter 8 – many phase III trials in head and neck cancer contain patients with hypopharyngeal cancers. Lefebvre JL, Andry G, Chevalier D, et al. Laryngeal preservation with induction chemotherapy for hypopharyngeal squamous cell carcinoma: 10-year results of EORTC trial 24891. Ann Oncol 2012;23:2708–2714.

INFORMATION SOURCES

Kwon DI, Miles BA, et al. Hypopharyngeal carcinoma: Do you know your guidelines? Head Neck 2019;41(3):569–576.

13

Nasopharynx

Indications for Radiotherapy

Curative

Radiotherapy is the principal treatment modality in nasopharyngeal cancer (NPC) and is usually combined with chemotherapy in advanced disease (stages IIb, III and IV). The role of surgery is confined to neck dissections for persistent or recurrent lymphadenopathy or, rarely, to salvage recurrent nasopharyngeal disease.

NPC is endemic in southern China, relatively common around the Mediterranean and uncommon in northern Europe and the USA. Endemic cases are usually associated with Epstein Barr Virus (EBV) infection, which is necessary but not sufficient to cause endemic NPC. Circulating EBV DNA levels at diagnosis can predict survival. Lymphadenopathy at presentation is common but EBV-associated NPC is relatively sensitive to chemotherapy and radiotherapy, so local control rates are good. Failure is often with metastases.

Human papilloma virus (HPV) can be a causative agent in nonendemic NPC. HPV and EBV infections are usually mutually exclusive. Keratinizing squamous cell carcinoma (formally known as WHO type 1) is EBV and HPV negative, is more common in the West but less common in endemic areas, and local control and survival are lower than for other subtypes. Because there is a relatively low incidence of occult cervical lymph node involvement in keratinizing NPC with no palpable lymphadenopathy, elective neck irradiation can be less extensive.

The most frequently used staging system is the UICC TNM. T staging reflects local invasion as described later. N staging criteria in the UICC system are different from those for other head and neck cancers to reflect the high incidence of lymphadenopathy and relative sensitivity to radiation (Table 13.1).

TABLE 13.1

Staging for Nasopharyngeal Cancer

Tx	Primary tumour cannot be assessed
Tis	Carcinoma in situ
T0	No primary tumour identified, but EBV-positive cervical node(s) involvement
T1	Tumour confined to the nasopharynx, or extension to oropharynx and/or nasal cavity without parapharyngeal involvement
T2	Tumour extends to parapharyngeal space and/or adjacent soft tissue involvement (medial pterygoid, lateral pterygoid, prevertebral muscles)
T3	Tumour infiltrates bony structures at skull base, cervical vertebrae, pterygoid structures (pterygoid plates, pterygomaxillary fissure, pterygopalatine fossa) and/or paranasal sinuses
T4	Tumour with intracranial extension, involvement of cranial nerves, hypopharynx, orbit, parotid gland and/or soft tissue extension beyond the lateral surface of the lateral pterygoid muscle
NX	Regional lymph nodes cannot be assessed
N0	No regional lymph node metastasis
N1	Unilateral metastasis in cervical lymph node(s) and/or unilateral or bilateral metastasis in retropharyngeal lymph node(s), 6 cm or smaller in greatest dimension, above the caudal border of the cricoid cartilage
N2	Bilateral metastasis in cervical lymph node(s), 6 cm or smaller in greatest dimension, above the caudal border of the cricoid cartilage
N3	Unilateral or bilateral metastasis in cervical lymph node(s), larger than 6 cm in greatest dimension, and/or extension below the caudal border of the cricoid cartilage

Source: Adapted from UICC TNM (8th edn, 2018).

DOI: 10.1201/9781315171562-13

TABLE 13.2

Stage Groupings for Nasopharyngeal Cancer

Stage 0	Tis, N0, M0
Stage I	T1, N0, M0
Stage II	T0/1, N1, M0
	T2, N0/1, M0
Stage III	T0/1/2, N2, M0
	T3, N0/1/2, M0
Stage IVA	T4, N0/1/2, M0
	Any T, N3, M0
Stage IVB	Any T, Any N, M1

Source: Adapted from UICC TNM (8th edn, 2018).

Overall five-year survival rates are 50–70 percent, but different staging systems, histological subtypes and case mix make comparisons between series difficult. T1/T2 N0/1 disease (stage I and II, Table 13.2) has a five-year local control rate of 70–90 percent with radiotherapy alone. Three-year local control rates of over 80 percent can be achieved in advanced EBV-associated NPC with the addition of chemotherapy to modern radiotherapy.

Local Recurrent Disease

Local recurrence in the nasopharynx is difficult to treat surgically. Brachytherapy with iodine-125 or gold-198 seeds can be used to treat small volume persistent or recurrent disease or can be combined with surgery. However, most local recurrences are detected when they are too large to be cured with brachytherapy.

Re-irradiation to a curative dose can be considered, particularly with smaller volume recurrence and an interval of more than two years from first treatment. It provides cure in 35 percent but must be balanced against the high rate (at least 30 percent) of serious late effects, including bone necrosis and temporal lobe damage.

Sequencing of Multimodality Therapy

The relative chemosensitivity of nasopharyngeal tumours has led to the addition of chemotherapy to try to improve local control and overall survival. Concomitant cisplatin is standard for stage III or IVA disease using either weekly or three-weekly regimens. The role of concomitant chemotherapy for stage II disease is more debated, but it is usually recommended for higher-risk stage II disease, for example with larger-volume lymph nodes.

Clinical trials of neoadjuvant or adjuvant chemotherapy based on cisplatin/5FU regimens have shown conflicting results, and their interpretation is complicated by the change in radiotherapy techniques over the last 20 years. A recent study of neoadjuvant gemcitabine-cisplatin chemotherapy with modern radiotherapy (IMRT) in locally advanced endemic disease has shown improvement in local control and overall survival. Acute but not long-term side effects were increased with this protocol.

Clinical and Radiological Anatomy

The nasopharynx is a mucosa-lined space behind the nasal cavities and above the oropharynx. Understanding the anatomy of this region helps correlate presenting symptoms with local invasion and is vital in order to define the CTV accurately (Figure 13.1). Tumours most commonly arise in the roof or lateral wall – often the fossa of Rosenmüller behind the Eustachian tube orifice. Tumour can spread via

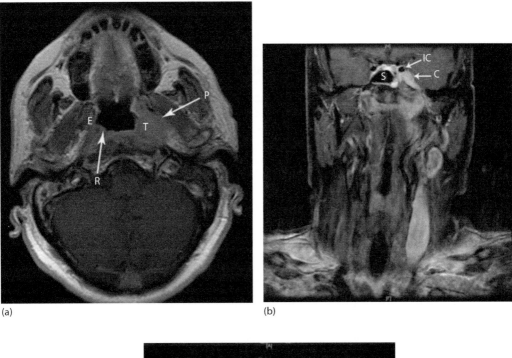

(a) (b)

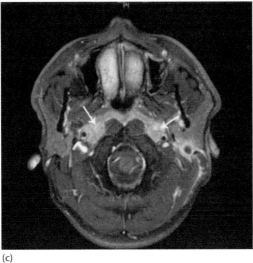

(c)

FIGURE 13.1 Diagnostic MR scans to illustrate nasopharyngeal anatomy and routes of tumour spread. (a) Axial T1-weighted contrast-enhanced MRI showing tumour (T) invading parapharyngeal space (P). The normal contralateral fossa of Rosenmüller (R) and normal Eustachian tube orifice (E) are also shown. (b) Coronal T1-weighted contrast-enhanced MRI showing cavernous sinus invasion (C), the sphenoid sinus (S) and internal carotid artery (IC). (c) Axial T1-weighted contrast-enhanced MRI showing bilateral retropharyngeal nodes (arrowed).

the mucosa or submucosa, to invade the nasal cavity anteriorly or the oropharynx inferiorly. Spread is often along neural pathways towards and involving skull base foramina.

The lateral wall is formed by the pharyngobasilar fascia, which offers relatively little resistance to tumour spread. Deep to the fascia is the parapharyngeal space containing the lateral retropharyngeal lymph nodes, cranial nerves IX–XII, carotid artery and internal jugular vein. Direct extension or nodal involvement can lead to IX–XII cranial nerve palsies. Tumour can grow out of the parapharyngeal space superiorly into the infratemporal fossa, foramen ovale and cavernous sinus. Anteriorly, spread can be into the pterygopalatine fossa foramen rotundum and the inferior orbital fissure towards the orbit.

The roof slopes downwards to become the posterior wall. Medially, it is formed by the sphenoid sinus and laterally by the foramen lacerum at the skull base. This provides relatively little barrier to local invasion into the cavernous sinus, which contains cranial nerves III–VI and the internal carotid artery. Skull base invasion occurs in 30 percent of cases.

The nasopharynx drains directly to both the lateral retropharyngeal nodes in the parapharyngeal space and to level II and upper level V nodes. Ipsilateral lymphadenopathy is detected in 60–90 percent of patients at diagnosis, and 50 percent have involved contralateral nodes. Skip metastases to lower neck nodes are uncommon.

Distant metastases are more common than in many head and neck subsites. PET-CT should be performed in people with T4 or N3 disease but is increasingly being used in all stage III and IV patients who are at highest risk of metastases at presentation. All patients should have at least a CT scan including the chest and liver, and an assessment of bone metastases, for example with a bone scan.

Assessment of Primary Disease

Careful clinical examination and cross-sectional imaging are required to assess local invasion and lymph node spread. Particular attention should be paid to sites where local invasion is suspected on the basis of clinical symptoms and signs. Clinical examination should include a nasendoscopy or EUA to assess mucosa, submucosa and extent of spread in the nasopharynx. Documentation of cranial neuropathies can direct imaging assessment. MRI is preferred to CT with contrast, as it provides better imaging of soft tissue invasion, particularly the parapharyngeal space and retropharyngeal lymph nodes. CT with bone windows is better for detecting bone involvement and may also be required if skull base invasion is suspected.

All patients should have a dental assessment and OPG, as xerostomia after treatment is common. A baseline audiogram is useful, as tumour, radiotherapy and chemotherapy can all contribute to hearing loss.

Data Acquisition

Immobilization

Patients are treated supine with head and shoulders immobilized in thermoplastic shell with at least five fixation points. If the primary GTV extends to the palate, a mouth bite may be used to depress the tongue away from the treated volume.

CT Scanning

CT scan slices no more than 3 mm thick are obtained from the skull vertex to the arch of the aorta inferiorly. Intravenous contrast helps the definition of both the primary site and cervical nodes. Reference marks are placed on the shell at the CT visit to aid verification.

Target Volume Definition

GTV

The GTVp and GTVn are contoured as separate structures on the planning CT using diagnostic images and clinical information. It may be helpful to fuse MRI images with the planning CT, particularly if there is skull base involvement. Retropharyngeal nodes 5 mm and cervical nodes 10 mm in short axis diameter are contoured as GTVn. If induction chemotherapy has been used, the GTV should reflect the initial sites of disease.

CTV

Three CTVs are defined: CTV_HIGH reflects the clinically apparent disease; CTV_MID reflects the high risk of local spread in and adjacent to the nasopharynx and in high-risk nodal levels; and a prophylactic CTV_LOW treats at-risk but clinically uninvolved nodes. It is easier to define each CTV for primary site and nodes separately and then to sum them together.

The GTVp is expanded isotropically by 5 mm to form the CTVp_HIGH, which is then edited from air and uninvolved bone, and to reflect natural tumour barriers.

Definition of the CTVp_MID is complicated and reflects likely paths of tumour spread, which differ depending on T stage of the tumour. It is formed by a 5 mm expansion from CTVp_HIGH, which is then edited extensively as shown in Table 13.3, based on the 2018 consensus guidelines. (See Figure 13.2.)

The CTVs as defined earlier will often come very close to OARs, making some compromise either in OAR doses or tumour coverage necessary. We recommend minimum margins of 1 mm from GTVp to CTVp_HIGH and 2 mm from GTV to CTVp_MID.

The GTVn is expanded by 5 mm and edited to reflect natural barriers like bone to form the CTVn_HIGH. A 10 mm margin is recommended where there is obvious extracapsular spread, and a 3 mm margin can be used for nodes less than 10 mm short axis which are suspicious for being involved.

The CTVn_MID should include the whole of any involved nodal level along with the bilateral retropharyngeal, retrostyloid, level II, III and Va nodes in all patients. Levels IVa and Vb should be included unless there are no nodes inferior to the hyoid on that side of the neck. Level 1b should be included if the primary tumour extends into the anterior nose or oral cavity of if there are level II nodes greater than 2 cm in size or with extracapsular spread (Figure 13.3).

The CTVn_LOW usually includes the rest of the bilateral neck (levels IVa, Vb, 1b). Level 1b can be omitted in the N0 neck. Lower neck nodes can be omitted in keratinizing squamous cell cancer with an N0 neck. The CTV_LOW should cover one nodal level beyond an involved level – so if there are nodes in IVa, level IVb should be treated.

PTV and OARs

A CTV-PTV margin is applied (usually 3–5 mm) based on measured setup errors assuming no tumour motion.

TABLE 13.3

Guidelines for CTVp_MID Definition in Nasopharyngeal Cancers

Site	All Patients	Select Patients
Superior	Include vomer and adjacent posterior-inferior ethmoid sinuses	Include superior posterior ethmoids if sphenoid sinus is involved; no need to include anterior or middle ethmoids
Sphenoid sinus	Include inferior portion	T3 and T4 – include whole sphenoid sinus
Cavernous sinus	–	T3 and T4 – include whole ipsilateral cavernous sinus
Skull base foramina	Bilateral foramen ovale, rotundum and lacerum	If there is extensive posterolateral infiltration or involvement of high adjacent nodes – jugular foramen and hypoglossal canal
Anterior	5 mm anterior to posterior choanae bilaterally to cover posterior nasal cavity 5 mm of posterior maxillary sinus bilaterally to cover pterygopalatine fossae and pterygomaxillary fissure	–
Lateral	Whole parapharyngeal space Pterygoid muscles if within 5+5 expansion	Whole lateral pterygoid only if there is direct tumour invasion of the muscle
Posterior	Anterior third of the clivus	Whole clivus if any of the clivus is involved

Source: Adapted from Lee et al. (2018).

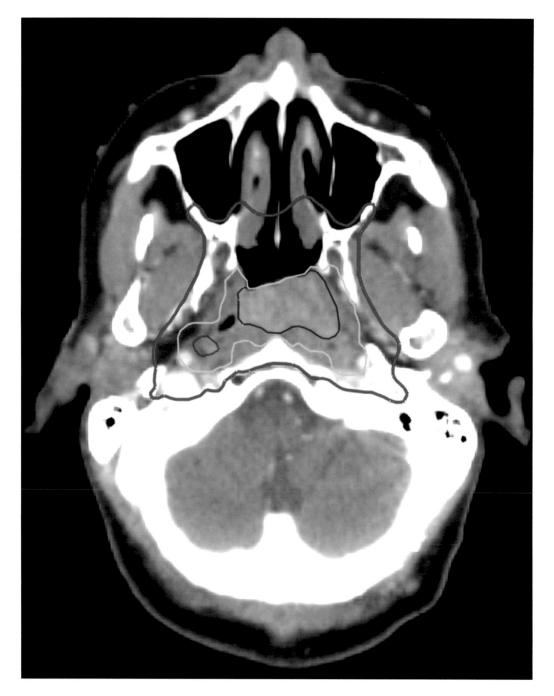

FIGURE 13.2 CTVs at level of nasopharynx for T1N2 nasopharynx cancer with bilateral retropharyngeal node involvement – GTV (dark blue), CTV_HIGH (cyan) and CTV_MID (magenta).

The brainstem, spinal cord and optic chiasm should be defined in all patients. The parotid glands, pituitary gland, temporomandibular joints (TMJs), each optic nerve, temporal lobes, middle ear apparatus (adjacent to the fossa of Rosenmüller) and cochlea should also be contoured as critical structures, as IMRT will allow some sparing of these structures though often only with some compromise to PTV coverage.

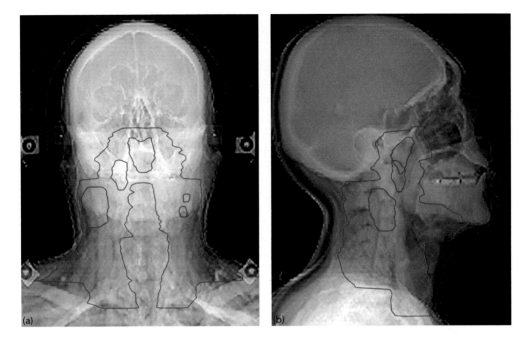

FIGURE 13.3 (a) Coronal and (b) sagittal projection of contours to show neck node levels included in CTV_MID for a T1N2 nasopharynx cancer – CTVn_MID (magenta) and GTV (blue).

Dose Solutions

Complex

The complex PTVs and adjacent critical normal structures make IMRT or VMAT almost essential to achieve reasonable PTV coverage with acceptable OAR sparing. Five or seven equally spaced coplanar IMRT beams or one or two arcs are usually employed. The CTV_LOW in the inferior neck can be included in the IMRT volume or treated with a matched anterior neck beam. While the dosimetric PTV coverage of a matched beam is less good, it can enable complete sparing of the larynx and hypopharynx, potentially reducing toxicity.

The proximity of the PTVs to OARs means compromise is usually necessary when producing a plan, as shown in Figure 13.4. It is widely accepted that spinal cord, brainstem and optic chiasm tolerances should not be exceeded, but that good PTV (and certainly GTV) coverage is more important than sparing other OARs. Daily cone beam CTs matched at the level of the primary tumour can be useful when agreeing such a compromise – for example to ensure GTV is always encompassed even if the PTV is not. The Lee et al. (2019) paper has a thorough discussion of all OARs in nasopharyngeal cancer with expert agreement on doses and priorities. It is important to involve patients in decisions where a balance is struck between ensuring coverage and not risking life-changing late effects.

As bilateral node involvement is relatively common, care must be taken not to compromise PTV coverage in level II for the sake of parotid sparing, as recurrences can occur in the high level II and retrostyloid regions close to the deep lobe of the parotid. If bilateral level II nodes are included in CTV_MID, the bilateral superficial parotid lobes should be contoured as one structure so that an attempt can be made to spare them while accepting more radiation to deep lobes close to the PTV.

Conformal

As the PTV includes both a midline tumour and bilateral cervical nodes, it is difficult to obtain adequate coverage conformally with anything other than opposing lateral photon beams. Conformal planning will at least allow MLC shielding to shape to PTVs rather than to bony anatomy. Treatment of the PTVs with a conformal plan will reduce the dose to adjacent critical structures such as the brainstem and temporal lobes.

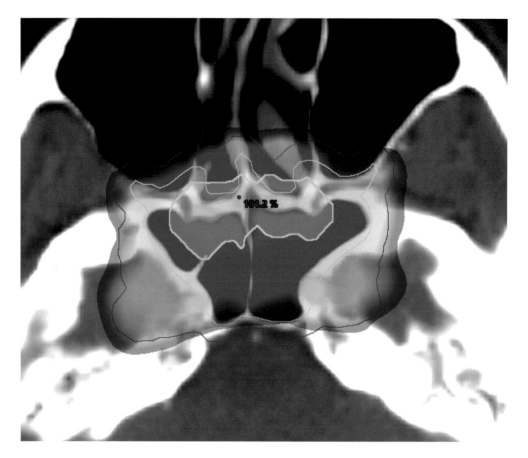

FIGURE 13.4 IMRT plan for nasopharyngeal cancer to illustrate compromise in coverage of PTV_MID (red) in order to spare brainstem to within tolerance. Note CTV_MID (cyan) is still covered. Daily cone beam CTs matched at this level will reduce the risk of underdoing the CTV. PTV_HIGH is shown in green.

PTV_LOW is initially treated to 40 Gy in 20 fractions with opposing lateral photon beams. MLC shielding is applied to oral cavity, orbit and brain. This is matched to a bilateral anterior neck beam with the match plane at least 10 mm below the nodal GTV.

The second phase treats the nasopharynx (PTV_MID) with a further 20 Gy in 10 fractions with a three-beam plan using an anterior infraorbital beam in addition to small lateral beams to reduce temporal lobe and TMJ dose. This arrangement is also used for the final 10 Gy in 5 fractions with additional shielding to reduce the treated volume if possible. The second phase also includes a matched anterior neck beam to cover lower neck nodes and matched electrons to posterior neck nodes.

An anterior neck beam prescribed to D_{max} will not cover all the cervical node PTV with the 95 percent isodose, but this arrangement has been used for decades without a high incidence of isolated nodal recurrence, so the dose delivered seems to be adequate for tumour control. If a higher dose to the nodes is required, for example when level V nodes are present, either the prescription point can be changed to 3 cm (which will produce a hot spot of 115 percent) or opposing anterior and posterior fields weighted anteriorly can be used (which will increase the volume of normal tissue treated to a high dose).

Conventional

Where resources are not available for conformal planning, conventional techniques may be unavoidable. Ho's technique describes a similar solution to the conformal one described earlier with bony landmarks used to define beam edges. For example beam borders for the first phase of treatment are: anterior – bisecting antrum; posterior – 2 cm posterior to nodes; superior – 5 mm above anterior clinoid.

Dose Fractionation

Simultaneous Boost IMRT/VMAT

- 70 Gy in 35 daily fractions given in seven weeks +/− concomitant cisplatin
  - PTV_HIGH receives 70 Gy in 35 fractions
  - PTV_MID receives 63 Gy in 35 fractions
  - PTV_LOW receives 56 Gy in 35 fractions
- 65 Gy in 30 daily fractions given in six weeks +/− concomitant cisplatin
  - PTV_HIGH receives 65 Gy in 30 fractions
  - PTV_MID receives 60 Gy in 30 fractions
  - PTV_LOW receives 54 Gy in 30 fractions

Conformal/Conventional

70 Gy in 35 daily fractions given in seven weeks +/− concomitant cisplatin to PTV_HIGH with 60 Gy in 30 fractions to PTV_MID and 50 Gy in 25 fractions to PTV_LOW.

Treatment Delivery and Patient Care

A dental assessment is carried out before radiotherapy because of the risk of long-term xerostomia. We recommend that a prophylactic feeding tube is inserted before radiotherapy in all patients with N2/3 disease and is considered for others thought to be at increased risk of weight loss during treatment.

See Chapter 8 for details.

Verification

See Chapter 8.

Key Trials

Al-Sarraf M, LeBlanc M, Giri PG, et al. Chemoradiotherapy versus radiotherapy in patients with advanced nasopharyngeal cancer: Phase III randomised intergroup study 0099. J Clin Oncol 1998;16:1310–1317.

Yang H, Chen X, Lin S, et al. Treatment outcomes after reduction of the target volume of intensity modulated radiotherapy following induction chemotherapy in patients with locoregionally advanced nasopharyngeal carcinoma: A prospective, multi-center, randomized clinical trial. Radiother Oncol 2018;126:37–42.

Zhang Y, Chen L, Guo-Qing H, et al. Gemcitabine and cisplatin induction chemotherapy in nasopharyngeal carcinoma. N Engl J Med 2019;381:1124–1135.

INFORMATION SOURCES

Blanchard P, Lee A, Marguet S, et al. Chemotherapy and radiotherapy in nasopharyngeal carcinoma: An update of the MAC-NPC meta-analysis. Lancet Oncol 2015;16:645–655.

Chua MLK, Wee JTS, Hui EP, et al. Nasopharyngeal carcinoma. Lancet 2016;387:1012–1024.

Ho's Technique. Treatment of Cancer, Halnan, K.E. (ed.). London: Chapman and Hall, 1982, pp. 249–268.

Lee AW, Ng WT, Pan JJ, et al. International guideline for the delineation of the clinical target volumes (CTV) for nasopharyngeal carcinoma. Radiother Oncol 2018;126:25–36.

Lee AW, Ng WT, Pan JJ, et al. International guideline on dose prioritization and acceptance criteria in radiation therapy planning for nasopharyngeal carcinoma. Int J Radiation Oncol Biol Phys 2019;105:567–580.

14

Larynx

Indications for Radiotherapy

Early-stage Squamous Cell Cancer of Glottic Larynx (T1/T2, N0)

Squamous cell carcinomas confined to the glottic larynx can be treated with either surgery (often laser excision) or radiotherapy. Large retrospective series suggest equivalent cure rates as long as radiotherapy is followed by close surveillance to detect and treat recurrences. Radiation alone gives five-year local control rates of 90 percent in T1 tumours and 75 percent in T2 tumours. Local surgical and radiotherapeutic expertise, patient choice, expected tolerability of treatment and likely voice quality after therapy all influence the treatment decision. If the anterior commissure is involved, voice quality with surgery may be worse as it can be more difficult to oppose the vocal cords after resection.

Early-stage Squamous Cell Cancer of Supraglottic Larynx (T1/T2, N0)

The supraglottic larynx has a richer lymphatic drainage than the glottic larynx. Although surgery and radiotherapy have equal cure rates, the ability to preserve organ function and to treat the adjacent neck nodes means radiotherapy is usually preferred.

Advanced Laryngeal Cancer (T3/T4, N+)

The preferred treatment for many years for advanced laryngeal cancer has been surgery (total laryngectomy and neck dissection) with adjuvant radiotherapy, sometimes with concomitant chemotherapy, in selected cases. In practice, adjuvant radiation is recommended to the primary site in T4 cancer or where resection margins are close or involved, and to the neck in N2–3 disease or in N1 disease with extracapsular nodal spread. Adjuvant radiotherapy is therefore recommended for the majority of patients who have a laryngectomy.

An alternative approach is organ preservation – initial radiotherapy, usually combined with chemotherapy, with laryngectomy reserved for recurrence. There are phase III data to support this approach in T3 and smaller-volume T4 tumours, provided there is careful follow-up to detect recurrence and offer salvage laryngectomy. Without this, (chemo)radiation will produce inferior cure rates compared with laryngectomy.

Organ preservation is recommended if the patient can tolerate concomitant chemotherapy, if speech and swallow before treatment are good, if the primary tumour does not invade through the laryngeal cartilage and if the patient is willing to commit to close follow-up so that salvage laryngectomy can be offered if there is residual or recurrent disease. In practice, many patients with advanced larynx cancer have comorbidities that make either a laryngectomy or radiation and concomitant chemotherapy a major challenge to complete successfully. A careful discussion about their preferences and the support from professionals including dietitians and speech and language therapists is key to making the right decision for an individual. Sometimes radiation alone is the only treatment option which people are able to tolerate.

Palliative Radiotherapy

If distant metastases are present initially or if the patient is not suitable for curative treatment, palliative radiotherapy may improve pain and reduce the chance of laryngeal obstruction or tumour ulceration in the neck.

DOI: 10.1201/9781315171562-14

Sequencing of Multimodality Therapy

Locally advanced laryngeal disease is often treated with surgery, radiotherapy and chemotherapy. Initial laryngectomy may be followed by adjuvant radiotherapy with concomitant chemotherapy for selected patients (see Chapter 8). Concomitant radiochemotherapy can be used as initial treatment with surgery (laryngectomy and/or neck dissection) for residual or recurrent disease.

Exophytic glottic and subglottic tumours may present with stridor. Even if organ preservation is the preferred treatment, surgical debulking may be required initially to preserve a clear airway if there is concern that radiation-induced oedema early in treatment might compromise the airway.

Clinical and Radiological Anatomy

The larynx is divided into three subsites: the supraglottic larynx (epiglottis, false cords, ventricles, ary-epiglottic folds and arytenoids), glottic larynx (true cords) and subglottic larynx (from the under surface of the cords to the inferior border of the cricoid cartilage) (Table 14.1 and Figure 14.1). Primary tumours can spread mucosally or submucosally between these subsites or to the adjacent oropharynx or hypo-pharynx. They can invade deep structures such as the laryngeal cartilages, pre-epiglottic and paraglottic fat, or into nearby structures such as the carotid sheath or prevertebral muscles.

The glottic larynx has very few lymphatics so early tumours confined to this site are usually N0 and adjacent nodes do not require treatment. The prelaryngeal (Delphian) node lies on the cricothyroid membrane and is usually included in radiotherapy treated volumes incidentally. Tumours originating in the supraglottic larynx can spread to adjacent level II or III nodes unilaterally or bilaterally if the primary tumour crosses the midline. Locally advanced cancers spread to adjacent level II–IV nodes. If there is subglottic involvement, tumours can spread to level IV or level VIb nodes.

TABLE 14.1

Tumour Staging for Supraglottic and Glottic Cancer

	Supraglottis	**Glottis**
Tx	Primary tumour cannot be assessed	Primary tumour cannot be assessed
Tis	Carcinoma in situ	Carcinoma in situ
T1	Tumour limited to one subsite of supraglottis with normal vocal cord mobility	Tumour limited to the vocal cord(s) (may involve anterior or posterior commissure) with normal mobility T1a – limited to one vocal cord T1b – involves both vocal cords
T2	Tumour invades mucosa of more than one adjacent subsite of supraglottis or glottis or region outside the supraglottis (e.g. mucosa of base of tongue, vallecula, medial wall of pyriform sinus) without fixation of the larynx	Tumour extends to supraglottis and/or subglottis, and/or with impaired vocal cord mobility
T3	Tumour limited to larynx with vocal cord fixation and/or invades any of the following: postcricoid area, pre-epiglottic space, paraglottic space and/or inner cortex of thyroid cartilage	Tumour limited to the larynx with vocal cord fixation and/or invasion of the paraglottic space and/or inner cortex of the thyroid cartilage
T4a	Moderately advanced local disease Tumour invades through the outer cortex of the thyroid cartilage and/or invades tissues beyond the larynx (e.g. trachea, soft tissues of the neck including deep extrinsic muscle of the tongue, strap muscles, thyroid or oesophagus	Moderately advanced local disease Tumour invades through the outer cortex of the thyroid cartilage and/or invades tissues beyond the larynx (e.g. trachea, cricoid cartilage, soft tissues of the neck including deep extrinsic muscle of the tongue, strap muscles, thyroid or oesophagus
T4b	Very advanced local disease Tumour invades prevertebral space, encases carotid artery, or invades mediastinal structures	Very advanced local disease Tumour invades prevertebral space, encases carotid artery, or invades mediastinal structures

Source: Adapted from UICC TNM (8th edn, 2018).

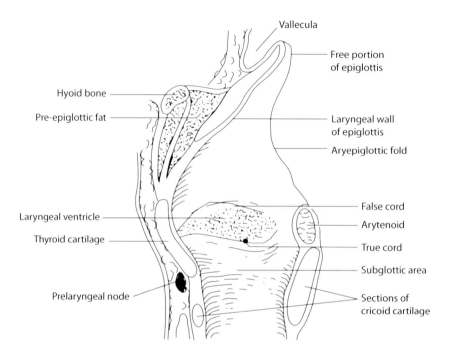

FIGURE 14.1   Midline sagittal view of the larynx.

Assessment of Primary Disease

For early disease, clinical assessment of local extent and vocal cord mobility is more important than cross-sectional imaging. Most patients have an EUA to obtain biopsies and to evaluate supraglottic and subglottic spread, although a transnasal oesophagoscopy can be used instead. Both oncologist and surgeon should examine the larynx with a nasendoscope to visualize the primary tumour and to assess vocal cord mobility (Figure 14.2).

T1aN0 glottic squamous cell cancer does not usually require cross-sectional imaging, as the risk of deep invasion or nodal spread is very small, though imaging should be performed in patients who are immunosuppressed where the risk of local spread and lymphadenopathy is higher. All other laryngeal cancer requires cross-sectional imaging with CT or MRI. Invasion of paraglottic fat and laryngeal

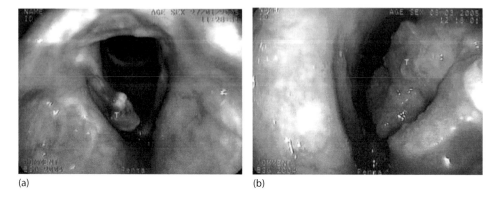

(a)   (b)

FIGURE 14.2   Nasendoscopy of the larynx. (a) T1a tumour (T) of the anterior half of the right vocal cord. (b) T3 tumour (T) of the left vocal cord extending into the supraglottic larynx.

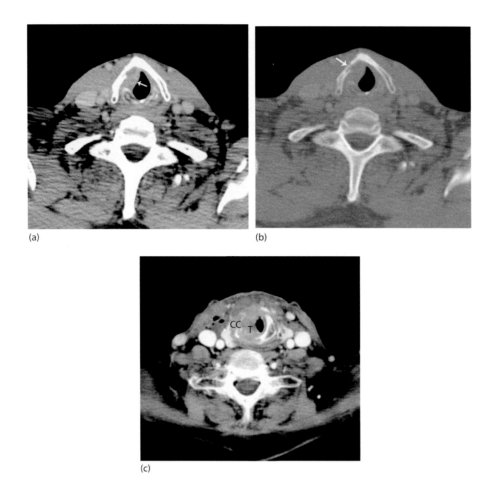

FIGURE 14.3 Cartilage invasion in laryngeal tumours. (a) Diagnostic CT scan showing tumour (arrowed) with possible invasion of the thyroid cartilage. (b) Same slice with window and level optimized for bone/cartilage to show cartilage invasion. (c) T4a tumour (T) invading through the cricoid cartilage (CC) into the soft tissues of the neck.

cartilages may be assessed by CT or MRI (Figure 14.3). Ultrasound can be useful particularly to help assess cartilage sclerosis where cartilage invasion is suspected but not proven with MRI or CT. As function is key to decision-making in T3 and T4 disease, dietetic and speech and language therapy assessments are important to assess nutrition, aspiration and voice quality.

Data Acquisition

Immobilization

All patients having radiotherapy should be immobilized in a rigid thermoplastic shell fixed to the couch in at least five places. The spine should be as straight as possible. The shoulders are immobilized in the shell as inferiorly as possible so that the shoulder tips are inferior to the lower border of the cricoid cartilage, thus permitting lateral radiation beams to treat the larynx without the need to angle them inferiorly. Grip bars on the side of the couch may help to achieve this.

CT Scanning

CT slices no more than 3 mm thick are obtained from the base of skull to the top of the aortic arch with the patient immobilized in the treatment position. As treatment of locally advanced glottic cancer or adjuvant radiation after a laryngectomy may require lateral beams angled inferiorly, the CT scan in these patients should be extended inferiorly to the carina.

Simulator

Radiotherapy for early (T1) glottic carcinomas with no extra-laryngeal disease can be planned on a simulator or using virtual simulation because the position of the primary tumour can be determined – the vocal cords extend horizontally from 10 mm below the thyroid promontory – and lymph nodes do not require treatment. The whole larynx can therefore be treated with opposing lateral beams with the following borders:

- Superior – mid-body of the hyoid
- Inferior – inferior margin of cricoid cartilage
- Anterior – to cover skin
- Posterior – anterior vertebral column

A 1-cm-thick tissue equivalent bolus should be applied anteriorly if tumour extends to the anterior commissure. As the larynx moves superiorly on swallowing, fluoroscopy can be used in the simulator to ensure that the glottis remains within the treated volume when the patient swallows.

Target Volume Definition

T1 N0 Glottic Larynx

Records and pictures from nasendoscopy and EUA should be available, as small primary vocal cord tumours can be difficult to see on CT scan. Many patients will have field change in the larynx with either bilateral cancer or in situ disease. While it is feasible to treat just the GTV with a 5 mm margin and to potentially spare the contralateral carotid artery, for many people having radiotherapy it makes more pragmatic sense to irradiate the whole glottic larynx. We recommend delineating the GTV and then contouring the soft tissues of the larynx on each axial slice up to the inner aspect of the thyroid and cricoid cartilages. The CTV should be extended at least 10 mm above and below the GTV to cover the inferior supraglottis and the upper part of the subglottic region. A 3–5 mm PTV margin is added.

Other Curative Radiotherapy

The GTVp is defined on the planning CT scan as the primary tumour with reference to nasendoscopy and diagnostic imaging. The CTVp_HIGH is formed by a 5 mm isotropic expansion from GTV, edited from air and uninvolved cartilage. The CTVp_MID includes adjacent parts of the larynx where local invasion or mucosal or submucosal spread is possible and is best created by applying a 10 mm expansion from GTV. This is then edited to reflect spread in each direction. Laterally, this should include the paraglottic space and adjacent thyroid or cricoid cartilages in all patients, the strap muscles if the cartilage is involved and the subcutaneous soft tissue lateral to the strap muscles if there is T4a disease. Medially, the contralateral larynx and hypopharynx mucosa is often included. Anteriorly and posteriorly, it is important to assess the risk of disease growing through the membranes separating the cartilages and adding at least a 10 mm margin in these areas. The posterior wall of the hypopharynx does not need to be included. Superiorly and inferiorly, the CTVp_MID should extend at least 10 mm from the GTV. For large tumours this often means the whole larynx and hypopharynx is included in the CTV_MID.

Any involved nodes are contoured as GTVn. The CTVn_HIGH is formed by a 5 mm isotropic expansion from GTV. A 10 mm margin can be used if there is extracapsular nodal spread of adjacent muscle invasion. The CTV_MID also includes lymph node regions that are at high risk of having microscopic tumour involvement – in practice this usually includes any involved nodal levels and the level III nodes immediately adjacent to the primary tumour (Figure 14.4).

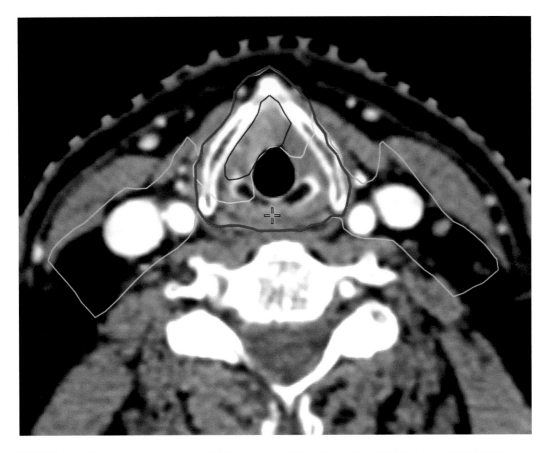

FIGURE 14.4 Radiotherapy contours for T2 N0 carcinoma of the right glottis – GTV (dark blue), CTV_HIGH (cyan), CTV_MID (magenta), CTV_LOW (green). Note whole larynx is included in CTV_MID. For a T3N0 tumour, the bilateral level 3 nodes may be included in CTV_MID.

The CTV_LOW in the patient with clinically negative nodes includes all nodes at risk for microscopic metastases as shown in Table 14.2. If adjacent structures are involved, the CTV_LOW must reflect their lymphatic drainage, e.g. level II nodes if there is tongue base invasion.

For T1/T2 N0 supraglottic tumours, the upper part of level II superior to the angle of the mandible is at low risk of micrometastases and can be excluded from the treated volume.

TABLE 14.2

Recommendations for the Selection of Low-risk Nodal Levels (CTV_LOW) for Hypopharyngeal Tumours

Nodal Status (TNM8)	Ipsilateral Neck	Contralateral Neck
N0-1	II, III, IVa Ib if level II is involved VIb if there is subglottic extension or involvement of the apex of the piriform sinus or postcricoid region	II, III, IVa VIb if there is subglottic extension or involvement of the apex of the piriform sinus or postcricoid region
N 2a-2b or N3	II, III, IVa, Va,b Ib if level II is involved IVb if level IVa is involved VIb if there is subglottic extension or involvement of the apex of the piriform sinus or postcricoid region VIIb if upper level II is involved	II, III, IVa VIb if there is subglottic extension or involvement of the apex of the piriform sinus or postcricoid region
N2c	According to N stage on each side of the neck	According to N stage on each side of the neck

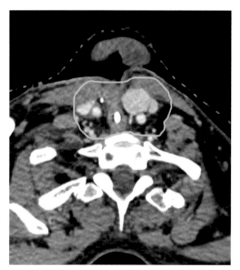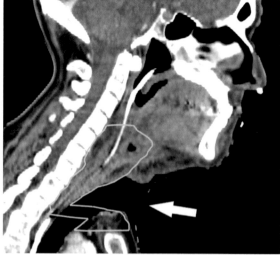

FIGURE 14.5 Adjuvant radiotherapy contours (CTV_HIGH) for a pT4N0 laryngeal tumour with R0 resection. (a) Axial view. Tissue planes can be difficult to define in the postoperative setting. (b) Sagittal view showing the stoma (arrowed) included within the target volume.

Adjuvant Radiotherapy

The CTV_HIGH after a laryngectomy is determined by the initial site of the tumour and which local structures were invaded, and by the pattern of lymph node spread found on initial imaging and at neck dissection. Preoperative imaging, clinicopathological correlation, a clear operation note and discussion with the surgeon can all be helpful, but, in practice, the neck anatomy looks so different after a laryngectomy that it can be very difficult to delineate anything other than the residual midline soft tissue. It can be helpful to define the superior and inferior extent of the pre-op tumour on the planning CT scan with reference to stable anatomical landmarks such as the vertebrae or carotid bifurcation. The CTV_HIGH should encompass the midline neck with at least a 15 mm margin longitudinally from the original GTVp location. Laterally, the contours should encompass the carotid artery in the pN0 neck. This should mean that any site of cartilage, strap muscle or thyrohyoid membrane involvement is treated with a margin. Subglottic tumour extension or an emergency tracheostomy before surgery predict for parastomal recurrence. In these cases, the stoma should be included in CTV_HIGH. (See Figure 14.5.)

For node positive disease, the CTV_HIGH should include all nodal levels which contained disease in the dissected neck. A separate CTV_LOW can be defined to treat dissected but uninvolved nodal levels, or to ensure that all nodal levels in Table 14.2 are included. As dissected nodal levels are hard to contour precisely, it can be easier to include all nodal levels to be treated in one dose level.

Dose Solutions

T1 N0 Glottic Larynx

Conformal

A homogeneous conformal dose distribution can usually be obtained by either using anterior oblique beams or lateral beams with the addition of an anterior beam. Bolus is usually needed to ensure adequate coverage over the anterior commissure as there is little subcutaneous soft tissue at this site. MLCs are used to conform each beam to the shape of the PTV and the beams can be modulated with IMRT to produce a more homogeneous dose distribution. In this way dose to the lateral neck is reduced, which may reduce the risk of damage to the carotid vessels. However, the adjacent lymph nodes will not receive a therapeutic dose as they would with an opposing beam arrangement (Figure 14.6). If there is any question of supra-glottic involvement, the adjacent nodes must be included in the CTV and the volume treated accordingly.

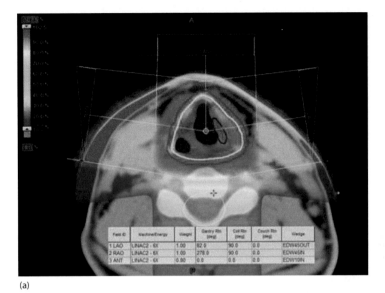

(a)

(b)

FIGURE 14.6 Conformal radiotherapy for T1a cancer of the left glottis with three beams. (a) Axial slice showing beams and dose distribution. (b) Sagittal slice. The superior beam border is the mid-body of the hyoid bone and the inferior border is the inferior margin of the cricoid cartilage.

Other Tumours

Complex

The complex midline contour shapes and adjacent critical structures mean IMRT or VMAT are preferred. An equispaced seven-beam coplanar IMRT arrangement is likely to produce the best plan, though five beams may be adequate. One or two arcs are sufficient if using VMAT. Unilateral or bilateral parotid sparing is usually possible. Care should be taken to ensure adequate coverage anteriorly where there is often little subcutaneous soft tissue between the PTV and air. A strip of bolus anteriorly may be required.

Dose Fractionation

T1/T2 N0 Glottic Larynx

- 55 Gy in 20 daily fractions given in four weeks
- 50 Gy in 16 daily fractions given in 22 days

Other Curative Treatments

- 70 Gy in 35 daily fractions given in seven weeks +/– concomitant cisplatin
  - PTV_HIGH receives 70 Gy in 35 fractions
  - PTV_MID receives 63 Gy in 35 fractions
  - PTV_LOW receives 56 Gy in 35 fractions
- 65 Gy in 30 daily fractions given in six weeks +/– concomitant cisplatin
  - PTV_HIGH receives 65 Gy in 30 fractions
  - PTV_MID receives 60 Gy in 30 fractions
  - PTV_LOW receives 54 Gy in 30 fractions

Adjuvant Treatment

- 60 Gy in 30 daily fractions given in six weeks +/– concomitant cisplatin
  - PTV_HIGH receives 60 Gy in 30 fractions
  - PTV_LOW receives 54 Gy in 30 fractions

Treatment Delivery and Patient Care

See Chapter 8.

Particular care of the tracheostomy site is needed if the stoma is included in the treated volume. Tracheitis will occur and may make it painful to replace a stoma button. Desquamation anteriorly can make fixing stoma devices difficult. These patients should be assessed weekly throughout treatment by a speech and language therapist. Patients having an intact larynx irradiated will develop varying degrees of laryngitis and need advice to rest their voice until acute effects subside.

Verification

See Chapter 8.

Forastiere AA, Zhang Q, Weber RS, et al. Long-term results of RTOG 91-11: A comparison of three nonsurgical treatment strategies to preserve the larynx in patients with locally advanced larynx cancer. J Clin Oncol 2013;31:845–852.

Henriques De Figueiredo B, Fortpied C, et al. Long-term update of the 24954 EORTC phase III trial on larynx preservation. Eur J Cancer 2016;65:109–112.

INFORMATION SOURCES

Abdurehim Y, Hua Z, Yasin Y, et al. Transoral laser surgery versus radiotherapy: Systematic review and meta-analysis for treatment options of T1a glottic cancer. Head Neck 2012;34:23–33.

Forastiere AA, Ismaila N, Lewin JS, et al. Use of larynx-preservation strategies in the treatment of laryngeal cancer: American Society of clinical oncology clinical practice guideline update. J Clin Oncol 2018;36:1143–1169.

15

Salivary Glands

Indications for Radiotherapy

Seventy percent of salivary gland tumours arise in the parotid glands, but over half of these are benign. Ten percent occur in the submandibular glands, but half of them are malignant. The remainder usually occur in the minor salivary glands and are almost always malignant. Most tumours are treated with surgery followed by postoperative radiotherapy when risk of locoregional recurrence is high. Retrospective series suggest the addition of radiotherapy can reduce local recurrence rates from 30 percent to 10 percent, but there is no effect on overall survival.

Patterns of local and metastatic spread vary with histological subtype. Careful pathological assessment is important to help predict risk of local and neck recurrence and the need for adjuvant radiotherapy. Pre- and postoperative discussions with the surgeon are useful to define the extent of surgery and likely sites of macroscopic or microscopic residual disease, though some tumours will only be found to be malignant at operation. Tumours close to the facial nerve within the parotid gland are often excised with positive or very close margins in order to preserve the nerve, with the expectation that adjuvant radiotherapy will be used. Primary skin cancers of the head and neck can metastasize to intraparotid lymph nodes. Radiotherapy for these cancers is considered separately in Chapter 9.

High-grade Tumours (e.g. Salivary Duct Adenocarcinoma, High-grade Mucoepidermoid Cancer, Carcinoma Arising from Pleomorphic Adenoma)

Adjuvant radiotherapy to the tumour bed is recommended for all high-grade salivary tumours except for T1 tumours completely excised with clear margins. Ipsilateral neck levels Ib, II and III should be treated prophylactically in view of the high risk of occult neck node metastases, unless a negative selective neck dissection has been performed. In node-positive patients, adjuvant neck radiotherapy is recommended for N2/3 disease or in the presence of extracapsular spread. Tumours of intermediate grade should be managed as high-grade cancers.

Low-grade Tumours (e.g. Low-grade Mucoepidermoid, Low-grade Adenocarcinoma, Acinic Cell Carcinoma)

Adjuvant radiotherapy is recommended where excision margins are positive or close (<5 mm) after discussion with the surgeon and pathologist. The deep excision margin close to the facial nerve is usually the closest. The risk of occult neck metastases is smaller than for high-grade tumours, so prophylactic treatment of the clinically N0 neck is not recommended.

Adenoid Cystic Carcinoma

These tumours have a relatively high local recurrence rate and a propensity for perineural spread. Adjuvant radiotherapy is recommended for all adenoid cystic cancers except in the rare situation of T1 tumours without pathological evidence of perineural invasion.

DOI: 10.1201/9781315171562-15

Pleomorphic Adenoma

See Chapter 38.

Sequencing of Multimodality Therapy

Adjuvant radiotherapy should ideally commence within six weeks after surgery as long as adequate wound healing has occurred. There is no proven role for concomitant chemotherapy.

Clinical and Radiological Anatomy

Parotid tumours usually arise in the portion of the gland lateral to the plane of the facial nerve – the superficial lobe – though there is no anatomical distinction between the superficial and deep lobes. They can invade locally throughout the gland, compromising facial nerve function if trunks of the nerve are invaded. Extraparotid extension can occur laterally into skin or medially into the pterygopalatine fossa and lateral parapharyngeal space, resulting in trismus or invasion of the carotid sheath. Bone invasion is uncommon. Adenoid cystic carcinomas in particular can invade nerve fibres spreading up the facial nerve in the parapharyngeal space towards the stylomastoid foramen or along the auriculotemporal nerve (a branch of the trigeminal nerve) to the foramen ovale.

The parotid gland contains several intraparotid lymph nodes. The superficial intraparotid nodes are on the external surface of the gland, and the deep nodes are found within the gland, mainly adjacent to the external carotid artery and external jugular vein. Parotid tumours can spread via the intraparotid nodes to the subparotid nodes in the retrostyloid space and thence to the retropharyngeal nodes, or directly to level II nodes (Figure 15.1).

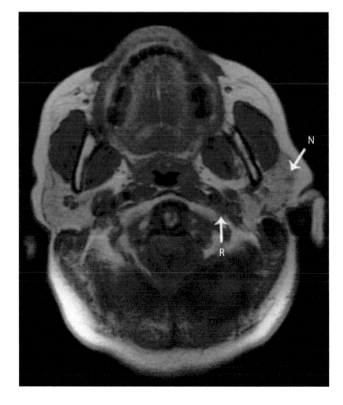

FIGURE 15.1   Axial T1-weighted MRI showing intraparotid lymph node (N) and the location of the subparotid nodes in the retrostyloid space (R).

Tumours of the submandibular salivary gland can invade locally or perineurally. Innervation of the gland is via the lingual nerve (a branch of mandibular division of the trigeminal nerve, V3) and the chorda tympani branches of the facial nerve, but spread via the chorda tympani is not common. The hypoglossal nerve lies close to the deep portion of the gland. Lymphatic drainage is to level Ib nodes lying adjacent to but not within the salivary gland and then to ipsilateral level II nodes.

There are minor salivary glands submucosally throughout the upper aerodigestive tract and malignant salivary tumours can occur in any site. The hard palate is the most common location for such tumours which spread to the same lymph nodes as squamous cell carcinomas at those sites.

Assessment of Primary Disease

Clinical examination can reveal invasion of local structures such as the skin, facial nerve (palsy) or pterygoid muscles (trismus), or spread to draining lymph nodes. Fine needle aspiration or core biopsy is usually performed under ultrasound guidance to provide confirmation of malignancy.

Cross-sectional imaging is performed to assess extent of the primary tumour particularly at the deep margin adjacent to the parapharyngeal space and to assess local lymph nodes. MRI is preferred to CT as primary tumours are better defined and nerve enhancement can be assessed. Scans should include imaging of the skull base. Preoperative cross-sectional imaging should be obtained in all patients suspected of having malignant tumours to enable more accurate postoperative volumes to be defined.

Data Acquisition

Immobilization

Patients should be immobilized lying supine with the neck slightly extended to move the orbits superiorly and reduce the chance of beams exiting through the eye. A thermoplastic shell with at least five fixation points should ideally be used even if the neck is not included in the treatment volume, as systematic and random errors will be smaller and CTV-PTV margins can be tighter.

CT Scanning

CT slices are obtained from the skull base to the hyoid in patients not requiring neck radiotherapy, or from the skull base to the arch of the aorta if the neck is to be irradiated. Slices should be 2–3 mm thick. Intravenous contrast will help define adjacent vascular structures and nodal volumes.

Fusion of planning MRI and CT images can be particularly helpful where there is extensive perineural invasion which necessitates inclusion of the skull base in the target volume.

Target Volume Definition

Parotid

The planning CT (and MRI if performed) should be carefully evaluated to detect macroscopic residual disease or lymphadenopathy. Preoperative imaging and discussions with the surgeon and pathologist are important. As radiotherapy is usually given as an adjuvant to surgery, no GTV is usually defined. It can be helpful to define the original extent of the tumour on the planning CT in order to help define the CTV. If there is macroscopic residual disease on the planning CT, or the site of an R1 resection or a node with ECS can be clearly defined as GTV, this can be expanded by 5 mm and treated to a higher dose than CTV_HIGH, e.g. 65 Gy in 30 fractions.

The CTV_HIGH is contoured as the sites of possible microscopic disease. Particular attention is given to the deep excision margin which is likely to be close or involved if the facial nerve has been preserved. As a minimum, the medial extent of the CTV_HIGH should be to the lateral surface of the internal jugular vein, but if the deep lobe of the parotid is thought to contain tumour, the parapharyngeal space should be included. The lateral extent of the CTV_HIGH will be close to the surface of the skin. The position of the contralateral parotid on the planning CT can be a useful guide to the superior and inferior limits of the CTV_HIGH.

In parotid tumours with microscopic perineural invasion, the CTV_HIGH should include the course of the facial nerve up to the stylomastoid foramen at the skull base. For adenoid cystic cancers, or any tumour with perineural invasion of large nerves, the course of the auriculotemporal nerve to the foramen ovale should also be covered. (See Figure 15.2.)

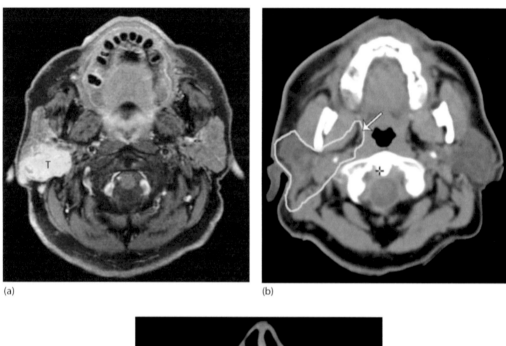

(a)   (b)

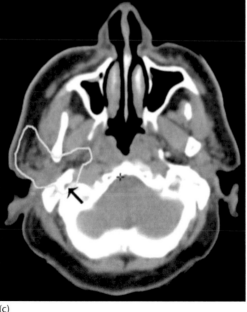

(c)

FIGURE 15.2 Target volume definition for an adenoid cystic tumour of the deep lobe of the parotid gland. (a) Axial T1-weighted contrast-enhanced MRI showing primary Tumour (T); (b) corresponding planning CT scan showing CTV including the parapharyngeal space (arrowed); (c) axial planning CT slice close to the skull base. The course of the facial nerve up to the stylomastoid foramen (arrowed) is included in the CTV.

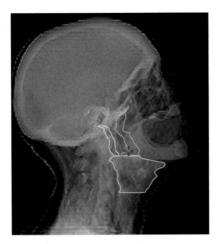

FIGURE 15.3 Lateral projection of adjuvant radiotherapy contours for a pT2N0 adenoid cystic cancer of the right submandibular gland. The course of the mandibular nerve (green) and hypoglossal nerve (yellow) are included in the CTV.

After a neck dissection, any nodal level with involved nodes should be included in the CTV_HIGH. There is no consensus on whether to include nodal levels that have been dissected but in which there were no involved nodes. We recommend including nodal levels immediately adjacent to those containing tumour – so if levels II and III are involved then include levels Ib, II, III, IVa, Va and retrostyloid nodes.

If a high-grade parotid tumour has been resected with no neck dissection, the ipsilateral level Ib, II and III nodes should be included in the treated volume. A separate CTV_LOW can be defined to give these sites a prophylactic dose, though they may also be included within CTV_HIGH if the risk of nodal relapse is felt to be high.

The CTV is expanded isotropically to form the PTV by a margin determined for each department by the observed random and systematic errors – usually 3–5 mm.

The contralateral parotid gland does not usually receive sufficient dose to cause xerostomia, but it should be contoured as an organ at risk if the mean dose to the gland is expected to be >24 Gy. The ipsilateral inner ear should be defined as an OAR, as reducing dose to the cochlear apparatus can reduce the risk of sensorineural hearing loss.

Other Sites

Similar principles can be applied for volume definition for tumours of the submandibular or minor salivary glands. In adenoid cystic carcinomas the nerve innervating the primary tumour site should be included up to the skull base.

In submandibular tumours with microscopic perineural invasion the course of the mandibular nerve to the foramen ovale should be included, with the course of the facial nerve to the stylomastoid foramen also included if there is macroscopic perineural invasion. The course of the hypoglossal nerve to the hypoglossal canal can be included if there is deep extraparenchymal extension. (See Figure 15.3.)

For tumours arising in or close to midline (e.g. hard palate), prophylactic lymph node volumes should be outlined bilaterally if lymph nodes are to be included in the CTV.

Dose Solutions

Complex

IMRT or VMAT are preferred in order to be able to treat the complex PTV shapes while minimizing dose to critical normal structures. Four to five ipsilateral IMRT beams or one/two arcs can provide excellent coverage while minimizing dose to contralateral structures. Using non-coplanar beams can also help

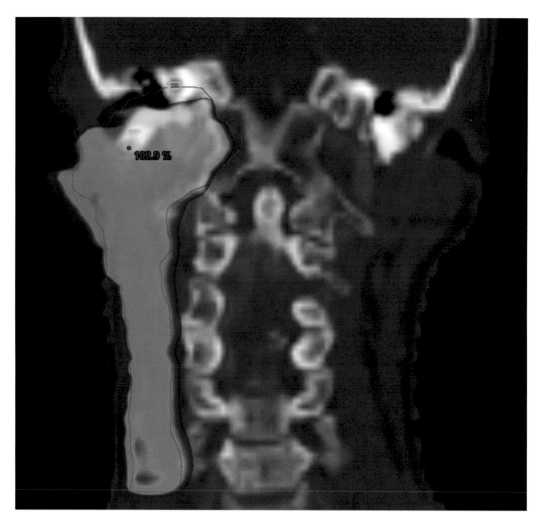

FIGURE 15.4 Adjuvant radiotherapy for a parotid tumour showing colour wash of 95 percent dose. Note how coverage of the PTV (red) has been compromised in this patient to spare the cochlea (green).

avoid critical structures and oral cavity mucosa. The PTV often comes close to the cochlea or inner ear, so compromise may be needed to either treat the PTV adequately or to avoid exceeding the ideal tolerance dose as shown in Figure 15.4. It is important to consider patient preferences and contralateral ear function when deciding this compromise, as some people are more willing to accept a risk of unilateral deafness than others. High dose in the temporomandibular joint (TMJ) should also be avoided if possible to reduce the risk of long-term TMJ dysfunction and trismus.

The PTV may come close to the skin surface, in which case it can be difficult to cover the lateral surface of the PTV unless tissue equivalent bolus is used. However, bolus is only recommended if there is a risk of microscopic residual disease in the skin. This is an uncommon situation, as involved skin is usually resected and a myocutaneous flap used to fill the defect. This new skin will not contain microscopic disease. The shell should not be cut out over the treated volume.

Conformal

Two or three ipsilateral photon beams will usually provide homogeneous dose distribution to the CTV without exceeding the tolerance of adjacent critical structures. The anterior oblique beam angle is chosen according to the shape of the anteromedial edge of the PTV while trying to minimize dose to the mucosa of the oral cavity and oropharynx. The posterior oblique angle is chosen according to the contour of the posterolateral edge of the PTV and should be lateral to the spinal cord and brainstem. The exit dose from this beam should be inferior to the contralateral eye. This is usually achieved by immobilizing the patient with the neck slightly extended, but half beam blocking may be needed if the PTV extends more superiorly. An additional lateral photon beam may provide a more homogeneous distribution but will increase dose to the contralateral parotid gland and possibly to the spinal cord. All beams should be shaped to the PTV contour with MLCs.

If level III and IV nodes are to be treated, an anterior neck beam matched to a parotid and upper neck plan can be used. The match plane should be inferior to any preoperative lymphadenopathy to avoid a junction through microscopic residual disease.

Dose Fractionation

Adjuvant

- 60 Gy in 30 daily fractions given in six weeks
  - PTV_HIGH receives 60 Gy in 30 fractions
  - PTV_LOW receives 54 Gy in 30 fractions

Verification

See Chapter 8.

Treatment Delivery and Patient Care

The amount of oral cavity and oropharynx included in the treatment volume may predict the degree of swallowing problems seen during treatment. Advice on jaw exercises can reduce the risk of trismus and TMJ dysfunction.

Conductive hearing loss due to middle ear effusions can occur during radiotherapy and take several months to improve after treatment has finished. If subjective hearing loss persists two months after treatment, an audiogram should be performed. If there is evidence of conductive hearing loss, a grommet may be indicated.

Key Trials

> Nutting CM, Morden JP, Beasley M, et al. Results of a multicentre randomised controlled trial of cochlear-sparing intensity-modulated radiotherapy versus conventional radiotherapy in patients with parotid cancer (COSTAR; CRUK/08/004). Eur J Cancer 2018;103:249–258.

INFORMATION SOURCES

Armstrong K, Ward J, Hughes NM, et al. Guidelines for clinical target volume definition for perineural spread of major salivary gland cancers. Clin Oncol 2018;30:773–779.

Ko HC, Gupta V, Mourad WF, et al. A contouring guide for head and neck cancers with perineural invasion. Pract Radiat Oncol 2014;4:247–258.

16

Sinuses: Maxilla, Ethmoid and Nasal Cavity Tumours

Indications for Radiotherapy

Tumours arising in the sinonasal region usually present with symptoms of local invasion, and the importance of local extent is reflected in the T stage (see Table 16.1).

Lymphatic spread and distant metastases are unusual, so surgery and radiotherapy to the primary site are the main treatments. Fifty percent of tumours appear to arise in the maxilla with 25 percent each in the nasal cavity and ethmoids. Primary tumours of the frontal or sphenoid sinus are very rare.

Squamous cell cancers are the commonest histological subtype (50 percent), and radiotherapy is often combined with chemotherapy in advanced disease on the basis that there is additional benefit from combined treatment in other head and neck squamous cell cancers.

There are many other tumour types that all have slightly different clinicopathological characteristics. Adenoid cystic cancers have a propensity for perineural spread, so radiotherapy volumes need to include the course of the relevant nerve to the skull base. Olfactory neuroblastomas (aesthesioneuroblastoma) arise in the olfactory epithelium of the superior nasal cavity and can invade the cribriform plate and anterior cranial fossa. This is important when planning both surgery (craniofacial resection) and radiotherapy. Adenocarcinomas usually start in the middle meatus or ethmoid sinus and are related to exposure to hardwood dust. Other rarer tumours include sinonasal undifferentiated carcinomas (SNUC) and chondrosarcomas.

TABLE 16.1

Tumour Staging for Nasal Cavity and Paranasal Sinuses Excluding Sinonasal Melanoma

	Maxilla	Nasal Cavity and Ethmoids
Tx	Primary tumour cannot be assessed	Primary tumour cannot be assessed
Tis	Carcinoma in situ	Carcinoma in situ
T1	Tumour limited to maxillary sinus mucosa with no erosion or destruction of bone	Tumour restricted to any one subsite, with or without bony invasion
T2	Tumour causing bone erosion or destruction including extension into the hard palate and/or middle nasal meatus, except extension to the posterior wall of maxillary sinus and pterygoid plates	Tumour invading two subsites in a single region or extending to involve an adjacent region within the nasoethmoidal complex, with or without bony invasion
T3	Tumour invades any of the following: bone of the posterior wall of maxillary sinus, subcutaneous tissues, floor or medial wall of orbit, pterygoid fossa, ethmoid sinuses	Tumour extends to invade the medial wall or floor of the orbit, maxillary sinus, palate or cribriform plate
T4a	Moderately advanced local disease. Tumour invades anterior orbital contents, skin of cheek, pterygoid plates, infratemporal fossa, cribriform plate, sphenoid or frontal sinuses	Moderately advanced local disease. Tumour invades any of the following: anterior orbital contents, skin of nose or cheek, minimal extension to anterior cranial fossa, pterygoid plates, sphenoid or frontal sinuses
T4b	Very advanced local disease. Tumour invades any of the following: orbital apex, dura, brain, middle cranial fossa, cranial nerves other than maxillary division of the trigeminal nerve (V2), nasopharynx or clivus	Very advanced local disease. Tumour invades any of the following: orbital apex, dura, brain, middle cranial fossa, cranial nerves other than maxillary division of the trigeminal nerve (V2), nasopharynx or clivus

Source: Adapted from UICC TNM (8th edn, 2018, with permission).

DOI: 10.1201/9781315171562-16

Malignant melanomas can arise from the nasal cavity mucosa, especially the lateral wall. Depth of invasion does not correlate well with prognosis. Sinonasal melanomas behave unpredictably but almost inevitably recur at some point, often locally. This means a more palliative approach should be considered in the elderly or those with poor performance status. Molecular genetic analysis for BRAF and C-KIT mutations should be performed to see if immunotherapy or target agents might be effective.

Adjuvant Radiotherapy

Surgery is the treatment of choice for almost all sinonasal malignancies, often with endoscopic endonasal resection. Adjuvant radiotherapy is recommended in most cases as it is difficult to resect these tumours en bloc with clear margins. There is nonrandomized trial evidence that radiotherapy improves local recurrence rates for all tumour types. The exception is completely resected T1 disease where recurrence rates are likely to be low. It may also be appropriate not to irradiate after surgery for sinonasal melanoma, reserving radiotherapy for the almost inevitable recurrence.

Combined surgery and postoperative radiotherapy lead to optimal five-year survival rates of 50 percent in maxillary sinus squamous cell cancers, 60 percent in ethmoid adenocarcinoma, 75 percent in olfactory neuroblastoma and 30 percent in sinonasal melanoma.

Primary Radiotherapy

If complete resection is considered impossible because of invasion of local structures (e.g. cranial fossa, masticator space) or if the patient declines surgery, primary radiotherapy can be used to obtain local control and, very occasionally, cure. There is no evidence supporting neoadjuvant radiotherapy as a way to downstage a tumour to reduce surgical morbidity.

Palliative Radiotherapy

Bleeding and pain can often be effectively palliated with short courses of palliative radiotherapy. This approach can be valuable in patients with poor performance status who are too frail to undergo curative treatment, or when the tumour has metastasized.

Sequencing of Multimodality Therapy

Adjuvant radiotherapy should begin after adequate surgical healing – usually about six weeks after surgery. Concomitant chemotherapy with cisplatin may be given in locally advanced squamous cell carcinomas, particularly if disease is unresectable or if excision margins are positive, though the evidence base for this is extrapolated from squamous cell cancer in other head and neck sites.

Neoadjuvant chemotherapy is sometimes used before radiation when an unresectable tumour is growing very quickly and is threatening sight.

Clinical and Radiological Anatomy

The nasal cavity, ethmoid sinuses and maxillary sinuses are interconnected mucosa-lined spaces in close proximity to the orbit and anterior cranial fossa (Figure 16.1). Most tumours present with symptoms from spread outside the sinuses. An understanding of the 3D anatomy is important to assess disease and to determine target volumes for radiotherapy.

Maxillary tumours can extend through the anterior wall to invade the cheek or posteriorly into the pterygopalatine fossa and masticator space (infratemporal fossa) causing trismus, and from there to the middle cranial fossa. Inferior extension into and through the floor of the maxilla may result in loose teeth or an oroantral fistula.

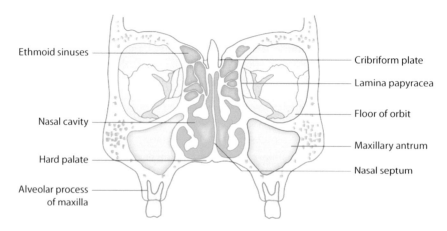

FIGURE 16.1   Anterior view of the paranasal sinuses.

It is relatively easy for tumour to grow into the orbit superiorly through the inferior orbital fissure, or for ethmoid tumour to grow into the orbit through the thin lamina papyracea. Ethmoid tumours can also grow superiorly through the cribriform plate and into the anterior cranial fossa, and anteriorly into the nasal cavity.

MRI with gadolinium enhancement is the imaging modality of choice as it can assess local extent and differentiate tumour from retained secretions. CT often provides additional information, particularly in assessing bone invasion if cribriform plate erosion or early orbital involvement is suspected.

Lymph node involvement is seen in less than 20 percent of tumours but the neck should be examined clinically and radiologically. Olfactory neuroblastomas have a higher rate of nodal involvement, and tumours invading the anterior nose and cheek have a higher risk of lymphatic spread than those contained within the sinuses. Lymphatic spread is also more common in tumours invading adjacent mucosal surfaces such as the nasopharynx. Level Ib and II nodes are most likely to be involved.

Metastases at presentation are uncommon but all patients should have a chest CT and appropriate investigation of symptoms suggestive of metastases.

Assessment of Primary Disease

Owing to the late presentation, it can be difficult to determine the exact primary site, so possible spread to all the sinonasal subsites should be assessed clinically and radiologically.

Clinical assessment includes nasendoscopy to assess the nasal cavity and examination of the oral cavity to check for inferior extension. Pterygopalatine fossa extension may lead to trismus, infraorbital canal involvement to facial pain and paraesthesia and orbital cavity spread to proptosis and diplopia, all of which should be sought.

Several surgical approaches are possible and need to be understood to define target volumes in the adjuvant setting.

Endoscopic techniques are used for many patients, as they have less morbidity than open surgery. Tumours are removed piecemeal but with multiple margin biopsies to assess completeness of excision. The technique is not suitable when the orbit and skull base are thought to be at risk.

A lateral rhinotomy allows access to the medial maxilla, the nasal cavity and the ethmoid, sphenoid and frontal sinuses. It has been superseded for many tumours by a midfacial degloving approach. In this operation, a sublabial incision allows the soft tissues of the face to be elevated to provide greater bilateral access, though access to the frontal sinus is more limited.

A craniofacial approach enables assessment and resection of the anterior skull base at the cribriform plate with en bloc resection of tumour involving the ethmoids. If there is tumour invading the medial wall of the orbit but not the periosteum (i.e. no tumour within the orbital cavity), part of the orbital periosteum can be resected. This enables the eye to be spared but presents a challenge in planning radiotherapy. Frozen sections are used to define margins of excision.

Data Acquisition

Immobilization

Patients should be immobilized supine in a thermoplastic shell. If the neck is not irradiated, the shoulders do not need to be immobilized.

A mouth bite is used if it can be tolerated, to depress the tongue and oral cavity away from the treated volume and reduce acute morbidity. Patients should be asked to look straight ahead to avoid rotating the lens or retina, particularly if the orbital cavity is included in the treated volume. Wax plugs in the nostrils are used if the tumour extends inferiorly in the nasal cavity to enable a more uniform dose distribution.

CT Scanning

A CT scan is performed with slices no more than 3 mm thick from the vertex to the hyoid bone (but extended to include the low neck if neck nodes are to be treated). Imaging the whole head is important if non-coplanar beams are to be used in the treatment plan (see more on this later in the chapter).

Fused CT-MRI images can be useful in the definition of the optic pathways and skull base. MRI also allows retained secretions to be differentiated from tumour where resection has been incomplete.

Target Volume Definition

Where resection is not possible or has been incomplete, the GTV is outlined, but defining the CTV is the most important step for most patients.

The proximity of these tumours to critical structures such as the optic nerves and chiasm, brainstem and lacrimal glands mandates meticulous CTV definition so that radiotherapy can be targeted to sites at highest risk of relapse in individual tumours and reduce the risk of long-term radiation damage. The importance of discussion between the surgeon, pathologist and radiation oncologist in defining sites at greatest risk of recurrence after surgery cannot be overemphasized. Preoperative imaging should be viewed beside the CT planning data set to ensure that initial sites of disease are adequately treated. It can be helpful to delineate the preoperative tumour extent on the planning CT.

The CTV should encompass all initial sites of disease (presurgery GTV), the mucosa of adjacent compartments of the sinonasal complex and at least a 10 mm margin from initial sites of GTV where no good bony barrier to invasion exists (e.g. masticator space, cribriform plate and infraorbital fissure) (Figure 16.2).

For most tumours, the CTV will include the ipsilateral maxillary sinus and nasal cavity and the ethmoid sinuses bilaterally. The superior extent can be modified for a very inferior tumour. Where the primary involved the maxilla, consideration should be given to including the pterygopalatine fossa and masticator space. When a maxillary tumour has invaded inferiorly, the hard palate should be included in the CTV so as to allow a 10 mm margin around the original disease.

The CTV for tumours involving the ethmoid sinuses should include the sphenoid sinus. Where initial disease came close to the orbit or invaded the lamina papyracea, the CTV should include that portion of the medial and inferior orbital wall (Figure 16.3). The orbital cavity should be included in the CTV if the orbital wall has been breached by tumour or if tumour has grown superiorly through the inferior orbital fissure. Where a craniofacial excision has been carried out, the CTV should extend 10 mm superior to the cribriform plate or 10 mm superior to initial sites of disease, whichever is greater. Olfactory neuroblastomas arise from the cribriform plate and particular attention should be paid to the CTV at this site.

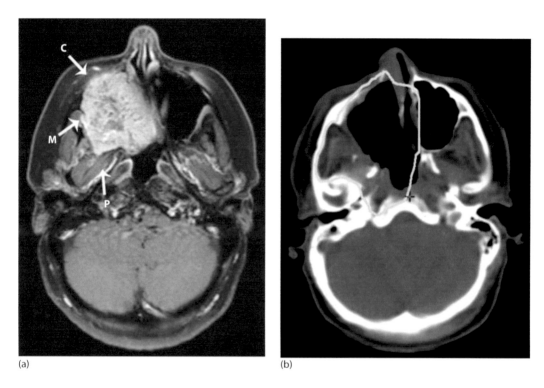

(a)   (b)

FIGURE 16.2 Definition of CTV for a pT4a carcinoma of the maxilla resected with clear margins. (a) Preoperative T1-weighted contrast-enhanced MRI showing primary tumour invading the cheek (C), masticator space (M) and lateral pterygoid muscle (P). (b) Corresponding planning CT slice showing CTV.

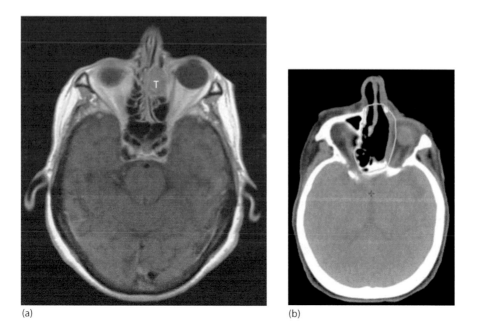

(a)   (b)

FIGURE 16.3 CTV for an olfactory neuroblastoma invading the lamina papyracea but not into the orbit. (a) Preoperative T1-weighted contrast-enhanced MRI showing primary Tumour (T) close to the left orbit. (b) Corresponding planning CT slice showing CTV including the medial portion of the orbital wall.

As local relapse in the primary site is usually the greatest risk, lateral neck nodes are often not treated in sinonasal tumours. Elective lymph node irradiation to ipsilateral levels 1b and II should be considered in tumours invading the oral cavity, pharynx or skin, or in T3/T4 maxillary squamous cell cancers. If the primary was close to or invading the nasopharynx, the adjacent ipsilateral retropharyngeal nodes should be also included in the CTV.

The CTV is expanded isotropically (usually by 3–5 mm but determined by local audit) to form the PTV.

Organs at risk to be outlined include the lenses, lacrimal glands (in the superolateral orbit and upper eyelid), optic nerves and chiasm, spinal cord, brainstem and pituitary gland. Many of these structures are easier to contour on fused MRI images than on the CT data set. In this case, the accuracy of image fusion needs to be carefully assessed. The optic nerves and chiasm are expanded by 2–3 mm to create a PRV to account for systematic and random errors.

Dose Solutions

Complex

IMRT or arc therapy provides the most conformal dose distribution to the unusual PTVs in sinonasal cancer, which are usually in close proximity to critical structures. A non-coplanar arrangement of three to five sagittal midline beams with right and left lateral beams avoids entry or exit of beams through the eyes and provides a more uniform dose distribution than a conformal plan (Figures 16.4–16.6). Five- or seven-field coplanar beams have been used, but these arrangements will increase dose to the orbital contents.

The course of the optic nerves becomes more medial at the posterior part of the orbital cavity as they exit through the optic canal. At this point, the nerves commonly overlap the PTV and there must still be either an acceptance of increased risk of blindness or a reduction in PTV coverage. We recommend not exceeding PRV tolerance doses unless there is thought to be a high risk of blindness from the tumour itself – for example in unresectable disease already compromising vision in that eye. It may be appropriate to accept a higher dose to one optic nerve if the other nerve is within tolerance and has good function. Other factors to consider in this compromise are the proportion of the optic apparatus that is over tolerance and, crucially, the patient's wishes.

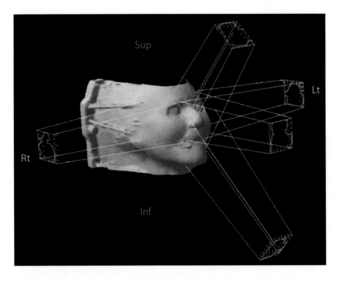

FIGURE 16.4 Beam arrangement for IMRT of sinonasal tumours.

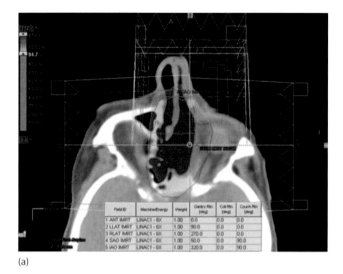

(a)

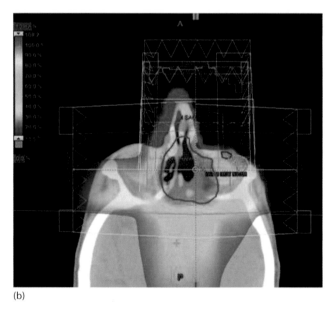

(b)

FIGURE 16.5 IMRT dose solution for a sinonasal tumour. (a) Note the more homogeneous coverage of the PTV than the conformal solution (Figure 16.7) provides. Colour wash scale is set from 95 percent. (b) Dose colour wash to illustrate relative sparing of the left lacrimal gland (pink) and lens (blue).

Beams should not enter, or ideally exit, through the eye. Lacrimal gland tolerance can almost always be maintained, but the relatively low dose at which damage occurs means the bilateral lacrimal glands should be contoured as organs at risk. Lens doses should be minimized, but a cataract is relatively easy to treat with surgery.

As with all plans, OAR doses, PTV coverage and dose homogeneity should also be reviewed and documented in the treatment planning system.

Conformal

The most common beam non-IMRT technique for sinonasal tumours uses an anterior beam to provide most of the dose, with an ipsilateral or bilateral wedged lateral beams added to provide extra dose to

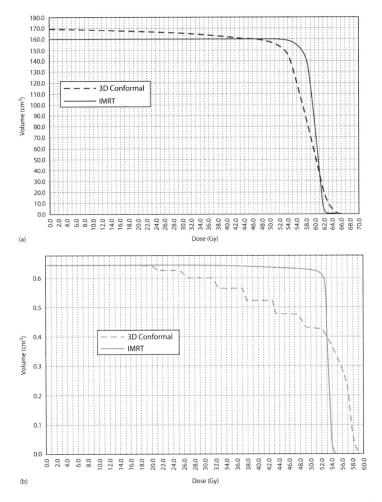

FIGURE 16.6 DVHs comparing plans shown in Figure 16.7 (3D conformal) and 16.5 (IMRT). Prescribed dose 60 Gy in 30 fractions. (a) PTV. (b) Ipsilateral (left) optic nerve. Note that in the conformal plan, dose to the nerve exceeds tolerance (55 Gy) and the prescribed dose would have to be reduced.

the posterior part of the PTV (Figure 16.7). MLCs are used to shape each beam to the PTV. The lateral fields have their anterior border behind the lens and can be angled 5° posteriorly to avoid exiting through the contralateral lens. As a result, not all the PTV will be within the lateral beams. This arrangement cannot provide a uniform dose distribution. Hot spots of >110 percent are usually found anteriorly, and inadequate posterior coverage occurs in spite of the lateral beams.

Dose Fractionation

Adjuvant

- 60 Gy in 30 fractions over six weeks with 54 Gy in 30 fractions to elective nodal volumes if treated.
- 66–70 Gy in 33–35 fractions over six and a half weeks if possible where there is residual or unresectable disease.

Palliative

- 30 Gy in 10 fractions over two weeks
- 30 Gy in 5 fractions of 6 Gy treating once weekly

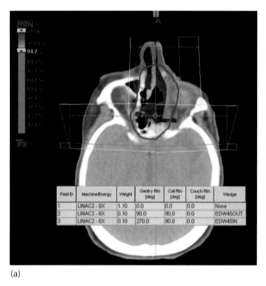

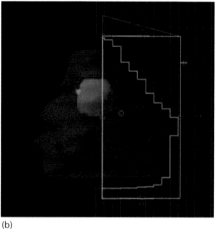

(a)   (b)

FIGURE 16.7   Conformal radiotherapy for sinonasal tumors. (a) Beam arrangement. Colour wash scale is set from 95 percent to demonstrate the hot spot anteriorly and the underdosing posteriorly. (b) BEV of left lateral beam. This beam is to add dose to the posterior part of the PTV only. Left eyeball green; lens yellow.

Verification

IGRT is essential for complex radiotherapy techniques used in sinonasal tumours, particularly when the target volumes are close to the brainstem and optic apparatus. Daily kV-CBCT imaging with online correction is recommended if resources are available.

Treatment Delivery and Patient Care

Patients are seen weekly during treatment in a multidisciplinary clinic. Exercises to reduce trismus (e.g. jaw stretching with spatulas or Therabite™) are recommended if there is preexisting trismus or where the masticator muscles are in the treated volume. Prophylactic feeding tubes are not usually required but should be considered when the patient is malnourished or has trismus and the treated volume includes a significant portion of the oral cavity (e.g. in maxillary sinus tumours). Careful oral hygiene is essential with prompt treatment of oral Candida infections.

   Where the cornea is within the treated volume, regular ophthalmic review should be carried out both during and after radiotherapy. Lubricating eye ointments can be applied during the day and at night. If there is a preexisting facial nerve palsy, the eyelid should be taped shut at night to avoid corneal abrasions.

   Pituitary function tests should be carried out annually during follow-up to evaluate late radiotherapy effects to the gland if it has received a mean dose of >20 Gy.

Key Trials   None in this rare cancer.

INFORMATION SOURCES

Dirix P, Vanstraelen B, Jorissen M, et al. Intensity-modulated radiotherapy for sinonasal cancer: Improved outcome compared to conventional radiotherapy. Int J Radiat Oncol Biol Phys 2010;78:998–1004.

Nenclares P, Ap Dafydd D, Bagwan I, et al. Head and neck mucosal melanoma: The United Kingdom national guidelines. Eur J Cancer 2020;138:11–18.

17

Orbit

Indications for Radiotherapy

Intraocular Tumours

Metastases to the vascular choroidal layer, which is part of the uvea, are the most common intraocular tumours. They usually present with reduced visual acuity and are treated with palliative external beam radiotherapy, which may need to be delivered urgently to help preserve vision. Breast and lung cancers are the most common primary tumours. Choroidal metastases usually indicate widespread disease and a poor prognosis except in some breast cancer patients.

The most frequent primary intraocular tumour is choroidal melanoma. Tumours arising in the choroid have a 30 per cent chance of metastasis at five years, usually to the liver, while rarer iris or conjunctival melanomas have a much lower risk. Liver metastases can also occur many years after initial therapy. Tumour size is the most important prognostic factor. Small melanomas are usually asymptomatic and can be difficult to differentiate from various benign conditions, so observation may be recommended at first.

Small tumours with minimal extraocular extension can be treated with plaque brachytherapy for example using ruthenium-106 or iodine-125. The plaque is temporarily sutured to the sclera underlying the melanoma and left in place for five to seven days. Doses 70–100 Gy to the apex of the tumour are usually used. Alternative treatment options include fractionated protons or stereotactic radiotherapy. Larger tumours are treated with enucleation or, occasionally, with eye-preserving surgery and adjuvant brachytherapy or external beam radiotherapy.

Radiotherapy can be used for cure of retinoblastoma but because there is a high incidence of second malignancies in heritable retinoblastoma, chemotherapy is now preferred, and radiation is only used when other treatment has not worked. Brachytherapy and protons are preferred to external beam radiotherapy to reduce dose to nearby structures.

Orbital lymphomas are usually low grade and confined to the conjunctiva or posterior orbital contents though they can also occur in the lacrimal glands. Fifteen per cent are bilateral, though the contralateral disease may occur some years later. Conjunctival lymphomas present as salmon-coloured patches on the sclera and can be treated with radiotherapy using electrons or superficial X-rays, though observation for very small tumours may be appropriate. Low-grade tumours in the orbit can cause exophthalmos or diplopia, and respond well to radiotherapy. In high-grade tumours or if there is systemic disease, initial chemotherapy followed by consolidation radiotherapy to the orbit is usually recommended.

Extraocular Tumours

Tumours arising from the skin or other structures close to the eye need careful multidisciplinary assessment. Local excision and reconstruction is usually preferred to radiotherapy for cosmetic and functional reasons, but radiotherapy has a 90 per cent cure rate for small basal and squamous cell carcinomas arising from the skin and lower eyelid. Superficial photons or electrons are used for early disease, whereas

DOI: 10.1201/9781315171562-17

EBRT can be used as an alternative to exenteration in more advanced disease, or can be considered following exenteration if excision margins are close or involved.

Primary lacrimal gland and nasolacrimal duct carcinomas are usually treated with excision and postoperative radiotherapy, preserving the eye if at all possible.

Clinical and Radiological Anatomy

The eye is composed of three layers. An outer fibrous layer is formed by the sclera posteriorly and the cornea anteriorly. The inner layer is the sensory retina with vision concentrated at the fovea, which is lateral to the optic nerve and directly posterior to the lens. In between these is the vascular layer – the uvea or choroid – which supplies the retina. The iris is the outer continuation of the vascular layer and the lens sits just behind it, suspended from the ciliary body. The eye has no lymphatic drainage (Figure 17.1).

The extraocular structures often need to be considered and contoured as critical structures in radiotherapy. The optic nerve can clearly be seen on cross-sectional imaging and leaves the orbit via the optic canal to form the optic chiasm. The lacrimal gland sits mainly in the lacrimal fossa – the undersurface of the orbital plate of the frontal bone – but also has a palpebral portion within the upper eyelid. It can be difficult to see on imaging. Tears from the eye drain through the nasolacrimal duct within the nasolacrimal canal, which runs from the lacrimal sac to the inferior nasal meatus between the inferior concha and nasal cavity floor. Tumour invasion, surgery or radiation to the duct can cause epiphora.

The conjunctiva is a clear epithelial membrane containing lymphoid tissue that covers the sclera and the inner surface of the eyelids, producing protective mucus and tears.

The orbit is conical and formed by the fusion of several bones, the thinnest of which is the lamina papyracea of the ethmoid bone, which forms part of the medial wall. Tumour can grow into the middle cranial fossa through the superior orbital fissure and optic canal or into the pterygopalatine fossa and masticator space via the inferior orbital fissure.

Only the eyelids, conjunctiva and lacrimal glands have lymphatic drainage, and they drain to the preauricular nodes.

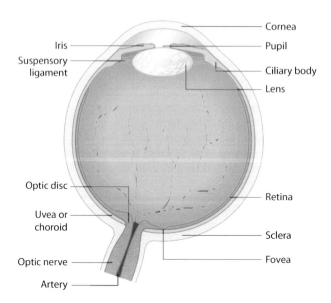

FIGURE 17.1   Anatomy of the eye.

Assessment of Primary Disease

The oncologist and ophthalmologist should jointly assess any intraocular tumour after the pupil has been dilated. Extraocular tumours are best assessed by cross-sectional imaging with MRI scans with coronal and sagittal reconstructions. CT may be complementary to MRI in assessing bone involvement. Clinical examination can also help define extraocular spread into the superior orbital fissure (which causes cranial nerve palsies of VI and then of III, IV and VI) or into the pterygopalatine fossa and masticator space via the inferior orbital fissure (causing trismus). Careful examination of eye movements can help distinguish invasion of the external ocular muscles from cranial neuropathies. Invasion of the ethmoid sinuses or the nasopharynx can be assessed at nasendoscopy.

Data Acquisition

Immobilisation

The proximity of target volumes to several critical normal structures means excellent immobilisation is vital. A custom-made thermoplastic shell is created with the patient supine, and the chin in a neutral position.

CT Scanning

Slices no more than 3 mm thick should be obtained with the patient immobilised. Radiotherapy for choroidal metastases can be planned with virtual simulation or on a simulator, as the target volume is usually the orbital contents. When individualised volumes are defined for extraocular tumours, the volume imaged should extend from the vertex of the skull to the hyoid bone, so non-coplanar beam arrangements may be used. Intravenous contrast is not usually necessary. Fused CT and MR images can be particularly helpful to define the optic chiasm and any skull base involvement.

Target Volume Definition

Intraocular Tumours

For choroidal metastases where the target volume is the whole of the orbit and the doses used are low, field borders rather than target volumes can be defined on a CT data set or in the simulator.

The dimensions of the eye vary by only 1–2 mm between subjects, with a vertical diameter of 23 mm and a slightly larger anteroposterior diameter. A 4×4 cm beam is defined with the anterior margin at the outer canthus, and the centre of the field in line with the pupil. The beam is angled posteriorly by 5° to avoid exit through the contralateral lens. Dose is either prescribed to D_{max} or to the depth of the metastasis if known from imaging (Figure 17.2). An alternative is to use a direct anterior 4×4 cm beam centred on the pupil and to treat with the eye open to minimise lens dose. For treatment of bilateral choroidal metastases, opposing beams are used, again angled 5° posteriorly.

Whilst a similar virtual simulation technique can be used for orbital lymphomas, especially when they are bilateral, formal target volume definition allows non-coplanar beams to be used to avoid dose to the contralateral eye. The CTV is the whole orbit as defined by the bony margins and includes the conjunctiva.

For lymphoma confined to the conjunctiva, the target volume is the entire conjunctiva including the reflection behind the eyelids. This is best treated with a direct anterior beam using electrons or orthovoltage photons to minimise dose to the posterior orbit. A 5-cm circular lead cut-out is used to define the

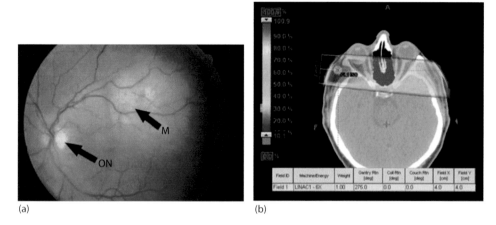

(a)   (b)

FIGURE 17.2 Palliative radiotherapy for choroidal metastasis. (a) Photograph of a choroidal metastasis (M) and optic nerve (ON) (both arrowed). (b) Dose colour wash illustrating the dose distribution created by a 4 × 4 cm lateral beam angled 5° posteriorly.

field edge. The eye should be shut during treatment, but bolus will also be required if electrons are used in order to bring up the surface dose. 6 MV photons can also be used but will give a higher exit dose to the brain (see Figure 17.3).

Extraocular Tumours

The principles of treatment for small BCCs and SqCCs close to the eye are similar to other skin cancers and are covered in the skin chapter. The target volume is the primary tumour with a 5–10 mm margin, depending on histological subtype, size and how well defined the tumour is. A lead cut-out is made to

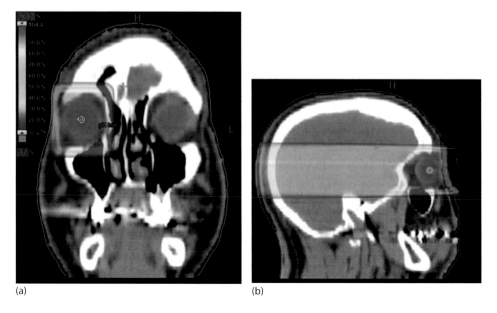

(a)   (b)

FIGURE 17.3 A 6-MV photon beam to treat conjunctival lymphoma. (a) Anterior view; (b) sagittal view. Note tissue equivalent bolus used to increase the surface dose.

define the field edge and shield adjacent structures. If the treated area is very close to the eye or involving the eyelid, an internal eye shield can be inserted for each treatment to protect the cornea and lens. The eye shield is essentially a lead contact lens inserted after local anaesthetic eye drops have been instilled. (See Figure 7.2.)

The variety of rare extraocular tumour types makes it difficult to give general recommendations for target volume definition for adjuvant external beam radiotherapy. Any residual disease is contoured as GTV. It may be helpful to define the preoperative site of disease on the planning CT scan and to expand this by 10 mm to ensure that microscopic residual disease is included. Discussion with the surgeon and pathologist may help to define locations at greatest risk of recurrence and possible patterns of spread. Elective treatment of draining lymph node regions is not necessary. A small isotropic margin is added to produce a PTV. With a good immobilisation technique, this should be 3–4 mm.

It is tempting to edit the target volumes away from critical structures with the assumption that tolerance of these structures will be exceeded unless the PTV size is reduced. The complexity of possible planning solutions with IMRT means that the compensation needed is hard to predict. We strongly recommend that tumour target volumes are not influenced by critical structures and vice versa. Any compromise needed can thus be assessed using dose distributions and DVHs to choose the plan providing the best solution. The optic nerves, chiasm, lenses, retinas, lacrimal glands and pituitary should all be contoured as OAR. See Chapter 16 for a further discussion of possible compromises.

The only motion possible with good immobilisation is that of the eye itself. Patients are usually scanned and treated with their eyes shut and eyes relaxed and looking forwards, as this is likely to be the most reproducible arrangement. Occasionally it may be helpful to ask people to look in one direction to move the fovea or lens away from radiation dose or to treat with the eye open to avoid the eyelid increasing the surface dose to the cornea.

Dose Solutions

Intraocular Tumours

For treatment to the choroid or posterior orbit, planning scan data can be used to create virtual simulation images to define the beam size and angle to minimise lens dose as just described. When the unilateral orbit is being treated in lymphoma, superior and inferior oblique beams provide good coverage of the conical PTV and avoid the contralateral eye.

Extraocular Tumours

Postoperative radiotherapy for carcinomas and sarcomas ideally requires doses of at least 60 Gy (66 Gy to sites of residual macroscopic disease), so the location and tolerance of critical structures needs to be considered from the start of the planning process.

Fractionated doses of more than 10 Gy have a high risk of inducing a cataract, but this late effect is treatable surgically. Lacrimal gland damage can occur with doses over 30 Gy and as a dry eye causes serious morbidity, great care should be taken to avoid this. Corneal ulceration is uncommon at doses below 48 Gy and can be minimised by patients being treated with the eye open to avoid any build-up effect of the overlying eyelid and by good eye care. Retinopathy can occur with doses over 30 Gy and is more common in diabetic patients. Particular care should be taken to avoid excess dose to the fovea. Optic nerve and chiasm doses should be kept below 55 Gy. It is usual for the oncologist to have to accept some compromise in PTV dose to keep all critical structures within tolerance or to accept an increased risk of late effects from delivering an adequate dose. This decision will be influenced by the risk and likely site of recurrence, and should be discussed with the radiotherapy team and the patient.

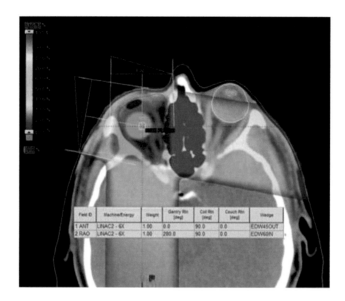

FIGURE 17.4   Conformal beam arrangement for adjuvant radiotherapy to the orbit after an enucleation. The lateral beam is angled to avoid the contralateral lens.

This trade-off between dose to the PTV and dose to many critical structures means inverse planned IMRT has some advantages over forward planned conformal therapy in these tumours. Non-coplanar beams are often used to minimise dose to the contralateral eye, with beam angles chosen to avoid ipsilateral critical structures such as the lens and lacrimal gland where possible. After an exenteration or enucleation, a simpler arrangement such as superior and inferior oblique beams with an anterior beam, or anterior and lateral beams, may be adequate (Figure 17.4).

Dose Fractionation

Choroidal Metastases

- 20 Gy in 5 fractions over one week

Low-Grade Orbital Lymphoma

- 24 Gy in 12 fractions over two and a half weeks

High-grade Lymphoma After Chemotherapy

- 30 Gy in 15 fractions over three weeks
- Doses of up to 40 Gy may be used if there is residual disease present or if chemotherapy is not used – see lymphoma chapter

Extraorbital Postoperative Radiotherapy

- 60 Gy in 30 fractions over six weeks
- Consider 66–70 Gy to any sites of macroscopic residual disease

Verification

See Chapter 8.

Treatment Delivery and Patient Care

Close liaison with the ophthalmic team during and after treatment is essential, and all patients should have a full ophthalmic assessment before radiotherapy begins. Patients should be advised on meticulous eye care and use of lubricating drops throughout treatment. There should be prompt assessment and treatment of any conjunctivitis or corneal damage.

> No randomised controlled trials in these rare tumours.

INFORMATION SOURCES

American Brachytherapy Society - Ophthalmic Oncology Task Force. The American brachytherapy society consensus guidelines for plaque brachytherapy of uveal melanoma and retinoblastoma. Brachytherapy 2014 Jan–Feb;13(1):1–14.

Nathan P, Cohen V, Coupland S, Curtis K, Damato B, et al. Uveal melanoma UK national guidelines. Eur J Cancer 2015 Nov;51(16):2404–2412.

Schwarcz RM, Coupland SE, Finger PT. Cancer of the orbit and adnexa. Am J Clin Oncol 2013 Apr;36(2):197–205.

Stannard C, Sauerwein W, Maree G, Lecuona K. Radiotherapy for ocular tumours. Eye (Lond) 2013 Feb;27(2):119–127.

Vasalaki M, Fabian ID, Reddy MA, Cohen VM, Sagoo MS. Ocular oncology: Advances in retinoblastoma, uveal melanoma and conjunctival melanoma. Br Med Bull 2017 Jan 1;121(1):107–119.

Yahalom J, Illidge T, Specht L, Hoppe RT, Li YX, et al. Modern radiation therapy for extranodal lymphomas: Field and dose guidelines from the international lymphoma radiation oncology group. Int J Radiat Oncol Biol Phys 2015 May 1;92(1):11–31.

18

Central Nervous System

Primary brain tumours are uncommon and comprise only 1.6 per cent of all primary cancers. Metastatic spread to the brain from primary cancers elsewhere in the body is more common, particularly as improvements in systemic therapy mean people are living longer with metastatic cancer. The variable behaviour of intracranial tumours depends on site and histology. Some cause problems by their intracranial extension alone (gliomas, meningiomas, pituitary tumours, metastases) while others (such as lymphomas, germ cell tumours and primitive neuroendocrine tumours [PNET]) have a predilection for leptomeningeal spread.

Primary brain tumours are classified by a combination of histology and molecular diagnostics to form an integrated diagnosis according to the WHO 2021 (CNS 5) classification. Furthermore, methylomics (using DNA methylation patterns across the genome) is increasingly used to aid classification in challenging cases. In addition to classification, molecular diagnostics provides prognostic information and is increasingly used to inform treatment options, particularly with chemotherapy. The majority of primary brain tumours are gliomas and two-thirds of these are glioblastomas. They arise from the supportive glial cells rather than the neurons themselves. Glial cells have a variety of functions, such as creating the myelin sheath around axons (oligodendrocytes), providing nutrients to enable repair (astrocytes) and producing CSF (ependymal cell). Tumours of mixed cell type can also occur. For the purposes of deciding radiotherapy dose and target volume, there are different approaches to low-grade and high-grade gliomas but not, at the moment, to different genetic variants.

This chapter also outlines radiotherapy approaches for meningioma, pituitary tumours and brain metastases in adults, and briefly discusses paediatric and rarer adult tumours.

High-Grade Glioma – Grade 3 and Grade 4 Glioma

Indications for Radiotherapy

The optimal initial treatment for high-grade glioma (HGG) is surgery. This provides immediate symptomatic relief, and the extent of resection that is achieved influences prognosis. As much of the tumour as possible is therefore usually resected whilst trying to maintain neurological function. Techniques such as fluorescent 5-aminolevulinic acid hydrochloride (5-ALA) guidance to highlight anaplastic foci of tumour and awake craniotomy with functional monitoring can be helpful in achieving this. Subsequent treatment depends on performance status, age and molecular histology.

The most common adult primary brain tumour is the glioblastoma (formerly known as glioblastoma multiforme, due to its heterogeneity, and often still abbreviated as GBM). They have a median age at diagnosis of 62 and are usually supratentorial. Mutations in the isocitrate dehydrogenase (IDH) genes define a subset of grade 4 tumours with a better prognosis. These were previously referred to as 'secondary GBMs' (as opposed to de novo IDH-wildtype GBM) but are now classed as 'astrocytoma, IDH-mutant (CNS WHO grade 4)'.

The DNA repair protein O^6-methylguanine-DNA methyltransferase (MGMT) rescues tumour cells from damage by alkylating agents such as temozolomide (TZ). Promoter methylation silences the gene resulting in reduced DNA repair activity and increased sensitivity to TZ. MGMT methylation can be assessed by PCR. The presence of methylation is a favourable prognostic factor but also indicates a higher response rate to TZ. This information is particularly relevant for older patients for whom combined RT and TZ is less well tolerated.

DOI: 10.1201/9781315171562-18

Grade 3 tumours are most commonly either oligodendrogliomas or astrocytomas, IDH mutant. Although they have different histologic appearances, the molecular signature of oligodendroglioma is the combined loss of the short arm of chromosome 1 and the long arm of chromosome 19 (1p/19q-codeletion). This confers a more favourable prognosis compared to IDH-mutant astrocytomas, which are 1p/19q-non-codeleted, with different chemotherapy regimens commonly used (PCV compared to TZ).

After maximal debulking surgery for GBM, radiotherapy is usually combined with concomitant and adjuvant temozolomide chemotherapy in patients with good performance status (KPS $\geq$ 70) who are aged around 70 or younger. This increases overall and median survival, and enables a small percentage of patients to live for many years.

In older patients, a shorter fractionation schedule such as 40 Gy in 15 fractions is often recommended, combined with concomitant and adjuvant TZ. TZ is especially effective in MGMT methylated tumours where radiotherapy is sometimes omitted.

For grade 3 tumours, maximal safe debulking surgery is the initial treatment if this is possible without compromising function. Radiotherapy is then recommended for all tumours if the patient is well enough to receive it (WHO PS 0–1).

If debulking surgery for HGG is not possible because of tumour location, symptoms or comorbidity, a biopsy will usually be performed to confirm the diagnosis and allow molecular testing. Radiotherapy is sometimes recommended as sole palliative treatment when maximal debulking surgery is not attempted but the patient is of good PS. For people with poor performance status, supportive care alone is usually the most appropriate approach, but hypofractionated radiotherapy (30 Gy in 6 fractions over two weeks) can sometimes provide useful palliation.

Sequencing of Multimodality Therapy

Surgery can be followed by radiotherapy within four to six weeks of uncomplicated recovery. For GBMs, radiotherapy following surgery extends median survival to 9–12 months. Dose escalation above 60 Gy does not improve outcomes. Chemotherapy with low-dose temozolomide (75 mg/m^2 daily) during radiotherapy and for six courses afterwards (150–200 mg/m^2 given for five days every 28 days) gives an increase in median and progression-free survival of two and a half months and survival at two years of 27.2 per cent, compared with 10.9 per cent with EBRT alone.

In grade 3 tumours, the addition of chemotherapy to radiotherapy depends on the molecular genetics of the tumour. If there is 1p/19q codeletion (oligodendroglioma) then radiotherapy and PCV chemotherapy (procarbazine, lomustine and vincristine) are both recommended. Radiotherapy is often given first followed by PCV, but there is no difference in tumour outcomes if PCV is given before radiotherapy. The choice should be discussed with the patient and may be influenced by factors such as time needed to explore fertility preservation options before chemotherapy.

In tumours without 1p/19q codeletion (astrocytoma), radiotherapy is followed by up to 12 cycles of adjuvant temozolomide.

Clinical and Radiological Anatomy

MRI should be performed at diagnosis in all patients unless it is contraindicated. T1 +/− gadolinium, T2 and FLAIR sequences are obtained. It can be helpful to repeat MRI imaging 48–72 hours after surgery to assess the extent of resection before reactive enhancement of the surgical cavity occurs, unless the patient has had a biopsy only.

Gliomas do not tend to spread to the contralateral hemisphere except via the corpus callosum. They tend to grow along the white matter tracts and do not invade the falx, tentorium or bone. Recurrences after radiotherapy tend to occur within 2 cm of the original GTV. Rarely, drop metastases can occur.

Assessment of Primary Disease

Patients should be seen as soon as they are recovered from surgery but ideally within four weeks to allow radiotherapy to start within six weeks if possible. Neurological function and performance status should be assessed. Steroid dose after surgery should be tapered as quickly as possible to reduce side effects. Patients do not need to routinely take steroids during radiotherapy. In people not able to have maximal debulking surgery, the potential benefits of palliative radiotherapy should be weighed against the likely side effects and the practical challenges of attending for multiple fractions of treatment. For some people, supportive care alone may be a more appropriate option.

Data Acquisition

The patient is immobilised supine in a thermoplastic mask. The angle of the head is usually that which is most comfortable for the patients but may be varied specifically to facilitate beam entry angles in some patients. Both CT and MRI images should be acquired with the patient in the treatment shell so that accurate fusion can be achieved, as MRI images are used to define target volumes. CT slices should be no more than 3 mm thick and obtained from the vertex of the skull to the inferior border of C3. Contrast is only necessary if there is a contraindication to MRI. T1 +/− contrast, T2 and FLAIR MRI sequences should be obtained and fused with the planning CT.

Target Volume Definition

GTV

The GTV is defined as the resection cavity, if present, and enhancing tumour on T1 + contrast MRI images. The peri-tumour oedema is not included. It can be helpful to compare post-op diffusion weighted imaging with pre-op scans to help identify postoperative vascular changes. IDH-mutant tumours can have a noncontrast enhancing component. Hyperintensity on T2 or FLAIR images can be used to identify this and include it as GTV.

CTV

An isotropic expansion of 20 mm is applied to the GTV to produce the CTV. This is then edited to take account of natural barriers to spread. The CTV can conform to the inner table of the skull. A 5-mm margin is used in the ventricles, falx, tentorium. No margin is required from GTV into brainstem or optic tracts as long as the tumour is distant to the white matter tracts that connect them. Tumours can still spread to the contralateral hemisphere via the corpus callosum, which should be included in the CTV if within the 20-mm expansion. Areas of peri-tumour oedema seen on T2 or FLAIR sequences do not need to be routinely included in CTV.

When using hypofractionated regimens in people with poor performance status, smaller GTV-CTV margins, e.g. 15 mm, can be used.

PTV

A 3–5-mm CTV-PTV expansion is performed depending on local audit of set-up errors. Tumour movement is negligible.

Dose Solutions

IMRT/VMAT or conformal beams are used, depending on the size and location of the PTV and the proximity to critical structures. The optic chiasm, optic structures and brainstem should be contoured in all patients, and tolerance doses should not be exceeded. Other organs at risk such as the cochlea or pituitary gland should be considered relative OARs, as dose to the PTV should not usually be compromised to spare them. As tolerance dose for both the optic chiasm and brainstem is <60 Gy (see OAR chapter), there will often need to be a compromise in PTV coverage when the PTV and OAR contours overlap. This is best achieved with an IMRT/VMAT plan which can limit dose to the overlapping region while trying to preserve dose to the rest of the PTV. The degree of compromise will need to be a clinical decision taking into account factors such as the expected prognosis of the patient and the proximity of gross tumour to the OAR. (See Figure 18.1.)

If IMRT is not available, two phases of treatment can be used to help spare OARs. 50GY in 25 fractions are prescribed to the whole PTV, with the final 10 Gy delivered to as much of the PTV as possible whilst not exceeding tolerance doses.

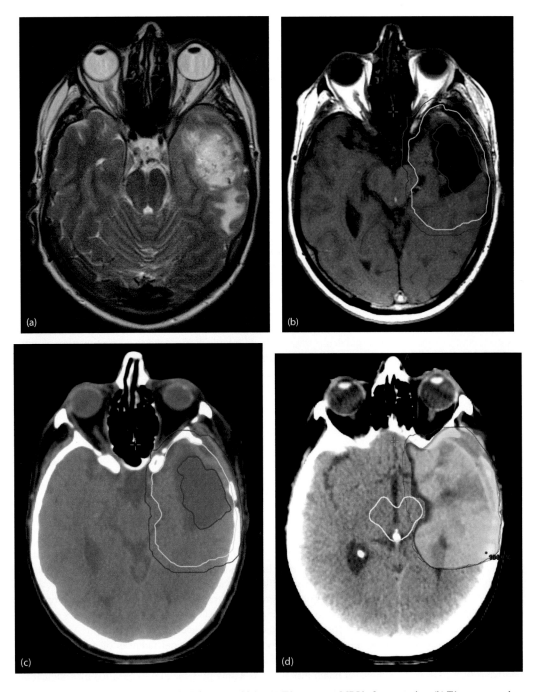

FIGURE 18.1 Glioblastoma multiforme left temporal lobe. (a) T1 + contrast MRI before resection; (b) T1 + contrast planning MRI; and (c) planning CT scan, after resection. The CT and MRI images are fused – GTV (blue), CTV (cyan) and PTV (red). (d) Ninety-five per cent dose colour wash from VMAT plan. Note how PTV (red) coverage is compromised in order to keep brainstem PRV (yellow) within tolerance.

If the GTV and OAR are very close, then it may be necessary to reduce the total dose to 54 Gy in 30 fractions, delivered in a single phase.

Dose Fractionation

GBM

- 60 Gy in 30 fractions over six weeks
- 40 Gy in 15 fractions over three weeks (elderly, good PS)

Grade 3 (with or without 1p/19q Codeletion)

- 59.4 Gy in 33 fractions over six and a half weeks

Poor Performance Status

- 30 Gy in 6 fractions over two weeks

Treatment Delivery and Patient Care

There may be an increase in peri-tumoural oedema during the first days of treatment, which may require low-dose steroids to prevent headache and vomiting. Antiemetics may also be required. Cutting out parts of the mask to reduce skin dose, for example over the ears, may help to prevent skin erythema and irritation, but adequate immobilisation must be maintained. Immobilisation may need to be adjusted with changes in steroid dose, which affect the amount of swelling of the patient's face. Hair loss from the irradiated area, including sites of exit of the beam, will start after about two weeks of treatment and will be permanent in the high-dose volumes.

Regular weekly review is essential to monitor response and check medication. This should include assessment of seizure control. Rapid deterioration during treatment may lead to discontinuation of radiotherapy. Patients and relatives often require considerable psychological support from the treatment team during this period. If temozolomide is used, blood counts should be checked weekly.

Verification

Daily cone beam CT imaging with online correction is recommended to help ensure optimal tumour coverage and OAR sparing.

Low-Grade Glioma

Indications for Radiotherapy

Low-grade gliomas (LGG) comprise a heterogeneous group of tumours which often occur at a younger age and present with more insidious symptoms than high-grade gliomas (HGG). Most are grade 2; grade 1 tumours are very rare in adults. Prognosis is variable and is adversely affected by age >40, size >5 cm, corpus callosum involvement and histology of astrocytoma rather than oligodendroglioma or mixed tumour. IDH-wildtype LGG tumours have a similar prognosis to GBM. IDH-mutant tumours are subdivided by chromosomal analysis into 1p/19q codeleted and non-codeleted groups.

Surgery is recommended for all LGG except those with radiological features of a very low-grade tumour where biopsy may be hazardous (e.g. optic pathway glioma). A maximal safe resection should be undertaken in order to remove as much tumour as is safely possible and to obtain a histological and molecular diagnosis. If a resection is not possible, a biopsy should be taken.

Initial radiotherapy is recommended in higher-risk tumours – when the patient is over 40 or a gross total resection has not been achieved. After radiotherapy, adjuvant PCV chemotherapy should be considered.

The evidence for this approach is stronger for 1p/19q codeleted tumours (oligodendroglioma) than non-codeleted (astrocytoma).

If biopsy or resection pathology and imaging show the tumour is very low grade or if an IDH-mutant tumour has been completely resected in a younger patient (age under about 40), active monitoring with MRI should be strongly considered rather than initial radiotherapy. Because LGG patients can live for many years, the possible late side effects of radiotherapy are important to consider and, where possible, to avoid. Trials of early versus delayed radiotherapy have shown similar outcomes, and the neuro-oncology team and the patient must weigh the risks and benefits of further treatment in each individual situation.

Neurological deficits caused by LGG can improve after radiotherapy, so it is still appropriate to consider radiotherapy for these patients, in contrast to HGG patients, who have a poor PS.

Sequencing of Multimodality Therapy

Radiotherapy can start within four to six weeks of surgery where recovery is uncomplicated. If PCV chemotherapy is used after radiotherapy, treatment should start four to six weeks after the end of radiotherapy.

Clinical and Radiological Anatomy

Low-grade gliomas can often be seen on CT as low-density areas, sometimes with calcification. On MRI, LGGs are best seen on T2 weighted or FLAIR MRI sequences.

Assessment of Primary Disease

As the management options for initial low-grade glioma include very different options from active monitoring to surgery, radiotherapy and chemotherapy, a multidisciplinary approach is very important. This should include psychological and rehabilitation support.

Data Acquisition

As for HGG.

Target Volume Definition

GTV is defined as the visible tumour on T2 weighted or FLAIR MRI fused with the planning CT. A 15-mm isotropic margin is added to create the CTV, which is edited from natural barriers as for HGG. A 3–5-mm PTV margin is added based on local setup variation analysis, assuming there is no movement of the tumour. (See Figure 18.2.)

Dose Solutions

As for HGG.

Dose Fractionation

- 50.4 Gy in 28 fractions over five and a half weeks
- 54 Gy in 30 fractions over six weeks for higher risk tumours

Treatment Delivery and Patient Care

As for HGG. Seizures are more common in LGG than HGG, and they may worsen during radiotherapy.

Verification

As for HGG.

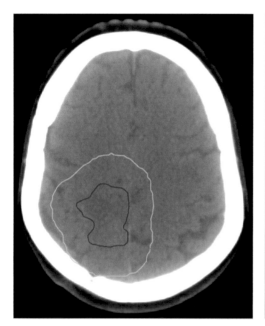
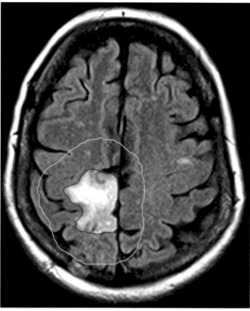

FIGURE 18.2   Grade 2 oligodendroglioma right parietal lobe (a) radiotherapy planning CT and (b) fused FLAIR MRI showing GTV (blue) and CTV (cyan). Note how much easier the tumour is to see on the FLAIR MRI image.

Meningioma

Indications for Radiotherapy

These tumours arise from the meninges, most commonly adjacent to the falx, along the sphenoid ridge, in the olfactory grooves, the sylvian region, cerebellopontine angle and the spinal cord. The WHO grade (1–3) is determined by local invasiveness and cellular atypia and is the most important determinant of treatment, including the timing of any radiotherapy.

Optimal treatment for grade 1 (benign) meningiomas is surgery, but observation may also be appropriate, particularly for incidentally detected meningiomas. Radiotherapy is indicated when tumours recur and there is no surgical option, or occasionally when surgery is not possible such as in optic nerve meningiomas.

Grade 2 (atypical) meningiomas have a higher risk of recurrence than grade 1 – 40 per cent at five years after surgery – so radiotherapy can be considered after surgery, though there is no phase 3 data to support this. The degree of resection (classified by Simpson grade) should be factored into individualised decision-making. Grade 3 (malignant) meningiomas should be treated with maximal debulking surgery and postoperative radiotherapy or with radiotherapy alone if surgery is not possible.

Clinical and Radiological Anatomy

Meningiomas are usually well defined and localised, although they may spread along the dura. They may lie flat along the meninges or be lobulated and indent the adjacent brain. Resectability is, in part, determined by the relationship to adjacent structures, particularly major blood vessels, such as the superior sagittal sinus, anterior and middle cerebral arteries and cavernous sinus, and must be evaluated for each site. Spread through bone and foramina into the orbit, temporal fossa and other sites may make radical excision very difficult.

CT scans usually show a well-defined hyperdense mass which enhances with intravenous contrast. Calcification is seen in about 25 per cent of tumours. Evidence of bone involvement may be seen.

Oedema may be a prominent feature. MRI is useful to demonstrate the attachment of the tumour to the dura and relationship to vascular structures. A tail of meningeal enhancement is common and does not necessarily indicate involvement, though thickened meninges should be considered involved.

Assessment of Primary Disease

Full clinical and radiological examination as just described is carried out to assess operability or need for radiotherapy. Tumours may be asymptomatic or may present with focal seizures, neurological impairment or, more rarely, with signs of raised intracranial pressure.

Data Acquisition

The patient is immobilised supine in a thermoplastic mask or relocatable stereotactic frame. CT and MRI images are helpful as for glioma. CT slices should be no more than 3 mm thick and obtained from the vertex of the skull to the inferior border of C3.

Target Volume Definition

The GTV is the enhancing tumour on MRI. The planning CT is useful to assess and include bone invasion.

CTVs are individualised depending on the grade, how invasive the tumour appears to be and possible meningeal involvement. It can be useful to co-register the preoperative MRI if surgery has been performed to ensure all the tumour bed is included. Adjacent hyperostotic bone should be included. Invasion into the brain is rare, so volume of brain tissue included in the CTV should be minimal. A variable margin (from 1–5 mm), which will increase with grade of tumour, should be added into brain to allow for microscopic spread. Meningeal invasion is more common, and adjacent meninges should be included with a margin from GTV varying from 5 mm in grade 1 tumours to 15 mm in grade 3. It may be helpful to review the neurosurgical operation note to identify areas of particular concern for residual tumour when deciding on a GTV. (See Figure 18.3.)

A PTV margin is added according to departmental protocols and measurements and is usually 3–5 mm. OAR are defined according to the primary site, and a PRV created and edited as appropriate.

Dose Solutions

Small meningiomas may be most appropriately treated by stereotactic techniques. For conventional radiotherapy, IMRT or VMAT should ideally be used to reduce dose to OARs.

Dose Fractionation

Grade 1

- 50.4–54 Gy in 28–30 fractions over five and a half to six weeks
- 50–55 Gy in 30–33 fractions over six to six and a half weeks if a lower dose per fraction is needed to reduce risk to OARs

Grade 2

- 54–60 Gy in 30 fractions over six weeks

Grade 3

- 60 Gy in 30 fractions over six weeks

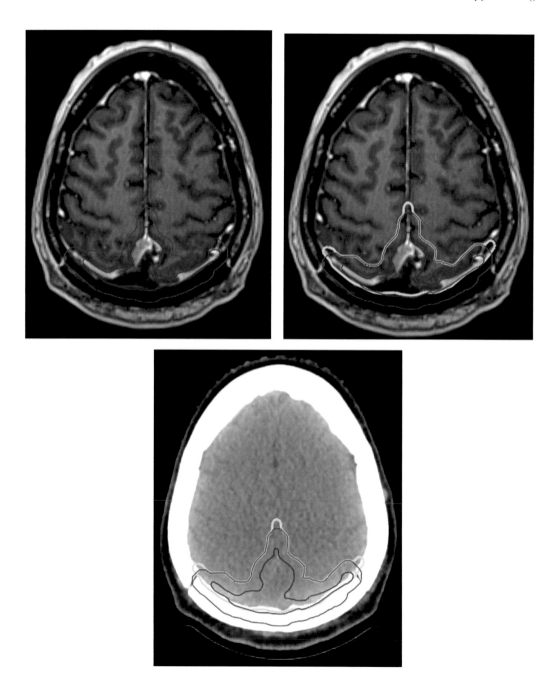

FIGURE 18.3 Postoperative radiotherapy for parafalcine atypical G2 meningioma. (a) Fused T1 + contrast MRI images showing post-op GTV (blue) and GTV with 5-mm isotropic margin (magenta); (b) as previous but including final CTV (cyan). Note CTV is extended along the meninges (c) planning CT scan. Note how CTV is excluded from bone.

Treatment Delivery and Patient Care

See general recommendations in the preceding HGG section. Nausea, headache or need for steroids are uncommon. Irradiating sphenoid wing meningiomas often causes otitis and glue ear symptoms. These usually resolve, but ENT assessment and grommets can be needed if they persist for months after radiotherapy.

Verification

Daily cone beam CT imaging with online correction is recommended to help ensure optimal tumour coverage and OAR sparing.

Pituitary Tumours

Pituitary Adenoma

Indications for Radiotherapy

Pituitary adenomas are benign and usually arise in the anterior pituitary. Secretory tumours produce an excess of growth hormone, ACTH or prolactin. Hormone levels can be controlled medically or surgically and fall very slowly after radiotherapy. Non-secretory tumours present with pressure symptoms, usually when the optic chiasm is compressed. Surgery, often endoscopic, provides rapid relief. Radiotherapy is indicated if the tumour extends laterally into the cavernous sinus where is cannot be resected.

When a tumour recurs after surgery, radiotherapy can be considered, though optimal timing of this will depend on local symptoms, pituitary function, and the age and preferences of the patient. Local control after radiotherapy is excellent – 90 per cent at 20 years – so possible long-term toxicity must be considered carefully.

Clinical and Radiological Anatomy

Contrast-enhanced MRI is the investigation of choice to demonstrate relationship to the optic chiasm superiorly and the sphenoid sinus inferiorly. Pituitary macroadenomas will show low signal on T1-weighted images but there may be high signal in areas of haemorrhage.

Assessment of Primary Disease

Patients are seen initially by an endocrinologist and neurosurgeon, and their assessment is discussed when appropriate in a multidisciplinary meeting with the oncologist. Before radiotherapy, there must be a full ophthalmological and endocrinological assessment and neurological examination.

Data Acquisition

The patient is immobilised supine in a thermoplastic mask or relocatable stereotactic frame. Co-registered CT and MRI images are used to define target volumes. CT slices should be no more than 3 mm thick and obtained from the vertex of the skull to the inferior border of C3.

Target Volume Definition

GTV is defined on T1 + contrast MRI images with particular attention to lateral (cavernous sinus) and suprasellar extension. CT is particularly helpful to outline the inferior floor of the pituitary fossa. GTV contours should be assessed on coronal and axial images.

No GTV to CTV margin is needed, as there is no microscopic spread.

A CTV to PTV margin is added according to departmental protocols, but is usually 3–5 mm. (See Figure 18.4.)

Dose Solutions

Fractionated radiotherapy with IMRT or VMAT is optimal. If conventional therapy is used, an anterior and two opposing lateral beams are chosen to cover the target volume, angled to avoid optic structures.

Single-fraction stereotactic treatment can be used if there is appropriate expertise and if the tumour is small and does not compress the optic chiasm.

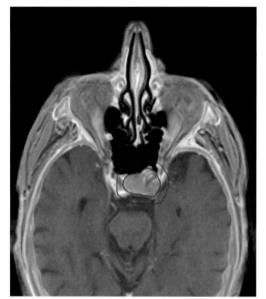

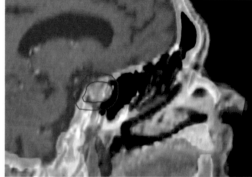

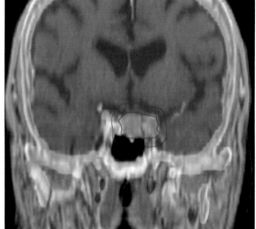

FIGURE 18.4 Radiotherapy for a pituitary adenoma. Fused planning CT and T1-weighted MRI images. GTV (blue) and PTV (red) shown in (a) axial; (b) sagittal; (c) coronal planes.

Dose Fractionation

- 45 Gy in 25 daily fractions of 1.8 Gy given in five weeks.

Treatment Delivery and Patient Care

If patients are on steroid replacement, the dose should be increased (usually doubled) during radiotherapy. Most patients will require hormone replacement after surgery and radiotherapy so they should be followed up in an endocrine clinic.

Verification

Daily cone beam CT imaging with online correction is recommended to help ensure optimal tumour coverage and OAR sparing.

Craniopharyngioma

Craniopharyngiomas are tumours of the sellar/suprasellar region comprising solid and often extensive cystic components. They are most common in children aged 5–15 or in adults aged 65–75 and usually present with symptoms of raised intracranial pressure, optic tract compression, hypopituitarism (including diabetes insipidus) or hypothalamic dysfunction. In adults, maximal safe resection is followed by radiotherapy using similar treatment techniques to pituitary tumours and doses of 50–55 Gy in 30–33 fractions. The CTV should include residual tumour after surgery, the location of the preoperative tumour (including any contact surfaces) and a 3–5-mm margin. The cystic component may recur after surgery, so if vision deteriorates at any point an urgent MRI should be performed and discussed with a neurosurgical team. As cystic progression may occur during radiotherapy, consideration should be given to planned re-imaging of tumours with a significant cystic residuum during a treatment course, with replanning if there is concern regarding tumour coverage.

Cerebral Metastases

Indications for Radiotherapy

More than 50 per cent of intracranial neoplasms are metastatic, arising in order of frequency from lung, breast, melanoma, renal, and colon cancers. They are increasing in frequency with improved treatment of the primary tumour leading to longer survival. Whole brain radiotherapy is no longer recommended for most patients due to improvement in resection and stereotactic radiotherapy techniques and improved systemic therapy which increases likely survival.

Focal treatment with surgery or stereotactic radiosurgery/radiotherapy (SRS/SRT) are options for single or few metastases in people likely to have a relatively good prognosis from their disease overall. Usually focal treatment is considered in people with one to three metastases where each is <3 cm in maximum diameter, but these limits are not absolute and depend on the preference of the patient, their symptoms and the location of the metastases. It will also be influenced by the predicted natural history of the underlying cancer, which will depend on systemic therapy options and by continued improvements in the available technology. The SRS commissioning criteria in the UK require that patients have a KPS of ≥70, a maximum tumour volume of 20 cc, and absent or controllable extracranial disease.

If focal treatment is an option, there is evidence that surgery and SRS offer equivalent overall survival, but SRS has a higher local control rate. SRS is preferred if the metastasis is in a location which makes surgery difficult. Surgery provides quicker control of symptoms such as hydrocephalus and enables pathological assessment, which can be particularly important if brain metastases are the initial presenting site of a cancer; it is also particularly helpful for pressure-related symptoms often in the posterior fossa. Surgery is also likely to enable a reduction in steroid use faster than SRS.

After resection, adjuvant cavity SRS should be considered. There is no evidence that adjuvant WBRT is helpful after focal treatment of a single metastasis.

Whole brain radiotherapy should be considered in people unable to have focal treatment, but the possible side effects and practicalities of treatment should be discussed with each individual, bearing in mind symptoms and life expectancy. Median survival after whole brain irradiation for multiple metastases is three to six months depending on the number of lesions and the tumour type along with performance status. The side effects of radiotherapy, which include hair loss and possibly headache, nausea, or other symptoms, are unfortunate with such a short survival period, but quality of life is nevertheless often much improved. There is evidence that WBRT should not be used in people with lung cancer and WHO PS ≥ 2 (QUARTZ).

Assessment of Disease

The treatment options for brain metastases must be assessed in the light of the extent of the primary tumour and other metastatic disease, and the general condition of the patient. MRI of the brain will reveal small metastases better than CT. Systemic staging appropriate to the primary tumour will help in predicting likely life expectancy and in deciding systemic therapy options. Management decisions should be discussed by a team with expertise in managing brain metastases along with the oncologist treating the primary tumour. Performance status and comorbidity should be carefully assessed. As with any preference-sensitive decision where there is more than one option available, the patient and the patient's family or carer should be fully engaged in the discussion.

Whole Brain Radiotherapy

Data Acquisition

The patient lies supine in a thermoplastic shell with the neck in a comfortable neutral position. Three-millimetre-thick CT slices are obtained from the vertex to the inferior level of C2. Contrast is not necessary.

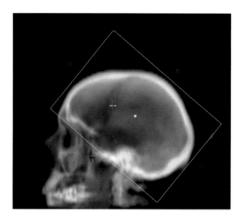

FIGURE 18.5   Lateral DRR with BEV for whole brain irradiation.

Target Volume Definition

The target volume is the whole brain, so fields are usually defined rather than volumes. This can be done on CT images as virtual simulation or in a simulator. Field borders are defined with appropriate MLC shielding to ensure that the eyes are spared. Care should be taken to ensure that the temporal lobes and anterior cranial fossa at the cribriform plate are appropriately treated. If beams are defined in the simulator, the whole skull is covered from the vertex to a line joining the external auditory meatus with the outer canthus of the orbit (Reid's base line). If there is any evidence of involvement of the skull base, this line will need to be 1–2 cm lower to ensure tumour is included in the treatment volume. (See Figure 18.5.)

Dose Solutions

Simple opposing lateral beam arrangements are used for whole brain irradiation with wedges to improve dose distribution if necessary.

Dose Fractionation

Whole brain irradiation:

- 12 Gy in 2 daily fractions given on consecutive days
- 20 Gy in 5 fractions of 4 Gy given in one week
- 30 Gy in 10 fractions of 3 Gy given in two weeks

Paediatric and Rare Adult Brain Tumours

While brain tumours are the most frequently occurring solid tumours in children, they are rare, with an age standardised incidence of 40 per million in the UK. They are a heterogeneous group of diseases and should be treated in specialised centres by experienced multidisciplinary teams and according to internationally agreed protocols. Late effects of treatment, and their often profound lifelong impact on the child following curative treatment, are a major challenge for those managing brain tumours. These include neurocognitive sequelae, damage to the hypothalamic-pituitary axis with growth hormone and other endocrine deficiencies, second malignancies, vasculopathies and direct inhibition of bone growth in the spine or skull. Paediatric brain tumour protocols may use chemotherapy to defer or avoid radiotherapy or to reduce the radiotherapy dose employed. Children should ideally have access to proton beam therapy, as results of dosimetric studies suggest the potential for a reduction in the late effects of treatment.

See Chapter 37 for a description of the principles of radiotherapy in children and useful websites for guidelines and protocols.

Medulloblastoma and Craniospinal Radiotherapy (CSRT)

Medulloblastomas are the most common malignant brain tumour in children. They are the most frequently occurring of the group of CNS embryonal tumours and arise in the posterior fossa. Other rare CNS embryonal tumours such as atypical teratoid/rhabdoid tumours (ATRT) and embryonal tumour with multilayered rosettes (ETMR) may arise at a number of other locations in the brain but are treated in a very similar way.

Medulloblastoma are stratified into standard and high-risk subgroups and management is risk adapted accordingly. It usually comprises a combination of surgery, radiotherapy and systemic therapy. Surgery should be as complete as possible without causing disability. Because of the risk of subarachnoid seeding of tumour, surgery is followed by CSRT with a boost to the posterior fossa or primary tumour bed, and by combination chemotherapy. Better understanding of the molecular subtypes of medulloblastomas has led to different subgroups being recognised. Trials for the worst-prognosis groups focus on more intensive treatment to improve outcomes, whilst radiation doses are being reduced in protocols to treat better prognosis tumours. Medulloblastomas in adults usually occur in people aged 20–40 and are treated in a similar way to those in children.

Craniospinal Radiotherapy Techniques

The target volume in CSRT is the whole cranial and spinal meninges – a very complex shape close to many other organs. Conventional 'field-based' solutions employed lateral beams to treat the head with one or two (depending on the height of the patient) matching posterior beams to treat the spine. A moving junction technique was used to reduce the likelihood of overdose or underdose at the level of the spinal cord.

Data Acquisition

The patient is immobilised supine with a thermoplastic head shell, and a vacuum-moulded bag is used to maintain body position. Two- to three-millimetre CT slices are obtained from the vertex of the head to the inferior sacrum.

Target Volume Definition

The CTV is the whole cranial and spinal meninges. The inferior border of the thecal sac varies and should be defined with the help of MRI images. Particular attention should be given to the cribriform fossa, the temporal lobes of the brain and the base of skull and nerve cranial foramina, which are common sites of relapse if not adequately treated. The middle and inner ears and optic structures should be contoured as OARs. In the spine, the meninges extend along the nerve roots so the intervertebral foramina should be included.

Dose Solutions

IMRT, VMAT and proton techniques with CTV delineation provide a more homogeneous and conformal dose than conventional matched beams. Although there is a move to IMRT/VMAT, there is concern about the whole body low-dose bath. As more patients are eligible for protons, centres have been reluctant to invest resources into developing alternative photon techniques.

Radiotherapy dose gradients across the vertebral bodies in children who have not reached final adult height may result in cosmetically and functionally significant kyphoscoliosis as a late effect. Anterior-posterior (A-P) gradients appear less significant than left-right (L-R) gradients. Conventional field-based CSRT inevitably results in an A-P gradient which does not appear to have resulted in clinically apparent spinal growth problems over many years of clinical experience. Protons, IMRT and VMAT enable a more flexible approach, and vertebral bodies should be outlined as an OAR to facilitate this. Where the patient has reached final adult height, sparing of vertebral bodies may be considered to reduce bone marrow dose and dose to the tissues anterior to the spinal volume. In patients who have yet to reach final adult height, for prescriptions of <25 Gy a maximum A-P dose gradient of <5 Gy should be the aim. If the prescription dose is >25 Gy, the vertebral bodies should be covered by a minimum of 20 Gy. It is assumed that negligible growth occurs beyond 20 Gy and hence larger dose gradients are acceptable beyond this. (See Figure 18.6.)

Dose Fractionation

Standard-risk

Medulloblastoma (classical, desmoplastic or MBEN histology; Chang stage M0 [no metastases]; ≤1.5 cm^2 of residual macroscopic disease; no MYC or MYCN gene amplification) when followed by adjuvant chemotherapy.

Phase 1 Craniospinal

- 23.4 Gy in 13 fractions given in two and a half weeks.

Where no chemotherapy is planned, the CSRT dose should be 36 Gy in 20 fractions given in four weeks.

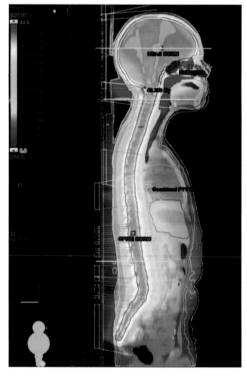

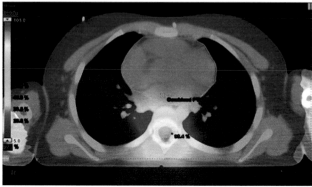

FIGURE 18.6   Craniospinal radiotherapy dose distributions to illustrate VMAT and 3D conformal techniques. (a) Sagittal VMAT; (b) axial VMAT. (*Continued*)

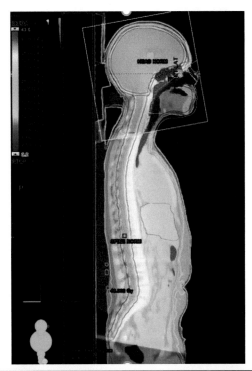

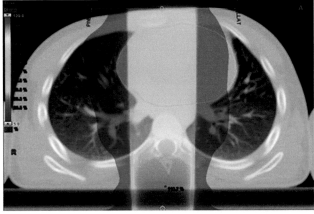

FIGURE 18.6 (*Continued*)   Craniospinal radiotherapy dose distributions to illustrate VMAT and 3D conformal techniques. (c) sagittal 3D conformal; (d) axial 3D conformal.

Phase 2 Tumour Bed Boost

- 30.6 Gy in 17 fractions given in three and a half weeks

High-risk

Medulloblastoma (large cell or anaplastic histology; Chang stage M1–3 [metastases in the CSF, intracranially or in the spinal subarachnoid space]; >1.5 cm^2 of residual macroscopic disease; MYC or MYCN gene amplification).

Phase 1 Craniospinal

- M0/M1 36 Gy in 20 fractions given in four weeks
- M2–3 39.6 Gy in 22 fractions given in four and a half weeks

Phase 2 Tumour Bed Boost

- To give a total dose of 54–55.8 Gy in 30–31 fractions given in six weeks.
- Consideration may be given to boosting areas of focal metastatic disease to 50.4 Gy in 28 fractions given in five and a half weeks.

CNS Germ Cell Tumours

CNS germ cell tumours (GCTs) arise in the suprasellar or pineal regions. They are subdivided into intracranial germinomas and non-germinomatous germ cell tumours (NGGCTs). Approximately 5–10 per cent of CNS GCTs present with synchronous suprasellar and pineal tumours, which are classed and managed as bifocal rather than metastatic disease. CNS GCTs can spread throughout the CNS axis. Seventy-five per cent occur in people aged 10–20.

Germinomas are very sensitive to chemotherapy and radiotherapy. In adults, radiotherapy alone is preferred, as cure rates are excellent. The whole craniospinal axis is given 25 Gy in 15 fractions, with a second phase of 15 Gy in 9 fractions to treat the primary site.

In children, a combination of chemotherapy and radiotherapy is used to reduce both radiation doses and volumes. This will minimise late radiation toxicity, particularly the effect of irradiating the whole spine on adult sitting height. Childhood germinomas are treated with chemotherapy followed by 24 Gy in 15 fractions to the whole ventricles and a boost to the primary of 16 Gy in 10 fractions. NGGCTs are less radiosensitive and require higher doses to the ventricles, boosting the primary to 54 Gy. CSRT is indicated for metastatic CNS GCTs.

Ependymomas

Ependymomas arise from ependymal cells lining the ventricular system and are more common in children than adults. They most commonly arise in the posterior fossa and present with obstructive symptoms. Extent of resection is the most important prognostic feature, and local recurrences are more common than leptomeningeal spread.

In children, surgery is followed by radiotherapy to the tumour bed giving a cumulative dose of 59.4 Gy in 33 fractions, respecting spinal cord and brainstem constraints. If an initial complete resection is not achieved, chemotherapy is used with the aim of enabling resection of residual disease and to obtain macroscopically clear scan prior to radiotherapy.

In adults, adjuvant radiotherapy is recommended after incomplete resection of grade II or III tumours. The CTV is the residual tumour and original site of disease with a 10–20 mm margin. Doses of 54–60 Gy in 30 fractions are used. There is no established role for chemotherapy in adults. Treatment techniques are similar to those used in gliomas.

Gliomas in Children

Low-grade gliomas include pilocytic astrocytomas and diffuse astrocytomas and are the most common CNS tumour in children. Initial management is dependent on the site and operability of disease and the age of the child. The aims of management are maximising survival, maintaining vision for optic pathway gliomas and minimising the risk of late effects.

Initial observation may be appropriate for some newly diagnosed tumours, for example in neurofibromatosis type 1 associated tumours or in asymptomatic tumours detected incidentally. Surgery is usually considered as the first line intervention, with operability depending on the site of disease. Near total or total resection is possible in up to 95 per cent of low-grade gliomas arising in the cerebellum. However surgery (including biopsy) for optic pathway and hypothalamic gliomas is potentially morbid, particularly for infants and young children, so alternative nonsurgical approaches may be considered. Systemic therapy is commonly employed as first-line therapy when surgery is not feasible, following incomplete resection or when there is progression on surveillance. Radiotherapy is usually reserved for older children (around eight to ten years and above) and where systemic and surgical options have been exhausted. Doses of 50.4 Gy in 28 fractions to 54 Gy in 30 fractions are used with complex techniques, including protons where available, to minimise dose to critical structures and hence reduce the risk of late effects.

High-grade gliomas are relatively infrequent in children and represent approximately 8–12 per cent of all paediatric CNS tumours. Prognosis is poor but is slightly better for some subgroups than adult entities. Management strategies comprise surgery, with gross total resection where safe and feasible, followed by focal (tumour bed) radiotherapy combined with systemic therapy. Adjuvant systemic therapy alone may be considered for very young children.

Diffuse midline gliomas (DMG) are high-grade tumours characterised by the H3K27M mutation, and include tumours previously referred to as diffuse intrinsic pontine glioma (DIPG), commonly seen in children between the ages of five and nine. They typically occur in the brainstem but can arise from other midline structures such as the thalamus and spinal cord. Prognosis is extremely poor, with a median survival of less than one year.

Surgery is usually not a feasible option due to the diffuse nature of these tumours and their brainstem location. Focal radiotherapy is the mainstay of treatment for these patients. It usually alleviates symptoms but is not curative. The CTV is the GTV as seen on MRI with a 20-mm margin. Historically, 54 Gy in 30 fractions has been prescribed, although there is evidence from a matched-cohort analysis demonstrating noninferiority of a hypofractionated approach of 39 Gy in 13 fractions given over three to four weeks. Re-irradiation using 20 Gy in 10 fractions can be considered if patients have responded to previous radiotherapy and have at least six months between the end of primary radiotherapy and disease progression. (See Figure 18.7.)

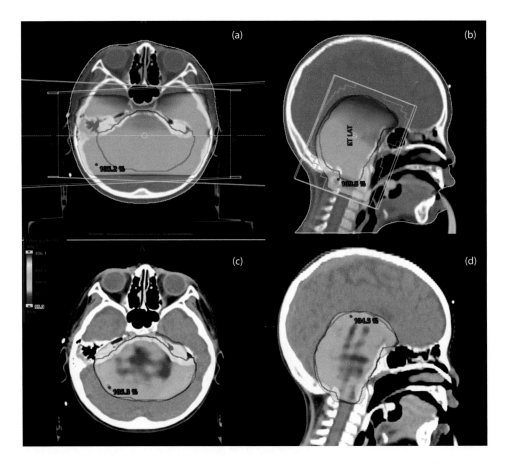

FIGURE 18.7 Radiotherapy plans at the 95 per cent dose colour wash for a patient with diffuse midline glioma of the brainstem. The midplane dose plan with MLC shielding is shown in the (a) axial and (b) sagittal planes and the intensity modulated arc therapy (IMAT) plan is shown in the (c) axial and (d) sagittal planes.

Key Trials

Calaminus G, Kortmann R, Worch J, et al. SIOP CNS GCT 96: Final report of outcome of a prospective, multinational nonrandomized trial for children and adults with intracranial germinoma, comparing craniospinal irradiation alone with chemotherapy followed by focal primary site irradiation for patients with localized disease. Neurooncology 2013;15:788–796.

Fangusaro J, Wu S, Macdonald S, et al. Phase II trial of response-based radiation therapy for patients with localized CNS nongerminomatous germ cell tumors: A children's oncology group study. J Clin Oncol 2019;37:3283–3290.

Gajjar A, Chintagumpala M, Ashley D, et al. Risk-adapted craniospinal radiotherapy followed by high-dose chemotherapy and stem-cell rescue in children with newly diagnosed medulloblastoma (St Jude medulloblastoma-96): Long-term results from a prospective, multicentre trial. Lancet Oncol 2006;7:813–820.

Janssens GO, Jansen MH, Selmer J, et al. Hypofractionation vs conventional radiation therapy for newly diagnosed diffuse intrinsic pontine glioma: A matched-cohort analysis. Int J Radiat Oncol Biol Phys 2013;85:315–320.

Mulvenna P, Nankivell M, Barton R, et al. Dexamethasone and supportive care with or without whole brain radiotherapy in treating patients with non-small cell lung cancer with brain metastases unsuitable for resection or stereotactic radiotherapy (QUARTZ): Results from a phase 3, non-inferiority randomized trial. Lancet 2016;388:2004–2014.

Packer RJ, Gajjar A, Vezina G, et al. Phase III study of craniospinal radiation therapy followed by adjuvant chemotherapy for newly diagnosed average-risk medulloblastoma. J Clin Onc 2006;24:4202–4208.

Perry JR, Laperriere N, O'Callaghan J, et al. Short-course radiation plus temozolomide in elderly patients with glioblastoma. N Eng J Med 2017;376:1027–1037.

Stupp R, Hegi ME, Mason WP, et al. Effects of radiotherapy with concomitant and adjuvant temozolomide versus radiotherapy alone on survival in glioblastoma in a randomised phase 3 study: 5-year analysis of the EORTC-NCIC trial. Lancet Oncol 2009;10:459–466.

van den Bent NJ, Afra D, de Witte O, et al. Long term efficacy of early versus delayed radiotherapy for low-grade astrocytoma and oligodendroglioma in adults: The EORTC 22845 randomised trial. Lancet 2005;366:985–990.

van den Bent MJ, Baumert B, Erridge SC, et al. Interim results from the CATNON trial (EORTC study 26053-22054) of treatment with concurrent and adjuvant temozolomide for 1p/19q non-co-deleted anaplastic glioma: A phase 3, randomised, open-label intergroup study. Lancet 2017;390:1645–1653.

INFORMATION SOURCES

Ajithkumar A, Horan G, Padovani L, et al. SIOPE - brain tumor group consensus guideline on craniospinal target volume delineation for high-precision radiotherapy. Radiother Oncol 2018;128:192–197.

Erridge SC, Conkey DS, Stockton D, et al. Radiotherapy for pituitary adenomas: Long-term efficacy and toxicity. Radiother Oncol 2009;93:597–601.

Lapointe S, Perry A, Butowski NA. Primary brain tumours in adults. Lancet 2018;392:432–446.

Louis DN, Perry A, Wesseling P, Brat DJ, Cree IA, Figarella-Branger D, et al. The 2021 WHO classification of tumors of the Central Nervous System: A summary. Neuro Oncol 2021 Aug 2;23(8):1231–1251.

Merchant TE, Bendel AE, Sabin ND, et al. Conformal radiation therapy for pediatric ependymoma, chemotherapy for incompletely resected ependymoma, and observation for completely resected, supratentorial ependymoma. J Clin Oncol 2019;37:974–983.

National Institute for Health and Care Excellence (NICE) (2021). Brain tumours (primary) and brain metastases in over 16s NG99.

Niyazi M, Brada M, Chalmers AJ, et al. ESTRO-ACROP guideline "target delineation of glioblastomas". Radiother Oncol 2016;118:35–42.

Taylor MD, Northcutt PA, Korshunov A, et al. Molecular subgroups of medulloblastoma: The current consensus. Acta Neuropathol 2012;123:465–472.

19

Thyroid and Thymoma

Thyroid

Indications for Radiotherapy

Papillary and Follicular Thyroid Cancers – Well-Differentiated Thyroid Cancer (WDTC)

Surgery and molecular radiotherapy with iodine-131 (I-131) are the main treatments used for papillary and follicular thyroid cancers. As most people are young at diagnosis and will be cured, there is a focus on reducing treatment intensity by performing a hemi- rather than a total thyroidectomy, and reducing the dose or omitting I-131 completely. The risk of recurrence can be monitored with serum thyroglobulin measurements. Metastatic tumours that are refractory to I-131 can respond to tyrosine kinase inhibitors such as lenvatinib, with an overall median survival of several years.

EBRT is therefore seldom used in the curative setting, but adjuvant radiotherapy does have a role in people with unresectable local disease after initial surgery, which might cause local symptoms such as recurrent laryngeal nerve palsy or dysphagia, particularly in cancers which are not iodine avid. The histology of these tumours is often a widely invasive follicular cancer or a papillary tumour with adverse features such as tall cell variant. As the natural history of these tumours is also to progress slowly, the possible late effects of radiotherapy should be carefully considered before advocating treatment.

Palliative local radiotherapy can be used in people with symptomatic, iodine refractory disease, particularly if it is enlarging. Palliative radiotherapy is effective at relieving the symptoms of metastases – usually in neck or mediastinal nodes or in bone.

Medullary Thyroid Cancer

Surgery is the principal treatment for medullary cancer. There is no role for iodine-131. Radiotherapy is indicated if there is inoperable or macroscopic residual local disease, unless there are uncontrollable distant metastases. It should also be considered in patients with microscopic residual disease, though careful follow-up with calcitonin and carcinoembryonic antigen measurements, and neck imaging, may be appropriate, as the natural history of the disease is very long in most people.

Anaplastic Thyroid Cancer

Many patients with anaplastic cancer are elderly and frail but have significant local symptoms. Lung metastases are very common at diagnosis or within the following few months. Good supportive and palliative care is paramount, but radiotherapy can be used for local control and to relieve or prevent compression of critical structures such as the trachea and oesophagus.

Occasionally, anaplastic carcinoma is operable, or a focus of anaplastic thyroid cancer is found in a thyroidectomy specimen removed for another reason. Adjuvant radiotherapy should then be considered to improve local control, as there are rare instances of long-term survival with this disease.

Sequencing of Multimodality Therapy

Follicular, papillary and medullary cancers tend to grow slowly so there is rarely an urgency to commence radiotherapy. If there is local disease present, surgery should be considered as the first option

DOI: 10.1201/9781315171562-19

before radiotherapy. In WDTC, EBRT should only be used if the tumour is not I-131 avid – which is best assessed by lack of uptake with a therapy dose of I-131.

In anaplastic cancer where surgery is possible, postoperative radiotherapy should begin as soon as possible. It may be followed by adjuvant doxorubicin-based chemotherapy to reduce the risk of distant metastases.

In the palliative setting, concurrent chemotherapy with radiation has been advocated in patients with good performance status and no distant metastases, but this approach increases acute toxicity without a proven survival advantage. When palliative radiotherapy is used to help local symptoms, palliative chemotherapy can be considered subsequently for distant metastases, though response rates are poor.

Clinical and Radiological Anatomy

Most WDTC is confined to the thyroid gland and is therefore completely excised at surgery. Tumours can invade beyond the gland into the soft tissues of the neck, trachea, oesophagus, larynx, neck vessels or recurrent laryngeal nerve, and in these tumours a microscopically complete excision is unusual. With anaplastic tumours, local structures have usually been invaded at presentation.

Lymphatic drainage is initially to the midline level VI nodes in the anterior neck, which extend from the hyoid to the suprasternal notch. Subsequent drainage is to levels III–V and then to the supraclavicular nodes, or inferiorly to nodes in the trachea-oesophageal groove or superior mediastinum. This region is sometimes termed level VII and extends from the suprasternal notch to the brachiocephalic veins. The term superior mediastinal nodes is used to avoid confusion due to the different numbering of mediastinal node levels and those in the neck (Figure 19.1). Papillary cancer has a relatively high risk of lymph node metastasis, though the prognostic significance of this is debated.

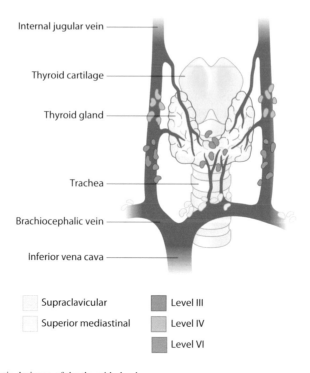

FIGURE 19.1   Lymphatic drainage of the thyroid gland.

Assessment of Primary Disease

Routine cross-sectional imaging is not required before surgery for WDTC unless there is clinical suspicion of local invasion or there is lymphadenopathy. A CT scan with or without contrast (iodinated contrast may inhibit uptake of therapeutic iodine-131) or MRI may then be of value to document local extent and help plan surgery and possible radiotherapy. If the patient is hoarse, nasendoscopy is used to assess vocal cord movement and hence involvement of the recurrent laryngeal nerve.

Medullary cancer should be treated in a centre with specialist expertise. Preoperative assessment should include genetic and biochemical tests to look for multiple endocrine neoplasia.

If treatment is contemplated for anaplastic cancer, a contrast-enhanced CT or MR scan of the neck should be performed along with a CT scan of the chest and mediastinum because of the high incidence of distant metastases.

All patients in whom radiotherapy is being considered should be discussed within a specialist thyroid multidisciplinary team. A full discussion with the surgeon is vital to be able to define sites at highest risk of local recurrence.

Data Acquisition

Immobilisation

Patients should be immobilised in a custom-made thermoplastic shell fixed to the couch top in at least five places. The neck is extended to move the oral cavity superiorly and to reduce dose to the mandible and salivary glands. The shoulders should be as low as possible.

CT Scanning

Slices no more than 3 mm thick are obtained from the base of skull to the carina to allow assessment of lymphadenopathy. If the target volume is smaller (for example the thyroid bed only) the extent of the scan can be reduced. Intravenous contrast can be helpful to delineate vascular structures.

Simulator

Rapidly growing anaplastic carcinomas may require urgent radiotherapy if there is tracheal compression, and though CT-based planning is preferred, field placement on a simulator can be used. Palpable disease is marked with lead wire, and parallel opposed anterior–posterior fields defined to cover the tumour.

Target Volume Definition

Papillary, Follicular and Medullary Cancer – Curative Dose

A careful discussion with the radiologist, surgeon and pathologist is essential to define the sites of macroscopic residual disease and those at highest risk of local recurrence. Any macroscopic residual disease is contoured as GTV. Any sites where tumour was excised with a known positive margin (e.g. tumour dissected from the trachea or vessels) should also be marked to facilitate CTV definition.

The CTV encompasses sites of macroscopic and microscopic residual disease with an appropriate margin of at least 10 mm and will usually include the thyroid bed, level VI nodal region and para-oesophageal and paratracheal spaces in the thyroid bed and superior mediastinum. It should cover the pre-op tumour volume. Elective nodal irradiation is not recommended, but mediastinal nodes can be hard to treat with surgery so the volume can be extended inferiorly to cover the superior mediastinal nodes. The CTV is edited from air and uninvolved bone or cartilage. A higher dose CTV can be defined to boost macroscopic residual disease with a 5-mm margin to 65 Gy in 30 fractions, or equivalent.

Papillary, Follicular and Medullary Cancer – Palliative Dose

The GTV is defined on the planning CT scan and is expanded by 5 mm to form a CTV which may then be extended to cover adjacent sites where local recurrence might cause further symptoms and be hard to treat, such as the paratracheal space.

The CTV is expanded by 3–5 mm to form the PTV, depending on local assessment of systematic and random errors and likely organ motion.

Anaplastic Thyroid Cancer

Most radiotherapy is palliative and needs to be started urgently in view of symptoms. There needs to be a careful balance between trying to cover all sites of possible disease and maintaining quality of life by minimising acute toxicity. The GTV is defined as the primary tumour and involved lymph nodes (more than 10-mm short-axis diameter). The GTV is expanded by 10 mm isotropically to form the CTV. This CTV is edited to reflect local patterns of tumour spread (e.g. including adjacent muscles if invaded but edited off bone and air).

In selected patients of good performance status with no evidence of metastases, a longer course of radiotherapy may be appropriate. Having defined the GTV, a high-dose CTV is created by a 10-mm expansion as just described. An elective dose can then be delivered to level II, IV, V, VI and VII nodal volumes bilaterally. There may be significant shrinkage of tumour during a long course of radiotherapy, so it may be necessary to redefine the CTV on a new planning CT scan during treatment.

If radiotherapy is adjuvant to surgery, the CTV is defined as for WDTC earlier, though consideration can be given to formally including levels III and IV and V in the neck and levels VI and VII in the superior mediastinum in an elective CTV. (See Figure 19.2.)

The CTV is expanded by 3–5 mm to form the PTV, depending on local assessment of systematic and random errors and likely organ motion.

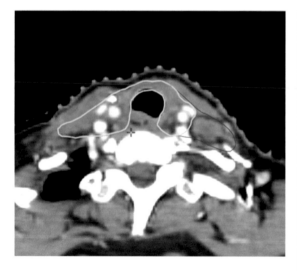

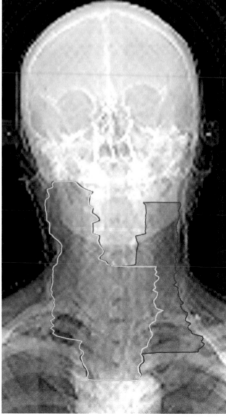

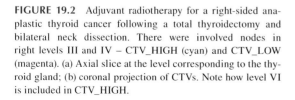

FIGURE 19.2 Adjuvant radiotherapy for a right-sided anaplastic thyroid cancer following a total thyroidectomy and bilateral neck dissection. There were involved nodes in right levels III and IV – CTV_HIGH (cyan) and CTV_LOW (magenta). (a) Axial slice at the level corresponding to the thyroid gland; (b) coronal projection of CTVs. Note how level VI is included in CTV_HIGH.

Dose Solutions

The proximity of the PTV to critical structures such as spinal cord and oesophagus makes a conformal approach with IMRT or arc therapy desirable in all patients with WDTC or medullary cancer and in anaplastic tumours where a high dose is used. Five or seven equispaced IMRT beams are often used in a similar approach to hypopharyngeal or cervical oesophageal cancer. PTV coverage may have to be compromised to keep the spinal cord within tolerance. The oesophagus and hypopharynx should be contoured to minimise dose to these structures where possible to help prevent dysphagia. IMRT should also be considered in palliative treatment of WDTC given the long natural history of the disease, which means re-treatment may be considered even years later.

Where a palliative dose is being given for anaplastic carcinoma, opposing anterior and posterior beams can be defined on the planning CT data set to cover the target volume with an appropriate margin to the beam edge. MLC shielding can reduce dose to adjacent normal structures. (See Figure 19.3.)

Dose Fractionation

WDTC or Medullary Cancer

Adjuvant

- 60 Gy in 30 daily fractions over six weeks

Palliative

- 20 Gy in 5 daily fractions over five to seven days
- 30 Gy in 10 daily fractions over two weeks

Anaplastic Cancer

- 20 Gy in 5 daily fractions over five to seven days
- 30 Gy in 6 fractions of 5 Gy given in two weeks
- 30 Gy in 10 daily fractions over two weeks
- 60 Gy in 30 daily fractions of 2 Gy given in six weeks if high dose treatment appropriate

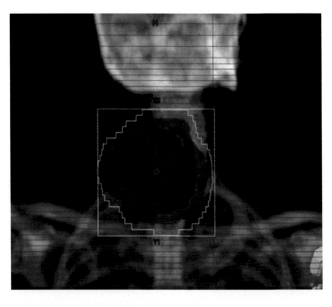

FIGURE 19.3 Palliative radiotherapy for anaplastic thyroid cancer. Anterior and posterior opposing beams with MLC shielding to reduce acute toxicity.

Treatment Delivery and Patient Care

Patients should be treated daily without hyperfractionation for missed treatments if they are receiving six weeks of treatment. Weekly review is critical to manage acute effects proactively. As mucositis of the pharynx and oesophagus are inevitable, dietetic advice should be provided to maintain weight and calorie intake throughout treatment. Enteral feeding with a nasogastric or gastrostomy tube may be necessary if weight falls more than 10 per cent from baseline. Pain should be managed with paracetamol, nonsteroidal anti-inflammatory drugs and oral or transdermal opiates as needed. Steroids are often necessary at the start of treatment in anaplastic cancer to reduce local oedema if the airway or swallowing are compromised, but the dose should be reduced to the lowest needed once radiotherapy begins.

Verification

As for head and neck cancers (see Chapter 8), if there is significant shrinkage of tumour, a repeat CT scan may be required to evaluate the 3D dose distribution of the original beam arrangement within the new contour. A new plan should be considered if there is an increased dose to critical structures or the PTV dose is reduced.

Thymus

Indications for Radiotherapy

Thymic tumours are usually clinically staged according to the Masaoka system (Table 19.1), which reflects local invasion. Pathological classification (WHO) separates thymic carcinomas (WHO C) from thymic epithelial tumours (WHO B – true thymoma) based on morphology and relative proportion of non-tumoural lymphocytic component. The most frequent subtype of thymic carcinomas is squamous cell carcinoma. Clinical staging is useful to predict prognosis and guide treatment decisions, which are outlined in Table 19.1.

Surgery is the treatment of choice for thymic tumours. Current practices in postoperative radiotherapy are highly variable. The majority of evidence is based on retrospective studies and includes pooled analyses. The global trend recently has been to not offer postoperative radiotherapy to all thymic epithelial tumours, but to keep radiotherapy in reserve for high-risk cases.

Sequencing of Multimodality Therapy

Combined modality treatment with surgery, radiotherapy and chemotherapy is recommended to provide optimal local control and survival in unresectable thymic tumours but the best sequence of treatment

TABLE 19.1

The Masaoka Clinical Staging System (with Permission) for Thymoma and Treatment Recommendations

Stage	Description	Treatment
I	Macroscopically and microscopically completely encapsulated (includes tumour invading into but not through the capsule)	Surgery Radiotherapy +/- chemotherapy can be considered for thymic carcinoma in patients unfit for an operation.
II	A microscopic transcapsular invasion B macroscopic invasion into the surrounding fatty tissue or grossly adherent to but not through mediastinal pleura or pericardium	Surgery. Routine adjuvant radiotherapy is not recommended. Adjuvant radiotherapy can be considered in patients at high risk of local recurrence, including close/positive surgical margins, capsular invasion or thymic carcinoma.
III	Macroscopic invasion into neighbouring organs (e.g. pericardium, great vessels, lung) A without invasion of great vessels B with invasion of great vessels	Often multimodality therapy. Discuss in a multidisciplinary setting with thoracic surgeons and oncologists. Neoadjuvant chemotherapy followed by surgery and postoperative radiotherapy can be considered.
IV	A pleural or pericardial dissemination B lymphogenous or haematogenous metastases	In unresectable disease, chemotherapy and radiotherapy are indicated followed by surgery where feasible.

is not known. Preoperative chemotherapy (usually CAP – cisplatin, doxorubicin and cyclophosphamide – or cisplatin and etoposide) may shrink a tumour to allow resection and postoperative radiotherapy. Preoperative radiation with or without chemotherapy has also been advocated to try to allow subsequent resection or as sole treatment. If resection is known to be incomplete, radio-opaque clips placed at sites of residual disease during surgery can be helpful for volume definition.

Clinical and Radiological Anatomy

The thymus sits in the anterior mediastinum behind the sternum. Fifty per cent of thymic tumours invade through the capsule and thence into local structures, including the mediastinal pleura, pericardium or great vessels. Lymph node spread is uncommon. Tumours can metastasize to the pleura or to distant sites.

Assessment of Primary Disease

CT or MRI imaging of the mediastinum is used to define local invasion. Mediastinoscopy can also be useful to assess resectability.

Data Acquisition

Immobilisation

Patients lie supine with their arms above the head immobilised with a T-bar or similar device. A custom-shaped vacuum bag can be used to aid immobilisation.

CT Scanning

Slices 3–5 mm thick are obtained from the inferior cricoid cartilage to the bottom of the thoracic cavity. Intravenous contrast can be helpful to delineate vascular structures in the mediastinum. Where available, a 4DCT acquisition technique should be used identical to that used for radical NSCLC patients. 4DCT acquisition should be identical to the technique used for NSCLC (as defined in Chapter 20).

Target Volume Definition

When adjuvant radiotherapy is used, discussion with the surgeon and pathologist is very important to define sites at risk of local recurrence. Surgeons will usually place surgical clips to help define the dimensions of the tumour bed. A GTV is defined if there is residual macroscopic disease. If there is no GTV, it can be helpful to contour any clips marking positive microscopic margins. The CTV traditionally covered the preoperative extent of disease, but now clinicians will usually define a more limited CTV using the surgical clips as a guide to encompass areas at risk of relapse. Particular attention should be paid to locations where there is felt to be an incomplete resection. After resection of a large tumour the postoperative anatomy may be very different from that on preoperative imaging (Figure 19.4).

If primary radiotherapy is the sole treatment for unresectable disease, the initial GTV is defined on the planning CT. If chemotherapy has been given, the CTV should incorporate all initial sites of disease and possible sites of microscopic invasion, which may include the mediastinum and adjacent mediastinal pleura and pericardium.

The CTV should be edited using the 4DCT data set to create an ITV to account for respiratory motion. The ITV is then expanded to form the PTV. The ITV-PTV margin depends on local assessment of systematic and random errors and is usually 5–10 mm.

Dose Solutions

Where possible, an IMRT solution should be used to achieve the optimum dose distribution to the target volume whilst keeping OAR doses to a minimum. Where IMRT is not available, a 3D conformal technique can be used. Three coplanar beams usually provide adequate PTV coverage without exceeding tolerance

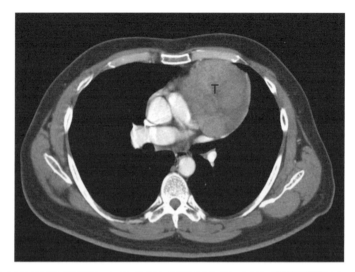

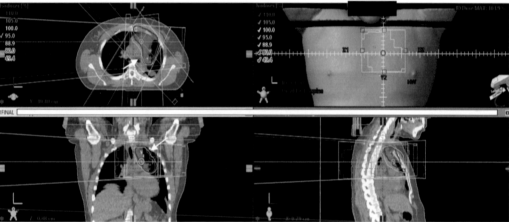

FIGURE 19.4 Adjuvant radiotherapy for thymoma. (a) Preoperative diagnostic CT showing thymoma (t); (b) planning CT showing 3D conformal beam arrangement, postoperative volume (PTV) and dose (95 per cent isodose). Note the radio-opaque surgical clips used to guide volume delineation (arrowed).

of the lungs, heart or spinal cord. Examples include two antero-oblique beams with an additional anterior or postero-oblique beam depending on the PTV. Doses below 54 Gy (1.8–2 Gy/#) are inadequate for gross residual disease. Acceptable dose-fractionation suggestions are listed in the following section.

Dose Fractionation

Adjuvant radiotherapy in stage II/III disease

- 50 Gy in 25 daily fractions given in five weeks
- 60–64 Gy in 30–32 daily fractions given in six weeks (for residual macroscopic disease)

Primary radiotherapy for unresectable disease

- 60–64 Gy in 30–32 daily fractions given in six weeks

Preoperative radiotherapy

- 45 Gy in 25 daily fractions of 1.8 Gy given in five weeks

Treatment Delivery and Patient Care

Treatment is usually well tolerated without severe acute effects, but oesophagitis can occur and should be managed with analgesia and dietary advice (see Chapter 24).

Verification

Cone beam CT images (CBCT) should be used according to local practice to assess for set-up errors. An example would be daily CBCT for first 3 fractions and weekly thereafter. Where CBCT is not available, portal images should be taken on days 1–3 and weekly thereafter to ensure any day-to-day set-up variation is within tolerance.

Key Trials

There are no data from prospective phase III trials of radiotherapy in these tumours. A multi-centre phase III trial (RADIORYTHMIC) is currently recruiting.

INFORMATION SOURCES

Thyroid

Filetti S, Durante C, Hartl D, et al. Thyroid cancer: ESMO clinical practice guidelines for diagnosis, treatment and follow-up. Ann Oncol 2019;1:1856–1883.

Haugen BR, Alexander EK, Bible KC, et al. 2015 American Thyroid Association Management guidelines for adult patients with thyroid nodules and differentiated thyroid cancer: The American Thyroid Association guidelines task force on thyroid nodules and differentiated thyroid cancer. Thyroid 2016;26:1–133.

Kiess AP, Agrawal N, Brierley JD, et al. External-beam radiotherapy for differentiated thyroid cancer locoregional control: A statement of the American Head and Neck Society. Head Neck 2016;38:493–498.

Perros P, Boelaert K, Colley S, et al. British Thyroid Association guidelines for the management of thyroid cancer. Clin Endocrinol 2014;81:1–122.

Smallridge RC, Ain KB, Asa SL, et al. American Thyroid Association guidelines for management of patients with anaplastic thyroid cancer. Thyroid 2012;22:1104–1139.

Thymoma

Falkson C, Bezjak A, Darling G, et al. The management of thymoma: A systematic review and practice guideline. J Thorac Oncol 2009;4:911–919.

Giaccone G. Treatment of malignant thymoma. Curr Opin Oncol 2005;17:140–146.

Girard N, Ruffini E, Marx A, et al. Thymic epithelial tumours: ESMO clinical practice guidelines for diagnosis, treatment and follow-up. Ann Oncol 2015;26(5):40–55.

Gomez D, Komaki R, Yu J, et al. Radiation therapy definitions and reporting guidelines for thymic malignancies. J Thorac Oncol 2011;6:S1743–S1748.

Gomez D, Komaki R. Technical advances of radiation therapy for thymic malignancies. J Thorac Oncol 2010;5:S336–S343.

Masaoka A, Monden Y, Nakahara K, et al. Follow-up study of thymomas with special reference to their clinical stages. Cancer 1981;48:2485–2492.

Zhu G, He S, Fu X, et al. Radiotherapy and prognostic factors for thymoma: A retrospective study of 175 patients. Int J Radiat Oncol Biol Phys 2004;60:1113–1119.

20

Lung

Indications for Radiotherapy

Non-Small Cell Lung Cancer

Curative Treatment – Stage I/II

Although surgery offers the best cure rates for earlystage non-small cell lung cancer (NSCLC), some patients may be medically unfit for surgery due to comorbidity (e.g. insufficient functional lung reserve for a lung resection) or may elect to have radiotherapy rather than surgery after an informed discussion. Inoperable patients with nodenegative disease should be considered for stereoablative radiotherapy (SABR) in the first instance. SABR offers a local control rate of approximately 95 per cent. Short-term mortality of SABR is <1 per cent compared to ~4 per cent with lobectomy/sublobar resection. There is a lack of randomised data comparing curative surgery to SABR in NSCLC. There are however many studies (single-institution and multi-institution) looking at propensity-matched studies, the results of which suggest similar conclusions for both treatments. Trials studying SABR vs surgery in patients at high risk for surgery are underway to attempt to answer this question. There are some patients not suitable for SABR; namely those with central tumours or tumours greater than 5 cm. These patients can be treated in the context of a clinical trial with a more conservative SABR fractionation, or treated with conventional radical radiotherapy alone. Curative radiotherapy alone gives a five-year survival of 20 per cent, although studies from single institutions report cure rates of up to 50 per cent. Cure is more likely for early stage or smaller tumours. WHO performance status >1 and significant weight loss (>10 per cent) predict for poorer outcome, presumably because they indicate occult distant metastases. There are no phase III trials comparing surgery with radiotherapy for these patients, and indirect comparisons are difficult because patients having radiotherapy are likely to have significant comorbidity and poorer performance status. There are also no phase III trials of curative radiotherapy compared to lower palliative dose radiation or observation. In patients with a short life expectancy for other reasons, both these alternatives should be considered.

In patients with poor lung function (FEV1 <1.0 l) a balance between attempting cure and maintaining lung function must be sought. Although there is no agreed lower cutoff below which conventional radiation is contraindicated, a curative dose of radiotherapy is likely to significantly impair lung function in patients with an FEV1 of <0.6 l or grade 4 dyspnoea on the MRC scale. SABR is extremely well tolerated by patients with poor lung function, and generally speaking there is no cutoff for not treating patients with SABR if the lung dose constraints can be met with a suitable radiotherapy planning technique. Patients with underlying pulmonary fibrosis should be treated with radiotherapy with extreme caution. Generally speaking, conventional radiotherapy is contraindicated unless the target volume is very small.

Curative Treatment – Stage IIIA/IIIB

Surgery is only possible for a minority of stage III patients. There are some data showing that surgery is beneficial in single-station N2 disease and can be considered, but for the majority of patients in this group, radiotherapy with chemotherapy is the mainstay of treatment. Curative radiotherapy is indicated

DOI: 10.1201/9781315171562-20

in patients with performance status 0–1 and <10 per cent weight loss in the preceding three months where disease can be safely encompassed in a radical radiotherapy volume. It produces two-year survival rates of 10–25 per cent. Contralateral mediastinal (IIIB) disease increases both the risk of occult distant metastases and the morbidity of radiotherapy. Curative radiotherapy should only be offered to patients in this category if they have good performance status, little comorbidity and relatively small volume disease. There are no firm pretreatment volume or functional indicators to predict which tumours can be encompassed, but radiotherapy should be attempted with caution in patients with stage III disease and FEV1 <1.0 l or MRC dyspnoea score of 3 or 4.

The addition of concomitant chemotherapy to radiation improves cure rates and should be considered in patients able to tolerate combined treatment. Sequential chemotherapy can be added to radical radiation in patients less fit but suitable for chemotherapy treatment. The outcome of sequential treatment is worse with concomitant treatment, offering a 5 per cent survival advantage over sequential. Hyperfractionated regimens such as the CHART protocol of 54 Gy in 36 fractions delivered with 3 fractions a day on 12 consecutive days offer a small advantage over conventional fractionation but have been difficult to implement.

There is mounting evidence that adjuvant immunotherapy post-concurrent chemoradiation shows benefit in stage III NSCLC and is given to patients with PDL positive NSCLC.

The brain is a common site of relapse in patients treated for IIIA/B disease, but prophylactic cranial radiotherapy is not widely used. There is evidence that it reduces the incidence of brain metastases, but there is no evidence that survival is improved.

Palliative Radiotherapy

The majority of patients treated with palliative radiotherapy for lung cancer obtain symptomatic benefit, particularly for cough, chest pain or haemoptysis. The optimal fractionation schedule is unclear, but longer regimens produce a more durable response and a small survival advantage compared to shorter regimens. They should be considered for patients with PS 0–1 who are not suitable for curative radiotherapy. Other patients should be treated with one or two fractions. There is no evidence to support the use of palliative radiotherapy in asymptomatic patients.

Intravascular stents relieve the symptoms of SVCO faster than radiation or chemotherapy and should be considered first. Nonetheless, SVCO is effectively palliated by EBRT in 60 per cent of patients with NSCLC and 80 per cent with SCLC. Palliative radiotherapy should also be considered for symptomatic distant metastases in sites such as bone, lung or skin.

Adjuvant Radiotherapy (Postoperative Radiotherapy – PORT)

Although for many cancers radiotherapy is used as an adjunct to surgery in patients at high risk of local recurrence, it is not recommended routinely in NSCLC. Meta-analyses have shown an improvement in local control but an adverse effect on overall survival, particularly in stage I/II disease. Most studies used nonconformal techniques and lower doses of radiotherapy than would be considered today, so the benefits of modern conformal radiotherapy as an adjunct to surgery were unclear. It was thought that there may be a modest benefit from radiotherapy in pathological N2 disease. The LungART trial was a Phase III study comparing postoperative conformal radiotherapy to no postoperative radiotherapy in patients with completely resected non-small cell lung cancer and mediastinal N2 involvement. Trial results were first reported in September 2020 and did not show a significant benefit in DFS or OS in the radiation arm. Significant cardiopulmonary toxicity was seen in patients receiving radiation. Adjuvant PORT should therefore not be recommended in pN2 patients.

PORT may be considered where there is macroscopic disease or microscopic residual disease (positive resection margins). It may also be considered in patients with bad prognostic factors such as extracapsular spread or lack of adjuvant chemotherapy due to fitness.

Neoadjuvant Radiotherapy

Some centres recommend radiotherapy in combination with chemotherapy for tumours that are border-line operable. However there are only two phase 3 trials (both from the 1970s) comparing the addition of preoperative radiation to surgery, and neither showed a benefit. There is no role for neoadjuvant radiotherapy outside a clinical trial.

Small Cell Lung Cancer

Curative Thoracic Radiotherapy

Radiotherapy should be considered for patients with small cell lung cancer (SCLC) who have tumour that can be encompassed within a curative radiotherapy volume. Four to six cycles of chemotherapy combined with radiotherapy are recommended because of the high incidence of systemic metastases and the relative chemosensitivity of SCLC. If patients are unable to tolerate chemotherapy, radiation alone is given if all sites of disease can be encompassed.

Thoracic radiotherapy has proven benefit (two-year survival improved from 13 to 19 per cent) if given after chemotherapy to patients with a partial or complete response with the aim of treating all sites of initial disease. In practice, this is mainly patients with limited stage disease, excluding those with a malignant pleural effusion. There is also a randomised controlled trial supporting the use of thoracic radiotherapy in extensive disease if there is a complete response outside the chest and a complete or partial response in the chest. Radiotherapy should therefore be considered in this situation.

There is also evidence to support starting thoracic radiotherapy early in the course of chemotherapy (concurrently with cycle 1 or 2) in patients with limited stage disease. The dose of radiation in this situation remains somewhat controversial, traditionally up to 50 Gy in 2 Gy/# terms has been utilised, however there is increasing evidence for higher doses (up to 70 Gy) showing improved outcomes. Turrisi et al. (1999) showed 45 Gy twice daily for three weeks was superior to 45 Gy once daily for five weeks. CONVERT trial results reported in 2017 showed similar results for b.d. delivery according to Turrisi regime to 66 Gy in 33# daily treatment. In addition, recent evidence is emerging to support a palliative dose of thoracic radiotherapy in patients with extensive stage SCLC showing a response to chemotherapy.

Smoking during thoracic radiotherapy for SCLC has been shown to affect outcomes adversely so cessation advice and support should be provided.

Palliative Thoracic Radiotherapy

There are emerging data from trials such as Slotman et al. (2015) looking at the benefit of palliative radiotherapy in SCLC. Based on these trials, patients with good PS who show a response to chemotherapy could be offered palliative thoracic radiotherapy (30 Gy in 10# or equivalent), however it should be noted that definite significant benefit has not yet been demonstrated. There are no data comparing palliative chemotherapy with palliative radiotherapy – treatment should be chosen on the basis of which is likely to provide better palliation for the individual patient.

Prophylactic Cranial Radiotherapy (PCI) in Patients with SCLC

In patients with limited-stage disease, PCI reduces the incidence of brain metastases and has a small benefit in overall survival. Late toxicity from whole brain radiotherapy includes cognitive function effects and should be considered when consenting patients for this treatment. The survival of patients with SCLC is limited, however some patients will achieve survival in excess of one year. It is given after curative chemotherapy and radiotherapy as long as there has been a complete or near-complete response. If thoracic radiation follows chemotherapy, the brain and chest can be irradiated at the same time.

The benefit of PCI in patients with extensive disease is unclear. Earlier trial data show a survival benefit, whereas more recent trials did not demonstrate a benefit (Takahasi et al., 2017). Patients should be considered carefully as the morbidity from PCI is significant, with potential long-term cognitive effects. If patients are not offered PCI, regular MRI surveillance imaging can be considered as an alternative. There are data reporting the use of SRS for limited brain metastases in some patients with SCLC and this may be a treatment option to consider in selected patients.

Sequencing of Multimodality Therapy

NSCLC Stage I/II Treated with Radiotherapy

Patients in this group undergoing radiotherapy will usually have single modality treatment, often SABR depending on location of the disease. Adjuvant chemotherapy after surgery confers a survival benefit in resected stage IB–IIIA disease. A similar benefit could be expected for the few patients with stage IB–II disease having potentially curative radiotherapy who are fit enough to undergo chemotherapy, but there is no clinical trial evidence to support this.

NSCLC Stage IIIA/B Treated with Radiotherapy and Chemotherapy

Chemotherapy and radiation can be combined concomitantly or sequentially. Concomitant regimens use cisplatin-based chemotherapy in various schedules concurrent with radiotherapy, and usually have further courses of chemotherapy either before or after concurrent treatment. Often, the dose of the second chemotherapy drug is reduced during radiation. The dose of cisplatin should remain at full dose.

No one regimen has been shown to be conclusively superior, although there are trials showing improved survival with concomitant compared to sequential regimens at the expense of increased acute toxicity (mainly oesophagitis and myelosuppression). Sequential regimens use three to four cycles of platinum-based chemotherapy followed three to four weeks later by radiotherapy. There are trials studying radiotherapy dose escalation in these stages of patients. The evidence is still not clear and radiation dose escalation should only be offered in the context of a clinical trial.

NSCLC Adjuvant Radiotherapy and Chemotherapy after Surgery

Where radiotherapy is indicated as an adjunct to surgery, it should ideally begin four to six weeks postoperatively or when wound healing is adequate. There are Phase 3 trial data to support the use of adjuvant chemotherapy in resected stage IB–IIIA NSCLC, and radiotherapy was given to some patients in these trials on a nonrandomised basis. For some patients, adjuvant chemotherapy and adjuvant radiotherapy may both be indicated, but there are no data on which to base sequencing of these treatments. The risks of local recurrence and systemic metastases should be assessed on an individual basis and radiotherapy or chemotherapy started first as appropriate. As the majority of patients having adjuvant radiotherapy will have positive excision margins, we recommend adjuvant radiotherapy should be given first, followed three to six weeks later by consideration of adjuvant chemotherapy if indicated.

NSCLC Palliative Therapy

Patients may have indications for both palliative chemotherapy and radiotherapy. Sequencing depends on the balance of local and systemic symptoms and the likely benefits of each treatment. If significant local symptoms exist, there is no good reason to delay radiotherapy, as the response is likely to be good.

Superior Sulcus (Pancoast) Tumours

Tumours in the superior sulcus are often considered separately from other lung cancers, and there is support for initial radiotherapy or radiotherapy with concomitant chemotherapy followed by surgery from several phase 2 studies or retrospective series, with five-year survival rates of 15–40 per cent. The optimal management of these tumours is unclear but there is no evidence that surgery improves cure rates when added to (chemo) radiotherapy in NSCLC overall. We therefore recommend managing patients with superior sulcus tumours in the same way as other NSCLC patients.

Small Cell Lung Cancer

The optimal timing of chemotherapy and radiotherapy for SCLC is still debated. Starting radiotherapy after chemotherapy will result in smaller treatment volumes and therefore reduced toxicity. It will also mean that patients who respond unusually poorly to chemotherapy will be spared the toxicity of radiation. There is, however, increasing evidence that starting radiotherapy early (concurrent with cycle 1 or 2) improves survival, suggesting that the overall treatment time may be important. We recommend radiation concurrent with cycle 2 in patients of excellent performance status with relatively small volume disease. The advantage of a shorter overall treatment time is only seen if optimal chemotherapy can still be given after the increased toxicity of early radiation.

Clinical and Radiological Anatomy

All pathological subtypes of lung cancer have a high rate of regional lymph node and distant metastases, so histology alone is not a good predictor of spread. Small cell cancer often presents with large volume mediastinal lymphadenopathy, and distant metastases are common. Squamous cell carcinomas are more frequently confined to the thorax than other subtypes and may cavitate.

Primary lung tumours spread within lung parenchyma where they are relatively asymptomatic. Satellite tumour nodules may be visible on imaging. Spread within major airways can cause obstruction and distal collapse or atelectasis, which can be difficult to differentiate from tumour (Figure 20.1). Tumour may invade the chest wall, mediastinal structures, major vessels or the heart. Although invasion does not preclude curative radiotherapy if the treated volume is small enough, it is a predictor for distant metastasis.

Lung tumours first spread to lymph nodes within the lung – the subsegmental, segmental, lobar and interlobar nodes which lie close to the division of bronchi, arteries or veins. These are rarely visible on imaging but are often removed at surgery when involvement may help define adjuvant radiotherapy volumes. Hilar nodes are situated at each hilum outside the reflection of the pleura. Adjacent tracheobronchial nodes are inside the reflection but cannot be differentiated from hilar nodes on CT.

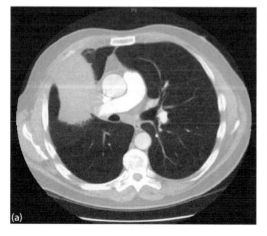 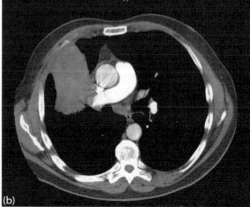

FIGURE 20.1 Tumour can be difficult to differentiate from distal collapse and consolidation on a contrast-enhanced CT scan with either (a) lung windowing or (b) soft tissue windowing.

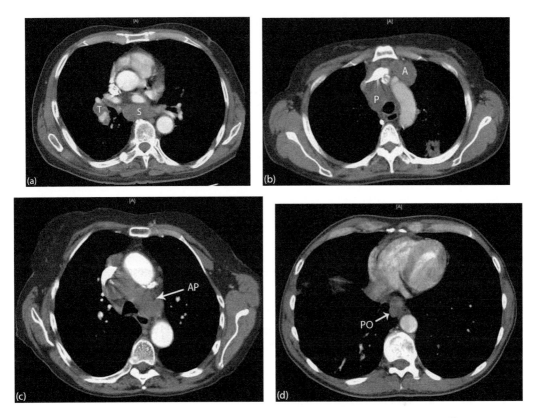

FIGURE 20.2 Enlarged mediastinal lymph nodes on diagnostic CT scans: (a) hilar (H) and subcarinal (S); (b) paratracheal (P) and anterior mediastinal (A); (c) aortopulmonary window (AP); (d) paraoesophageal (PO).

The lymph node stations of the mediastinum are best divided into tracheobronchial, paratracheal, aortopulmonary, anterior mediastinal, subcarinal and paraoesophageal nodes (Figure 20.2). There are numerical classification systems for mediastinal nodes based on surgical series.

N staging in the TNM system reflects involvement of ipsilateral hilar (N1), ipsilateral mediastinal (N2) or contralateral mediastinal or supraclavicular (N3) nodes (Table 20.1a and b).

The right lung drains systematically to hilar and adjacent mediastinal nodes (e.g. right upper paratracheal for upper lobe tumours, right lower paratracheal and subcarinal for middle and lower lobes). Left lower lobe tumours drain to the paraoesophageal, subcarinal, left paratracheal and aortopulmonary nodes. In contrast, the left upper lobe can also drain to the right paratracheal nodes. Skip metastases to the mediastinal nodes when hilar nodes are negative occur in up to 15 per cent of tumours.

The criterion for nodal involvement on CT is a short axis diameter of ≥10 mm, but 15 per cent of nodes smaller than 10 mm contain tumour if removed, and more than 30 per cent of 2-cm nodes are pathologically negative. The likely pattern of nodal spread, number of enlarged nodes, node shape and presence of obstructive pneumonitis or other lung pathology (e.g. sarcoidosis) all need to be considered when assessing nodes on cross-sectional imaging, along with size. Primary tumour size is also correlated with Nstage. See Table 20.1.

Assessment of Primary Disease

Initial assessment and imaging aims to identify disease that is either operable or treatable within a curative radiotherapy volume. The primary tumour is imaged with chest radiograph and contrast-enhanced CT with particular attention to differentiating tumour from distal collapsed lung and to

TABLE 20.1A

Staging of Lung Cancer

T0	No primary tumour
Tis	Carcinoma in situ
T1	Tumour 3 cm or less in greatest dimension
T1a	Superficial spreading tumour in central airways
T1a	Tumour less than 1 cm
T1b	Tumour >1 but <2 cm
T1c	Tumour >2 cm but ≤ 3 cm
T2	Tumour >3 cm but ≤ 5 cm or tumour involving visceral pleura, main bronchus (not
T2a	carina), atelectasis to hilum
T2b	Tumour >3 cm but ≤ 4 cm
	Tumour >4 cm but ≤ 5 cm
T3	Tumour >5 cm but ≤ 7 cm or invading chest wall, pericardium, phrenic nerve;
	Or separate tumour nodule(s) in the same lobe
T4	Tumour > 7cm or tumour invading mediastinum, diaphragm, heart, great vessels,
	recurrent laryngeal nerve, carina, trachea, oesophagus, spine;
	Or tumour nodule(s) in a different ipsilateral lobe
N0	No regional nodal metastasis
N1	Metastasis to ipsilateral pulmonary or hilar lymph nodes
N2	Metastasis to ipsilateral mediastinal and/or subcarinal lymph nodes
N3	Metastasis to contralateral mediastinal, contralateral hilar or supraclavicular lymph node(s)
M0	No distant metastasis
M1a	Malignant pleural/pericardial effusion or pleural/pericardial nodules;
	Or separate tumour nodule(s) in a contralateral lobe
M1b	Single extrathoracic metastasis
M1c	Multiple extrathoracic metastases (1 or >1 organ)

Source: UICC TNM (8th edn, 2017).

assessing mediastinal invasion. CT imaging for staging should include the low neck nodes, liver and adrenal glands. MRI may be useful to look for local invasion of the brachial plexus in superior sulcus tumours. A flexible or rigid bronchoscopy is used to determine endobronchial tumour extent and to obtain histology. Cytological confirmation of a possibly malignant effusion may be necessary, if it would alter management.

CT will allow assessment of mediastinal lymph nodes on size criteria but this has relatively high false negative (40 per cent) and false positive (20 per cent) rates. The number of visible nodes, their

TABLE 20.1B

Stage Groupings for Lung Cancer

T/M	Label	N0	N1	N2	N3
T1	T1a	IA1	IIB	IIIA	IIIB
	T1b	IA2	IIB	IIIA	IIIB
	T1c	IA3	IIB	IIIA	IIIB
T2	T2a (central/visceral pleura)	IB	IIB	IIIA	IIIB
	T2a (>3–4 cm)	IB	IIB	IIIA	IIIB
	T2b (>4–5 cm)	IIA	IIB	IIIA	IIIB
T3	T3	IIB	IIIA	IIIB	IIIC
T4	T4	IIIA	IIIA	IIIB	IIIC
M1	M1a	IVA	IVA	IVA	IVA
	M1b	IVA	IVA	IVA	IVA
	M1c	IVB	IVB	IVB	IVB

Source: UICC TNM (8th edn, 2017).

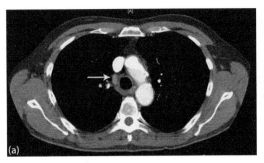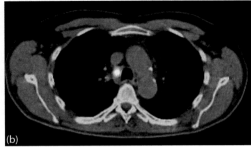

FIGURE 20.3 Diagnostic PET-CT can change treatment volumes by identifying involved mediastinal lymph nodes. (a) Contrast-enhanced CT showing a right paratracheal node 9 mm in short axis diameter; (b) corresponding slice on PET-CT showing abnormal increased uptake. This node should be contoured as GTV.

shape and location can provide further information. If available, a PET-CT can be used to assess enlarged mediastinal nodes and distant metastases, and should be considered in all patients eligible for curative treatment for NSCLC (Figure 20.3). Enlarged mediastinal nodes that are visible on PET-CT should ideally be confirmed on cytology/biopsy via endobronchial ultrasound (EBUS) or mediastinoscopy, as there is still a significant false positive rate, though the false negative rate is small. If a NSCLC is N0 on CT, a staging PET will still detect occult mediastinal nodes in some patients. Overall PET-CT will change the treatment in patients eligible for curative radiotherapy in up to 40 per cent of cases.

Distant metastases in the liver, adrenals or bones are assessed using the staging CT scan and PET-CT if performed. Bone scans and brain imaging are useful in the presence of unexplained bone pain or neurological symptoms but are not performed routinely.

There is an emerging concept of an oligometastatic state in lung cancer. The premise of this hypothesis is that newer more sophisticated imaging techniques such as PET will upstage patients with non-symptomatic low-volume metastatic disease (typically between three and five sites) and that this state behaves differently to widespread metastatic disease. There are clinical trials studying a more radical approach to oligometastatic disease in NSCLC and patients can be considered for these where available.

Three-Dimensional Data Acquisition

Immobilisation

Patients should be positioned supine with arms immobilised above the head in a comfortable, reproducible position to allow a greater choice of beam angle. The patient holds on to a T-bar device with their elbows supported laterally (Figure 20.4). A knee support provides a more comfortable and therefore reproducible setup. If treatment delivery is prolonged (e.g. with respiratory gating or stereotactic radiotherapy) a vacuum bag should be used to reduce movement.

Simulator/Virtual Simulation

If anterior-posterior beams are to be used for palliation, the borders can be defined in the simulator or on CT in the case of virtual simulation. The beam centre is marked with a reference tattoo and a photograph of the borders, drawn on the skin/specified on CT. Fluoroscopy can be used in the simulator to view tumour movement, but the accuracy of assessment in two dimensions is not enough to predict margins required.

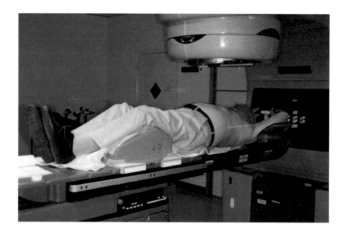

FIGURE 20.4   Immobilisation for thoracic radiotherapy with a T-bar devise, lateral elbow supports and a knee rest.

CT Scanning

CT scans are obtained from the cricoid cartilage to the superior aspect of the L2 vertebra to allow the lung DVH to be calculated. Ideally, 3–5 mm slices are used both to aid volume definition and to create high-quality DRRs to aid verification. A separate simulator verification visit can then be omitted. An isocentre is tattooed in the CT scanner, as are lateral reference points. Intravenous contrast may help define mediastinal extent of disease.

A co-registered PET scan can be used to aid volume definition. Defining volumes on a PET-CT image may help distinguish tumour from collapsed lung. Relatively poor spatial resolution, movement artefact and difficulty in defining the edge of a PET positive mass make this an experimental technique at present.

Techniques to Account for Tumour and Lung Motion

A free-breathing 'slow' CT scan with a single slice scanner is the simplest method of acquiring 3D data for planning. Depending on the speed of image acquisition, some motion will be accounted for with a single CT data set. Target volumes are then defined taking into account possible organ motion based on population studies.

Whilst some tumours move several centimetres in one or more plane in a respiratory cycle, others are relatively stationary. Moreover, it is difficult to predict from the location of a tumour how much movement there will be. There are several ways to account for individual tumour motion: imaging the tumour at extremes of motion thus incorporating motion into the CT data, limiting mobility by breath-holding or diaphragmatic compression, tracking respiration with respiratory gating and tracking the tumour itself with IGRT.

A very slow CT data set (four seconds per slice) taken during normal breathing will effectively provide a composite image of the tumour as it moves so that volumes defined on the CT scan already take motion into account. Image quality may be reduced, making accurate GTV definition more difficult. Fast images taken at maximum inspiration and expiration can be co-registered with a free-breathing scan, enabling margins of tumour movement in each plane to be determined so that extremes of motion are encompassed. These techniques allow individualisation of margins whilst the patient is treated breathing normally.

The most commonly used motion correction technique is a 4D CT acquisition scan. A 4D CT scan uses a fast multislice scanner correlated to the respiratory cycle. Several CT data sets are therefore obtained, each at a different point in the respiratory cycle. A fiducial marker can be placed in the tumour to track its position in the respiratory cycle, or an external surrogate placed on the patients' torso tracks the position of the skin/chest wall movement and can be correlated to position in the respiratory cycle.

The process of correlating the external surrogate with the CT data sets obtained is known as retrospective binning and will produce a moving image of the tumour and thorax contents over a composite breathing cycle. A GTV or CTV is edited over the phases of respiration to create an ITV that includes all positions of the tumour in the respiratory cycle, allowing individual tumour motion to be accounted for in volume definition.

Several techniques to limit respiratory movement have been researched, including breath-holding and abdominal compression, but they can be difficult to reproduce reliably for each fraction of treatment and may be poorly tolerated by patients. In addition, this approach may require patient education with audio and/or visual cues. These additional techniques can be useful for patients identified likely to have significant respiratory motion, e.g. lower lobe tumours.

Respiratory gating uses a fiducial marker or surrogate marker on the chest wall to switch the linear accelerator on in a certain phase of respiration. The external surrogate approach assumes that an external marker of respiration correlates with internal tumour movement, which is not always the case. The gold standard is to use an internal fiducial marker placed in the tumour, however this requires a separate invasive intervention and procedure for the patient and may not always be possible. The baseline thoracic volume can also vary from day to day, so a relative measure of tidal volume may not correlate with an absolute position of a tumour.

Several ways of managing respiratory motion are available, and each patient should be considered individually to optimise both the acquisition of CT data and to accurately manage tumour motion during treatment.

Target Volume Definition

Curative

To define the GTV accurately it is important to have all diagnostic imaging including PET-CT available – ideally on a separate workstation adjacent to the planning computer (Figure 20.8a and b). Clinical information and bronchoscopy, EBUS or mediastinoscopy reports should be available. In the case of adjuvant radiotherapy, a discussion with the surgeon and pathologist is essential to define sites at highest risk of relapse. Clips placed at surgery at sites of incomplete excision are valuable but must not be confused with clips used to ligate vessels. Uncertainty in GTV definition can be reduced by a radiologist and oncologist collaborating to define the GTV.

The parenchymal extent of the GTV should be defined with CT images viewed on a standardised lung window setting (Figure 20.5). The spiculated edge of the tumour is included within the GTV. Anatomical knowledge, contrast CT scans and radiologist input can help differentiate tumour from normal structures

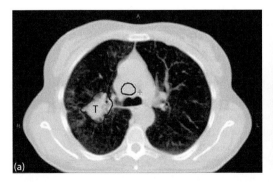
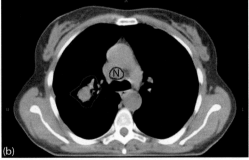

FIGURE 20.5 GTV definition with the appropriate window setting on a planning CT. (a) Lung window setting to define the primary tumour within the lung; (b) same slice on mediastinal window setting to define invasion into the mediastinum and involved nodes. Note the apparent smaller size of the primary tumour.

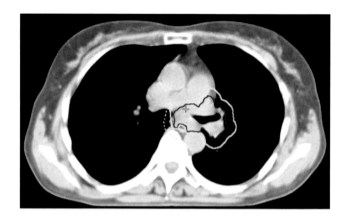

FIGURE 20.6 Defining the CTV in lung cancer. The GTV is grown isotropically (dashed line) and then edited to take account of natural tumour barriers and likely patterns of spread to create the final CTV.

such as pulmonary vasculature and the azygous vein. Tumour can be very difficult to differentiate from adjacent lung collapse or atelectasis.

CT images should be viewed on a mediastinal window setting to define mediastinal extent of disease and any involved lymph nodes. Contrast-enhanced images (planning or diagnostic scan) and PET-CT, if available, may help define local mediastinal extent.

If chemotherapy is used before radiation, the GTV should include all sites of disease at presentation – e.g. any enlarged nodes that have shrunk to less than 10 mm with treatment.

The GTV is grown isotropically to produce a CTV. The margin added to GTV to create the CTV varies at different institutions. Up to 5-mm margin from GTV to CTV is considered adequate to cover microscopic disease in lung tissue. The CTV is edited to take account of natural barriers to tumour spread (e.g. uninvolved bone or great vessels). It is extended to encompass likely patterns of spread and to encompass the original GTV if neo-adjuvant chemotherapy has been used. In practice, this usually produces a variable GTV-CTV margin throughout the volume, but adding an isotropic margin which is then edited will be less prone to systematic errors than manually defining the CTV (Figure 20.6). Elective nodal irradiation is not recommended, as most recurrences after radiotherapy are within the primary tumour or as distant metastases rather than as isolated nodal recurrences.

The CTV is then edited over the phases of respiration (on a 4D CT data set) to cover the movement of the tumour and its excursion through the respiratory cycle. This creates the ITV. ITV to PTV margins depend on tumour motion and day-to-day setup errors. The latter should be measured in each department and should be 5–10 mm in each direction. The margin added for tumour motion will vary from zero in the case of perfect IGRT using implanted fiducial markers to a standard solution if individual motion is not accounted for. While this may not reflect extremes of movement for all tumours, larger margins may make it difficult to keep within dose constraints for critical normal structures. The point of expansion of the volume to allow for respiratory motion can differ according to clinician preference and may be added to GTV to create a 4D GTV data set. CTV and PTV margins can then be added to the 4D GTV as just described.

The spinal cord is contoured on axial slices throughout the PTV and an isotropic 5-mm margin applied to produce a PRV. Other OARs such as oesophagus, brachial plexus and heart are contoured throughout the PTV if the tumour is close to them. Automatic contouring tools can be used to contour the lungs. A lung minus GTV structure is then constructed by subtraction.

Palliative

If CT planning is used, the GTV is defined as previously described, and a 10-mm margin applied to produce a PTV on the basis that larger margins would reduce the therapeutic ratio in the palliative setting.

If beams are defined on the simulator, the diagnostic CT images can still be used to define a virtual GTV, which can be superimposed onto the simulator radiograph. A 15-mm margin from this virtual GTV to the beam edge will give the same effect.

Dose Solutions

Simple

Palliative therapy given in one or two fractions can be defined in the simulator as described earlier. Anterior and posterior photon beams are used with dose prescribed to the midplane. MLC shielding may reduce the dose to normal lung tissue. 6MV photons are adequate unless the separation at the centre is more than 28 cm, in which case a higher energy (e.g. 10 MV) is needed.

Conformal

There are several challenges to covering the PTV within ICRU targets whilst maintaining toxicity at acceptable levels. The location and size of the PTV and its proximity to critical structures, particularly the oesophagus and spinal cord, often necessitate a compromise in choosing the most acceptable plan for an individual patient.

When curative radiotherapy is used for stage I or II disease, a three-field conformal plan is acceptable. Many tumours are closer to the chest wall than to the mediastinum, and ipsilateral beams will minimise the dose to contralateral normal lung tissue and normally provide a homogeneous dose distribution (Figure 20.7). Beam angles are chosen to reduce lung dose, with an anterior oblique, posterior oblique and lateral beams often used. Wedges compensate for the obliquity of the beams in relation to the chest wall, and MLC shielding is used to conform each beam shape to the PTV. Three-dimensional conformal plans may also be used with dose calculated with inhomogeneity correction. The beam arrangement should be selected to conform the 95 per cent isodose to the PTV and produce the lowest lung dose, notwithstanding other dose constraints.

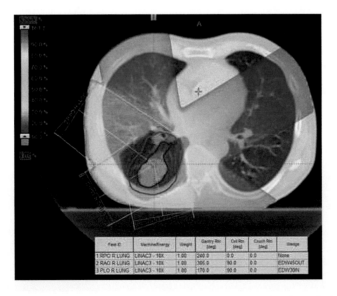

FIGURE 20.7 Beam arrangement and dose colour wash with 3D conformal technique for a T2N0 lung cancer situated posteriorly in the right lower lobe. Lung windowing is used to demonstrate the primary tumour more clearly.

More modern planning systems use IMRT and arc therapy to produce better dose distribution to the tumour and minimise the doses to organs at risk (Figure 20.8c and d).

In stage IIIA disease, a similar three-field conformal plan is often used. The beam angles are chosen using the beam's eye view tool whilst viewing the PTV, spinal cord PRV and oesophagus contour so as to reduce dose to the spinal cord and oesophagus as much as possible and with the aim of minimising lung dose.

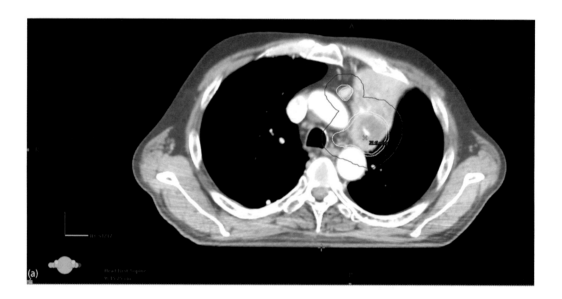

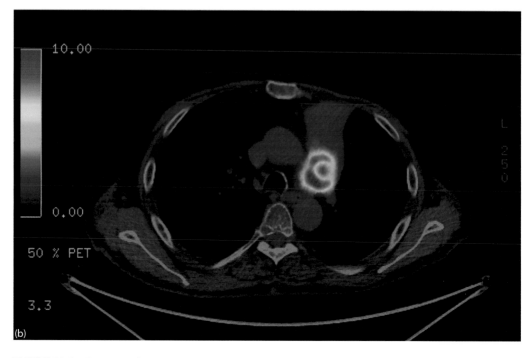

FIGURE 20.8 Treatment of a large T3N2 NSCLC with a VMAT IMRT technique. (a) CTV, ITV and PTV volumes; (b) colour wash dose distribution. (*Continued*)

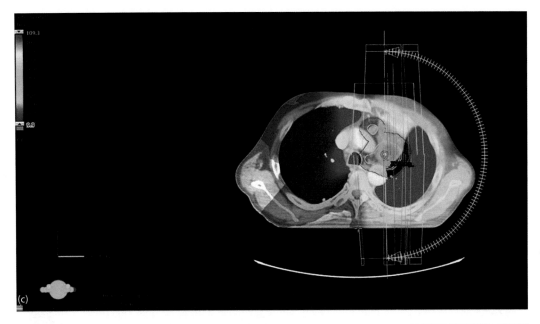

(c)

Fields | Dose | ☐ Field Alignments | ☑ Plan Objectives | ☐ Optimization Objectives | Dose Statistics | Reference Points | Calculation Models | Plan Sum

Primary	Prescription			Fraction Dose [Gy]	Total Dose [Gy]	Actual Total Dose [Gy]
☑ PTV	At least	50.0	% receives more than	2.000	64.000	64.000
☐ Spinal Cord	Maximum dose		is less than	1.438	46.000	21.320
☐ SCPRV3mm	Maximum dose		is less than	1.563	50.000	24.976
☐ Lungs-CTV	Mean dose		is less than	0.563	18.000	9.136
☐ Oesophagus	Maximum dose		is less than	2.000	64.000	63.991

Structure	Index		Target Value	Actual Value
ITV	D98.00 [Gy]	is more than	59.52	62.88
ITV	D95.00 [Gy]	is more than	60.80	63.26
ITV	D5.00 [Gy]	is less than	67.20	65.11
ITV	D2.00 [Gy]	is less than	68.48	65.65
PTV	D98.00 [Gy]	is more than	59.52	59.57
PTV	D95.00 [Gy]	is more than	60.80	60.88
PTV	D5.00 [Gy]	is less than	67.20	65.57
PTV	D2.00 [Gy]	is less than	68.48	66.06
Spinal Cord	D0.10cc [Gy]	is less than	44.00	20.24
SCPRV3mm	D0.10cc [Gy]	is less than	48.00	22.00
Lungs-CTV	V5.00Gy [% of volume]	is less than	60.00	45.30
Lungs-CTV	V20.00Gy [% of volume]	is less than	25.00	15.29
Heart	V30.00Gy [% of volume]	is less than	50.00	0.00
Heart	V40.00Gy [% of volume]	is less than	30.00	0.00

(d)

FIGURE 20.8 (*Continued*) Treatment of a large T3N2 NSCLC with a VMAT IMRT technique. (c) half-arc VMAT technique for optimum dose distribution to PTV and to minimise OAR dose; (d) plan objectives data evaluating target volume coverage and OAR dose.

For larger tumours, in particular those crossing the midline in the mediastinum, it is more difficult to cover the medial extent of the tumour with ipsilateral beams. Adding a contralateral beam will significantly increase the dose to normal lung.

Primary tumours close to the spinal cord may have a PTV that is very close to, or even overlaps the spinal cord PRV. These can be treated in two phases for treatment accepting full dose to the cord for phase 1 with the addition of MLCs to shield the cord from at least two beams in phase 2. However, with modern planning techniques, this approach is no longer recommended and patients should be treated with a single phase using IMRT to shape the beams around the spinal cord to cord tolerance. A radical dose is normally achievable in most cases.

In small cell lung cancers or non-small cell tumours with N2 disease, the PTV will often be very close to the oesophagus. The risk of grade 3 acute toxicity or long-term oesophageal stricture is related to the length of oesophagus in the treated volume, and ideally this is kept below 8 cm by choosing beam angles carefully. For some patients, it may be appropriate to accept some underdosing of the PTV to achieve this. Concomitant chemotherapy in either non-small cell or small cell disease increases the risk of oesophagitis.

Complex

The principal challenges in lung cancer radiotherapy are volume definition and accounting for motion. Complex treatment dose solutions should only be used when tumour motion is also accounted for. In such circumstances, IMRT may produce more conformal dose distributions, particularly for tumours close to the spinal cord.

IMRT plans should achieve the following parameters for PTV coverage:

- No more than 5 per cent of any PTV will receive < 95 per cent or >105 per cent of the prescription dose.
- No more than 2 per cent of any PTV will receive < 93 per cent of the prescription dose.
- No more than 2 per cent of the primary PTV will receive > 107 per cent of the prescription dose.

ICRU 83 recommends a dose-volume-based specification of absorbed dose. The D50 per cent, the median absorbed dose, should be reported. The report also recommends that the near-minimum absorbed dose is reported. This is the D98 per cent, also called the near minimum dose (minimum absorbed dose that covers 98 per cent of the PTV). The D2 per cent should also be reported.

The plan should be assessed carefully by the oncologist. In vivo the risk of radiation pneumonitis depends not only on the dose absorbed but also on the use of concomitant chemotherapy, preexisting lung disease, the lobe being treated and vascular perfusion. Table 20.2 illustrates an example of planning parameters that may be used, but patient factors should also be taken into account when deciding the best plan. Brachial plexus, stomach and liver doses should also be considered in patients whose tumours are in close proximity to these structures. A V20 of <32 per cent is a useful target, but for patients with poor lung function, a lower target may be needed, while for those with good lung function a value closer to 35 per cent may be acceptable. It is therefore difficult to use one value in assessing all plans. With modern radiotherapy planning techniques, it is much easier to achieve acceptable values for OARs and the toxicity to the patient is considerably less.

Similarly, there are several parameters of the oesophageal DVH identified that correlate with the risk of grade 3 or 4 acute oesophagitis or the risk of strictures. We recommend aiming to keep the length of oesophagus within the treated volume to less than 8 cm where possible and certainly to less than 12 cm. Other variables, including the V40 or V50, have also been shown to correlate with toxicity in some series.

Beam energies above 10 MV should be avoided because secondary electrons have a greater range in lung tissue, so higher energy photon beams have a wider penumbra. Modern dose calculation engines

TABLE 20.2

Basic Planning Parameters for OARs in Radical Lung Treatment

| OAR | α/β | Parameter | 60–64 Gy/30–32# | | 55 Gy/20# | |
			Optimal	Mandatory	Optimal	Mandatory
Total lungs GTV	10	$V_{20/17}$	V_{20} <25%	V_{20} <35%	V_{17} <25%	V_{17} <32%
		V_5	60%	60% to contralateral lung	60%	60% to contralateral lung
		D_{mean}	12 Gy	18 Gy	11 Gy	17 Gy
Spinal cord	1.5	D_{max}	47 Gy	47 Gy	42 Gy	42 Gy
Spinal cord PRV	1.5	D_{max}	50 Gy	50 Gy	43 Gy	43 Gy
Oesophagus	10	D_{max}	60 Gy	65 Gy	52 Gy	55 Gy
		D_{mean}	34 Gy		32 Gy	
Heart	3	D100%		44 Gy		36 Gy
		D67%		52 Gy		44 Gy
		D33%		59 Gy		57 Gy
		V_{40}	30%			
		V_{30}	40%			
		D_{mean}	26 Gy	32 Gy	22 Gy	

such as voxel Monte Carlo will produce more accurate dose calculations within the lung than the older pencil beam convolution algorithms implemented in most planning systems.

SABR – Target Volume Definition and Dose Solutions

SABR takes considerably more time to deliver than conventional radiotherapy. It is therefore essential that the patient positioning is comfortable and reproducible between treatments. If a patient is unable to comply with acceptable immobilisation criteria they will be deemed unsuitable for SABR.

Patients should have a 4D CT scan identical to the radical lung radiotherapy technique described earlier.

Delineation of Target Volumes

Various additional data sets can be created using the 4D images to help with accurate target volume definition. Examples are time-averaged data sets or amplitude-based data sets.

Volumes are contoured on the appropriate data set derived from information from all respiratory phases of the 4D CT radiotherapy planning scan.

The GTV is defined as the radiologically visible tumour in the lung, contoured using lung windows (Figure 20.9). As with conventional lung radiotherapy, mediastinal windows may be suitable for defining tumour borders adjacent to the chest wall. Information from other imaging modalities should be used to aid delineation of the GTV.

CTV = GTV, as no margin for microscopic disease extension is added.

The ITV is the tumour volume across all phases of respiration, defined as tumour contoured using information from each phase of a 4D CT scan.

The expansion from ITV to Planning Target Volume (PTV) is up to 5 mm in all directions.

To achieve adequate target coverage using SABR whilst sparing critical organs at risk (OAR), including the skin surface, plans are typically generated with an IMRT/VMAT technique using 6 MV photons.

Organs at Risk

For SABR planning dose to OAR evaluation is critical. All surrounding structures should be contoured and dose constraints calculated. Typical OAR contouring for lung SABR patients includes spinal cord, oesophagus, brachial plexus, heart, trachea and bronchial tree.

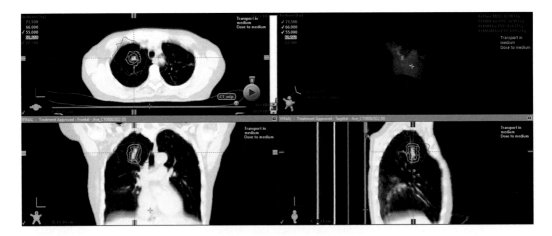

FIGURE 20.9 Treatment of lung cancer with SABR 55 Gy/5# planned on time-averaged data set showing ITV (green) and PTV (red).

Timmerman et al. (2006) noted excessive toxicity when treating centrally located tumours with SABR and subsequently coined the term 'No fly zone' which proposed outlining central airways and avoiding treating tumours in this region. Trachea and proximal bronchial tree are contoured as separate structures using lung windows:

- *Proximal trachea*: contours begin at the more superior of (i) 10 cm superior to superior extent of PTV or (ii) 5 cm superior to the carina and continue inferiorly to the superior aspect of the proximal bronchial tree.
- *Proximal bronchial tree*: contours include the distal 2 cm of trachea and bilateral proximal airways. The following airways are included: distal 2 cm trachea, carina, right and left main bronchi, right and left upper lobe bronchi, the bronchus intermedius, right middle lobe bronchus, lingular bronchus and the right and left lower lobe bronchi. Contouring of the lobar bronchi must end immediately at the site of a segmental bifurcation.

'No-fly zone': a 2-cm expansion of the trachea and proximal tree in all directions is named the 'no-fly zone'. If the ITV falls within this artificial structure, caution must be taken, and the patient's suitability for standard SABR dose schedules reconsidered. There have been reports of significant tracheal/central bronchial toxicity in patients with centrally located tumours receiving the large doses of radiation in SABR. The delineation of the no-fly zone ensures that patients with central tumours aren't treated with SABR.

Whole lung: left and right lungs should be contoured using a pulmonary window level. All inflated and collapsed lung must be included. However, ITV and trachea/ipsilateral bronchus as defined earlier must not be included. The lungs-ITV must be kept within normal tissue dose constraints listed later in the chapter.

Skin and bone: the OAR must be inspected to ensure that wherever a treatment beam traverses the OAR, it has been contoured. The body contour must also be contoured wherever the beams traverse it. The skin contour must be inspected to ensure that beams do not overlap, producing excessive skin dose, especially where there is a skin fold.

Chest wall: the ipsilateral ribs and soft tissue to a depth of 2 cm beyond pleura surrounding the PTV should be volumed.

Dose Solutions

All dose calculations should be performed using a superposition algorithm or equivalent. In the case of new planning software or upgrades being installed, the beam models should be revalidated, including small field and heterogeneity measurements.

Analysis of the dose-volume histogram (DVH) for the PTV and critical normal structures forms the basis for selecting a particular treatment plan. It is therefore recommended that plans be calculated on a fine dose grid, with a separation no greater than 2.5 mm, to ensure the accuracy of DVH calculations.

Dose Distribution Requirements

Successful treatment planning will require accomplishment of the following criteria:

- The dose must be prescribed to an isodose line encompassing the PTV (typically 100 per cent isodose).
- Dose constraints to OARs should also be optimised, and acceptable tolerance doses adhered to. An example of typical planning parameters can be seen in 2022 UK Consensus on Normal Tissue Dose-Volume Constraints for Oligometastatic, Primary Lung and Hepatocellular Carcinoma Stereotactic Ablative Radiotherapy.

Dose Fractionation

Non-Small Cell Lung Cancer

Curative NSCLC-SABR Doses

- 55 Gy in 5 fractions on alternate days
- 54 Gy in 3 fractions on alternate days
- 60 Gy in 8 fractions on alternate days

Curative NSCLC – Conventional Doses

- 55 Gy in 20 daily fractions of 2.75 Gy given in four weeks
- 64–66 Gy in 32–33 daily fractions given in six and a half weeks

Adjuvant NSCLC

- 50 Gy in 20 daily fractions of 2.5 Gy given in four weeks
- 60 Gy in 30 daily fractions given in six weeks

Curative Small Cell Lung Cancer

- 40 Gy in 15 daily fractions of 2.67 Gy given in three weeks

Consider

- 66 Gy in 33 daily fractions given in six and a half weeks
- 45 Gy in 30 fractions of 1.5 Gy treating twice daily given in three weeks

Palliative

- 10 Gy in 1 fraction
- 16 Gy in 2 fractions of 8 Gy a week apart
- (the dose has been reduced from 17 Gy in 2 fractions to minimize the risk of spinal cord damage if survival is prolonged)

If PS0–1 and life expectancy is greater than six months, consider

- 20 Gy in 5 fractions of 4 Gy given in one week

or

- 36 Gy in 12 fractions of 3 Gy given in four weeks
- (39 Gy in 13 fractions if 3D conformal plan or spinal cord not in treated volume)

Prophylactic Cranial Irradiation

- 25 Gy in 10 daily fractions of 2.5 Gy given in two weeks

Treatment Delivery and Patient Care

Patients should be reviewed weekly by a trained radiographer or physician so that acute side effects are treated proactively. A mild increase in dyspnoea or cough is common but rarely needs treatment, though intercurrent infections should be excluded. Advice on skin care is given. When the oesophagus is within the treated volume, pain on swallowing and dysphagia usually begin in the third week of treatment. Systemic analgesia, topical local anaesthetic agents and advice on soft and high-calorie diets from a dietician should be available.

Verification

Ideally the treatment isocentre on a DRR from the CT simulation is compared with portal images of the isocentre on the treatment machines using electronic portal imaging. Offline correction protocols are used for standard conformal treatment. Images are taken on days 1–3 and weekly thereafter with a correction made if the mean error in any one plane is >5 mm. If stereotactic radiation or IGRT are used, online correction protocols are necessary.

Other Points

A single fraction of high-dose-rate brachytherapy can provide useful palliation in NSCLC. Other local treatments such as stent insertion, laser debulking and cryotherapy can produce similar results, and the choice of treatment depends largely on local expertise. External beam radiotherapy is likely to be more effective in patients who have not had radiation before, but brachytherapy can offer good palliation after curative radiotherapy.

<table>
<tr><td rowspan="7">Key Trials</td><td>Antonia SJ, et al. Overall survival with durvalumab after chemoradiotherapy in stage III NSCLC. N Eng J Med 2018;379:2342–2350.</td></tr>
<tr><td>Faivre-Finn Corinne, Snee Michael, Ashcroft Linda, et al. Concurrent once-daily versus twice daily chemoradiotherapy in patients with limited-stage small-cell lung cancer (CONVERT): An open-label, phase 3 randomised, superiority trial. Lancet Oncol 2017;18:1116–1125.</td></tr>
<tr><td>Le Pechoux Cecile, Pourel Nicolas, Barlesi Fabrice, et al. Postoperative radiotherapy versus no postoperative radiotherapy in patients with completely resected non-small-cell lung cancer and proven mediastinal N2 involvement (lung ART): An open-label, randomised, phase 3 trial. Lancet Oncol 2022;23:104–114.</td></tr>
<tr><td>Saunders M, Dische S, Barrett A, et al. Continuous, hyperfractionated, accelerated radiotherapy (CHART) versus conventional radiotherapy in non-small cell lung cancer: Mature data from the randomised multicentre trial. CHART Steering Committee. Radiother Oncol 1999;52(2):137–148.</td></tr>
<tr><td>Takahashi S, et al. Prophylactic cranial irradiation versus observation in patients with extensive-disease small-cell lung cancer: A multicentre, randomised, open-label, phase 3 trial. Lancet Oncol 2017;18:663–671.</td></tr>
<tr><td>Turrisi AT 3rd, Kim K, Blum R, et al. Twice-daily compared with once daily thoracic radiotherapy in limited small-cell lung cancer treated concurrently with cisplatin and etoposide. N Engl J Med 1999;340:265–271.</td></tr>
</table>

INFORMATION SOURCES

Alberts WM. Diagnosis and management of lung cancer executive summary: ACCP evidence-based clinical practice guidelines (2nd edition). Chest 2007;132(3 Suppl):1S–19S.

Auperin A, Arriagada R, Pignon JP, et al. Prophylactic cranial irradiation for patients with small-cell lung cancer in complete remission. Prophylactic cranial irradiation overview collaborative group. N Engl J Med 1999;341:476–484.

Bradley J, et al. Standard dose vs high-dose conformal radiotherapy with concurrent and consolidation carboplatin/paclitaxel with or without cetuximab for patients with stage IIIA or IIIB NSCLC (RTOG 0617). Lancet Oncol 2015;16:187–199.

Chapet O, Kong FM, Quint LE, Chang AC, et al. CT-based definition of thoracic lymph node stations: An atlas from the University of Michigan. Int J Radiat Oncol Biol Phys 2005;63(1):170–178.

De Ruysscher D, Pijls-Johannesma M, Bentzen SM, et al. Time between the first day of chemotherapy and the last day of chest radiation is the most important predictor of survival in limited-disease small-cell lung cancer. J Clin Oncol 2006;24:1057–1063.

Diez P, Hanna GG, Aitken KL, et al. UK 2022 consensus on normal tissue dose-volume constraints for oligo-metastatic, primary lung and hepatocellular carcinoma stereotactic ablative radiotherapy. Clin Oncol. 2022;34(5):288–300.

Lester JF, Macbeth FR, Toy E, Coles B. Palliative radiotherapy regimens for non-small cell lung cancer. Cochrane Database Syst Rev 2006;4:CD002143.

National Collaborating Centre for Acute Care, London. http://www.nice.org.uk.

NICE clinical guideline 24 February 2005; Diagnosis and treatment of lung cancer.

Pignon JP, Arriagada R, Ihde DC, et al. A meta-analysis of thoracic radiotherapy for small-cell lung cancer. N Engl J Med 1992;327(23):1618–1624.

Okawara G, Ung YC, Markman BR, et al. Postoperative radiotherapy in stage II or IIIA completely resected non-small cell lung cancer: A systematic review and practice guideline. Lung Cancer 2004 Apr; 44(1):1–11.

Rowell NP, O'Rourke NP. Concurrent chemoradiotherapy in non-small cell lung cancer. Cochrane Database Syst Rev 2004;4:CD002140.

Rowell NP, Williams CJ. Radical radiotherapy for stage I/II non-small cell lung cancer in patients not sufficiently fit for or declining surgery (medically inoperable). Cochrane Database of Syst Rev 2001;2:Art No.:CD002935.

Scottish Intercollegiate Guidelines Network Guidance 80. Management of patients with lung cancer. A National Clinical Guideline (no. 80), 2005. http://www.sign.ac.uk.

Senan S, De Ruysscher D, Giraud P, et al. Literature-based recommendations for treatment planning and execution in high-dose radiotherapy for lung cancer. Radiother Oncol 2004;71(2):139–146.

Slotman B, Faivre-Finn C, Kramer G, et al. Prophylactic cranial irradiation in extensive small-cell lung cancer. N Eng J Med 2007;357:644–672.

Slotman B, et al. Use of thoracic radiotherapy for extensive stage small-cell lung cancer: A phase 3 randomised controlled trial. The Lancet 2015;385(9962):36–42.

Stereotactic Ablative Body Radiation Therapy (SABR): A Resource SABR UK consortium, 2019. https://www.sabr.org.uk.

Timmerman R, McGarry R, Yiannoutsos C, et al. Excessive toxicity when treating central tumors in a phase II study of stereotactic body radiation therapy for medically inoperable early-stage lung cancer. J Clin Oncol 2006;24:4833–4839.

21

Mesothelioma

Indications for Radiotherapy

Mesothelioma is a challenging disease to treat, and a number of treatment strategies have been tried over the years. Various clinical trials have been carried out, some of which are multimodality and some purely radiotherapy based. Current evidence does not favour major surgery in the form of extra pleural pneumonectomy (EPP). Trials including this treatment have also utilised chemotherapy and radiotherapy. Other surgical techniques include pleurectomy and decortication, often accompanied by (neo) adjuvant chemotherapy and radiotherapy. In addition, prophylactic radiotherapy (PORT-site) can be used along with palliative radiotherapy to painful pleural deposits.

Prophylactic Radiotherapy

Radiotherapy has been given to prevent painful subcutaneous masses from forming at sites of transthoracic interventions such as pleural biopsies or chest drains. Seeding of malignant cells along such needle tracts is reported to occur in 15–50 per cent of sites, but there is no good evidence that such masses are symptomatic in most patients. The simultaneous modulated accelerated radiation therapy (SMART) trial randomised patients who had a large-bore intervention procedures such as pleural drains or VATS biopsy to immediate port-site radiotherapy vs delaying treatment till track metastasis had occurred. The trial showed no significant benefit for prophylactic treatment with a trend towards benefit in epithelioid tumours who were deemed not fit enough for systemic therapy. We recommend considering prophylactic radiotherapy for patients of PS 0–1 in this subset of patients only (Figure 21.1). Ideally it is performed within two weeks of the intervention.

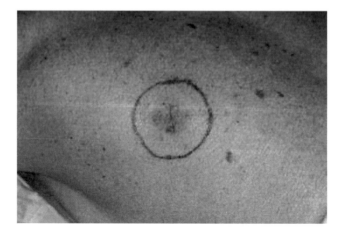

FIGURE 21.1 Prophylactic radiotherapy with 12 MeV electrons to the site of a chest drain. The beam edge is marked in pen – 2 cm from the drain site.

DOI: 10.1201/9781315171562-21

Palliative Radiotherapy

Palliative radiotherapy can help alleviate chest wall pain in mesothelioma. Several small single centre series suggest response rates of 20–70 per cent, but the doses used and methods of response evaluation were very variable. There is no good evidence of a dose–response relationship. Mesothelioma often presents as diffuse pleural disease and it can be difficult to decide which part of the pleural disease should be targeted with palliative radiotherapy. Radiotherapy is best considered as one method of pain control, alongside opiates, antineuropathic agents and cordotomy.

Adjuvant Radiotherapy

A few patients with good PS (WHO 0–1), low comorbidity and early-stage disease confined to the thoracic pleural surface are treated with combined modality therapy with curative intent. This comprises chemotherapy, surgery (extrapleural pneumonectomy [EPP] – en bloc removal of the parietal pleura, lung, diaphragm and pericardium) and adjuvant radiotherapy. a systematic review of trimodality therapy (chemotherapy, EPP, adjuvant radiotherapy) concluded that selected patients may benefit from this treatment and also that treatment should be carried out by experts in specialist centres for the best outcomes. Eligible patients should be included in phase III studies where possible or at least treated at centres with experience of this programme. To irradiate one hemithorax while minimising dose to critical structures (heart, spinal cord, liver, kidneys and contralateral lung) presents a major radiotherapeutic challenge. The lowest local recurrence rates with acceptable toxicity have been achieved by treating the hemithorax to 54 Gy. Comparative series suggest that lower doses are less effective.

Sequencing of Multimodality Therapy

If radiotherapy is used as part of multimodality therapy, it should follow neoadjuvant chemotherapy and surgery, ideally commencing eight to ten weeks postoperatively. We recommend that this should be in the context of a clinical trial.

Clinical and Radiological Anatomy

Mesothelioma usually spreads locally within the pleural space on the parietal and mediastinal pleural surfaces and can invade the chest wall and mediastinum. A contrast-enhanced CT scan of the thorax and upper abdomen is used to assess the degree of pleural space involvement and mediastinal lymphadenopathy.

Assessment of Primary Disease

If multimodality therapy is to be attempted, careful patient selection is very important. All such patients should have a mediastinoscopy to evaluate mediastinal lymph nodes, and a staging PET scan to exclude patients with inoperable disease. Patients should be assessed by a multidisciplinary team including medical oncologist, surgeon and radiation oncologist before commencing the treatment programme to ensure they are eligible for all modalities involved.

If palliative radiotherapy is to be of value, it needs to be targeted to a site likely to be causing pain, and this can be difficult to assess given the diffuse nature of mesothelioma. A careful history and clinical examination are most useful, but chest radiographs or CT scans can show rib or vertebral destruction, which may correlate with sites of pain.

Data Acquisition

Immobilisation

For adjuvant radiotherapy, patients should be supine with arms above the head in a comfortable and reproducible position. A head rest, knee pillow and arm support may be helpful, and a vacuum bag for the thorax should be considered.

Patients for prophylactic or palliative electron treatment should be placed in a comfortable position on the simulator couch which allows skin apposition of the electron applicator.

CT Scanning

For adjuvant radiotherapy, drain sites and all chest incisions other than the median sternotomy scar are marked with radio-opaque wire. CT slices no more than 5 mm thick are obtained from the cricoid cartilage to the iliac crests. A treatment isocentre is tattooed at the time of CT scanning in order to reduce systematic setup errors.

Simulator

Palliative radiotherapy can be planned on a simulator if a single electron beam or parallel opposing photon beams are used. Painful chest wall masses or sites of origin of pain are marked with radio-opaque wire before screening.

Target Volume Definition

Adjuvant Radiotherapy

The entire pleural cavity should be marked with radio-opaque clips at the time of surgery to facilitate CTV definition. Clips at the insertion of the diaphragm and on the pleural reflections are especially useful. Volumes are defined after consultation with the surgeon and pathologist to identify high-risk sites in the hemithorax such as residual macroscopic or microscopic disease or locations where there was tumour on the mediastinal pleural surface.

The GTV is residual macroscopic disease if present. The CTV1 comprises the GTV with a minimum 10-mm margin in each plane and any sites of microscopic residual disease (positive resection margins). The CTV2 is defined as the entire ipsilateral thoracic cavity from lung apex to insertion of the diaphragm, ipsilateral mediastinal pleura, mediastinal tissues at sites where there was evidence for tumour invasion, the ipsilateral pericardial surface, and full thickness of the thorax at the sites of thoracotomy and chest tube incisions. It is very challenging to treat all the CTV2 to 54 Gy so some dose compromise to this large volume may be unavoidable. It can be very helpful to review the CTVs with the thoracic surgeon once they have been defined.

The CTVs are grown by at least 10 mm to produce the PTVs, but this margin should be adjusted according to measured departmental errors for hemithoracic radiation.

The spinal cord with a 5-mm margin, contralateral lung, heart, liver, oesophagus and kidneys are contoured as OAR volumes.

Prophylactic Radiotherapy

As electrons or 300 kV photons are used and the beam border marked onto the patient's skin, GTV, CTV and PTV are not defined. A 2-cm margin from the edge of the scar being treated to the 50 per cent electron beam edge is recommended to account for the shape of isodoses at depth. This will usually mean a 6-cm circle-shaped field for simple drain sites, with larger fields for patients who have had a thoracotomy for a video-assisted thoracoscopic pleurodesis or a decortication.

Palliative Radiotherapy

As beams are usually defined on the simulator, GTV, CTV and PTV are not defined. A 1-cm margin from the edge of any masses to the beam edge is recommended.

Dose Solutions

Conformal – Adjuvant Radiotherapy

It is a major challenge to produce a conformal plan to treat the PTV uniformly to 54 Gy while maintaining critical organ tolerance (Figure 21.2). Table 21.1 gives suggested OAR tolerance doses when the dose prescribed to the PTV is given in 1.8 Gy fractions.

Dose to the PTV2 can be compromised to achieve target doses to the spinal cord, contralateral lung, contralateral kidney and liver. The minimum dose to PTV2 should be 45 Gy and the PTV1 should receive the prescribed dose of 54 Gy.

The large circumferential CTV and multiple OAR mean the best conformal solution is a pair of anterior and posterior photon beams with MLC shielding to the liver, kidneys, heart and spinal cord added during the treatment course, depending on their tolerance. The shielded areas within the target volume are then treated with electrons matched as well as possible to the photon fields.

Complex – Adjuvant Radiotherapy

In view of the difficulties of producing a conformal plan that adequately treats the PTV while achieving the dose constraints in Table 21.1, IMRT has been used in this setting. A potential disadvantage of IMRT

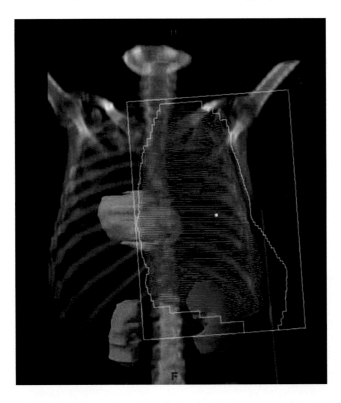

FIGURE 21.2   Target volume for adjuvant radiotherapy after extrapleural pneumonectomy. A DRR showing the overlap of PTV2 (red) with the kidney, spinal cord and heart. It is impossible to treat this volume to 54 Gy with conventional photon fields while keeping to critical organ tolerance doses.

TABLE 21.1

Suggested Tolerance Doses for OAR in Adjuvant Radiotherapy for Mesothelioma[a]

OAR	Target
Spinal cord + 5 mm	50 Gy
Contralateral lung	V20 ≤ 15 per cent. Some centres also recommend constraints on mean lung dose (e.g. MLD <9.5 Gy) and V5 (e.g. V5 <60 per cent)
Contralateral kidney	D80 per cent <15 Gy
Ipsilateral kidney	As low as possible
Heart	D70 per cent <45 Gy and D_{max} <60 Gy. These limits may be exceeded if residual disease is present close to the heart.
Liver	Mean dose <35 Gy
Oesophagus	Less than 12 cm length in treated volume

[a] Taken from the MARS trial with permission of Dr. Senan.

is the increased dose to the remaining lung, with small single centre series reporting death rates from pneumonitis as high as 50 per cent. To reduce this risk, the gantry angles for IMRT should be chosen to minimise exit through the contralateral lung.

The IMRT beams can also be restricted so that the superior part of the PTV is treated with just a few beams thus avoiding exit doses to the contralateral lung and reducing pulmonary toxicity. The inferior portion near the heart or liver is treated with all beams to maximise the advantage of highly conformal dose in this part of the volume.

Another possible solution is to use combined photon IMRT and electron beams – using the electrons to produce a conformal dose at depth to the more superficial part of the PTV, and IMRT to produce conformality in other planes.

Simple – Prophylactic and Palliative Radiotherapy

In prophylactic treatment, electrons are preferred, with the energy chosen to treat from the skin surface down to the pleura within the 90 per cent isodose. The depth of the pleura is best measured on diagnostic CT scans but can be estimated clinically. In practice, 9–12 MeV electrons with 5-mm tissue equivalent bolus are frequently used. While standard cutouts are used for drain sites, a patient-specific cutout is usually required for larger scars that follow more complex procedures. If electrons are not available, 300 kV photons can be used, but this technique will not produce adequate coverage of the tract close to the pleural surface.

Palliative radiotherapy for painful masses can be achieved with a direct electron beam or with parallel opposed photon beams. Photons are often more appropriate given the depth of painful lesions, particularly when the mass extends around the curved chest wall.

Dose Fractionation

Adjuvant

PTV1

- 54 Gy in 30 daily fractions of 1.8 Gy given in six weeks
- The plan chosen must deliver a minimum dose of 45 Gy to PTV2

Prophylactic

- 21 Gy in 3 daily fractions of 7 Gy given in three days

Palliative

- 8 Gy in 1 fraction
- 20 Gy in 5 fractions of 4 Gy given in one week

Treatment Delivery and Patient Care

Adjuvant Radiotherapy

Cardiac function (ejection fraction must be >40 per cent) and contralateral renal function (serum creatinine or glomerular filtration rate [GFR] estimation and evaluation of differential renal function) should be assessed before treatment.

A dietetic assessment before radiotherapy is desirable to initiate high calorie supplements if necessary. Patients should be advised about good skin care (gentle washing with simple soap, and application of aqueous cream) and management of esophagitis (see Chapter 19). Codeine linctus or oral opiates may help alleviate cough. Five-HT antagonists may be required to prevent emesis.

A careful discussion with the patient about the potential benefits and possible late effects of radiotherapy is essential. Patients are treated daily with no compensation for missed days.

Palliative/Prophylactic Radiotherapy

Patients should be instructed in skin care – the use of simple soaps and aqueous cream to keep the skin moisturised. Bright erythema is usual when 21 Gy in 3 fractions over three days is used, and some long-term pigmentation of the skin is common.

Verification

Treatment is verified using the protocol described for lung cancer in Chapter 20.

Key Trials

Boutin C, Rey F, Viallat JR. Prevention of malignant seeding after invasive diagnostic procedures in patients with pleural mesothelioma. Chest 1995;108:754–758.

Clive O, et al. Prophylactic radiotherapy for the prevention of procedure-tract metastases after surgical and large bore procedures in malignant mesothelioma (SMART): A multicentre open label phase 3 randomised controlled trial. Lancet Oncol 2016;17(8):1094–1104.

MARS (Mesothelioma and Radical Surgery) trial. Three Cycles of Chemotherapy Followed Either by EPP and Radiotherapy or by No Surgery or Radiotherapy. ICR, Scientific Principal Investigator Prof Julian Peto. Closed 2008.

O'Rourke N, Garcia JC, Paul J, et al. A randomised controlled trial of intervention site radiotherapy in malignant pleural mesothelioma. Radiother Oncol 2007;84:18–22.

SAKK 17/04 study. Neoadjuvant Chemotherapy and Extrapleural Pneumonectomy of Malignant Pleural Mesothelioma With or Without Hemithoracic Radiotherapy. A randomised multicentre phase II trial. Swiss trial aiming to recruit over 150 patients.

INFORMATION SOURCES

Allen AA, Schofield D, Hacker F, et al. Restricted field IMRT dramatically enhances IMRT planning for mesothelioma. Int J Radiat Oncol Biol Phys 2007;69:1587–1592.

Waite K, Gilligan D. The role of radiotherapy in the treatment of malignant pleural mesothelioma. Clin Oncol 2007;19:182–187.

22

Breast

Indications for Radiotherapy

Breast Radiotherapy

Adjuvant radiotherapy given following surgery for primary carcinoma of the breast has been shown to reduce the incidence of locoregional recurrence from 30 per cent to 10.5 per cent at 20 years and breast cancer deaths by 5.4 per cent at 20 years.

Radiotherapy is standard treatment after complete local excision of ductal carcinoma in situ (DCIS), and current trials are evaluating its role in 'low-risk' patients compared with surgery alone.

Clinical T1, T2 less than 3 cm, N0 invasive breast cancers are treated by wide local excision (WLE) followed by radiotherapy with comparable local control rates to mastectomy, both combined with axillary surgery. The tumour site, size, histological type, grade and extent of in situ disease, along with the size of the breast, all influence choice of treatment, as does consideration of the expected cosmetic result and patient preference. Radiotherapy is indicated for all patients after conservative surgery. There have been trials aiming to identify a 'low-risk' group where surgery alone gives adequate local control and radiotherapy may be omitted. PRIME 2 trial studied women over the age of 65 with low risk, node-negative, ER-positive invasive cancer following WLE. The results showed that although there was a significant but modest reduction in local recurrence in the radiotherapy arm, there was no effect on overall survival. Therefore omission of adjuvant radiotherapy in this group of women may be considered. Contraindications to conservative surgery include multifocal breast tumours, patients with a known TP53 mutation, extensive DCIS, central tumours in a small breast and incomplete excision. Significant preexisting cardiac or lung disease, scleroderma and limited shoulder mobility may prevent the use of radiotherapy. Patients with operable tumours which are 3–4 cm or more in diameter have a higher local recurrence rate with conservative surgery and radiotherapy, and may be offered primary systemic therapy. Long-term results of this strategy, which aims to downstage the tumour and avoid mastectomy in many patients, are awaited. After primary chemotherapy, indications for locoregional radiotherapy are determined by high risk factors at presentation and preoperative clinical staging rather than postoperative pathological staging.

Accelerated Dose Fractionation for Breast Radiotherapy

The Early Breast Cancer Trialists' Collaborative Group systematic overview confirms the role of adjuvant radiotherapy after primary surgery in early-stage breast cancer. Initially, the dose delivered was 50 Gy in 25 fractions over five weeks. The START trial showed that 40 Gy in 15 fractions gave no difference in locoregional relapse and is standard fractionation in UK. The FastForward trial has recently reported five-year follow-up showing non-inferiority of 26 Gy in 5 fractions over one week compared to 40 Gy in 15 fractions in terms of local recurrence and normal tissue effects. Patients included in the trial were pT1-3, pN0-1, M0.

Primary lymphoma of the breast is commonly high grade and treated by primary chemotherapy followed by local radiotherapy. For malignant phyllodes tumours and sarcomas of the breast, mastectomy is the treatment of choice.

Patients with bilateral tumours are treated according to the indications for each individual tumour site.

DOI: 10.1201/9781315171562-22

Tumour Bed Boost Radiotherapy

After complete excision, the decision to use a 'boost' dose to the tumour bed should balance the individual's risk of local recurrence (dependent on factors such as age, tumour grade and size, lymphovascular invasion, margin status, endocrine receptor status, and use of systemic therapy) against the risk of late effects (e.g. cardiac or lung damage because of shallow breast tissue over heart or ribs). EORTC 22881 showed that in patients younger than 40, a boost dose of 16 Gy in 8 fractions resulted in a greater reduction of local failure than for other age groups, but the relative risk reduction was similar for all ages. All patients who have microscopic tumour present within 1 mm of resection margin, and where re-excision or mastectomy is declined, should be considered for boost radiotherapy.

Post-mastectomy Radiotherapy

More patients are having immediate breast reconstruction after mastectomy using either microvascular techniques or an implant. Subsequent radiotherapy may lead to a risk of late fibrosis and outcomes are being monitored. Post-mastectomy radiotherapy is recommended for patients with T3, T4 tumours and those with four or more positive axillary nodes who have a high risk of local recurrence (around 30 per cent), which is reduced by at least two-thirds. The Danish Breast Cancer Trials Group (DBCG) reported a 9 per cent absolute increase in survival rate at 15 years after post-mastectomy radiotherapy in all groups of node positive patients. Therefore patients with one to three nodes, and, for example, young patients and those with one or more risk factors including large T2–3 tumours, grade III, oestrogen receptor negative, lymphovascular invasion or lobular histology with an estimated 10–20 per cent local recurrence risk at ten years, may also be considered for chest wall radiotherapy. Local guidelines must be developed with a threshold chosen for the level of risk of local recurrence that merits treatment until further trial data are available.

For inoperable T3 and T4 tumours, primary systemic therapy is given before combined local treatment with surgery and locoregional radiotherapy, the sequence depending on tumour regression, staging and prognostic factors.

Lymph Node Irradiation

Axillary node surgery can vary from a sample of nodes to complete axillary node dissection depending on the clinical situation. Lymph node irradiation also varies depending on the type of surgery performed and the number of nodes containing malignancy.

Sentinel node biopsy allows selective axillary dissection for patients with a positive node biopsy. NSABP-32 trial shows that no additional advantage is seen with axillary lymph node dissection over sentinel lymph node biopsy in node-negative patients. A number of trials have reported assessing management of the axilla after positive sentinel node biopsy. Trials to date studying this scenario have been criticised due to protocol violations, lack of radiotherapy consistency and underpowered study. POSNOC is a UK trial studying axillary radiotherapy versus axillary lymph node dissection versus no further treatment in the event of a positive sentinel lymph node biopsy. We await the results of this trial. Until this and similar trials have reported, we recommend that patients with a macrometastasis at sentinel lymph node biopsy in a fewer-than-three-node sample should have further surgery to clear the axilla. If further surgery is not possible, axillary radiotherapy can be given as per AMAROS trial. Where sentinel node biopsy is not available, lymph node irradiation is unnecessary if an axillary dissection up to the lateral border of the pectoralis minor (level I) is negative.

If level I axillary nodes are involved, there is a >5 per cent risk of subsequent supraclavicular fossa (SCF) recurrence, so irradiation may be given to levels II and III axillary and SCF nodes. When four or more nodes, a single node >2 cm or level III nodes are involved, the risk of SCF involvement is 15–20 per cent and radiotherapy is indicated. After axillary dissection to level III with positive nodes, axillary radiotherapy is associated with considerable morbidity and should be avoided unless there is known residual disease, but SCF treatment is given. Nodal radiotherapy is indicated for locally advanced disease after primary systemic treatment, where surgery is not possible.

Radiotherapy to the internal mammary nodes should be considered in patients at high risk of locoregional recurrence. A 3–5 per cent disease-free survival benefit was seen in MA20 & EORTC 22922/10925 trials. Internal mammary node irradiation increases lung and cardiac toxicity and scanning in deep inspiratory breath hold position (DIBH) and planning with IMRT or arc therapy to reduce dose to organs at risk may be considered. The internal mammary chain should be outlined on the RT planning scan.

Improved adjuvant systemic therapies such as anthracyclines, taxanes and trastuzumab alter the risk versus benefit analysis of breast and lymph node irradiation because of the risk of cardiac toxicity. Gene expression profiling of primary breast cancer will be used to individualise indications for radiotherapy in the future, based on predictions of risk of locoregional recurrence.

Partial Breast Irradiation

A number of recent trials have been studying partial breast irradiation (with and without acceleration) with a variety of techniques including external beam photon therapy, interstitial brachytherapy, intraoperative therapy. These trials have shown promising results with better cosmesis and can be considered for patients who cannot undergo conventional EBRT and are not suitable for mastectomy. There are now local control and long-term survival data with some of these techniques but they are not yet routine practice.

Palliative Radiotherapy

Radiotherapy has a major role in the palliation of locally advanced and fungating breast tumours and in treating symptomatic metastases at sites such as bone, brain, skin, lymph nodes, choroid and meninges.

Prognostic factors, PS and patient preference all affect the final decision made by the multidisciplinary team.

Sequencing of Multimodality Treatment

In the adjuvant setting, chemotherapy is given before radiotherapy to reduce side effects. This may mean that radiotherapy is delayed by four to six months. The optimal sequencing of chemo- and radiotherapy was the subject of the SECRAB trial where treatment was randomised to a sequential versus synchronous schedule of chemo- and radiotherapy. There was no difference in the locoregional recurrence rate between the two arms, and a subgroup analysis limited to local recurrence revealed a small statistically significant advantage in favour of synchronous therapy. Synchronous therapy did not have a negative impact on survival or radiation-induced skin toxicity. Primary chemotherapy for operable breast cancer is followed by surgery and then subsequent radiotherapy. For locally advanced disease, primary chemotherapy or endocrine therapy may be followed by surgery if technically feasible, or further downstaging using locoregional radiotherapy may be attempted, reserving surgery for excision of residual disease if restaging is clear.

Clinical and Radiological Anatomy

Breast cancer spreads locally by direct infiltration of the surrounding parenchyma and may extend to underlying muscle and overlying skin, including the nipple. A dense network of lymphatics in the skin may facilitate widespread cutaneous permeation by tumour.

Lymphatics drain laterally to the axilla, medially to internal mammary nodes and superiorly to the supraclavicular fossa (Figure 22.1). Lymphatic vessels from the whole breast drain to the internal mammary nodes, which communicate with the contralateral chain superiorly. The internal mammary nodes lie on the internal surface of the anterior chest wall closely applied to the internal mammary artery. Although the anatomical drainage pattern is complex, involvement by tumour is most commonly found in the axillary lymph nodes. These are divided into levels I–III, which are used to guide surgical axillary

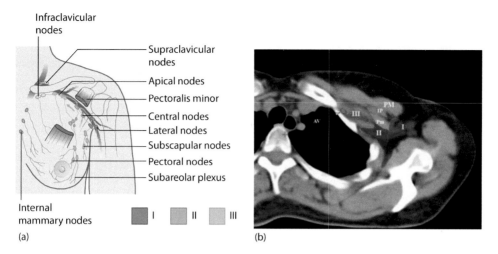

FIGURE 22.1 (a) Diagram of lymphatic drainage of the breast. (b) Transverse CT scan of the left axilla (patient with arms up) both showing position of levels I–III axillary lymph nodes. AV, axillary vessels; Pm, pectoralis minor; PM, pectoralis major; IP, inter-pectoral nodes.

node dissection. Levels are described in relation to the pectoralis minor muscle. Level I nodes lie infero-lateral to its lateral border, level II posteriorly between its medial and lateral borders, and level III medial to the medial border of pectoralis minor adjacent to the axillary vein and first rib. Level III nodes are continuous with the supraclavicular nodes medially and anteriorly and also with the infraclavicular nodes.

Assessment of Primary Disease

Ideally, the radiation oncologist should examine the patient preoperatively. Breast examination includes inspection for nipple or skin retraction, discharge, ulceration or asymmetry, and palpation for size and site of the lump and fixation to adjacent structures. Glandular drainage areas are also assessed and TNM staging recorded on an accurate diagram. A photograph may be used to show the exact position of the lesion. Mammography is performed to demonstrate the tumour and to detect calcification, multifocal or in situ disease and bilateral involvement. Ultrasound is used to measure the size of the lesion and to guide fine needle aspiration cytology and/or core biopsy for histology. MRI can be used to exclude multifocal disease prior to conservative surgery, particularly for large tumours in a radiographically dense breast and for lobular cancers. MRI is also used to monitor response to therapy where primary chemotherapy is used. Axillary node status may be assessed using ultrasound and guided fine needle aspiration (FNA), or, where there is palpable disease, with CT as part of a staging procedure for more advanced disease. Examination of the surgical specimen should define the size, site and local extent of the primary lesion with macroscopic margins and the number and position of axillary nodes in the specimen. Histological review determines size, type of tumour, grade, microscopic assessment of excision margins, lymphovascular invasion, oestrogen, progesterone and HER2 receptor status, number of lymph nodes involved and removed and any extracapsular extension. Many oncoplastic techniques place the surgical scar at a distance from the tumour bed and this relation should be shown in an accurate operative diagram. Details of the level of any axillary dissection, any residual disease and the placement of titanium clips or gold seeds in the tumour bed should all be recorded. When inoperable primary tumours remain palpable after systemic therapy, they can be assessed by palpation and ultrasound, the dimensions marked on the skin, and a photograph taken.

All patients are discussed in multidisciplinary meetings, with review of imaging and histopathology. If the radial or superficial margins are incomplete, re-excision is advised, although usually the deep margin has been cleared down to pectoral fascia. Extensive DCIS is an indication for mastectomy, but minor focal margin involvement by DCIS may be dealt with by re-excision or a tumour bed boost, according to risk factors. Severe lung or cardiac disease, scleroderma, other significant comorbidity or immobility that would contraindicate radiotherapy should be identified so that mastectomy can be considered instead of conservative surgery.

Data Acquisition

Immobilisation

The position of the patient must remain identical for localisation on a CT scanner or simulator and during subsequent treatment. Most commonly, the patient is treated supine using an immobilisation device which secures both arms above the head, as this lifts the breast superiorly, reducing cardiac doses, and also provides symmetry if contralateral breast irradiation is required later. A headrest, elbow and armrests, knee supports and a footboard provide stability. Care must be taken at data acquisition to adapt all the supporting devices to the individual patient's size and shape to maximise comfort, and so aid reproducibility for subsequent treatment. These recorded parameters, with a system of medial and lateral tattoos and orthogonal laser lights, ensure alignment of the patient and consistency of setup (Figure 22.2). Often, an inclined plane is used with fixed angle positions. This brings the chest wall parallel to the treatment couch and may reduce the need for collimator angulation. The inclination is limited to a 10–15° angle for 70 cm, and 17.5–20° for larger 85-cm aperture CT scanners or simulator planning. Some centres treat the patient lying flat on the couch top, without an incline, with a similar immobilisation system but using collimator rotation.

Patients with large or pendulous breasts treated supine require a breast support, either with a thermoplastic shell or breast cup, which can be used to bring the lateral and inferior part of the breast anteriorly away from the heart, lung and abdomen. It is important to avoid displacing the breast too far superiorly over the neck. Increased erythema due to loss of skin sparing by the shell may be offset by reduced severity of skin reaction in the inframammary fold. Alternatively, patients with pendulous breasts can be treated in the prone position, which reduces mean lung and cardiac doses and produces a more homogeneous dose distribution (Figure 22.3). This may improve cosmesis, but risks underdosage at the medial and lateral borders of the PTV close to the chest wall, and should be avoided for primary tumours in

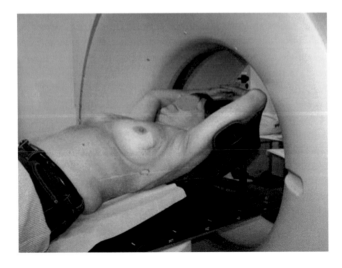

FIGURE 22.2   Large-bore CT scanner with patient immobilised on system using inclined plane, arms up, with reference points outlined with radio-opaque material and aligned with laser lights.

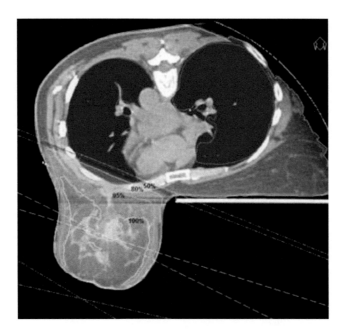

FIGURE 22.3 CT dose distribution to right breast with patient in the prone position (6 MV [gantry 296° and 107°], weighting 100 per cent lat/105 per cent med. 15.6 [W] 19 [L]). (Courtesy of Greg Rattray, Royal Brisbane and Women's Hospital.)

these situations. This technique cannot be combined with lymph node irradiation but can be used to treat bilateral tumours.

Whole Breast

CT Scanning

Where available, CT scanning has become standard for planning breast radiotherapy. After palpation, the breast CTV and surgical breast scar are marked with radio-opaque material before scanning. The upper and lower limits of the CT scan are chosen so that CT data are acquired superiorly from above the shoulder to include the neck and inferiorly to include all of the ipsilateral lung and 5 cm below breast tissue. CT data of the whole breast and critical structures such as lung and heart are needed for DVH calculations and to position lymph node beams. Slice thickness should be sufficient (usually 2–3 mm but dependent on agreed local CT protocols) to produce good quality images for target volume and OAR definition and to create DRRs for accurate portal image comparison. Three reference tattoos are placed on the central slice and in the medial and lateral positions on right and left sides so that measurements can be made to subsequent beam centres.

The volumetric CT data are exported to the treatment planning system (TPS) and a virtual simulation package can be used to define medial and lateral tangential beams to encompass the breast CTV. These can be adapted by viewing the posterior border of the CTV on all CT slices to ensure coverage of the tumour bed as delineated by titanium clips or gold seeds on CT. Central lung distance (CLD) should be less than 2 cm to avoid symptomatic pneumonitis. The heart, especially the left anterior descending artery, should be excluded. Where this is impossible, maximum heart distance (MHD) must be kept to less than 1 cm. CT also helps distinguish glandular from adipose tissue, especially at the posterolateral aspect of the breast. If the heart cannot be excluded completely from the target volume without compromising the tumour bed CTV, techniques such as deep inspiratory breath-hold (DIBH) and/or localised cardiac shielding can be introduced at the dose planning stage. During DIBH setup the patient is instructed to inspire to a specified threshold and the radiation planning scan is performed. The patient is

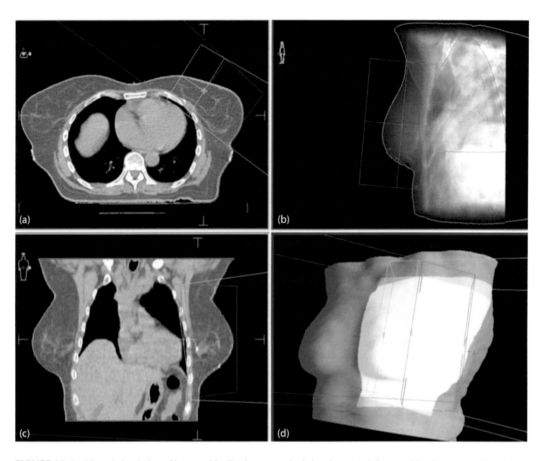

FIGURE 22.4 Virtual simulation of breast with clips in tumour bed showing (a) axial scan with adjustment of beam border anteriorly from skin markers to avoid heart; (b) sagittal; (c) coronal; (d) rendered image of tangential beams.

then required to hold the same level of inspiration during each radiation treatment. A number of studies have confirmed reduction in mean cardiac dose with DIBH. The final virtual simulation is performed by a radiographer, usually with an oncologist, and diagrams, DRRs and virtual simulation rendered images are created before the dose plan is produced (Figure 22.4). Alternatively, the breast CTV and PTV can be outlined on each CT image with full 3D delineation of the target volume. This is more time-consuming but has advantages where more advanced or inoperable tumours are visualised or when inverse planned IMRT is used. The lung is contoured in its entirety for all 3D dose planning and DVHs.

Target Volume Definition

CTV Breast

For adjuvant whole breast radiotherapy after surgical excision of tumour there is no GTV, and the whole breast is the CTV. The aim is to treat all the glandular breast tissue down to deep fascia, but not the underlying muscle, rib cage, overlying skin or excision scar. A CTV-PTV margin is added to account for respiration, variations in patient position, both intra- and inter-fractionally, breast swelling and setup uncertainties. For partial breast irradiation, the GTV is outlined by the surgical clips placed at the time of surgery and a typical GTV-CTV margin for PBI is 15 mm with a CTV-PTV margin of 10 mm. Each department should measure its systematic and random errors using a verification programme comparing simulator or DRR images with EPIs. Most departments record standard deviations for systematic errors of around 2–5 mm, and an additional margin of 5 mm is reported as sufficient to account for respiratory motion. This gives a CTV-PTV margin of 10 mm for a standard breast target volume. When implanted clips are viewed in the tumour bed at CT, the proposed CTV and PTV margins may need to be repositioned to ensure adequate coverage of the tumour bed. During virtual simulation, the tangential beams can be redesigned to encompass the CT-derived CTV and PTV and to reduce the amount of lung and heart included in the treatment volume.

GTV Breast

For inoperable tumours and following partial regression after primary systemic therapy where surgery is still not feasible, the gross tumour is present. This can be defined with the patient in the treatment position using palpation, CT or ultrasound to design boost volumes.

CTV-Reconstructed Breast or Chest Wall

The target volume is the skin flaps and scar and any subcutaneous tissues down to the deep fascia overlying muscles. In locally advanced breast cancer with skin infiltration, skin is included in the target volume. The extreme ends of the surgical scar may be excluded medially or laterally to reduce dose to underlying heart and lung to tolerance limits. It is important to know the site of the primary tumour within the breast at presentation and histological details of the surgical specimen when adjusting beams in this way at virtual simulation.

Simulator

Conventionally, a simulator has been used to localise the breast with the previously described immobilisation system and the patient aligned with two laterals and a sagittal laser light. Field borders rather than target volumes are defined by palpating the entire breast and adding a 1.5 cm margin which includes penumbra. The superior border covers as much of the breast as possible and lies at about the level of the suprasternal notch medially, and just below the level of the abducted arm laterally to allow beam entry. The inferior border lies 1.5 cm below the breast, or more if the tumour bed is situated very inferiorly. The medial border is usually in the midline and the lateral border 1.5 cm from the lateral border of the breast. However, these borders should be modified, both to ensure good coverage of the tumour bed and also to reduce heart (MHD <1 cm) and lung doses (CLD <2 cm), even if in some patients this means compromising coverage of peripheral breast tissue sited away from the tumour bed (Figure 22.5).

Using the simulator, an isocentric technique of medial and lateral tangential fields is constructed. The anterior border of the field in free air should be at least 1.5 cm from the skin surface to ensure a satisfactory dose distribution. The borders of the medial and lateral fields are then marked on the skin. Two reference tattoos are made at medial and lateral field centres over reproducible stable sites with a third one made on the contralateral side of the body to align with lasers to prevent rotation. An external contour of a transverse cross section of the patient is taken in 2D through the centre of the fields. Where a simulator CT is available, three CT outlines may be taken at different levels for lung correction and superior–inferior dose compensation.

Beam divergence into the lung at the posterior border of the field can be reduced by using either independent collimators to block the posterior half of the beam, or an appropriate gantry angle to align the opposing posterior field borders.

Breast Tumour Bed

Target Volume

Using CT data, the tumour bed can be visualised in 3D by using clips placed in pairs (to identify migration) at surgery around the wall of the surgical cavity to mark its posterior, lateral, medial,

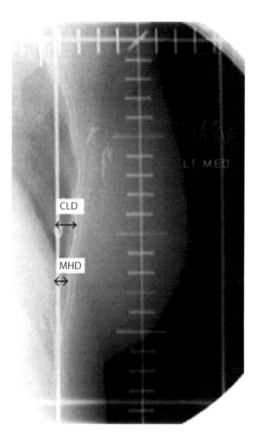

FIGURE 22.5   Simulator film of left medial tangential field with CLD, MHD and clips in the tumour bed.

superior and inferior borders (Figure 22.6) and any changes in surrounding tissue architecture on CT felt clinically to be included in the target. The anterior border of the cavity should also be marked with clips if the surgical scar is not located anterior to the tumour bed. The CTV (tumour bed) then includes the tumour bed, and an anisotropic margin of 5 mm in the direction of the close surgical margins should be added. A further margin is also necessary if there are no clips marking the excision cavity. This will be determined on an individual patient basis and should be a rare occurrence. The CTV should be modified if the volume produced is felt to be clinically inappropriately large and could potentially increase the risk of late normal tissue complications. The planning target volume (PTV) includes the tumour bed CTV plus a uniform 5 mm margin. An anisotropic margin of 5 mm in the direction of the close surgical margins should be added. A further margin is also necessary if there are no clips marking the excision cavity. This will be determined on an individual patient basis and should be a rare occurrence. The CTV should be modified if the volume produced is felt to be clinically inappropriately large and could potentially increase the risk of late normal tissue complications. The planning target volume (PTV) includes the tumour bed CTV plus a uniform 5 mm margin, editing 5 mm from the skin and lung surfaces. Both CT scanning and the use of clips have been shown to improve accuracy of localisation of the volume, depth of the tumour bed and choice of electron energy compared with clinical assessment alone.

Commonly, boost radiotherapy to the tumour bed is given with electron therapy. To aid treatment delivery, rendered images can be produced to show the position of the electron beam in relation to the surface scar. If the boost volume is too deep for treatment with electrons a photon boost can be used to achieve optimal PTV using smaller beams in a 3D conformal beam arrangement. A simultaneous integrated boost technique with photons may also be used. The whole breast and boost volume are planned

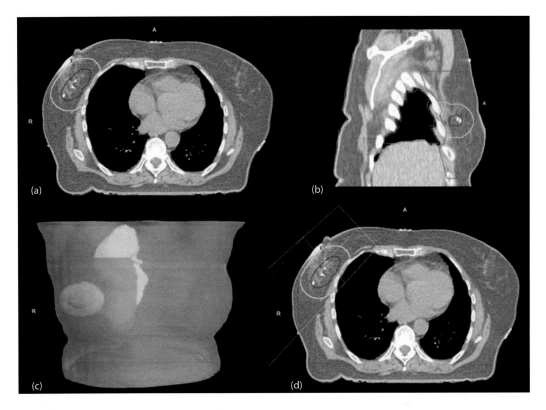

FIGURE 22.6 (a) Axial CT scan with clips in the tumour bed (dark blue), boost CTV (cyan) and whole breast PTV (red); (b) sagittal view; (c) 3D image (lung in green); (d) axial CT scan with beams for whole breast EBRT (6 MV, gantry 221° and 47°, 9.5[W] 20[L]).

together with photons (Figure 22.7). The heart and lung doses should be measured and kept below tolerances reported in the literature, e.g. IMPORT High trial tolerances (Table 22.1).

Axillary and Supraclavicular Lymph Nodes

CT Scanning

A CT protocol is used similar to that described for whole breast. Axillary surgical clips may aid localisation, but uninvolved nodes are not seen on CT. CT scanning can be used to design a mono-isocentric technique for combined breast and lymph node irradiation where a single isocentre is set up at depth on the match line of the tangential and anterior nodal fields (Figure 22.8).

TABLE 22.1

Planning Parameters for OARs Treated with Photon Boost

OAR	Mandatory	Optimum
Ipsilateral lung V18 Gy	15	10
Contralateral lung V2.5 Gy	15	3
Heart V13 Gy	10	2
Ipsilateral lung mean dose	6	–
Contralateral lung mean dose	1	–
Heart mean dose	3	1.7

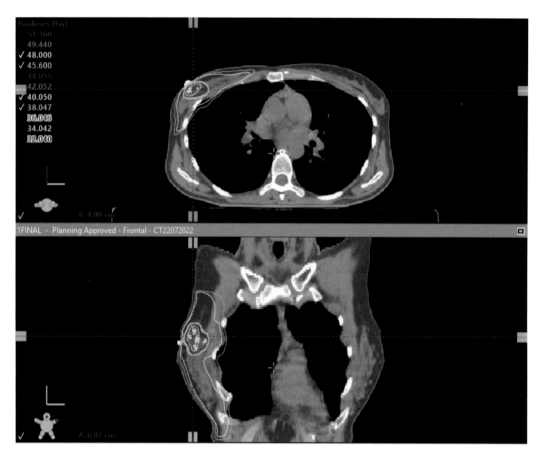

FIGURE 22.7   A simultaneous integrated photon boost technique (Breast dose 40 Gy, boost dose 48 Gy).

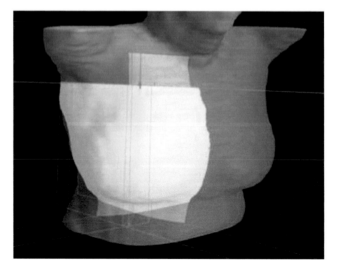

FIGURE 22.8   Single isocentric technique for EBRT to treat breast, axillary and supraclavicular lymph nodes shown with 3D rendered CT image.

Target Volume

The lymphatic drainage to the axillary and supraclavicular nodes forms an irregular volume with its upper border lying anteriorly in the supraclavicular fossa, and extending more posteriorly at the lower border to include all groups of axillary nodes (see Figure 22.1, p. 258).

CT studies have shown that axillary nodes lie at a mean depth of 3–5 cm and are anterior to the mid-axillary line. Supraclavicular nodes lie at a mean depth of 4 cm. Internal mammary lymph nodes lie 2–4 cm lateral and deep to the midline in the first three intercostal spaces. CT scanning can be used to locate the internal mammary arteries which are closely applied to the nodes to help delineate the target volume. Studies show that level I axillary nodes may not be routinely included in the standard breast CTV, and great care must be used to delineate these nodes marked with surgical clips in the axillary tail of the breast CTV when treatment is indicated.

The irregular target volume of the breast or chest wall and regional lymph nodes makes it technically difficult to deliver an equal and adequate dose to all areas and to spare the lungs, heart, brachial plexus and spinal cord.

Simulator

Immobilisation, patient positioning and alignment are as described for breast radiotherapy. An anterior field is used to include level II and III axillary and supraclavicular nodes in the target volume. The medial border is placed 1 cm lateral to the midline or at the midline with a 10° gantry angle away from the larynx and spinal cord. The lateral border lies at the outer edge of the head of the humerus. The superior border extends at least 3 cm above the medial end of the clavicle, but laterally leaves a 1–2-cm margin of skin clear superiorly to avoid excessive skin reaction. Using a mono-isocentric technique to treat breast and lymph nodes, the inferior border is on line with the superior border of the tangential fields through the match line with the isocentre at depth. Shielding of the acromioclavicular joint and humeral head is important to avoid fibrosis and maintain shoulder mobility. Shielding to the apex of the lung should be applied with care as it may shield level II and/or III nodes which may be part of the target volume. Where level III nodes have been removed, an anterior field to the supraclavicular fossa nodes only is used, with the lateral border altered to lie at the coracoid process (see Figure 8.7, p. 101). Placement of surgical clips may mark the level II and III axillary lymph node areas and should be used to design the nodal field borders.

Dose Solutions

Breast and Reconstructed Breast

For most patients, 6 MV (range 4–8 MV) photons are chosen as optimal. However, with increased breast volume and separation, higher energies (commonly 10 MV) may produce better homogeneity. Because of the increased skin sparing of higher energy beams, care should be taken to check that superficial cavity wall margins and scars of reconstructed breasts receive adequate dose.

Conformal or Complex

Using virtual simulation, beams have been optimised and CT data are used to correct for lung density. A significant number of plans fail to achieve a homogeneous 3D dose distribution (–5 per cent, +7 per cent) when the 2D tangential technique is calculated in 3D (Figure 22.9). Forward planned 3D dose compensation can be achieved using a variety of methods. A randomised clinical trial has shown that patients treated with IMRT and improved 3D dose homogeneity have significantly better breast cosmesis (Figure 22.10). Inverse planned dose solutions aim at optimisation to a set of dose volume constraints and may improve homogeneity still further. This is particularly important for the reconstructed breast.

The position of the left anterior descending coronary artery (LAD) can be seen on CT to lie within the target volume for many patients having left-sided breast radiotherapy. Full dose to this segment of artery

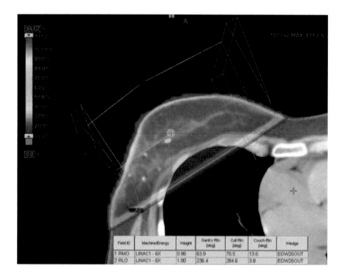

FIGURE 22.9   Dose colour wash for 3D conventional tangential plan through isocentre, off axis dose maximum 111.7 per cent.

may be the cause of increased cardiac mortality from left breast radiotherapy reported in the literature. Modern planning techniques reduce dose to the heart, and it is anticipated that in the future this will translate into decreased cardiac mortality and increase in overall survival with breast radiotherapy. With forward planned dose compensation, MLC leaves can be used to shield the heart (Figure 22.11) and left anterior descending coronary artery for one or both beams, without shielding the tumour bed site which has been marked with clips and is clearly seen in 3D with CT planning. Doses to the contralateral breast may also be lower, reducing the risk of secondary malignancies.

Respiratory motion may affect the dosimetry of dynamic MLC/IMRT techniques, and hence gated therapy or ABC devices to suspend respiration may have advantages in this situation.

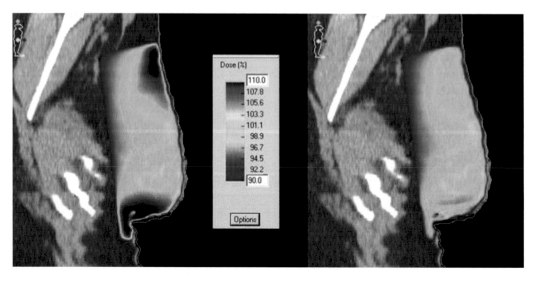

FIGURE 22.10   Sagittal dose distributions of conventional breast radiotherapy (left) compared with dose-compensated IMRT (right) with dose ranges.

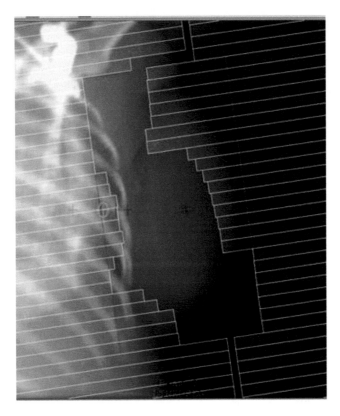

FIGURE 22.11   Sagittal DRR with segmented fields for dose-compensated IMRT with cardiac shielding. Clips seen in the tumour bed and axilla (within shielding).

Conventional

A 2D outline with centres of field borders marked is used to prepare a dose distribution with opposing medial and lateral tangential fields and wedges used as missing tissue compensators. The presence of lung tissue increases dose to the medial and lateral aspects of the breast, and although the amount varies, it is important to incorporate lung corrections. An estimation of lung tissue is marked on the outline from the simulator film and a correction factor (range 0.2–0.3) is applied and a dose solution produced, aiming at a homogeneous dose distribution on a single slice of –5 per cent, +7 per cent (ICRU50). This does not give information at superior or inferior levels of the target volume where dose inhomogeneities of up to 10–15 per cent can occur, especially in large patients. Ideally these patients should have at least three outlines taken through the centre, superior and inferior levels of the volume using a simulator CT facility or camera based outlining system. Dose distributions can then be produced at multiple levels and tissue compensators used to improve homogeneity. Cardiac shielding using blocks or MLC leaves can be used in both beams, although care must be taken with inferior quadrant tumours where the tumour bed may overlie the heart. A risk versus benefit analysis then has to be made, and the MHD reduced to less than 1 cm by altering the posterior field border or partial shielding if possible.

Chest Wall

Conventional planning uses opposing tangential fields but dosimetry is rarely optimal because of the thin target volume of the chest wall surrounded by air and lung. Skin doses cannot be calculated or measured accurately and the role of bolus to the skin remains controversial. Selective use of bolus in high-risk disease after excision of local recurrence or extensive lymphovascular invasion may be considered, usually for the first half of the treatment so that it can be removed if the skin reaction is excessive.

Electron fields have the advantage of avoiding the lung and heart, but CT or ultrasound should be used to measure thickness of the chest wall, which may vary throughout its volume, making choice of electron energy difficult. If the chest wall is very convex in shape, standoff may occur at the medial and lateral field edges with reduction of dose at these sites. Electrons to the chest wall may be combined with photons to the axilla and supraclavicular nodes, as used in the Danish Breast Cancer Group studies.

Where immediate breast reconstruction has taken place, conformal or IMRT techniques should be used to optimise homogeneity of dose, and bolus should be avoided if possible to maintain good cosmesis. Higher energies (e.g. 10 MV) should be avoided because of the risk of low skin dose due to increased skin sparing.

Tumour Bed

Electron beams are commonly used for tumour bed boost irradiation. The target volume should be delineated and is usually 5–8 cm in diameter, requiring an electron applicator of 7–10 cm to allow for lateral penumbra. The electron energy is chosen using CT, simulator-CT or ultrasound to measure depth of the target volume, which should be encompassed by the 90 per cent isodose (ICRU71).

Electrons of 4–15 MeV may be required, but exit doses to the heart should be avoided. For larger volumes or where gross tumour is present, small tangential beams with CT planning or interstitial brachytherapy may be preferable.

Axillary and Supraclavicular Lymph Node Irradiation

A single anterior beam alone is recommended for adjuvant radiotherapy to supraclavicular and axillary lymph nodes. For advanced palpable axillary disease, extensive extranodal involvement or residual axillary disease, an additional posterior axillary beam may be needed to give adequate tumour dose. When the axillary separation exceeds 15 cm, the MPD to the axilla for a single anterior beam falls below 80 per cent for 6 MV photons. An adequate MPD to the axilla can be achieved using a posterior axillary beam every day and weighted according to the separation in the axilla (e.g. for 16–18 cm, 1:10 weighting of posterior: anterior beam applied doses). However, the dose to D_{max} increases for larger separations to 110 per cent and care must be taken to stay within the tolerance of the brachial plexus situated at 2–3 cm depth. A dose distribution must be produced for each patient when this technique is used. Placement of the posterior axillary beam is difficult and should be by CT and/or clinical palpation for macroscopic tumour and the use of surgical clips marking residual or extranodal extension of disease. Three-dimensional conformal treatment volumes are optimal to achieve best dose plan conformality in these situations.

Internal Mammary Node Irradiation

Megavoltage anterior beams are no longer used to treat internal mammary lymph nodes because of the exit dose to the heart. For medial quadrant disease, the tumour bed may lie so close to the internal mammary nodes that it is impossible to treat both target volumes homogeneously. Treatment may then have to be given to the primary tumour alone, by moving the tangential beam further across the midline on to the contralateral side. Studies show that standard fields do not encompass internal mammary nodes (IMN) consistently and often overtreat normal tissues. CT planning is therefore mandatory for internal mammary node irradiation. The internal mammary node chain should be outlined on the Planning CT, and a 5-mm margin added for CTV-PTV. Left-sided breast cancers should be scanned in DIBH to reduce cardiac dose. Electron or combined electron/photon beams can be used to treat internal mammary nodes as in the EORTC 22922/10925 trial protocol. Alternatively, wide tangential fields with cardiac and lung shielding may be used, as in the NCIC CTG MA20 trial. Care must be taken to ensure homogeneity of dose to the primary tumour bed, and a match must be made of the internal mammary node fields to adjacent tangential breast fields. Arc therapy such as VMAT can also be used as an alternative, especially if

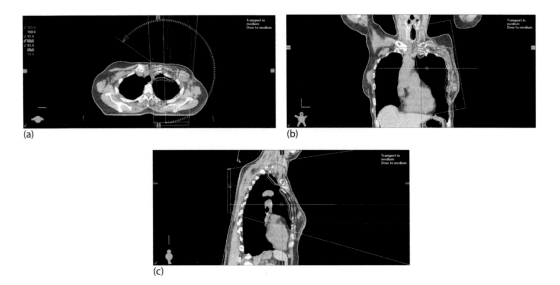

FIGURE 22.12 Six MV VMAT plan for Chest wall + Internal mammary chain (IMC) + supraclavicular fossa showing (a) VMAT arcs; (b) coronal view illustrating dose conformality; (c) IMC PTV outlined in red.

constraints cannot be met by other techniques (Figure 22.12). RCR postoperative radiotherapy for breast cancer: UK consensus states constraints as follows whilst aiming for 90 per cent coverage of IMN PTV with 90 per cent isodose:

- Heart V17 Gy <10 per cent
- Mean heart dose <6 Gy
- Ipsilateral lung V17 Gy <35 per cent
- Mean contralateral lung dose <4 Gy
- Total lung V5 Gy <45 per cent
- Mean contralateral breast dose <3.5 Gy

Combined Breast/Chest Wall and Nodal Irradiation

The inferior border of the nodal beam has to be matched to the superior border of the tangential beams to avoid underdosage or overdosage. This can be achieved by half-beam blocking the inferior border of the nodal beam and rotating the collimator and couch to eliminate the divergence of the superior border of the tangential beams at the match line.

A technique with a single isocentre at depth on the match plane uses asymmetric collimation, but restricts the maximum wedged length of the breast tangential beams. However, it is the preferred technique, as it avoids couch and collimator rotations with risk of collisions and errors and reduces treatment time. When nodal irradiation is required for relapse after breast radiotherapy, a gap can be left between fields to allow for divergence of the superior tangential beams.

Bilateral Breast Irradiation

When bilateral breast irradiation is indicated, both arms are immobilised above the head as illustrated in Figure 22.2 (p. 259). An appropriate gap of 1–1.5 cm should be left in the midline between the tangential fields to avoid overlap.

When radiotherapy is later required for a primary tumour in the contralateral breast, it is important to use the same immobilisation device as for the first tumour treatment to keep the patient position constant.

Previous radiotherapy should be reconstructed to avoid overlap of treatment, especially in the midline and supraclavicular regions, and dose to the underlying spinal cord should be estimated.

Partial Breast Irradiation

Studies show that around 85 per cent of local recurrences after surgery and radiotherapy for operable breast cancer occur in the same quadrant as the primary tumour. A risk-adapted strategy for breast radiotherapy has led to the investigation of partial breast irradiation (PBI) treating the volume around the primary tumour site only. Techniques include external beam radiotherapy with or without concomitant IMRT boost, low- and high-dose brachytherapy, balloon catheter brachytherapy (Ammonite device), kV X-ray applicators (Intrabeam) and intraoperative electron therapy. Clinical trials are being carried out to test PBI using these different modalities. Protocols defining the tumour bed, CTV and PTV for PBI use radio-opaque markers and a careful quality assurance programme which will ensure accurate treatment delivery. Data highlighted that using these techniques shows promising results, however there are low numbers of events reported in the trials and relatively short follow-up to date. The UK IMPORT LOW trial has reported five-year follow-up with PBI using an EBRT technique and shown noninferiority of the technique compared to standard whole breast radiotherapy in terms of local relapse, and equivalent or fewer late normal-tissue adverse effects. PBI with EBRT can therefore be considered in patients over 50 with G1–2 invasive ductal cancers, ≤ 3 cm ER positive and node negative with clear margins and no adverse risk factors. In selected cases, interstitial brachytherapy may be considered in centres set up to use this technique.

Dose Fractionation

Breast, Reconstructed Breast and Chest Wall

- 40 Gy in 15 daily fractions of 2.67 Gy given in three weeks
- 42.5 Gy in 16 daily fractions of 2.66 Gy given in three and a half weeks
- 50 Gy in 25 daily fractions given in five weeks
- 26 Gy in 5 daily fractions in one week as per FastForward trial

All these regimens have been tested in randomised trials with good results. The same fractionation regimens can be used to treat DCIS, as there is no evidence that it has a different radiosensitivity from invasive disease.

Breast Boost Irradiation

Tumour Bed

- 16 Gy in 8 daily fractions given in one and a half weeks
- 10 Gy in 5 daily fractions given in one week
- 13.35 Gy daily fractions given in one week

Doses are prescribed using electron therapy to D_{max} or using photons to the ICRU point at the centre of the target volume; 16 Gy in 8 daily fractions has been shown in the EORTC trial 22881 to reduce local failure by a factor of two compared with no boost. Ten Gy in 5 daily fractions may be used in patients with lower risk of local recurrence.

Incomplete Excision or Residual Primary Tumour

- 20–26 Gy in 10–13 daily fractions given in two to two-and-a-half weeks

Interstitial implantation may also be considered for tumour bed boost irradiation.

Lymph Node Irradiation

- 40 Gy in 15 daily fractions of 2.67 Gy given in three weeks
- 50 Gy in 25 daily fractions given in five weeks

Doses are prescribed at D_{max} (e.g. at 1.5 cm for 6 MV photons).

Palliative Radiotherapy

Patients with breast cancer often live many years with metastatic disease, especially in bone. Care must be taken to check sites of previous irradiation and to match fields carefully to avoid overdosage and unwanted toxicity.

- 8 Gy single fraction for most bone metastases for relief of pain.
- 20 Gy in 5 daily fractions of 4 Gy given in one week may be used for sites such as cervical spine, meningeal disease and nodal masses.
- 36 Gy in 6 fractions of 6 Gy once or twice weekly, given in six weeks for fungating primary tumors, especially in frail patients.

Treatment Delivery and Patient Care

Treatment delivery will vary according to available technology. Where manual wedges, physical compensators or couch rotation are used, the overall time for each treatment fraction is longer. IMRT with wedged tangential beams and additional MLC shaped dose compensating segments has been shown to take very little longer to deliver than conventional tangential fields.

Patients are instructed to avoid abrasion of the irradiated skin when washing and to use simple soap. Aqueous cream is applied twice daily at least 2 hours before or after treatment to keep the skin moisturised. One per cent hydrocortisone cream may be used to relieve the irritation of dry desquamation. If moist desquamation occurs, treatment is temporarily stopped and Atrauman gauze with a pad or hydrogel sheet or foam dressing is applied until healing occurs. Tight-fitting clothes should be avoided as much as possible to reduce friction and abrasion of the skin. Loose cotton garments are recommended. Gentle arm exercises started after surgery are continued.

Later side effects may include breast oedema, shrinkage, pain and tenderness, rib fracture, skin telangiectasia, symptomatic lung fibrosis, cardiac morbidity or late malignancy when radiotherapy is combined with chemotherapy. After nodal radiotherapy, there is a risk of arm lymphoedema, shoulder stiffness or nerve complications.

Verification

The immobilisation device, room laser lights, setup instructions and rendered images are all used to ensure an identical patient position and accurate treatment delivery. Portal imaging should be undertaken using locally agreed evidence-based imaging protocols. This typically consists of imaging the first three daily fractions and then weekly checks, with images being compared with the CT-generated DRR or simulator films and a +/- 5-mm tolerance accepted in the CLD/isocentre position. Consideration should be given to any change in soft tissue contour where forward planned IMRT is used to ensure the delivery of a homogeneous dose distribution. In vivo dosimetry using a diode or TLD measurement is carried out on day 1 in all patients to ensure delivery of the planned dose to each field/segment. To ensure true readings, consideration should be given to the positioning of the diode/TLD for the smaller dose compensation segments used in forward planned techniques. IGRT can be used to match the position of titanium clips in the tumour bed for pretreatment verification.

Key Trials

EORTC 22922/10925: Breast Internal Mammary-medial SCF Node Irradiation for Selected High Risk Group Patients. http://astro2005.abstractsnet.com/handouts/000156_ASTRO_Meeting__September_2005.pdf (Accessed 5 December 2008).

EORTC 22881/10882: Boost Versus No Boost Tumour Bed RT. See Antonini et al. Below (www.ncbi.nlm.nih.gov/pubmed/17126434).

Coles CE, et al. Partial-breast radiotherapy after breast conservation surgery for patients with early breast cancer (UK IMPORT LOW trial): 5-year results from a multicentre, randomised, controlled, phase 3, non-inferiority trial. The Lancet 2017;390(10099):1048–1060.

Dose-escalated simultaneous integrated boost radiotherapy in early breast cancer (IMPORT HIGH): a multicentre, phase 3, non-inferiority, open-label, randomised controlled trial Prof Charlotte E Coles, Joanne S Haviland, Anna M Kirby, et al. The Lancet 401 p 2124–2137.

Donker M, van Tienhoven, G, Straver ME, et al. Radiotherapy or surgery of the axilla after a positive sentinel node in breast cancer (EORTC 10981-22023 AMAROS): A randomised, multicentre, open-label, phase 3 non-inferiority. Lancet Oncol 2014 Nov;15(12):1303–1310.

Hypofractionated breast radiotherapy for 1 week versus 3 weeks (FAST-Forward): 5-year efficacy and late normal tissue effects results from a multicentre, non-inferiority, randomised, phase 3 trial Prof Adrian Murray Brunt, Joanne S Haviland, Duncan A Wheatley et al The Lancet 2017;390(10099):1048–1060.

Partial-breast radiotherapy after breast conservation surgery for patients with early breast cancer (UK IMPORT LOW trial): 5-year results from a multicentre, randomised, controlled, phase 3, non-inferiority trial Dr Charlotte E Coles, Clare L Griffin, Anna M Kirby, et al. The Lancet 390 p1048–1060.

SECRAB: Sequencing of Chemotherapy and Radiotherapy in Adjuvant Breast Cancer. See Bowden et al. Below.

START Trials A and B: Fractionation Study of Breast RT (See Below).

SUPREMO (Selective Use of Post Operative Radiotherapy After Mastectomy): Mastectomy Chest Wall RT for Intermediate Risk Patients. www.supremo-trial.com/ (Accessed 5 December 2008).

INFORMATION SOURCES

Adlard JW, Bundred NJ. Radiotherapy for ductal carcinoma in situ. Clin Oncol 2006;18:179–184.

Antonini N, Jones H, Horiot JC, et al. Effect of age and radiation dose on local control after breast conserving treatment: EORTC trial 22881-10882. Radiother Oncol 2007;82:265–271.

Bowden SJ, Fernando IN, Burton A. Delaying radiotherapy for the delivery of adjuvant chemotherapy in the combined modality treatment of early breast cancer: Is it disadvantageous and could combined treatment be the answer? Clin Oncol 2006;18:247–256.

Brunt AM, et al. Hypofractionated breast radiotherapy for 1 week versus 3 weeks (FAST-forward): 5-year efficacy and late normal tissue effects results from a multicentre, non-inferiority, randomised, phase 3 trial. The Lancet 2020;395(10237):1613–1626.

Dobbs HJ, Greener AJ, Driver D. Geometric Uncertainties in Radiotherapy of Breast Cancer. In: Geometric Uncertainties in Radiotherapy: Defining the Planning Target Volume. BIR Report, BIR Publications Dept, London, UK, 2003.

Donovan E, Bleakley N, Denholm E, et al. On behalf of the Breast Technology Group (UK) randomised trial of standard 2D radiotherapy versus intensity modulated radiotherapy in patients prescribed breast radiotherapy. Radiother Oncol 2007;82:254–264.

Early Breast Cancer Trialists' Collaborative Group (EBCTCG). Effects of radiotherapy and of differences in the extent of surgery for early breast cancer on local recurrence and 15 year survival: An overview of the randomised trials. Lancet 2005;366:2087–2106.

Goodman RL, Grann A, Saracco P, et al. The relationship between radiation fields and regional lymph nodes in carcinoma of the breast. Int J Radiat Oncol Biol Phys 2001;50:99–105.

https://www.rcr.ac.uk/clinical-oncology/service-delivery/postoperative-radiotherapy-breast-cancer-uk-consensus-statements

Hurkmans CW, Borger JH, Pieters BR, et al. Variability in target volume delineation on CT scans of the breast. Int J Radiat Oncol Biol Phys 2001;50:1366–1372.

Krag DN, et al. Sentinel lymph node resection compared with conventional axillary lymph nodes dissection in clinically node-negative patients with breast cancer: Overall survival findings from the NSABP B-32 randomised phase 3 trial. Lancet Oncol 2010;11:927–933.

Kunkler IH, et al. PRIME II investigators. Breast-conserving surgery with or without irradiation in women aged 65 years or older with early breast cancer (PRIME II): A randomised controlled trial. Lancet Oncol 2015 Mar;16(3):266–273.

Lievens Y, Poortmans P, Van den Bogaert W. A glance on quality assurance in EORTC study 22922 evaluating techniques for internal mammary and supraclavicular lymph node chain irradiation in breast cancer. Radiother Oncol 2001;60:257–265.

Overgaard M, Nielsen HM, Overgaard J. Is the benefit of postmastectomy irradiation limited to patients with four or more positive nodes, as recommended in international consensus reports? A subgroup analysis of the DBCG 82 b and c randomised trials. Radiother Oncol 2007;82:247–253.

Owen JR, Ashton A, Bliss JM, et al. Effect of radiotherapy fraction size on tumour control in patients with early breast cancer after local excision: Long term results of a randomised trial. Lancet Oncol 2006;7:467–471.

Radiotherapy of breast cancer: Special issue. Radiother Oncol 2007;82:243–357.

Ragaz J, Olivotto IA, Spinelli JJ, et al. Loco regional radiation therapy in patients with high risk breast cancer receiving adjuvant chemotherapy: 20 year results of the British Columbia randomised trial. J Natl Cancer Inst 2005;97:116–126.

RCR Breast Cancer Consensus Guidelines Links. https://www.rcr.ac.uk/publication/postoperative-radiotherapy-breast-cancer-hypofractionation-rcr-consensus-statements

Recht A, Edge SB, Solin LJ, et al. Post mastectomy radiotherapy: Clinical practice guidelines of the American Society of Clinical Oncology. J Clin Oncol 2001;19:1539–1569.

START Trialists' Group. The UK standardisation of breast radiotherapy (START) trial B of radiotherapy hypofractionation for treatment of early breast cancer: A randomised trial. Lancet 2008;371:1098–1107.

START Trialists' Group. The UK standardisation of breast radiotherapy (START) trial A of radiotherapy hypofractionation for treatment of early breast cancer: A randomised trial. Lancet Oncol 2008;9:331–341.

Whelan T, Mackenzie R, Julian J, et al. Randomised trial of breast irradiation schedules after lumpectomy for women with lymph node-negative breast cancer. J Natl Cancer Inst 2002;94:1143–1150.

23

Haematological Malignancies

LYMPHOMA

Indications for Radiotherapy

Hodgkin Lymphoma

Classical Hodgkin lymphoma most commonly affects young adults aged 20–40 years. Staging is performed using the Lugano classification. The current standard of care for limited-stage (stage I/II) Hodgkin lymphoma with no risk factors (favourable group) is two to three cycles of ABVD (doxorubicin, bleomycin, vinblastine and dacarbazine) followed by consolidation radiotherapy. Those with limited-stage disease and one or more risk factors (large mediastinal mass >10 cm, extranodal involvement, elevated ESR, three or more lymph node regions involved and B symptoms) (unfavourable group) are treated with four cycles of ABVD or two cycles of BEACOPP (bleomycin, etoposide, doxorubicin, cyclophosphamide, vincristine, procarbazine and prednisolone) followed by consolidation radiotherapy. Even in patients with a complete metabolic response on assessment PET, consolidation radiotherapy after ABVD reduces the risk of subsequent disease relapse. However, in the RAPID trial, the absolute reduction in progressive-free survival with no consolidation radiotherapy was only 4 per cent at three years for this group of patients. Hence, consolidation radiotherapy can be omitted in those with a complete metabolic response following ABVD if the risk of late radiation toxicity outweighs the potential benefit of improved tumour control. In patients with residual PET-avid disease after two cycles of ABVD, treatment intensification using two cycles of escalated BEACOPP is recommended prior to consolidation radiotherapy. Radiotherapy alone may be administered in patients with limited-stage Hodgkin lymphoma if they are not candidates for systemic chemotherapy. Advanced-stage (stage III/IV) Hodgkin lymphoma is usually treated with chemotherapy alone with six cycles of ABVD or four to six cycles of escalated BEACOPP. Additional radiotherapy is only used in those with PET-avid residual disease following chemotherapy.

Most patients with primary refractory or relapsed Hodgkin lymphoma are managed with salvage chemotherapy to reduce the tumour burden and mobilise stem cells prior to high-dose chemotherapy (HDCT) and autologous stem cell transplantation (ASCT). Radiotherapy may be indicated in patients with single site PET-avid disease after salvage chemotherapy and prior to HDCT and ASCT. In patients with stage IA nodular lymphocyte predominant Hodgkin lymphoma (NLPHL) and no clinical risk factors, the standard treatment is radiotherapy alone. All other stages of NLPHL are managed in the same way as classical Hodgkin lymphoma. The prognosis of patients with Hodgkin lymphoma has improved substantially over the past three decades. Eighty to ninety per cent of patients now achieve permanent remission following treatment.

Non-Hodgkin Lymphoma

The most common type of high-grade non-Hodgkin lymphoma is the diffuse large B-cell lymphoma (DLBCL). It accounts for 30–60 per cent of all non-Hodgkin lymphomas. Most DLBCLs originate in lymph nodes, but they may also arise from extranodal sites, the most common of which is the

DOI: 10.1201/9781315171562-23

gastrointestinal tract. Other extranodal sites include the mediastinum, breast, testes and the central nervous system (CNS). In patients with early-stage (stage I/II) DLBCL, the treatment options include systemic therapy alone with six to eight cycles of R-CHOP (rituximab, cyclophosphamide, doxorubicin, vincristine and prednisolone) or three to four cycles of R-CHOP followed by consolidation radiotherapy. Factors to take into account when considering consolidation radiotherapy include the initial tumour bulk ($\geq$10 cm), magnitude of response to systemic therapy and the likely morbidity of radiotherapy. Radiotherapy alone can be considered in patients with localised DLBCL not suitable or too frail for systemic therapy. Patients with advanced-stage (stage III/IV) DLBCL are treated primarily with intensive systemic therapy. This may be followed by consolidation radiotherapy to sites of initial bulky disease, PET-negative residual masses or isolated residual PET-avid disease post-systemic therapy. The prognosis of patients with relapsed or primary refractory DLBCL is generally poor. Those with disease that responds to salvage chemotherapy will benefit from HDCT and ASCT. For patients not eligible for HDCT and ASCT, radiotherapy can provide effective palliation and perhaps longer-term disease control if the relapsed/refractory disease is localised.

Primary mediastinal large B-cell lymphoma most commonly occurs in women in their third to fourth decades of life. Patients usually present with a bulky tumour in the anterior mediastinum causing local compressive symptoms. Standard treatment consists of combination systemic therapy followed by consolidation mediastinal radiotherapy in responders. Primary testicular lymphomas usually present as a unilateral testicular mass. CNS relapses may occur in up to 30 per cent of these patients. Standard treatment includes an orchidectomy, six to eight cycles of R-CHOP and CNS prophylaxis with either intrathecal chemotherapy or high-dose intravenous methotrexate. If orchidectomy is not performed, consolidation radiotherapy is given to the involved testis. Prophylactic radiotherapy to the contralateral testis will also reduce testicular relapses. For primary breast lymphomas, the recommended treatment is six cycles of R-CHOP followed by consolidation radiotherapy to the entire ipsilateral breast. Mantle cell lymphoma is an aggressive rare form of non-Hodgkin lymphoma with a poor prognosis. For the small subset of patients with non-bulky stage I/II disease and no adverse prognostic features, treatment comprises systemic therapy followed by consolidation radiotherapy in an approach similar to that for early-stage DLBCL.

Low-grade non-Hodgkin lymphoma includes follicular lymphoma, marginal zone lymphoma and small lymphocytic lymphoma. Low-grade follicular lymphoma presents as localised stage I and II disease in approximately 20 per cent of cases. They are managed with potentially curative radiotherapy. Marginal zone lymphoma comprises extranodal marginal zone lymphoma of mucosa-associated lymphoid tissue, also known as MALT lymphoma, splenic marginal zone lymphoma and nodal marginal zone lymphoma. MALT lymphoma can arise at any extranodal site. It occurs most commonly in the stomach, followed by the orbital adnexa, lung, salivary gland, thyroid and other soft tissues. It usually remains localised within its tissue of origin for a prolonged period of time. Concomitant involvement of multiple mucosal sites and regional lymph nodes may occur. Gastric MALT lymphoma is usually multifocal. It is generally associated with Helicobacter pylori infection. Helicobacter pylori eradication therapy is recommended as the initial treatment for all patients with gastric MALT lymphoma regardless of stage. This can induce lymphoma regression and result in long-term disease control in 75 per cent of cases. For those whose disease fails to regress or recurs after Helicobacter pylori eradication therapy, radiotherapy to the stomach and perigastric nodes can be considered, with treatment response and local control rates exceeding 90 per cent. Radiotherapy is also the preferred treatment option for patients with localised stage IE or IIE MALT lymphoma affecting other sites, with ten-year survival rates of 70–80 per cent.

Patients with stage III and IV low-grade follicular lymphoma may be asymptomatic with low disease burden; such patients can be managed with active surveillance, and systemic therapy is deferred until symptomatic disease progression. Less than 50 per cent of patients on active surveillance require treatment within six years of diagnosis. The disease is not curable and relapses are frequent. The monoclonal antibody rituximab, given in combination with chemotherapy and as maintenance therapy after initial treatment, has improved response rates, progression-free survival and overall survival. Radiotherapy can provide effective palliation and control of localised symptomatic disease. The FoRT trial is a randomised non-inferiority study comparing the standard radiation dose of 24 Gy in 12 fractions with low-dose radiation comprising 4 Gy in 2 fractions in patients with low-grade non-Hodgkin lymphoma. The local progression-free rate at five years was 89.9 per cent with 24 Gy, and 70.4 per cent with 4 Gy.

Cutaneous lymphomas and their management are discussed in Chapter 7.

Clinical and Radiological Anatomy

Lymphomas can affect any lymph node site within the body as well as extranodal sites such as the Waldeyer's ring, gastrointestinal tract, CNS, testes, breast, bone and skin. The staging system for lymphomas is the Lugano classification, which is based on the older Ann Arbor system. Spread occurs to contiguous lymph nodes and via the bloodstream to the spleen, liver, lungs or bone marrow, with extranodal involvement occurring more commonly with non-Hodgkin lymphoma. Lymphomas affecting the paranasal sinuses and testes have a predilection for CNS spread.

Assessment of Primary Disease

Patients are assessed for performance status, comorbidities and B symptoms. Physical examination should include the Waldeyer's ring, liver, spleen and all peripheral lymph node regions with measurement of any palpable involved nodes. An image-guided core biopsy is performed for histological diagnosis. Chest X-ray can identify gross mediastinal lymphadenopathy. A diagnostic contrast-enhanced CT scan of the neck, chest, abdomen and pelvis is performed. MRI is indicated for CNS and extradural lymphomas, along with primary lymphoma of the bone and orbit. Lumbar puncture is performed in patients at high risk of CNS involvement. Radioisotope bone scan or PET scan is required in patients with primary lymphoma of the bone to exclude other skeletal lesions, as multifocal disease is common. Bone marrow aspiration and trephine is performed as part of the diagnostic workup in selected patients.

[18F] 2-fluoro-2-deoxy-D-glucose PET-CT (PET-CT) has a sensitivity of greater than 90 per cent for the detection of most types of lymphoma, with the exception of marginal zone lymphoma and small lymphocytic lymphoma. It is the most accurate method for assessing the disease extent in Hodgkin and non-Hodgkin lymphoma. It is thus an essential staging investigation and it permits accurate identification of sites of involvement before treatment. It should be performed whenever possible in the radiotherapy treatment position so that the scans can be used for subsequent image registration for treatment planning. PET-CT can also be repeated following two or three cycles of chemotherapy for treatment response assessment (Figure 23.1). PET is more sensitive than contrast-enhanced CT at identifying residual disease following chemotherapy. It may identify a subgroup of patients who may benefit from consolidation radiotherapy.

Data Acquisition

Patients are scanned supine with immobilisation devices appropriate for the anatomical site to be treated. For cervical nodal irradiation, a customised thermoplastic shell is used with reference marks on the shell for alignment with lasers.

As lymphomas occur at a wide variety of anatomical sites, decisions regarding treatment techniques are made before CT scanning to ensure that the most appropriate CT protocol is used. The scan should include the entire volume of critical organs of interest such as the lung, heart and kidneys for dose-volume histogram (DVH) assessment. CT scans of 3-mm slice thickness are acquired using intravenous contrast to aid identification and delineation of lymph nodes adjacent to vascular structures and enhance soft tissue definition.

PET-CT scan taken ideally in the treatment position is co-registered with the planning CT scan for target volume delineation.

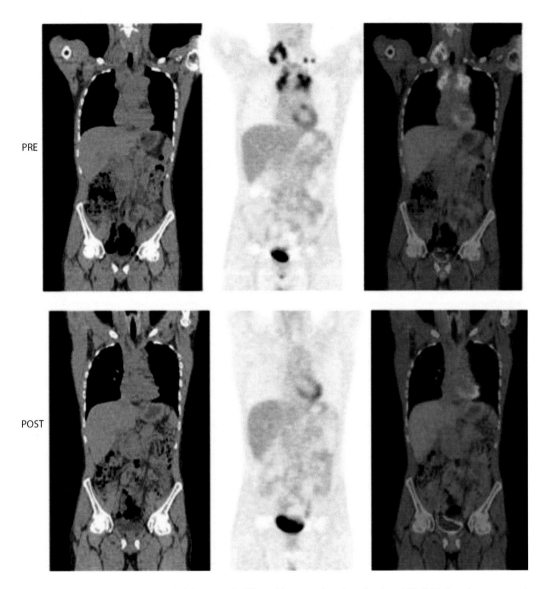

FIGURE 23.1 PET scan of a patient with stage IIA (bilateral lower neck and mediastinum) Hodgkin lymphoma pre- and post-chemotherapy.

If organ motion is likely to be significant during treatment, 4D-CT scans can be used to determine the margins for the internal target volume (ITV). Deep inspiration breath-hold and intensity-modulated radiotherapy (IMRT) or volumetric-modulated arc therapy (VMAT) allow significant sparing of the lungs and heart from radiation and are recommended for the treatment of mediastinal lymphomas.

Target Volume Definition

Traditionally, extended-field radiotherapy techniques such as 'Mantle' and 'Inverted Y' were used as primary treatment for lymphomas, with good cure rates but also relatively high rates of late toxicity, particularly to the heart, lungs and breasts. With treatments now combining chemotherapy and consolidation radiotherapy, data has accumulated to support the use of smaller radiotherapy treatment volumes to minimise toxicity and normal tissue exposure.

Since lymphatic spread first involves nodes adjacent to the primary disease site, locoregional treatment that involves elective irradiation of the first nodal stations may be given. This is known as involved field radiotherapy (IFRT), with the CTV comprising the GTV and adjacent uninvolved nodes. The concept of involved node radiotherapy (INRT) was introduced by the European Organization for Research and Treatment of Cancer (EORTC) in 2006 with the aim of using the smallest effective radiotherapy treatment volume comprising only the disease sites involved by lymphoma, with chemotherapy controlling the adjacent potential microscopic disease. INRT can thus potentially reduce the toxicity risks associated with IFRT. Its efficacy has been confirmed in prospective randomised clinical trials.

The INRT principle of using the smallest effective radiotherapy treatment volume requires optimal imaging for accurate disease localisation and precise co-registration of baseline imaging with the radiotherapy planning CT scan. This is not often possible in routine clinical practice. The baseline imaging may be suboptimal or difficult to co-register with the planning CT due to altered patient position or anatomic changes following chemotherapy. Involved site radiotherapy (ISRT) was thus introduced by the International Lymphoma Radiation Oncology Group (ILROG) in 2014 with a slightly larger treatment volume to account for these uncertainties. It is now the standard of care for lymphoma radiotherapy.

Extended-Field Radiotherapy

Extended-field radiotherapy was historically used in the treatment of Hodgkin lymphoma. Total lymphoid irradiation involves treating all the major lymphoid areas and comprises the Mantle and Inverted Y fields along with the Waldeyer's ring. The Mantle field includes all the major lymph node regions above the diaphragm and it encompasses the cervical, supraclavicular, axillary, hilar and mediastinal nodes, whereas the Inverted Y covers the nodal regions below the diaphragm such as the spleen, para-aortic, pelvic and inguinofemoral nodes. Subtotal nodal irradiation comprises the Mantle field plus the spleen and para-aortic nodes. Extended-field radiotherapy has now been replaced by smaller treatment fields.

IFRT

When radiotherapy is given as the sole treatment modality without chemotherapy, such as in stage I and II indolent non-Hodgkin lymphoma, nodular lymphocyte-predominant Hodgkin lymphoma or patients with localised Hodgkin lymphoma or aggressive nodal non-Hodgkin lymphoma who are not suitable candidates for systemic chemotherapy, larger CTV margins than those used in ISRT are required to include subclinical disease. IFRT is thus used. It encompasses within its CTV the initial volume of involved lymph nodes, the clinically involved lymph node region(s) and the adjacent uninvolved first echelon lymph node station (Figures 23.2 and 23.3). A CTV-PTV margin is added to account for daily setup variations and organ motion, which will vary for different disease sites.

ISRT

For radiotherapy as part of combined modality treatment, the ISRT target volume is based on the pre-chemotherapy macroscopic disease extent, as it assumes that the adjacent microscopic disease has been eradicated by chemotherapy. A pre-chemotherapy PET-CT is required for accurate disease localisation. This is fused with the post-chemotherapy planning CT scan. A pre-chemotherapy GTV is defined using information from both the CT and PET components of the pre-chemotherapy PET-CT. This is then modified to take into account anatomical changes as a result of chemotherapy-induced tumour shrinkage. The GTV thus comprises the original sites of disease modified for normal tissue boundaries.

The pre-chemotherapy GTV is expanded by 15 mm cranio-caudally in the direction of lymphatic spread to form the superior and inferior extent of the CTV while the transverse plane extends up to the

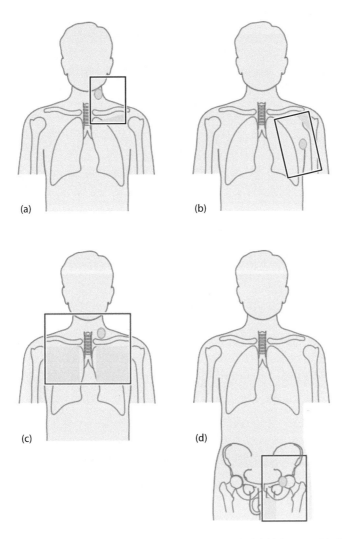

FIGURE 23.2 Diagrams of opposing fields for IFRT. (a) Unilateral cervical field for stage IA disease involving high cervical node with shielding to the lung apex; (b) axillary field with shielding of the humeral head; (c) neck and mediastinal field with lung shielding; (d) inguinal field with shielding of the testes.

boundaries of the nodal compartment. Encompassing the entire nodal region is not necessary. In cases where the treatment volume is affected by significant internal organ motion, an ITV can be added to the CTV using data from 4D-CT scans (Figure 23.4).

When radiotherapy is used to treat residual lymphoma after chemotherapy, a post-chemotherapy GTV comprising the residual PET-positive lesion and any other residual masses is defined on the planning CT scan. A 15-mm margin is added to the GTV to create the CTV. This is then edited to stay within the boundaries of the nodal compartment and to exclude natural barriers and uninvolved organs. The residual PET-positive areas can be treated to a higher dose using simultaneous integrated boost.

Extranodal Sites

When primary radiotherapy is given for extranodal non-Hodgkin lymphoma, the GTV is the part of the organ/structure involved by lymphoma at diagnosis. The pre-chemotherapy GTV is used when radiotherapy follows a course of chemotherapy. In many organs such as the stomach, the lymphoma is multifocal and the GTV thus encompasses the entire involved organ. Table 23.1 shows the CTV definition for stage

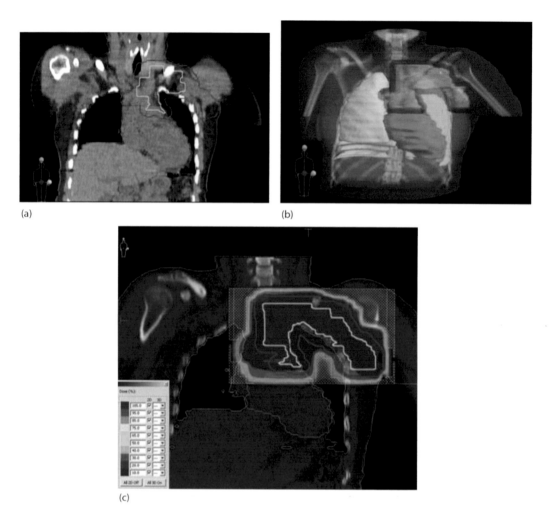

(a)

(b)

(c)

FIGURE 23.3 IFRT for a patient with stage IIA Hodgkin lymphoma showing radiotherapy to the mediastinum, left supraclavicular fossa and left axilla. (a) Coronal CT scan with target volumes; (b) 3D image; (c) dose distribution using anterior and posterior beams with multi-leaf collimators. Lungs green, heart yellow, spinal cord light yellow; (b) and (c) are at different slice level to (a).

TABLE 23.1

CTV Definition for Stage IE Non-Hodgkin Lymphoma

	CTV
Orbital adnexal	Entire bony orbit including extraorbital extensions Entire conjunctival sac if disease is limited to conjunctiva + local extensions to eyelid
Waldeyer's ring	Whole tonsillar fossa from the level of the soft palate to the level of the vallecula
Salivary glands	Entire unilateral salivary gland
Thyroid	Whole thyroid
Breast	Entire ipsilateral breast
Stomach	Entire stomach volume from the gastro-oesophageal junction to beyond the duodenal bulb; perigastric nodes are included if visible
Testes	Involved testis if not resected and the contralateral testis and scrotum in diffuse large B-cell lymphoma

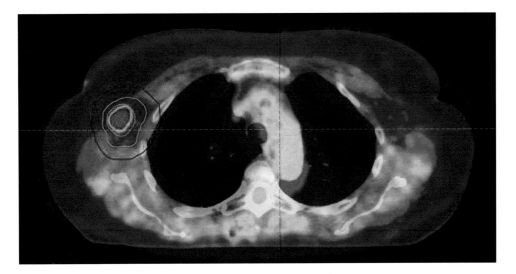

FIGURE 23.4 ISRT for patient with stage 1A diffuse large B-cell non-Hodgkin lymphoma showing treatment to right axillary lymph nodes. The pre-chemotherapy PET-CT was fused with the planning CT scan, and the GTV (orange), CTV (pink) and PTV (red) were delineated.

IE non-Hodgkin lymphoma for a range of extranodal sites. CTV-PTV margins vary according to the mobility of the organ and immobilisation device used. For the stomach, a 20-mm cranio-caudal margin may be required to account for respiratory motion (Figure 23.5).

The organs-at-risk dose constraints used for epithelial malignancies are less relevant in lymphoma, as the prescribed doses are often lower than the conventional constraints. However, important late

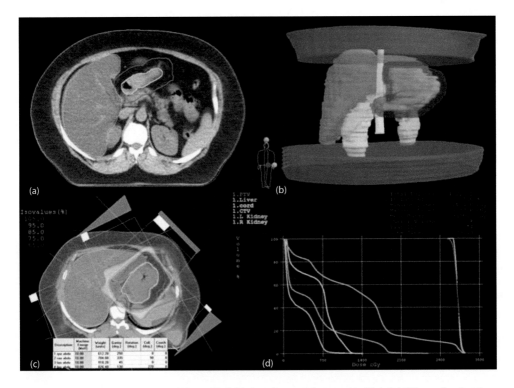

FIGURE 23.5 Patient with stage IE MALT non-Hodgkin lymphoma of the stomach. (a) Axial CT scan showing the target volume; (b) 3D image; (c) conformal plan; (d) DVH with liver (yellow), kidneys (green) and spinal cord (light yellow).

TABLE 23.2

Dose Constraints for Mediastinal Radiotherapy

Organ	Metric	Optimal (Small-Volume, Early-Stage Lymphoma)	Acceptable (Bulky Mediastinal Disease)	If Necessary (Relapsed/ Refractory Disease)
Heart (avoid the coronary arteries and left ventricle)	Mean dose	<5 Gy	5–10 Gy	10–18 Gy
	V15 Gy	<10%	10–25%	25–35%
	V30 Gy		<15%	15–20%
Lung	Mean dose	<8 Gy	8–12 Gy	12–15 Gy
	V5 Gy	<35%	35–45%	45–55%
	V20 Gy	<20%	20–28%	28–35%
Breast	Mean	<4 Gy	4–15 Gy	
	V4 Gy	<10%	10–20%	
	V10 Gy		<10%	

toxicities may still occur in long-term survivors of lymphoma; therefore, it is vital to keep radiation doses to critical organs at risk as low as reasonably achievable. The dose constraints for mediastinal radiotherapy as recommended by the International Lymphoma Radiation Oncology Group are shown in Table 23.2.

Palliative Radiotherapy

Planning CT scans are performed. The GTV is contoured. An isotropic margin of 1–2 cm is added to the GTV to create the PTV. Virtual simulation is used to design beams to encompass the PTV. Shielding of the organs at risk is achieved through appropriate MLC configurations. A simple arrangement of anterior and posterior opposing beams is often used.

Dose Solutions

Choose the treatment technique that provides optimal PTV coverage and offers the lowest risk of significant long-term toxicity and complication. IMRT and VMAT are often used to achieve these objectives. Using CT planning, the most appropriate multi-beam plan is prepared with radiation doses to the normal structures kept as low as possible. If the involved nodes are more than 5 cm apart, separate treatment fields may be required. Butterfly VMAT/IMRT comprises two coplanar arcs of 60° using gantry starting angles of 150° and 330° and one non-coplanar arc of 60° using gantry starting angles of 330° at a couch angle of 90°. This technique is useful in young women with mediastinal disease, as it lessens the low dose bath to the lungs and breast tissue, thus minimising the risk of a second malignancy. 4D-CT and deep-inspiration breath-hold techniques should be considered when using VMAT/IMRT for the mediastinum or disease sites significantly affected by respiratory motion. For mediastinal radiotherapy, deep-inspiration breath-hold results in a significant reduction in the radiation dose to the lungs and heart. Less often, an anterior and posterior parallel-opposed field arrangement is used, shaped using MLCs to minimise the volume of normal tissue irradiated.

Dose Fractionation

Classical Hodgkin Lymphoma

Limited stage disease, favourable group with a complete response to chemotherapy

- 20 Gy in 10 daily fractions given in two weeks

Limited stage disease, favourable group with an incomplete response to chemotherapy

- 30 Gy in 15 daily fractions given in three weeks

Limited stage disease, unfavourable group

- 30 Gy in 15 daily fractions given in three weeks

Advanced stage disease with residual PET-positive lymphoma and salvage radiotherapy in relapsed disease

- 30–40 Gy in 15–20 daily fractions given in three to four weeks

Nodular Lymphocyte Predominant Hodgkin Lymphoma

As sole therapy in early-stage disease

- 30 Gy in 15 daily fractions given in three weeks

High-Grade Non-Hodgkin Lymphoma

Early-stage disease as part of combined modality treatment

- 30 Gy in 15 daily fractions given in three weeks

Consolidation radiotherapy in advanced stage disease

- 30–36 Gy in 15–18 daily fractions given in three to three and a half weeks

Consolidation radiotherapy for primary mediastinal and extranodal high-grade non-Hodgkin lymphoma

- 30–36 Gy in 15–18 daily fractions given in three to three and a half weeks

Radiotherapy for PET-positive residual disease and salvage radiotherapy in relapsed disease

- 30–40 Gy in 15–20 daily fractions given in three to four weeks

Low-Grade Non-Hodgkin Lymphoma

Radiotherapy as single modality treatment for stage I/II disease

- 24–30 Gy in 12–15 daily fractions given in two and a half to three weeks

Splenic Irradiation

Localised low-grade splenic lymphoma

- 24 Gy in 12 daily fractions given in two and a half weeks

Palliative splenic irradiation

- 4–10 Gy in fractions of 0.5–1.0 Gy given up to three times per week

In cases of symptomatic hypersplenism or when the spleen is an organ of extramedullary haematopoiesis such as in chronic myeloproliferative disorders, a full blood count should be obtained before each fraction of radiotherapy. If blood counts are initially very low, treatment should be commenced cautiously with low doses given once a week. Radiotherapy should be postponed if there is a significant drop in counts.

Palliative Radiotherapy

- 4 Gy in 2 daily fractions (short-term palliation for low-grade non-Hodgkin lymphoma)
- 8 Gy as a single fraction
- 20 Gy in 5 daily fractions given in one week
- 24 Gy in 12 daily fractions given in two and a half weeks (durable palliation for advanced stage low-grade non-Hodgkin lymphoma)
- 30 Gy in 10 daily fractions given in two weeks

Treatment Delivery and Patient Care

Acute side effects depend on the anatomical site being treated. Skin reactions and other acute side effects are usually mild and occur less frequently, as radiotherapy doses used for lymphomas are lower than those used for other malignancies. Brisker skin reactions may occur in the axilla, groin and perineum. Aqueous or 1 per cent hydrocortisone cream can be used. Sore throat, dysphonia and dysphagia may occur with lower cervical nodal radiotherapy. Dry cough and dyspnoea due to radiation pneumonitis may occur with mediastinal radiotherapy. Pelvic nodal treatment may cause acute cystitis and diarrhoea. Bone marrow suppression may occur, especially with the use of large pelvic radiotherapy fields following chemotherapy, and blood counts should be monitored. Loss of fertility and early menopause may also occur with pelvic radiotherapy.

Extended mantle radiotherapy was used to treat Hodgkin lymphoma. This led to an increased incidence of second malignancies among survivors, particularly breast cancer in patients treated in adolescence and young adulthood. Long-term results have shown that the use of involved field or involved site radiotherapy, with its reduced dose to the breast and lungs, has led to fewer second malignancies. Nonetheless, breast cancer screening should be performed in all female patients who have received mediastinal radiotherapy before the age of 36. Breast cancer screening should commence eight years after radiotherapy or at the age of 30, whichever occurs later.

Verification

ISRT requires accurate treatment delivery and verification with daily portal imaging or cone beam CT depending on the area treated.

SOLITARY PLASMACYTOMA AND MULTIPLE MYELOMA

Indications for Radiotherapy

Plasma cell neoplasms are mature B-cell malignancies comprising clonal plasma cells characterised by immunoglobulin secretion. They are radiation-sensitive tumours. The majority are multiple myeloma, which tend to affect older adults. Systemic chemotherapy is the mainstay of treatment for multiple myeloma. Osteolytic lesions are present in 70–80 per cent of patients with multiple myeloma at diagnosis.

These can manifest as bone pain, pathological fractures and neurological compromise due to spinal cord or nerve root compression. Palliative radiotherapy is effective at relieving the symptoms associated with myeloma osteolytic lesions.

Approximately 5 per cent of plasma cell neoplasms will present as a solitary plasmacytoma of the bone or extramedullary tissues with no systemic involvement. Solitary bone plasmacytoma occurs most commonly in the axial skeleton. It has a high risk of progression to multiple myeloma. Solitary extramedullary plasmacytoma is less common than solitary bone plasmacytoma. They occur most frequently in the head and neck region. Solitary plasmacytomas are usually treated with definitive radiotherapy with the aim of achieving durable remission and even cure. The cure rate with radiotherapy is higher for solitary extramedullary plasmacytoma. Radiotherapy can also provide long-term local tumour control in 80–90 per cent of these cases. Occasionally, surgical stabilisation of the spine or weight-bearing long bones or decompressive surgery for malignant spinal cord compression is required prior to definitive radiotherapy.

Sequencing of Multimodality Therapy

If surgical stabilisation or decompressive surgery is required for solitary plasmacytoma, definitive radiotherapy should commence as soon as adequate wound healing has occurred.

Assessment of Primary Disease

All suspected cases of plasma cell neoplasm should undergo investigations with a full blood count, peripheral blood film, serum electrolytes, creatinine, calcium, lactate dehydrogenase, β2-microglobulin, serum light chain levels, serum and urine electrophoresis along with bone marrow aspirate and trephine biopsy. An image-guided needle biopsy may be required in solitary plasmacytoma for histological confirmation of diagnosis.

Imaging studies include skeletal survey and cross-sectional imaging such as CT and MRI to define the local extent of the plasmacytoma. CT scans in general can't detect diffuse bone marrow infiltration and they may miss small extraosseous lesions. MRI on the other hand is routinely performed in the staging workup of plasma cell neoplasms. It permits improved visualisation of the medullary cavity and bone marrow and is particularly useful for solitary extramedullary plasmacytomas of the head and neck region, lesions involving the spine and epidural space and to exclude spinal cord or nerve root compression. Plasmacytomas enhance with contrast and are typically hypointense on T1-weighted MRI images and hyperintense on T2-weighted and STIR sequences.

PET-CT is highly sensitive at detecting myeloma deposits. It is therefore a useful screening tool for myeloma lesions, and it can detect additional lesions in 30 per cent of patients diagnosed with a solitary plasmacytoma on MRI. PET-CT can also clarify ambiguous MRI findings and it should be performed as part of the standard workup of patients with suspected solitary plasmacytoma.

Data Acquisition

Patients are scanned supine with immobilisation devices appropriate for the anatomical site to be treated. For head and neck irradiation, a customised thermoplastic shell is used with reference marks on the shell for alignment with lasers.

As plasma cell neoplasms occur at a wide variety of anatomical sites, decisions regarding treatment techniques are made before CT scanning to ensure that the most appropriate CT protocol is used. For definitive radiotherapy of solitary plasmacytoma, the scan should include the entire volume of the organs of interest for DVH assessment. Co-registration of the planning CT with the diagnostic MRI or PET-CT may aid GTV delineation.

Target Volume Definition

The GTV is defined. The CTV is created by adding isotropic margins of 1–1.5 cm to the GTV. A smaller GTV-CTV margin of 0.5–1 cm may be appropriate for solitary extramedullary plasmacytoma of the head and neck. However, larger proximal and distal margins of 2–3 cm will be required for solitary plasmacytoma of a long bone. Anatomical boundaries to tumour spread should be respected. If there is uncertainty regarding the extent of bone involvement on imaging, the entire bone should be included in the CTV. In patients who have undergone surgery prior to definitive radiotherapy, the CTV should include any residual tumour, the preoperative disease extent with 0.5–1-cm margin and all areas at risk of surgical seeding of malignant cells, such as the full extent of the intramedullary nail used to manage a pathological fracture of the femur.

Regional nodal disease is present in 25 per cent of solitary extramedullary plasmacytoma of the head and neck at presentation. For these patients, prophylactic irradiation of the adjacent at-risk nodes, such as the uninvolved ipsilateral cervical neck nodes, should be considered. However, prophylactic nodal irradiation is not required in node-negative cases.

CTV-PTV margins will vary according to organ motion and the immobilisation device used.

Dose Solutions

Choose the treatment technique that provides optimal PTV coverage and offers the lowest risk of significant long-term toxicity and complication. IMRT and VMAT are often used to achieve these objectives. Using CT planning, the most appropriate multi-beam plan is prepared with radiation doses to the normal structures kept as low as possible. Less often, an anterior and posterior parallel-opposed field arrangement is used, sometimes shaped using MLC to minimise the volume of normal tissue irradiated.

Dose Fractionation

Solitary Bone Plasmacytoma

- 45–50 Gy in 25 daily fractions given in five weeks

Solitary Extramedullary Plasmacytoma

- 45–50 Gy in 25 daily fractions given in five weeks

Palliative Radiotherapy

- 8 Gy as a single fraction
- 20 Gy in 5 daily fractions given in one week
- 30 Gy in 10 daily fractions given in two weeks

For large treatment volumes or re-irradiation:

- 20 Gy in 10 daily fractions given in two weeks
- 30 Gy in 15 daily fractions given in three weeks

Verification

Daily portal imaging or cone beam CT depending on the treatment area.

SYSTEMIC IRRADIATION

Indications for Systemic Irradiation

Total Body Irradiation

With the development of more effective systemic treatments, the use of total body irradiation (TBI) as part of conditioning pre stem cell transplant (SCT) is decreasing. There is also greater awareness of the long-term complications of TBI, particularly in the paediatric population. The main indication for TBI-based conditioning is adult leukaemia. There are potential advantages of including radiotherapy in a conditioning regimen. Unlike chemotherapy, the treatment is not affected by pharmacokinetic factors. TBI may treat chemo-resistant clones of cells, and also reaches sanctuary sites such as the brain and the testes. In addition, there is the possibility of delivering synchronous or sequential boosts to sites of refractory disease.

TBI may be part of a myeloablative (MA) or nonmyeloablative (NMA) conditioning schedule. In MA conditioning, the aim is to eradicate any residual tumour cells as well as suppress the recipient's immune system to allow engraftment. The dose delivered needs to be high enough to achieve tumour control without excessive toxicity and MA TBI is usually given in a fractionated schedule. Due to the morbidity of allogeneic-SCT (allo-SCT) with MA conditioning, it is rarely performed in patients older than 55–60 years.

In NMA conditioning, the primary aim is immunosuppression. TBI may be given to increase the chance of successful engraftment of the donor stem cells. A lower dose of radiotherapy (typically 2–4 Gy) can be used in this situation, often in a single fraction. The development of such reduced intensity conditioning (RIC) schedules has opened allo-SCT to an older population, and it is now not uncommon to transplant patients up to the age of 70.

With the increased use of IMRT, novel techniques targeting only the bone marrow, known as 'total marrow irradiation', have been developed and are being tested in clinical trials. It is currently unknown whether targeting only the bone marrow could replace TBI and whether excluding the liver, spleen, lymph nodes and peripheral blood is safe for both cytoreduction and immunosuppression.

Current indications for allo-SCT with TBI conditioning include:

Myeloablative

- Acute myeloid leukaemia (AML) with intermediate or poor risk molecular or cytogenetic features in first remission
- Standard risk AML in second remission
- Standard risk acute lymphoid leukaemia (ALL) in second remission
- Philadelphia positive ALL
- Childhood AML/ALL in second remission

Nonmyeloablative

- Patients meeting above criteria but not fit for MA conditioning
- Lymphomas – relapse post autologous stem cell transplant
- Chronic lymphocytic leukaemia
- Myelodysplastic syndrome
- Myelofibrosis
- Bone marrow failure including aplastic anaemia

Assessment of Disease and Pretreatment Investigations

Patients are treated according to national and international protocols. The radiation oncologist must have access to these protocols and to the relevant multidisciplinary team to ensure that radiation is given appropriately and at the correct time. Remission of the disease should be obtained where possible before TBI and SCT. For patients with ALL, boosts may be given in conjunction with TBI to sanctuary sites, either prophylactically or when there has been a previous relapse at these areas.

Patients with lymphoma who achieve a good response after chemotherapy but who have residual tumour at sites of initial bulky disease can also be treated with local boosts to these areas. However, TBI is less commonly used for these patients nowadays. TBI given after previous mediastinal or cranial irradiation can be associated with a higher rate of complications.

In other situations, boosts may be given safely and conveniently in a few treatments before TBI. Total doses are determined according to the age of the patient, the time interval since previous irradiation and the type and amount of previous chemotherapy. Young age, short time interval since previous irradiation and high doses of chemotherapy are generally associated with increased toxicity.

As the chemotherapy component of conditioning may vary from one drug (such as cyclophosphamide or melphalan) to various drugs in combination, the oncologist must be familiar with local haematological protocols and take into account any potential interactions with radiotherapy.

Prior to TBI, patients should be evaluated for any preexisting conditions that may affect lung, hepatic or renal function. Baseline thyroid function should be measured. Fertility preservation should have been considered before treatment of the underlying condition; this is not always possible to perform due to the urgency to commence treatment. In all cases, the effect of TBI on fertility, hormonal function and menopause in female patients should be discussed.

Data Acquisition

Conventional

There is wide variation between treating centres in the techniques used for TBI. Patients may be treated supine, in a sitting position, on their side or in a standing position. In a recent survey of UK centres, a reclined sitting or supine setup were most commonly used.

The following describes TBI delivered in a semi-reclined sitting position using two lateral opposed fields (Figure 23.6). The patient is positioned in the centre of a mobile treatment couch with tilted back-rest and knees bent. It is important that the patient is comfortable so that they remain in the desired position over the course of treatment. Additional knee and foot supports may be used to improve comfort.

Measurements of lateral body separation are taken at multiple sites (head, neck, shoulders, upper and lower thorax, waist, hips, pelvis, thigh, ankles) to assess the amount of bolus or compensation required at each level.

Complex

For treatment using 3D conformal radiotherapy, IMRT or tomotherapy technique, a CT scan of the whole body should be obtained, with the patient lying supine with a knee support and footrest.

Target Volume Definition

Conventional

There is no GTV if the patient is treated in complete clinical remission and the CTV is the whole body. Radiation beams are used which extend beyond the patient at all points, and as such a PTV is not defined.

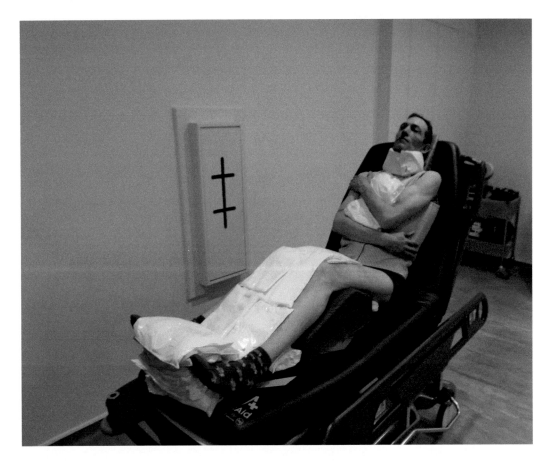

FIGURE 23.6 Patient in a semi-reclined position on a mobile treatment couch.

Complex

For complex treatment solutions, the external body contour is delineated. This will be the CTV. OARs such as the lungs, kidneys and eyes should be contoured to obtain DVHs and design MLC shielding.

If additional radiation is to be given to sites at high risk of microscopic residual disease such as the testes, brain or mediastinum, these may be designated as additional CTVs with a dose specified.

Dose Solutions

Conventional

The treatment couch is positioned at an extended source to skin surface distance (SSD) from the linear accelerator to allow a single beam to cover the whole body (Figure 23.7). Typical SSDs of 4–5 m are used depending on the size of the treatment bunker. The collimator is usually rotated so that the increased projection size of the diagonal of the beam can be utilised.

A Perspex screen is placed at the edge of the treatment couch between the patient and the linear accelerator to remove any skin buildup (Figure 23.8). As leukaemic cells may infiltrate the skin, skin sparing

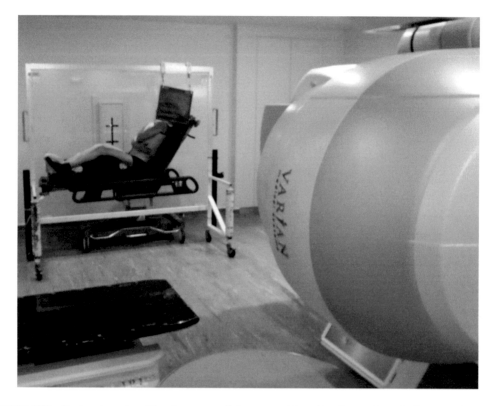

FIGURE 23.7   Treatment couch positioned at an extended source to skin surface distance from the linear accelerator.

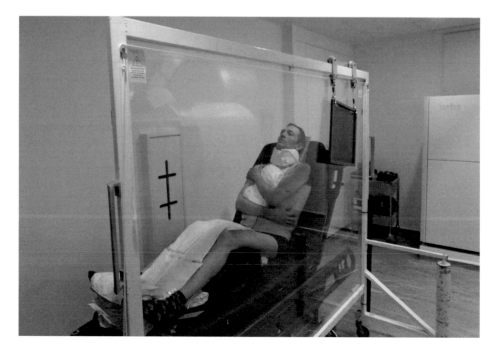

FIGURE 23.8   Perspex screen placed at the edge of the treatment couch between the patient and the linear accelerator to remove skin buildup.

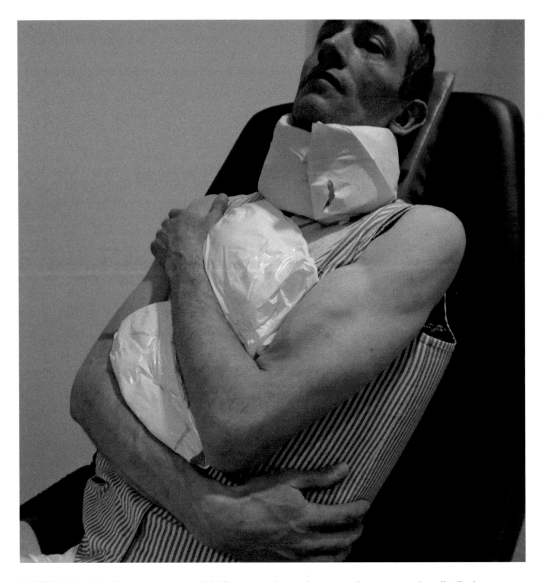

FIGURE 23.9 Bolus/tissue compensators/shielding are used to produce a more homogeneous dose distribution.

is undesirable. The required thickness of the Perspex screen depends on the treatment energy, and it will be typically 10–15 mm.

Differences in separation along the length of the patient, together with variation in tissue density can lead to dose heterogeneity exceeding 10–20 per cent. The maximum dose is found in the head and neck and the ankles, and the lowest dose in the abdomen and pelvis. Lung doses are relatively high due to the low density of lung tissue. A combination of bolus, tissue compensators and shielding can be used to produce a more homogeneous dose distribution (Figure 23.9). The patient's arms may also be positioned so as to increase separation and reduce lung doses.

Shielding may also be used to spare the lungs and kidneys. Pneumonitis is a common and potentially severe complication of TBI and the lungs are the dose limiting OAR. Some centres use shielding to keep lung doses below 8–12 Gy. Others do not shield, but set the prescription point as the maximum lung dose.

Renal function needs to be preserved as much as possible, as many nephrotoxic drugs are used in these patients. However, shielding at extended SSD in a patient who is not well immobilised may lead to undesired shielding of potential sites of leukaemic cell infiltration.

Opposing open lateral beams are used to achieve adequate mid-plane dose. For the second field, the couch is rotated 180 degrees and the setup repeated in reverse.

Complex

CT planned 3D conformal or IMRT techniques for TBI are becoming increasingly commonplace, with the aim of delivering an optimised homogenous dose across the body, and to allow more accurate shielding of OARs. Techniques range from parallel opposed fields with field in field MLC lung shielding, to advanced IMRT techniques including helical tomotherapy. The latter is particularly well suited to TBI, as treatment can be delivered under standard isocentric conditions, without the need for any field matching. Multi-isocentric VMAT techniques have also been developed and are used in some centres. IMRT techniques allow the reduction of dose to certain OARs (due to toxicity concerns) or to certain parts of the body (due to previous radiotherapy). Such modern techniques not only have the benefit of improved dosimetry, but they also reduce the need for cumbersome equipment such as compensators and lead blocks.

Dose Fractionation

Myeloablative TBI

Using a 6–10 MV linear accelerator beam at extended SSD, or rotational therapy:

- 13.2 Gy in 8 fractions of 1.65 Gy specified as the mid-plane dose at the level of the umbilicus or the maximum lung dose, given twice daily over four days with a minimum six-hour interval between fractions

If previous radiotherapy or concern regarding toxicity:

- 12 Gy in 6 fractions, given over three days with a minimum six-hour interval between fractions

Nonmyeloablative TBI

- 2–8 Gy in 1–4 fractions of 2 Gy given over one to two days with a minimum six-hour interval between fractions

Boosts

Where there has been no previous cranial or testicular irradiation and a full prophylactic dose is indicated, a boost may be given in the three days preceding total body irradiation.

Cranial Boost

Opposing lateral beams are used without shielding, using Reid's baseline (external outer canthus of the eye to the external auditory meatus) since subsequent cataract is likely anyway from TBI.

- 5.4–6 Gy in 3 fractions given over three days

Testicular Boost

A single direct beam of orthovoltage radiation or electrons is used with the penis taped as far out of the field as possible and legs apart to avoid the skin of the thighs.

- 5.4–6 Gy in 3 fractions given over three days

Mediastinal Boost (Bulk Disease with Residuum After Chemotherapy – No Previous Radiation)

This should be CT planned to ensure optimal coverage of the target volume and sparing of organs at risk.

- 10–10.8 Gy in five to six daily fractions

Treatment Delivery and Patient Care

Due to the scheduling of the conditioning regimen and the patient's complex medical needs, TBI is usually delivered on an inpatient basis. Before treatment, the patients should remove any jewellery and all clothing apart from underwear and a non-wired vest.

During the first fraction of TBI, diodes or thermoluminescent dosimeters (TLDs) are placed on the patient. These remain in place throughout the first fraction and on subsequent fractions when dose measurement is required.

Although these patients are immunosuppressed and at risk of infection, special sterile precautions have been shown to be unnecessary. Premedication with steroid and antiemetics given 30 minutes before each fraction will reduce nausea and vomiting. Parotid swelling is common within the first 24 hours of irradiation but subsides spontaneously. Subsequent dry mouth and disturbance of taste may persist for up to a year. Mild diarrhoea occurs from four to five days after the start of treatment. The skin may feel sore, particularly in folds and where bolus is placed. Reversible hair loss, if not already present, starts after 10–14 days. Recovery of engrafted cells begins from day 7–21. A somnolence syndrome of anorexia, lassitude, nausea or headache may occur from six to eight weeks after treatment and is self-limiting. Single-dose NMA TBI appears to be very well tolerated, with minimal acute toxicity.

Pneumonitis presenting with cough and breathlessness occurs in 10–30 per cent of patients following allo-SCT with TBI. It is often multifactorial, with the most common causes being infection and acute graft versus host disease, in addition to the effect of radiotherapy on the lung tissue. The development of pneumonitis is associated with significantly increased mortality within one year of transplant, and accurate diagnosis is essential for successful treatment.

Sterility may be expected but is not absolutely inevitable, and patients should be counselled accordingly. Hormone replacement therapy may be needed for many patients. Cataract is usual after several years. Thyroid function should be monitored. The incidence of second malignancies after TBI and stem cell transplantation increases with each year of survival and lifetime surveillance is essential.

Verification

In vivo dosimetry is used to verify TBI treatment delivery. Diodes or TLDs are placed on the sides of the patient in the positions as shown in Figures 23.10 and 23.11. They measure exit and entry doses and allow calculation of the midline dose delivered. Dose is measured during the first fraction and specified fractions thereafter to confirm accuracy of delivery and to monitor specific sites of interest as required. Diodes have the advantage of allowing real-time assessment of dose, meaning that if measured doses are not within tolerance (e.g. -10% -/+10%), treatment can be modified before the next fraction, by adjusting the number of monitor units delivered, or by altering bolus or shielding. Prior to TBI, a test dose

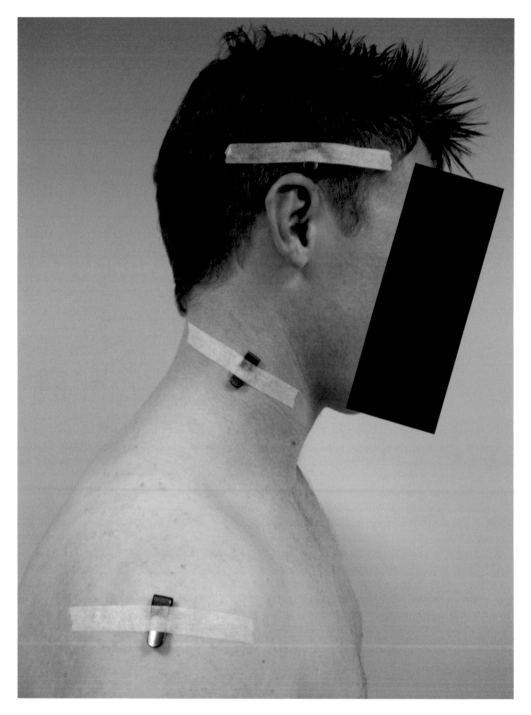

FIGURE 23.10   Thermoluminescent dosimeters on the head, neck and shoulder.

treatment is often given. This simulates the actual treatment but delivers a much-reduced dose, typically <0.2 Gy. The delivered test dose, measured using diodes or TLDs, is then scaled to accurately determine the required machine monitor units for the actual treatment along with appropriate bolus, shielding or compensation at different levels. A test dose is particularly important for single fraction treatments where subsequent adjustments are not possible.

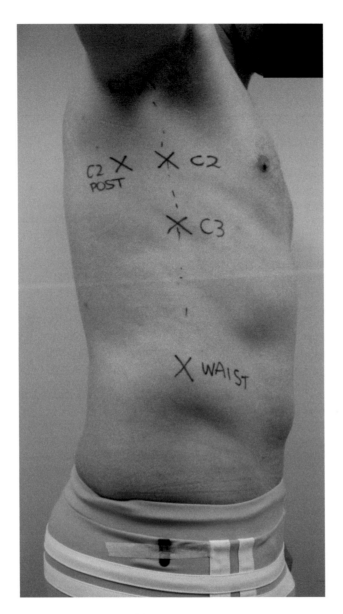

FIGURE 23.11   Thermoluminescent dosimeter positions.

Key Trials

Eich HT, Diehl V, Gorgen H, et al. Intensified chemotherapy and dose-reduced involved-field radiotherapy in patients with early unfavorable Hodgkin's lymphoma: Final analysis of the German
Hodgkin study group HD11 trial. J Clin Oncol 2010;28:4199–4206.

Engert A, Plutschow A, Eich HT, et al. Reduced treatment intensity in patients with early-stage
Hodgkin's lymphoma. N Engl J Med 2010;363:640–652.

Held G, Murawski N, Ziepert M, et al. Role of radiotherapy to bulky disease in elderly patients with
aggressive B-cell lymphoma. J Clin Oncol 2014;32:1112–1118.

Hoskin PJ, Kirkwood AA, Popova B, et al. 4Gy versus 24Gy radiotherapy for patients with indolent
lymphoma (FORT): A randomised phase 3 non-inferiority trial. Lancet Oncol 2014;15:457–463.

Lowry L, Smith P, Qian W, et al. Reduced dose radiotherapy for local control in non-Hodgkin lymphoma: A randomised phase III trial. Radiother Oncol 2011;100:86–92.

Miller TP, Dahlberg S, Cassady JR, et al. Chemotherapy alone compared with chemotherapy plus radiotherapy for localized intermediate- and high-grade non-Hodgkin's lymphoma. N Engl J Med 1998;339:21–26.

Radford J, Illidge T, Counsell N, et al. Results of a trial of PET-directed therapy for early-stage Hodgkin's lymphoma. N Engl J Med 2015;372:1598–1607.

INFORMATION SOURCES

Bird D, Patel C, Scarsbrook AF, et al. Evaluation of clinical target volume expansion required for involved site neck radiotherapy for lymphoma to account for the absence of a pre-chemotherapy PET-CT in the radiotherapy treatment position. Radiother Oncol 2017;124:161–167.

Esiashvili N, Lu X, Ulin K, et al. Higher reported lung dose received during total body irradiation for allogeneic hematopoietic stem cell transplantation in children with acute lymphoblastic leukemia is associated with inferior survival: A report from the children's oncology group. Int J Radiat Oncol Biol Phys 2019;104:513–521.

Hegenbart U, Niederwieser D, Sandmaier BM, et al. Treatment for acute myelogenous leukemia by low-dose, total-body, irradiation-based conditioning and hematopoietic cell transplantation from related and unrelated donors. J Clin Oncol 2006;24:444–453.

Illidge T, Specht L, Yahalom J, et al. Modern radiation therapy for nodal non-Hodgkin lymphoma – target definition and dose guidelines from the International Lymphoma Radiation Oncology Group. Int J Radiat Oncol Biol Phys 2014;89:49–58.

Leiper AD. Late effects of total body irradiation. Arch Dis Child 1995;72:382–385.

Mikhaeel NG, Milgrom SA, Terezakis S, et al. The optimal use of imaging in radiation therapy for lymphoma: Guidelines from the International Lymphoma Radiation Oncology Group (ILROG). Int J Radiat Oncol Biol Phys 2019;104:501–512.

Ng AK, Dabaja BS, Hoppe RT, et al. Re-examining the role of radiation therapy for diffuse large B-cell lymphoma in the modern era. J Clin Oncol 2016;34:1443–1447.

Nogova L, Reineke T, Eich HT, et al. Extended field radiotherapy, combined modality treatment or involved field radiotherapy for patients with stage IA lymphocyte-predominant Hodgkin's lymphoma: A retrospective analysis from the German Hodgkin Study Group (GHSG). Ann Oncol 2005;16:1683–1687.

Patel RP, Warry AJ, Eaton DJ, et al. In vivo dosimetry for total body irradiation: Five-year results and technique comparison. J Appl Clin Med Phys 2014;15:306–315.

Specht L, Yahalom J, Illidge T, et al. Modern radiation therapy for Hodgkin lymphoma: Field and dose guidelines from the International Lymphoma Radiation Oncology Group (ILROG). Int J Radiat Oncol Biol Phys 2014;89:854–862.

Thomas ED, Clift RA, Hersman J, et al. Marrow transplantation for acute nonlymphoblastic leukemia in first remission using fractionated or single-dose irradiation. Int J Radiat Oncol Biol Phys 1982;8:817–821.

Tsang RW, Campbell BA, Goda JS, et al. Radiation therapy for solitary plasmacytoma and multiple myeloma: Guidelines from the International Lymphoma Radiation Oncology Group. Int J Radiat Oncol Biol Phys 2018;101:794–808.

Wilhelm-Buchstab T, Leitzen C, Schmeel LC, et al. Total body irradiation: Significant dose sparing of lung tissue achievable by helical tomotherapy. Z Med Phys 2020;30:17–23.

Wirth A, Mikhaeel NG, Aleman BMP, et al. Involved site radiation therapy in adult lymphomas: An overview of International Lymphoma Radiation Oncology Group Guidelines. Int J Radiat Oncol Biol Phys 2020;107:909–933.

Wirth A, Yuen K, Barton M, et al. Long-term outcome after radiotherapy alone for lymphocyte-predominant Hodgkin lymphoma. A retrospective multicenter study of the Australasian Radiation Oncology Lymphoma Group. Cancer 2005;104:1221–1229.

Wong JYC, Filippi AR, Dabaja BS, et al. Total body irradiation: Guidelines from the International Lymphoma Radiation Oncology Group (ILROG). Int J Radiat Oncol Biol Phys 2018;101:521–529.

Yahalom J. Radiotherapy of follicular lymphoma: Updated role and new rules. Curr Treat Options Oncol 2014;15:262–268.

Yahalom J, Illidge T, Specht L, et al. Modern radiation therapy for extranodal lymphomas: Field and dose guidelines from the International Lymphoma Radiation Oncology Group. Int J Radiat Oncol Biol Phys 2015;92:11–31.

24

Oesophagus and Stomach

Indications for Radiotherapy

The oesophagus connects the pharynx to the stomach. It extends from the lower border of the cricoid cartilage at the level of the sixth cervical vertebra to the cardiac orifice of the stomach at the level of T11. It is arbitrarily divided into the cervical portion and the intrathoracic portion. The cervical oesophageal segment begins at the cricopharyngeus and ends at the suprasternal notch while the intrathoracic segment is further subdivided into the upper, middle and lower thirds.

Gastro-oesophageal junction (GOJ) cancer usually includes adenocarcinomas of the lower oesophagus and gastric cardia along with the true junction between the two. Traditionally, the Siewert classification is used to plan management of tumours arising from the GOJ. Tumours whose epicentre is in the distal oesophagus are considered Siewert I, those arising at the GOJ are grouped as Siewert II whereas tumours of the gastric fundus are called Siewert III. According to the 8th edition of TNM, tumours with epicentre no more than 2 cm into the proximal stomach with involvement of the GOJ (Siewert types I/II) are classified as oesophageal cancers while those with epicentre more than 2 cm away (even if they involve the GOJ) and all cardiac tumours not involving the GOJ (even if their epicentre is within 2 cm of the GOJ) are classified as gastric cancers. More than half of oesophageal cancers and the majority of gastric cancers in the Western world are adenocarcinomas. The rest are mostly squamous cell carcinomas.

Oesophagus

Surgery is a principal curative treatment for oesophageal cancer. Randomised trials have demonstrated overall survival benefit with the addition of preoperative chemotherapy (two cycles of cisplatin and fluorouracil in the OEO2 trial) and perioperative chemotherapy (three preoperative and three postoperative cycles of epirubicin, cisplatin and fluorouracil [ECF] in the MAGIC trial) compared with surgery alone. Docetaxel, oxaliplatin and fluorouracil plus leucovorin (FLOT) has now replaced ECF as the perioperative chemotherapy of choice, with the FLOT4 trial demonstrating improved median survival compared with ECF in patients with resectable GOJ or gastric adenocarcinoma. In addition to perioperative chemotherapy, preoperative radiotherapy with concomitant chemotherapy (CRT) (radiotherapy to 41.4 Gy with five concomitant weekly cycles of paclitaxel and carboplatin in the CROSS trial) has also been shown to improve overall survival compared with surgery alone in patients with oesophageal or GOJ cancer. With preoperative CRT in the CROSS trial, more R0 resections were achieved with no increase in postoperative complications or mortality. Overall pathological complete response rate was 29 per cent with preoperative CRT. Preoperative CRT benefited both squamous cell carcinomas and adenocarcinomas, although higher rates of pathological complete response and better survival outcomes were observed with squamous cell carcinomas (pathological complete response rate of 49 per cent for squamous cell carcinoma and 23 per cent for adenocarcinoma; median survival of 81.6 months for squamous cell carcinoma, 45 months for adenocarcinoma and 24 months with surgery alone). These data confirm the higher sensitivity of oesophageal squamous cell carcinoma to radiation-based treatments, and challenges the need for planned oesophagectomy following CRT in this group of patients. Stahl et al. randomised patients with locally advanced squamous cell carcinoma of the oesophagus to either CRT to 40 Gy followed by surgery or CRT to at least 65 Gy without surgery after induction chemotherapy. Although local progression-free survival was significantly better with the addition of surgery, treatment-related

DOI: 10.1201/9781315171562-24

mortality was also significantly higher and overall survival was equivalent between the two groups. The NEEDS trial is a randomised controlled phase III study with a noninferiority design with regard to the primary endpoint of overall survival. It will compare the CROSS approach of neoadjuvant CRT and subsequent oesophagectomy with definitive CRT followed by surveillance and salvage oesophagectomy only in those with persistent disease or isolated local tumour recurrence. As for oesophageal and GOJ adenocarcinomas, preliminary results from the Neo-AEGIS trial showed that perioperative chemotherapy was noninferior to preoperative CRT in terms of the estimated survival probability at three years, despite higher rates of R0 resection margin, pathological complete response and tumour regression with preoperative CRT. Perioperative chemotherapy and preoperative CRT are therefore both valid treatment options in patients with oesophageal and GOJ adenocarcinoma.

In patients treated with preoperative CRT followed by surgery, adjuvant nivolumab should be considered if there is residual pathological disease in the oesophagectomy specimen despite preoperative CRT. This is based on the results of the CheckMate 577 trial, which demonstrated a significant improvement in median disease-free survival with adjuvant nivolumab regardless of programmed death ligand 1 (PDL1) status.

There is currently no good evidence to support the routine use of postoperative radiotherapy or CRT in oesophageal cancer. However, postoperative CRT can be considered in selected patients in whom the risk of local recurrence is high and exceeds that of distant metastases and whose prognosis is likely to be influenced by local relapse, such as those with node-negative tumours and involved resection margins.

Definitive CRT can be considered an alternative to surgery in patients with locally advanced oesophageal squamous cell carcinoma and those with oesophageal adenocarcinoma who are medically inoperable, decline surgery or have locally advanced disease where surgical cure is felt unlikely. CRT with cisplatin and fluorouracil/capecitabine has been shown to improve survival compared to radiotherapy alone. Most regimens also include two cycles of chemotherapy either before or after CRT. The ARTDECO study examined radiotherapy dose escalation with definitive CRT and weekly carboplatin and paclitaxel in oesophageal cancer. There was no significant difference in the three-year local progression-free survival with radiation dose escalation to 61.6 Gy to the primary tumour compared with a standard dose of 50.4 Gy, regardless of histology. The SCOPE2 trial also aims to assess the role of CRT dose escalation from the standard 50 Gy to 60 Gy (to the gross tumour) using simultaneous integrated boost in locally advanced oesophageal cancer along with systemic concomitant therapy adaptation using PET response after one cycle of induction chemotherapy. Radiotherapy alone is usually reserved for patients with localised disease who are unable to tolerate surgery or CRT or in whom the use of concomitant chemotherapy is contraindicated. For cervical oesophageal squamous cell cancers, resection usually requires a laryngo-oesophagectomy. Definitive CRT is therefore the preferred treatment modality for this group of patients. Some centres use two cycles of induction cisplatin and capecitabine followed by CRT with two further cycles of concomitant cisplatin and capecitabine while others adopt an approach similar to that of CRT in head and neck squamous cell carcinoma with concomitant weekly cisplatin. Table 24.1 summaries the key randomised controlled trials in oesophageal cancer.

Many patients with oesophageal cancer are elderly, of poor performance status or have distant metastases at presentation. Radiotherapy is useful in the palliation of dysphagia and pain but it rarely relieves complete dysphagia. Other ways of palliating dysphagia include expandable metal stents and high dose rate intraluminal brachytherapy. A Cochrane review has shown that intraluminal brachytherapy for dysphagia is associated with fewer requirements for re-intervention, improved survival and better quality of life compared with self-expanding metal stents.

Stomach

Surgery is the treatment of choice for resectable gastric cancers. The extent of surgery is important. A D2 resection (extended lymphadenectomy involving the removal of stations I–XI nodes) produces better locoregional tumour control than a D1 resection (limited lymphadenectomy confined only to the perigastric nodes). The Intergroup 0116 trial demonstrated an improvement in three-year survival rates from 41 per cent to 50 per cent with postoperative CRT. However, only 10 per cent of patients in this

TABLE 24.1

Key Randomised Controlled Trials in Oesophageal Cancer

Trial	Treatment Arms	Histology	Results	Conclusion
RTOG 85-01 Cooper et al. (1999)	CRT 50 Gy in 25 fractions over five weeks + cisplatin and fluorouracil vs radiotherapy alone 64 Gy in 32 fractions over six and a half weeks	Oesophageal squamous cell carcinoma + adenocarcinoma	Five-year overall survival: 26% vs 0%	CRT improves overall survival compared to radiotherapy alone
Stahl et al. (2005)	Induction chemotherapy followed by CRT to 40 Gy and surgery vs the same induction chemotherapy followed by CRT to at least 65 Gy without surgery	Oesophageal squamous cell carcinoma	Overall survival equivalent between the two groups Two-year progression-free survival: 64.3% vs 40.7% (p=0.003) Treatment-related mortality: 12.8% vs 3.5% (p=0.03)	Adding surgery to CRT improves local tumour control but not overall survival
MAGIC Cunningham et al. (2006)	Perioperative ECF + surgery vs surgery alone	Lower oesophageal and GOJ adenocarcinoma	Five-year overall survival: 36% vs 23% (p=0.009)	Perioperative chemotherapy improves overall survival
MRC OEO2 Allum et al. (2009)	Preoperative CF + surgery vs surgery alone	Oesophageal and GOJ squamous cell carcinoma + adenocarcinoma	pCR rate with preoperative CF: 4% R0 resection rate: 60% vs 54% (p=0.001) Five-year overall survival: 23% vs 17% (p=0.03)	Preoperative chemotherapy improves overall survival
FNCLCC/ FFCD Ychou et al. (2011)	Perioperative CF + surgery vs surgery alone	Lower oesophageal, GOJ and gastric adenocarcinoma	R0 resection rate: 84% vs 73% (p=0.04) pCR rate with CF: 3% Five-year overall survival: 38% vs 24% (p=0.02)	Perioperative chemotherapy increases R0 resection rate and improves overall survival
CROSS Van Hagen et al. (2012)	Preoperative CRT (41.4 Gy with weekly carboplatin + paclitaxel) + surgery vs surgery alone	Oesophageal and GOJ squamous cell carcinoma + adenocarcinoma	R0 resection rate: 92% vs 69% (p<0.001) pCR rate with preoperative CRT: 29% Median overall survival: 49 months vs 24 months (p=0.003) Five-year overall survival: 47% vs 34%	Preoperative CRT improves overall survival
AIO-FLOT4 Al-Batran et al. (2019)	Perioperative FLOT vs perioperative ECF/ECX	GOJ or gastric adenocarcinoma	R0 resection rate: 84% vs 77% (p=0.011) pCR rate: 16% vs 6% (p=0.02) Median overall survival: 50 months vs 35 months Five-year overall survival: 45% vs 36% (p=0.012)	Perioperative FLOT improves overall survival compared with perioperative ECF/ECX
Neo-AEGIS Reynolds et al. (2021)	Preoperative CRT + surgery (CROSS protocol) vs perioperative chemotherapy (ECF/ECX/EOF/EOX/FLOT) + surgery	Oesophageal and GOJ adenocarcinoma	Three-year estimated survival probability: 56% vs 57% (NS)	Perioperative chemotherapy not inferior to preoperative CRT
CheckMate 577 Kelly et al. (2021)	Adjuvant nivolumab versus placebo in patients with residual pathological disease following preoperative CRT and R0 resection	Oesophageal and GOJ squamous cell carcinoma + adenocarcinoma	Median disease-free survival: 22.4 months vs 11.0 months (p<0.001)	Disease-free survival was significantly improved with adjuvant nivolumab

(Continued)

TABLE 24.1 (*Continued*)

Key Randomised Controlled Trials in Oesophageal Cancer

Trial	Treatment Arms	Histology	Results	Conclusion
ARTDECO Hulshof et al. (2021)	CRT to 50.4 Gy vs CRT to 61.6 Gy to the primary tumour	Oesophageal squamous cell carcinoma + adenocarcinoma	Three-year local progression-free survival: 70% vs 73% (NS)	No significant improvement in local tumour control with radiation dose escalation to 61.6 Gy, regardless of histology

Abbreviations: CF = cisplatin and fluorouracil, CRT = radiotherapy with concomitant chemotherapy, ECF = epirubicin, cisplatin and fluorouracil, ECX = epirubicin, cisplatin and capecitabine, EOF = epirubicin, oxaliplatin and fluorouracil, EOX = epirubicin, oxaliplatin and capecitabine, FLOT = docetaxel, fluorouracil and oxaliplatin, GOJ = gastro-oesophageal junction, NS = not significant, pCR = pathological complete response.

trial had a D2 resection. Fifty-four per cent had less than a D1 resection, and this might account for the high relapse rate in the surgery-only arm of the trial. Postoperative CRT might thus be compensating for inadequate surgery. Combined pre- and postoperative chemotherapy has also been shown to improve survival in patients with resectable gastric cancer. Preoperative chemotherapy allows down-staging of locoregionally advanced tumours prior to surgery and early treatment of micrometastases. Significantly higher R0 resection rates are achieved with no adverse impact on perioperative mortality or postoperative complications. Patients can be spared the morbidity of an unnecessary gastrectomy if distant metastases develop during or after preoperative therapy. Perioperative chemotherapy is now the standard of care in the management of locoregionally advanced resectable gastric cancer. Postoperative CRT with concomitant capecitabine or fluorouracil can be considered in patients at high risk of relapse who did not undergo preoperative chemotherapy and a D2 resection. Finally, CRITICS was a randomised phase III trial comparing postoperative chemotherapy versus CRT following surgical resection and preoperative chemotherapy. No survival benefit was observed with postoperative CRT over chemotherapy alone. A recent meta-analysis also failed to demonstrate a survival benefit with postoperative CRT over chemotherapy alone in patients with resected gastric cancer. In the palliative setting, radiotherapy can be used to relieve persistent bleeding from gastric cancers.

Sequencing of Multimodality Therapy

Perioperative chemotherapy comprises four cycles of FLOT before surgery and a further four cycles of FLOT after surgery. Preoperative CRT for oesophageal cancer consists of radiotherapy with concomitant weekly carboplatin and paclitaxel. Surgery should be performed four to six weeks after preoperative FLOT or eight to ten weeks after preoperative CRT. Following R0 resection, those with residual pathological disease in the resected specimen despite preoperative CRT should receive adjuvant nivolumab. Postoperative chemotherapy or CRT should be initiated within 6–12 weeks after surgery as soon as adequate wound healing has occurred.

Patients with oesophageal cancer managed with definitive CRT will receive two cycles of induction cisplatin and capecitabine followed by radiotherapy with two further cycles of concomitant cisplatin and capecitabine every three weeks. Induction chemotherapy may be omitted in those with small-volume disease.

Clinical and Radiological Anatomy

Oesophageal cancers can invade through the wall of the oesophagus. The lack of a serosal barrier allows tumours to invade adjacent structures such as the tracheobronchial tree. Skip metastases are intramural tumour deposits distant from the primary disease. They are formed through tumuor extravasation from

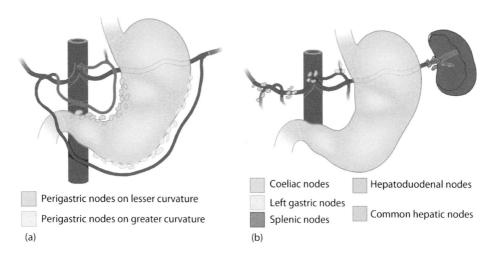

Perigastric nodes on lesser curvature

Perigastric nodes on greater curvature

(a)

Coeliac nodes

Left gastric nodes

Splenic nodes

Hepatoduodenal nodes

Common hepatic nodes

(b)

FIGURE 24.1 Lymphatic drainage of the stomach. (a) Perigastric nodes. (b) Stomach removed to show nodes along the branches of the coeliac axis.

the network of submucosal lymphatics. The submucosal lymphatics of the oesophagus enable longitudinal flow of lymph both proximally and distally before it drains into the adjacent lymph nodes deep to the muscularis layer. It accounts for the high incidence of involved nodes in oesophageal cancer. It also allows tumour spread to distant nodes relatively early in the course of the disease. The cervical oesophagus drains first to the deep cervical nodes medial to the internal jugular vein and then to nodes lateral to the vein in the supraclavicular fossa. The middle third of the oesophagus drains first to the para-oesophageal nodes and then to the mediastinal nodes. More inferior tumours involve the lymph nodes around the superior branch of the left gastric artery, the left gastric nodes and the lesser curvature nodes before spreading to those around the coeliac axis. The risk of nodal spread increases with T stage.

The stomach is divided arbitrarily into the fundus (cardia), body and pylorus (antrum). As in the oesophagus, there are extensive submucosal lymphatics that facilitate intramural tumour spread. Lymphatic drainage is initially to the perigastric nodes on the greater and lesser curvatures of the stomach followed by nodes along the branches of the coeliac axis (Figure 24.1). Proximal gastric tumours can also spread to the para-oesophageal nodes.

Assessment of Primary Disease

Most tumours are diagnosed at gastroscopy and the superior and inferior tumour extent is usually documented as the distance from the incisor teeth. A biopsy is obtained for histological confirmation of diagnosis. All patients should have contrast-enhanced CT scan of the thorax, abdomen and pelvis to assess the primary tumour, look for involved nodes and exclude distant metastases. A repeat CT should also be considered prior to postoperative radiotherapy. [18F] 2-fluoro-2-deoxy-D-glucose PET-CT (PET-CT) allows detection of metastatic disease that may otherwise not be identifiable with other techniques, and it should be performed in all patients with oesophageal and GOJ cancer undergoing potentially curative treatment. Endoscopic ultrasound (EUS) may be used to further evaluate the primary tumour and regional nodes if it helps guide ongoing management. Staging laparoscopy should be performed for all locally advanced GOJ tumours infiltrating the cardia and gastric cancers to exclude peritoneal metastases. Bronchoscopy or vocal cord assessment is required if tumour invasion of the tracheobronchial tree or recurrent laryngeal nerve is suspected.

The patient's nutritional status should be assessed and nutritional support provided if indicated. Patients scheduled for multimodality treatment, and surgery should also undergo lung function assessment and cardiac investigation.

Data Acquisition

For curative radiotherapy of cervical and upper third oesophageal tumours, the patient is positioned supine, arms down with knee support and immobilised using a thermoplastic shell in the same way as for hypopharyngeal tumours. For tumours of the mid and distal oesophagus and stomach, the patient is planned and treated supine with arms above the head, knee support and immobilised using a vacuum-formed polystyrene bag.

Contrast-enhanced 3D-CT with a minimum slice thickness of 3 mm is obtained from the base of skull to the lung bases for cervical and upper third oesophageal tumours and from the lung apex to the inferior border of L4 vertebral body for tumours of the mid and distal oesophagus and stomach to ensure inclusion of all organs at risk. For tumours involving the stomach or causing significant oesophageal obstruction, the patient will be required to fast for two hours prior to CT acquisition and treatment. For postoperative gastric radiotherapy, the planning CT should extend from the carina to the iliac crests. 4D-CT for treatment planning should be considered for lower oesophageal, GOJ and gastric tumours due to significant organ motion secondary to respiration. By taking into account patient-specific variation in organ motion over the course of a respiratory cycle, 4D-CT has the potential to reduce the risk of a geographical miss. Abdominal compression may help to reduce intra-fraction respiratory-induced organ motion.

Target Volume Definition

Preoperative and Definitive Radiotherapy in Oesophageal Cancer

The GTV consists of the primary tumour, all involved nodes and the entire circumference of the intervening oesophagus (with the exception of involved nodes located >3 cm from the primary tumour), taking into account all available diagnostic information. PET-CT findings should not be used to reduce the tumour volume defined using information from CT and EUS. Involved nodes below the diaphragm/oesophagus and those located >3 cm from the primary tumour are outlined as separate structures. If the diagnostic modalities produce discordant results, the GTV should encompass the greatest apparent tumour extent from all investigations.

The CTV is produced by expanding the GTV 2 cm superiorly and inferiorly along the axis of the oesophagus. This is then edited to include the adjacent mediastinum where there may be microscopic disease, ensuring a minimum margin of 0.5 cm from the primary tumour GTV (Figure 24.2). The CTV margin for involved nodes below the diaphragm and those located >3 cm from the primary tumour is 0.5 cm isotropically. For distal oesophageal tumours, the CTV is manually defined below the level of the GOJ to include the fat space below the diaphragm, around the cardia and gastro-hepatic ligament, between the lesser curve of the stomach and medial liver edge and nodal regions at significant risk of microscopic involvement along the lesser curve of the stomach and around the left gastric artery and coeliac region if they lie within 2 cm of the inferior extent of the primary tumour GTV. The CTV should also include the adjacent mucosa of the lesser curve of the stomach (Figure 24.3). It is edited in the axial plane from the adjacent normal structures, such as the lung, heart, major vessels, trachea, main bronchus, liver and vertebrae, as they act as natural barriers to tumour spread. However, the CTV should not be edited away from areas where there is T4 disease, such as the left lung in cases where there is left pleural involvement by tumour.

The para-oesophageal nodes in the superior mediastinum are located posterior to the trachea and to the left and right of the oesophagus. More inferiorly, they are found adjacent to the thoracic duct and aorta. In practice, these nodes will be included within the CTV as defined earlier.

There is data demonstrating a low rate of relapse in the adjacent clinically uninvolved nodes when prophylactic nodal radiotherapy is not performed. The majority of relapses are within the radiotherapy target volumes. Some centres nevertheless perform elective irradiation of the bilateral supraclavicular nodes for cervical oesophageal tumours.

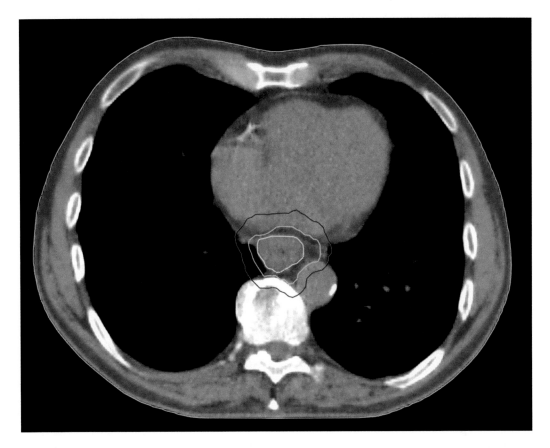

FIGURE 24.2 Volume definition for a T3N0 carcinoma of the thoracic oesophagus showing the GTV (cyan), CTV (green) and PTV (red).

The CTV is grown by a minimum margin of 0.5 cm axially and 1 cm superior-inferiorly to produce the PTV. For tumours involving the distal oesophagus and GOJ, a larger inferior PTV margin of 1.5 cm should be considered. 4D-CT enables tumour motion to be captured over a respiratory cycle and allows the creation of patient-specific target volumes which takes into account physiological organ motion. It may be useful for lower oesophageal and GOJ tumours. An internal target volume (ITV) is generated using 4D-CT data sets. The PTV is derived by growing the ITV using 0.5-cm isotropic margins. Respiratory gating or exhale breath-hold can also be considered for respiratory motion management.

Postoperative Radiotherapy in Oesophageal Cancer

The location and extent of the original tumour is determined by fusing the preoperative diagnostic CT or PET-CT with the planning CT images. The postoperative tumour bed is defined as the area within the mediastinum surrounded by the vertebra posteriorly, the lungs laterally and the heart, major blood vessels and liver anteriorly. Areas at highest risk of relapse are identified using information from the operation notes and histopathology report.

Postoperative Radiotherapy in Gastric Cancer

The CTV includes the tumour bed, remnant stomach and anastomosis with a 2-cm margin along with the perigastric nodes on the greater and lesser curvature of the stomach. The Intergroup 0116 trial also

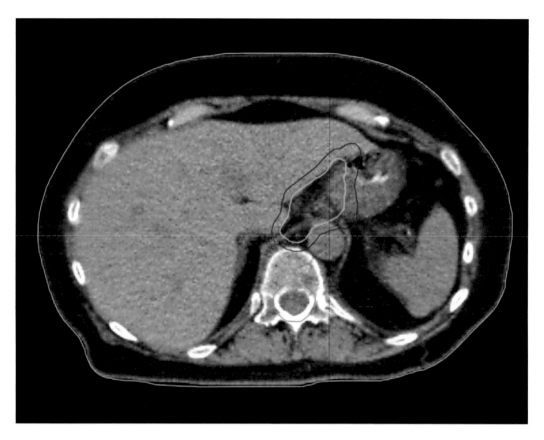

FIGURE 24.3 CTV (green) manually edited below the level of the gastro-oesophageal junction to include the fat space between the lesser curve of the stomach and medial liver edge and around the cardia and gastro-hepatic ligament. The CTV should also include the adjacent mucosa of the lesser curve of the stomach.

included the coeliac, para-aortic, splenic, hepato-duodenal and pancreatico-duodenal nodes within the CTV. For tumours of the fundus, the lower para-oesophageal nodes should be included, but the pancreatico-duodenal nodes can be omitted. For antral tumours, the splenic nodes can be omitted. An isotropic 1-cm margin is added to the CTV to produce the PTV.

Palliative Radiotherapy

The GTV is contoured. A 1-cm axial and 1–2-cm cranio-caudal margin is added to the GTV to create the PTV.

Organs at Risk

The organs at risk include the spinal cord, lungs, heart, liver, kidneys, stomach and spleen. Dose constraints are shown in Table 24.2.

Dose Solutions

Complex

IMRT is now often used in the treatment of both oesophageal and gastric cancer, as it improves dose conformity and reduces radiation exposure of organs at risks (Figure 24.4).

TABLE 24.2

Organs at Risk Dose Constraints

Structure	Constraint	Optimal	Mandatory
Spinal cord PRV	D0.1 cc	<40 Gy	<42 Gy
Combined lungs	Mean dose	<17 Gy	<19 Gy
	V20 Gy	<20%	≤25%
Heart	Mean dose	<25 Gy	<30 Gy
	V25 Gy	<50%	
	V30 Gy	<45%	
	V40 Gy	<30%	
Individual kidneys	V20 Gy	<25%	≤30%
Liver	Mean dose	≤28 Gy	≤30 Gy
	V30 Gy	<30%	<60%
Stomach excluding PTV	V50 Gy	<16 cc	<25 cc
Spleen	Mean dose	<10 Gy	

Conformal

Thoracic oesophageal volumes can be treated using an anterior and two posterior oblique beams or four equispaced beams. Both these beam arrangements spare the spinal cord but deliver more dose to the lung compared with opposing anterior-posterior beams (Figure 24.5). Angles for the posterior oblique beams are chosen to avoid the spinal cord PRV. Treatment plans can be tailored according to comorbidity. For example, in a patient with respiratory disease, it may be appropriate to choose a solution that minimises lung dose at the expense of increased dose to the spinal cord PRV and heart. A two-phase approach is used with opposing anterior-posterior beams to 30 Gy followed by a three- or four-beam conformal

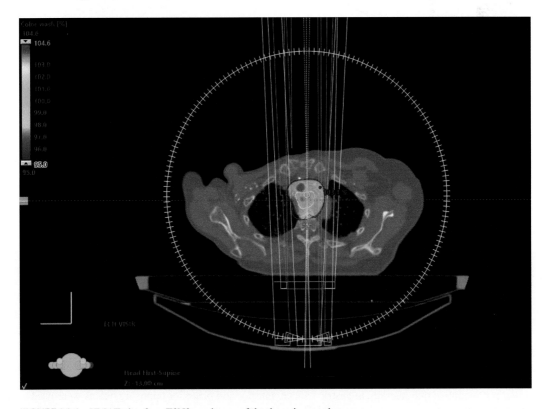

FIGURE 24.4 VMAT plan for a T3N0 carcinoma of the thoracic oesophagus.

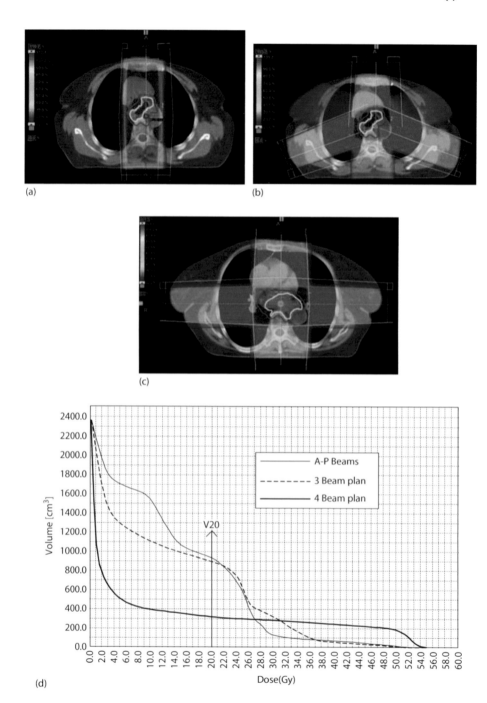

(a)

(b)

(c)

(d)

FIGURE 24.5 Conformal beam arrangements for a T3N1 carcinoma of the thoracic oesophagus. (a) Plan with anterior and posterior beams – minimal lung dose but higher dose to the spinal cord and heart. (b) Three-beam plan for the same volume – lower spinal cord dose but higher lung dose than a four-beam solution. (c) Four-beam plan for the same volume. (d) DVHs for lungs minus PTV for each plan, treated to 50 Gy in 25 fractions.

arrangement. Tumours of the cervical oesophagus are located more anteriorly and the anterior beam can be supplemented by right and left anterior oblique beams.

For postoperative radiotherapy in gastric cancer, anterior and posterior opposing beams were used to cover the target volume in the Intergroup 0116 trial but more conformal volume-based techniques have been described using five coplanar or four non-coplanar beams.

Simple

For simple palliative treatments, parallel-opposed anterior and posterior fields may give a satisfactory dose distribution.

Dose Fractionation

Oesophagus

Preoperative Radiotherapy with Concomitant Chemotherapy

- 41.4 Gy in 23 daily fractions given in four and a half weeks
- 45 Gy in 25 daily fractions given in five weeks

Definitive Radiotherapy with Concomitant Chemotherapy

- 50 Gy in 25 daily fractions given in five weeks
- 60–65 Gy in 30 daily fractions given in six weeks (for squamous cell carcinoma of the cervical oesophagus)

Definitive Radiotherapy Alone

- 50 Gy in 16 daily fractions given in three weeks (for tumours 5 cm or less in length in patients with adequate lung function)
- 55 Gy in 20 daily fractions given in four weeks
- 60 Gy in 30 daily fractions given in six weeks

Postoperative Radiotherapy +/- Concomitant Chemotherapy

- 45 Gy in 25 daily fractions given in five weeks (with concomitant chemotherapy)
- 50 Gy in 20 daily fractions given in four weeks (radiotherapy alone)

Palliative Radiotherapy

- 8 Gy as a single fraction
- 20 Gy in 5 daily fractions given in one week
- 27 Gy in 6 fractions given in three weeks
- 30 Gy in 10 daily fractions given in two weeks
- 40 Gy in 15 daily fractions given in three weeks

Palliative Brachytherapy

- 12 Gy as a single fraction
- 12–16 Gy in 2 fractions

Stomach

Postoperative Radiotherapy with Concomitant Chemotherapy

- 45 Gy in 25 daily fractions given in five weeks

Palliative Radiotherapy

- 8 Gy in a single fraction
- 20 Gy in 5 daily fractions given in one week
- 30 Gy in 10 daily fractions given in two weeks

Treatment Delivery and Patient Care

Patients receiving curative oesophageal radiotherapy are classified as Category 1 patients and compensation should be made for missed fractions. Oesophagitis and odynophagia are prominent symptoms of oesophageal radiotherapy and they should be managed proactively with analgesia, proton-pump inhibitor, steroids, dietary advice and nutritional support. Other acute toxicities may include dermatitis, lethargy, mucous production, loss of appetite, indigestion, nausea and vomiting, abdominal discomfort, dysphonia and inflammation of the lungs leading to cough and breathlessness. It is important to ensure that patient's nutritional intake is adequate before treatment begins. All patients should be weighed and assessed weekly during treatment. High calorie supplement drinks may be required to maintain adequate nutritional intake. Nasogastric or naso-jejunal tube feeding should be considered if the patient continues to experience significant weight loss due to poor oral calorie intake. Regular blood monitoring is required when concomitant chemotherapy is administered. Many patients receiving adjuvant CRT for gastric cancer will experience grade 3 or 4 nausea. They should be given prophylactic 5HT-antagonist antiemetics. Possible late or long-term side effects of oesophagogastric radiotherapy may include chronic fatigue, skin changes within the treatment area, fibrosis of the underlying lung, oesophageal dysmotility, need for long-term nutritional support via a feeding tube, oesophageal stricture formation requiring endoscopic dilatation, oesophageal fistula formation, cardiac toxicity and oesophageal or gastric ulceration, bleeding and perforation.

Verification

Cone-beam CT imaging encompassing the entire PTV with online correction using bone and soft tissue match is performed daily. Daily kV imaging is used if cone-beam CT is not available.

Key Trials

Al-Batran SE, Homann N, Pauligk C, et al. Perioperative chemotherapy with fluorouracil plus leucovorin, oxaliplatin, and docetaxel versus fluorouracil or capecitabine plus cisplatin and epirubicin for locally advanced, resectable gastric or gastro-oesophageal junction adenocarcinoma (FLOT4): A randomised, phase 2/3 trial. Lancet 2019;393:1948–1957.

Allum WH, Stenning SP, Bancewicz J, et al. Long-term results of a randomized trial of surgery with or without preoperative chemotherapy in esophageal cancer. J Clin Oncol 2009;27:5062–5067.

Cooper JS, Guo MD, Herskovic A, et al. Chemoradiotherapy of locally advanced esophageal cancer: Long-term follow-up of a prospective randomized trial (RTOG 85-01). Radiation Therapy Oncology Group. JAMA 1999;281:1623–1627.

Cunningham D, Allum WH, Stenning SP, et al. Perioperative chemotherapy versus surgery alone for resectable gastroesophageal cancer. N Engl J Med 2006;355:11–20.

Hulshoft MCCM, Geijsen ED, Rozema T, et al. Randomized study on dose escalation in definitive chemoradiation for patients with locally advanced esophageal cancer (ARTDECO) study. J Clin Oncol 2021;39:2816–2824.

Kelly RJ, Ajani JA, Kuzdzal J, et al. Adjuvant nivolumab in resected esophageal or gastroesophageal junction cancer. N Engl J Med 2021;384:1191–1203.

Macdonald JS, Smalley SR, Benedetti J, et al. Chemoradiotherapy after surgery compared with surgery alone for adenocarcinoma of the stomach or gastroesophageal junction. N Engl J Med 2001;345:725–730.

Minsky BD, Pajak TF, Ginsberg RJ, et al. INT 0123 (Radiation Therapy Oncology Group 94-05) phase III trial of combined-modality therapy for esophageal cancer: High-dose versus standard-dose radiation therapy. J Clin Oncol 2002;20:1167–1174.

Park SH, Sohn TS, Lee J, et al. Phase III trial to compare adjuvant chemotherapy with capecitabine and cisplatin versus concurrent chemoradiotherapy in gastric cancer: Final report of the adjuvant chemoradiotherapy in stomach tumors trial, including survival and subset analyses. J Clin Oncol 2015;28:3130–3136.

Reynolds JV, Preston SR, O'Neill B, et al. Neo-AEGIS (Neoadjuvant trial in Adenocarcinoma of the Esophagus and Esophago-Gastric Junction International Study): Preliminary results of phase III RCT of CROSS versus perioperative chemotherapy (Modified MAGIC or FLOT protocol). (NCT01726452). J Clin Oncol 2021;39:4004.

Shapiro J, van Lanschot JJB, Hulshof MCCM, et al. Neoadjuvant chemoradiotherapy plus surgery versus surgery alone for oesophageal or junctional cancer (CROSS): Long-term results of a randomised controlled trial. Lancet Oncol 2015;16:1090–1098.

Stahl M, Stuschke M, Lehmann N, et al. Chemoradiation with and without surgery in patients with locally advanced squamous cell carcinoma of the esophagus. J Clin Oncol 2005;23: 2310–2317.

van Hagen P, Hulshof MCCM, van Lanschot JJB, et al. Preoperative chemoradiotherapy for esophageal or junctional cancer. N Engl J Med 2012;366:2074–2084.

Ychou M, Boige V, Pignon J, et al. Perioperative chemotherapy compared with surgery alone for resectable gastroesophageal adenocarcinoma: an FNCLCC and FFCD multicenter phase III trial. J Clin Oncol 2011;29:1715–1721.

INFORMATION SOURCES

Button MR, Morgan CA, Croydon ES, et al. Study to determine adequate margins in radiotherapy planning for esophageal carcinoma by detailing patterns of recurrence after definitive chemoradiotherapy. Int J Radiat Oncol Biol Phys 2009;73:818–823.

Crosby T, Hurt CN, Falk S, et al. Chemoradiotherapy with or without cetuximab in patients with oesophageal cancer (SCOPE1): A multicentre, phase 2/3 randomised trial. Lancet Oncol 2013;14:627–637.

Gwynne S, Falk S, Gollins S, et al. Oesophageal chemoradiotherapy in the UK – Current practice and future directions. Clin Oncol (R Coll Radiol) 2013;25:368–377.

Hoeben A, Polak J, Van De Voorde, et al. Cervical esophageal cancer: A gap in cancer knowledge. Ann Oncol 2016;27:1664–1674.

Jabbour SK, Hashem SA, Bosch W, et al. Upper abdominal normal organ contouring guidelines and atlas: A Radiation Therapy Oncology Group consensus. Pract Radiat Oncol 2014;4:82–89.

Lordick F, Mariette C, Haustermans K, et al. Oesophageal cancer: ESMO clinical practice guidelines for diagnosis, treatment and follow-up. Ann Oncol 2016;27:v50–v57.

Matzinger O, Gerber E, Bernstein Z, et al. EORTC-ROG expert opinion: Radiotherapy volume and treatment guidelines for neoadjuvant radiation of adenocarcinomas of the gastroesophageal junction and the stomach. Radiother Oncol 2009;92:164–175.

Mukherjee S, Hurt CN, Gwynne S, et al. NEOSCOPE: A randomised phase II study of induction chemotherapy followed by oxaliplatin/capecitabine or carboplatin/paclitaxel based pre-operative chemoradiation for resectable oesophageal adenocarcinoma. Eur J Cancer 2017;74:38–46.

National Institute for Health and Care Excellence. Oesophago-gastric cancer: Assessment and management in adults, 2018. https://www.nice.org.uk/guidance/ng83.

Smalley SR, Gunderson L, Tepper J, et al. Gastric surgical adjuvant radiotherapy consensus report: Rationale and treatment implementation. Int J Radiat Oncol Biol Phys 2002;52:283–293.

Wu AJ, Bosch WR, Chang DT, et al. Expert consensus contouring guidelines for IMRT in esophageal and gastroesophageal junction cancer. Int J Radiat Oncol Biol Phys 2015;92:911–920.

25

Pancreas and Liver

PANCREAS

Indications for Radiotherapy

Carcinoma of the pancreas is the fourth and fifth most common cause of cancer-related deaths among men and women in the UK respectively. Incidence rates are highest in those aged 75 years and over. Ninety per cent of cases are ductal adenocarcinomas. Late presentation is common, as initial symptoms are often non-specific and insidious in onset.

Surgical resection is the only potentially curative treatment option for pancreatic cancer. Tumours are considered operable if there is limited or no involvement of the superior mesenteric vein and artery, portal vein and hepatic artery, and no evidence of distant metastases. Only 20 per cent of pancreatic cancers are suitable for curative surgical resection at diagnosis. This is then followed by adjuvant chemotherapy for six months. Adjuvant radiotherapy has not yet been shown to improve outcomes. RTOG 0848 is a phase III randomised trial seeking to determine whether the addition of radiotherapy with concurrent fluoropyrimidine to standard adjuvant chemotherapy further enhances the survival of patients with resected head of pancreas adenocarcinoma and no evidence of disease progression after five months of adjuvant chemotherapy. Despite surgery and adjuvant chemotherapy, prognosis remains poor and the five-year survival rate is 30 per cent for node-negative disease and 10 per cent for node-positive tumours.

Thirty per cent of patients with pancreatic cancer have locally advanced non-metastatic borderline resectable or unresectable tumour at diagnosis, and a further 50 per cent have distant metastases. The definition of borderline resectability varies. This group of patients may be candidates for neoadjuvant therapy. The potential benefits of neoadjuvant therapy include early treatment of micrometastatic disease, improvement in the rates of margin-negative surgical resection and better patient selection for radical surgery. This approach was investigated in the ESPAC-5F trial, which was a prospective randomised feasibility Phase II study comparing immediate surgical exploration with neoadjuvant treatments using either chemotherapy alone (gemcitabine/capecitabine or FOLFIRINOX) or capecitabine-based chemoradiotherapy (CRT) in patients with borderline resectable pancreatic cancer. The primary end point of this study was the rate of surgical resection. Although there was no difference in the resection rate between the study arms, there was a significant survival benefit at one year with neoadjuvant therapy compared with immediate surgery.

For patients with locally advanced non-metastatic unresectable pancreatic cancer (LANPC), the current treatment options include chemotherapy only or induction chemotherapy followed by definitive CRT. The role of radiotherapy in LANPC remains controversial. The LAP07 trial comparing chemotherapy alone with the same chemotherapy regimen for four months followed by CRT failed to demonstrate an improvement in median overall survival with the addition of radiotherapy. The UK SCALOP study randomised patients with non-progressive disease following four months of induction gemcitabine and capecitabine to CRT with either concurrent gemcitabine or capecitabine. This study suggested a better median overall survival with capecitabine-based CRT. Severe treatment-related toxicities also appeared lower with capecitabine-based CRT. SCALOP therefore established capecitabine as the preferred

DOI: 10.1201/9781315171562-25

radiosensitiser for CRT in patients with LANPC. It has long been assumed that pancreatic cancer is a systemic disease. However, studies have shown local disease progression, rather than distant metastases, to be the principal cause of death in a significant proportion of patients with LANPC. Thus, there may be a role for CRT in the treatment of LANPC. The UK SCALOP-2 trial is a 5-arm randomised study, looking at whether radiotherapy dose escalation and/or the addition of nelfinavir to CRT following four cycles of induction gemcitabine/nab-paclitaxel improves overall and progression-free survival in patients with LANPC. This study also includes a chemotherapy-only arm.

Definitive radiotherapy or CRT are also treatment options in patients with non-metastatic pancreatic cancer who are unsuitable for surgical resection due to medical comorbidities and those with isolated local tumour recurrence following primary surgery. An alternative to CRT in the treatment of patients with localised pancreatic cancer is stereotactic ablative body radiotherapy (SABR). Its role currently remains undefined, as there is no trial data comparing its efficacy against CRT. Intraoperative radiotherapy is at present not considered standard practice in the management of LANPC due to a lack of randomised trial evidence demonstrating its benefit.

In patients with incurable pancreatic cancer, a short course of radiotherapy may also be useful in the palliation of pain and bleeding from duodenal infiltration.

Sequencing of Multimodality Therapy

Adjuvant chemotherapy is recommended for all patients with pancreatic cancer following successful surgical resection, including those with T1N0 disease. This is usually initiated within 12 weeks of surgery. For patients with LANPC, CRT can be considered following three to six months of systemic chemotherapy in those with responding or stable disease and performance status of 0–1 whose tumour is encompassible within a radically treatable radiotherapy volume (pancreatic tumour of 6 cm or less in diameter).

Clinical and Radiological Anatomy

The pancreas is a retroperitoneal structure situated within the four parts of the duodenum. Developmentally, it forms from the ventral and dorsal outgrowths of the foregut which fuse around the vessels that later become the superior mesenteric artery and vein. The head of the pancreas lies anterior to the inferior vena cava, overlying the first to third lumbar vertebral bodies. The body of the pancreas passes obliquely to the left overlying the aorta, the left psoas muscle and the splenic artery and vein, while the tail extends in front of the left kidney to the hilum of the spleen (Figure 25.1).

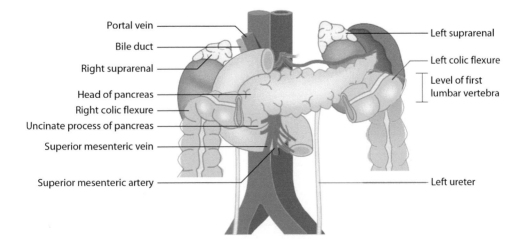

FIGURE 25.1 Relationships of the pancreas.

Assessment of Primary Disease

Pretreatment evaluation should include an assessment of the patient's symptom burden, general medical condition, performance status, comorbidities, psychological status and social support. The goals of treatment should be discussed, taking into account patient preferences. Histological confirmation of diagnosis and adequate blood parameters are required before treatment initiation. Endoscopic ultrasound (EUS)-guided fine needle biopsy is the preferred method for obtaining histology, especially in patients with non-metastatic disease, as it is associated with a lower risk of peritoneal tumour seeding than percutaneous biopsy. CT is the diagnostic modality most commonly used in the evaluation of pancreatic cancer. Intravenous contrast is administered and a 1000 ml of water is also given orally as negative intraluminal contrast. The typical CT appearance of ductal adenocarcinoma is an ill-defined hypoattenuating mass within the pancreas. Other signs include contour abnormalities, dilatation of the common bile duct or pancreatic duct and pancreatic parenchymal atrophy. CT is helpful in assessing the anatomic relationships and extent of the primary tumour and in determining involvement of the adjacent arteries or veins (Figure 25.2). It can also detect lymph node enlargement, distant metastases and bile duct obstruction. If the pancreatic lesion is not visible on CT, then further assessment with EUS or MRI may be required. MRI does not offer an advantage over CT for local staging of pancreatic tumours. Neither CT nor MRI is good at accurately assessing the margins of tumour extension, detecting peritoneal spread or predicting lymph node involvement. [18F] 2-fluoro-2-deoxy-D-glucose PET-CT (PET-CT) scan should be performed to look for occult metastases before considering surgery or high dose radiotherapy for localised disease. In patients with tumours involving the body or tail of the pancreas in close proximity to the left kidney, a MAG3 renogram or DMSA scan is sometimes required to assess differential renal function prior to CRT.

Data Acquisition

Patients should be positioned supine with knee support and with both arms immobilised above the head using either a T-bar device with arm rests or a vacuum moulded polystyrene bag.

CT scans are acquired with intravenous contrast and a slice thickness of 3 mm from at least 5 cm above the dome of the diaphragm to the lower border of L4 vertebrae to ensure inclusion of all organs at risk. To aid visualisation of the upper gastrointestinal tract, patients should drink 150–200 ml of water 15 minutes prior to scan acquisition. Patients should also drink the same amount of water prior to each treatment to ensure reproducibility. CT acquisition with the patient in exhale breath-hold may improve visualisation of the

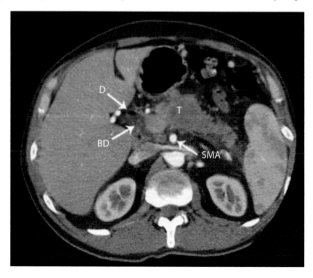

FIGURE 25.2   Axial CT scan showing tumour of pancreatic body. T, tumour; SMA, superior mesenteric artery; BD, bile duct; D, duodenum.

abdominal organs. CT-MRI fusion may be useful in cases where MR scanning provides additional information that will aid target volume definition. PET-CT may be useful in distinguishing pancreatic tumour from duodenum or in identifying disease not visible on CT. However, the use of PET-CT in treatment planning should not result in a reduction of the GTV unless the structure has clearly been identified as uninvolved on PET-CT (such as the duodenum). Pancreatic tumours may move by up to 1–2 cm secondary to respiration. 4D-CT can be used to quantify this respiration-induced tumour motion and is mandatory in SABR.

Target Volume Definition

Due to the difficulty in accurately defining the tumour margins, joint delineation of the GTV between the radiation oncologist and an upper GI/pancreatic radiologist is recommended, taking into account information derived from all available imaging. If the imaging modalities produce discordant results, the GTV should encompass the greatest apparent tumour extent. If MRI is available, deformable co-registration with the planning CT may help to improve GTV delineation. The GTV should therefore include the visible macroscopic primary pancreatic tumour and all locoregional lymph nodes greater than 1 cm in short-axis diameter. Any peri-tumoural node of less than 1 cm in dimension should also be included within the GTV if the radiologist felt that they are highly likely to be malignant, such as those with necrotic centres. The GTV should in addition encompass all FDG-avid lymph nodes (SUV >2.5) on staging PET-CT irrespective of size. Where tumour abuts or involves vessels, the entire circumference of such vessels should be included in the GTV. The GTV is expanded using a 0.5-cm isotropic margin to form the CTV. This is then edited to exclude areas of overlap with the uninvolved gastrointestinal tract. Prophylactic regional nodal irradiation is not required. PTV margins are 1.5 cm cranio-caudally (free breathing) and 1.0 cm in the AP and lateral directions to take into account organ movement with respiration and gut motion, along with setup variations (Figure 25.3). PTV margins may be reduced if exhale breath-hold techniques, gating or 4D-CT are used.

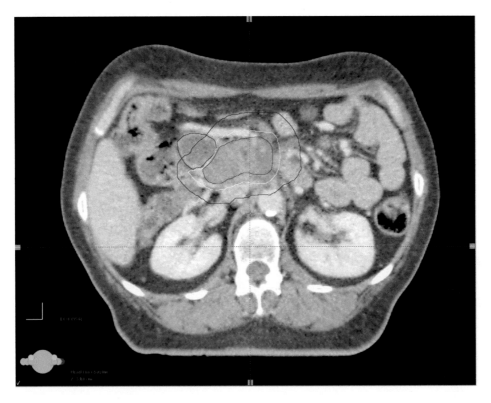

FIGURE 25.3 Axial free-breathing planning CT scan showing GTV (brown), CTV (yellow) edited to exclude uninvolved duodenum (blue) and PTV (red).

TABLE 25.1

OAR Constraints for Conventional Fractionation Pancreatic Radiotherapy

Structure Name	Constraint	Optimal	Mandatory
Duodenum	D_{max} (0.1 cc)	≤58 Gy	≤60 Gy
	V50 Gy	<10 cc	-
	V15 Gy	<60 cc	-
Stomach	D_{max} (0.1 cc)	≤58 Gy	≤60 Gy
	V50 Gy	<5 cc	-
	V45 Gy	<75 cc	-
Small bowel	D_{max} (0.1 cc)	≤58 Gy	≤60 Gy
	V50 Gy	<10 cc	-
	V15 Gy	<120 cc	-
Liver	V30 Gy	-	≤30%
	Mean	≤28 Gy	≤30 Gy
Kidney receiving higher dose	V20 Gy	≤40%	≤45%
Combined kidneys	V20 Gy	≤30%	≤35%
Spleen	Mean	10 Gy	-
Spinal cord PRV	D_{max} (0.1 cc)	-	≤45 Gy

For treatment planning using 4D-CT, a composite GTV (ITV) is created ensuring that it adequately covers the involved tumour and nodes on all phases of the 4D-CT data sets. CTV definition is the same as that just described. An isotropic margin of 0.5 cm is added to this CTV to produce the PTV.

OARs include the spinal cord, liver, kidneys, stomach, duodenum, small bowel and spleen. The entire organ should be outlined for DVH assessment except the spinal cord and small bowel, which are outlined on all slices from 2 cm above to 2 cm below the PTV. The kidneys should be outlined separately. A PRV of a margin of 0.5 cm is added to the spinal cord. OAR constraints are shown in Table 25.1.

For SABR, the GTV and ITV are defined in the same way as treatment planning using 4D-CT as described earlier. An isotropic margin of 5 mm is added to the ITV to create the PTV.

For palliative radiotherapy, the PTV is obtained by growing the GTV isotropically with a 2-cm margin.

Dose Solutions

Conformal

Three-field coplanar conformal plan with an anterior and two lateral wedged beams using 6–10 MV photons, forward planning using multi-leaf collimators to reduce the radiation dose to the OARs.

Complex

Inverse-planned intensity-modulated radiotherapy allows escalation of the radiation dose to the PTV using a five- (three anterior/two lateral) or seven-beam plan while minimising the dose to the OARs (Figure 25.4).

Simple

For palliative treatments, parallel-opposed anterior and posterior fields will give a satisfactory dose distribution.

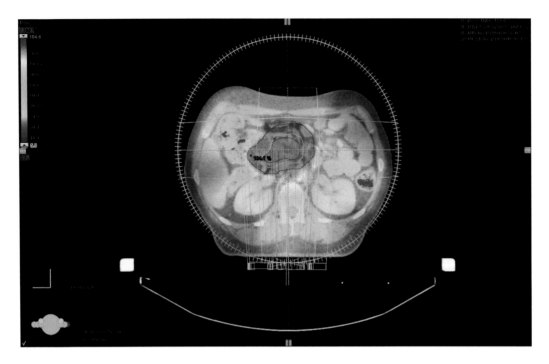

FIGURE 25.4   Dose distribution for IMRT of pancreatic body tumour.

Dose Fractionation

Radical (in Combination with Capecitabine Chemotherapy)

- 45 Gy in 25 fractions of 1.8 Gy, given once daily, five days per week over five weeks
- 50.4 Gy in 28 fractions of 1.8 Gy, given once daily, five days per week over five and a half weeks
- 54 Gy in 30 fractions of 1.8 Gy, given once daily, five days per week over six weeks

SABR

- 33–40 Gy in 5 fractions, given once daily, 3–5 fractions per week

Palliative

- 8 Gy as a single fraction
- 20 Gy in 5 fractions of 4 Gy, given once daily, five days per week over one week
- 30 Gy in 10 fractions of 3 Gy, given once daily, five days per week over two weeks

Treatment Delivery and Patient Care

Early or short-term side effects include fatigue, dermatitis, nausea and vomiting, diarrhoea, loss of appetite, weight loss, indigestion as a result of gastric irritation, abdominal discomfort, cramping and bloating along with ulceration and bleeding from the stomach and small bowel. Nausea and vomiting are controlled with 5-HT antagonist antiemetics such as ondansetron 8 mg at least 30 minutes prior to radiotherapy. All patients should take a daily proton pump inhibitor starting on the first day of radiotherapy. This should be continued until six weeks after radiotherapy completion. Special attention should be given to maintaining adequate nutrition and hydration. Suspected gastrointestinal bleed should be investigated with a gastroscopy. Concurrent chemotherapy may result in bone marrow suppression. Patients should be seen weekly for close monitoring and symptom management.

Verification

For radiotherapy using conventional fractionation, daily volumetric imaging verification with cone beam CT and online correction should be performed. For SABR, daily image-guidance using cone beam CT is essential to ensure correct patient setup and to verify the position of the PTV prior to and during treatment delivery.

LIVER TUMOURS

Indications for Radiotherapy

Hepatocellular Carcinoma

Hepatocellular carcinoma (HCC) is the fifth most common cancer in the world and is four times more frequent in Asia than in Europe and the United States. It is the third leading cause of cancer-related deaths worldwide. The majority of cases are related to exposure to the hepatitis B and C viruses. Other risk factors include alcohol, aflatoxins, autoimmune hepatitis and primary biliary cirrhosis. Radical surgical resection, where feasible, is the treatment of choice. Partial hepatectomy is recommended in patients with a solitary tumour, adequate liver reserve and no evidence of gross vascular invasion. Liver transplantation is considered in those who meet the Milan criteria. More than two-thirds of cases are not suitable for curative options at the time of diagnosis due to underlying liver disease or advanced tumour. For inoperable disease, treatment options include radiofrequency ablation, percutaneous ethanol injection, trans-arterial chemoembolisation (TACE) and systemic therapy. Historically, radiotherapy is seldom used in HCC due to concerns over radiation-induced damage to the adjacent normal liver tissue. Recent studies however have reported favourable response rates and clinical outcomes with the use of modern radiotherapy techniques such as IMRT, SABR, proton therapy and selective internal radiotherapy (SIRT) using radioisotopes such as Yttrium-90 or Iodine-131. Yttrium-90 radio-embolisation has also been used as a bridge to transplant and to downstage large tumours and bring them within transplantable criteria. SABR can be considered in patients with adequate performance status who are unsuitable candidates for surgical resection, liver transplantation or TACE or whose disease is refractory to TACE. The exclusion criteria for SABR in HCC include direct tumour extension into the stomach, duodenum, small or large bowel, lesion greater than 6 cm in dimension, more than five discrete lesions, evidence of extrahepatic metastases or malignant nodes, presence of clinically apparent ascites, active hepatitis or clinically significant liver failure such as portal hypertension, oesophageal varices or hepatic encephalopathy, prior liver transplantation and Child-Pugh Class B and C liver cirrhosis.

Liver Metastases

Surgical resection is the treatment of choice for liver metastases. Patients unsuitable for surgical resection may be managed with radiofrequency ablation, cryotherapy or SABR. Ideal candidates for SABR are those with performance status of 0–1, adequate liver function (Child-Pugh Class A), controlled or absent extrahepatic disease, three or fewer liver lesions each with a diameter of 3 cm or less and an uninvolved liver volume of 1000 cc or greater. Local control rates of 60–90 per cent at two years have been reported. Treatment is well tolerated, and severe toxicities are uncommon.

Assessment of Primary Disease

HCCs may be classified as unifocal expansive, infiltrating or multifocal. They invade the portal vein and spread thence to the lungs. They commonly present with non-specific symptoms of abdominal pain, malaise, fever and weight loss, although rupture and haemorrhage may occur. Diagnosis and staging is by dynamic multiphasic contrast-enhanced CT and MRI imaging. HCC classically demonstrates arterial phase enhancement. This is followed by washout in the portal venous and/or delayed phase. Tumour thrombosis of the portal vein can alter the imaging features of HCC. The appearances of HCC on MRI are variable. Most HCCs are mildly hyperintense or isointense on T2-weighted images. They are mostly hypointense on T1-weighted images and hyperintense on diffusion-weighted MR imaging. Biopsy is recommended but imaging findings are often characteristic. Identification of the target volume for SABR in liver metastases is aided by contrast-enhanced CT and/or MRI co-registered to the planning CT data set. A pretreatment DMSA renal scan is required if the right kidney is located close to the tumour.

Target Volume Definition

SABR requires precise target volume definition, treatment planning and delivery. The use of individualised immobilisation devices, 4D-CT and image guidance to verify the position of the PTV before and during treatment delivery are essential. Abdominal compression can help to reduce the magnitude of respiratory liver motion. MRI and PET-CT may aid target volume definition. An ITV is delineated encompassing all GTVs in the various phases of the respiratory cycle. A PTV margin is then applied to the ITV to take into account setup uncertainties. Implantation of fiducial markers may help target localisation and guide treatment delivery.

Dose Solutions

These treatments require complex solutions with stereotaxis and should be carried out in centres with appropriate equipment and expertise.

Dose Fractionation

Hepatocellular Carcinoma

- 40–50 Gy in 5 fractions (treating 3 fractions per week)

Liver Metastases

- 48 Gy or higher in 3–5 fractions, depending on normal tissue constraints

Verification

For SABR, image guidance is essential to ensure correct patient setup and to verify the position of the PTV prior to and during treatment delivery. This can be in the form of cone beam CT.

Key Trials

Mukherjee S, Hurt CN, Bridgewater J, et al. Gemcitabine-based or capecitabine-based chemoradiotherapy for locally advanced pancreatic cancer (SCALOP): A multicentre, randomised, phase 2 trial. Lancet Oncol 2013;14:317–326.

Neoptolemos JP, Stocken DD, Friess H, et al. A randomized trial of chemoradiotherapy and chemotherapy after resection of pancreatic cancer. N Engl J Med 2004;350:1200–1210.

Neoptolemos JP, Stocken DD, Bassi C, et al. Adjuvant chemotherapy with fluorouracil plus folinic acid versus gemcitabine following pancreatic cancer resection: A randomized controlled trial. JAMA 2010;304:1073–1081.

Neoptolemos JP, Palmer DH, Ghaneh P, et al. Comparison of adjuvant gemcitabine and capecitabine with gemcitabine monotherapy in patients with resected pancreatic cancer (ESPAC-4): A multicentre, open-label, randomised, phase 3 trial. Lancet 2017;389:1011–1024.

Oettle H, Neuhaus P, Hochhaus A, et al. Adjuvant chemotherapy with gemcitabine and long-term outcomes among patients with resected pancreatic cancer: The CONKO-001 randomized trial. JAMA 2013;310:1473–1481.

Regine WF, Winter KA, Abrams R, et al. Fluorouracil-based chemoradiation with either gemcitabine or fluorouracil chemotherapy after resection of pancreatic adenocarcinoma: 5-year analysis of the U.S. Intergroup/RTOG 9704 phase III trial. Ann Surg Oncol 2011;18:1319–1326.

INFORMATION SOURCES

Pancreas

Goodman KA, Regine WF, Dawson LA, et al. Radiation Therapy Oncology Group consensus panel guidelines for the delineation of the clinical target volume in the postoperative treatment of pancreatic head cancer. Int J Radiat Oncol Biol Phys 2012;83:901–908.

Hurt CN, Mukherjee S, Bridgewater J, et al. Health-related quality of life in SCALOP, a randomized phase 2 trial comparing chemoradiation therapy regimens in locally advanced pancreatic cancer. Int J Radiat Oncol Biol Phys 2015;93:810–818.

Hurt CN, Falk S, Crosby T, et al. Long-term results and recurrence patterns from SCALOP: A phase II randomised trial of gemcitabine- or capecitabine-based chemoradiation for locally advanced pancreatic cancer. Br J Cancer 2017;116:1264–1270.

Van Laethem J, Hammel P, Mornex F, et al. Adjuvant gemcitabine alone versus gemcitabine-based chemoradiotherapy after curative resection for pancreatic cancer: A randomized EORTC-40013-22012/FFCD-9203/GERCOR phase II study. J Clin Oncol 2010;28:4450–4456.

Liver Tumours

Heimbach JK, Kulik LM, Finn RS, et al. AASLD guidelines for the treatment of hepatocellular carcinoma. Hepatology 2018;67:358–380.

Hoyer M, Swaminath A, Bydder S, et al. Radiotherapy for liver metastases: A review of evidence. Int J Radiat Oncol Biol Phys 2012;82:1047–1057.

Sanuki N, Takeda A, Kunieda E. Role of stereotactic body radiation therapy for hepatocellular carcinoma. World J Gastroenterol 2014;20:3100–3111.

Scorsetti M, Clerici E, Comito T. Stereotactic body radiation therapy for liver metastases. J Gastrointest Oncol 2014;5:190–197.

26

Rectum

Indications for Radiotherapy

Colorectal cancer is the fourth most common cancer in the UK, with more than 40,000 new cases diagnosed each year. Colorectal cancer is more common in men and its incidence is related to age, with a sharp increase in age-specific rates from 50 years onwards. Incidence peaks between 85 and 89 years of age. Unlike anal cancer, where the incidence has doubled, over the past ten years the incidence of colorectal cancer has remained stable. Of the bowel cancer sub-sites, rectal cancer is the largest group, representing 32 per cent of male and 23 per cent of female bowel cancers. When diagnosed at an earlier stage, bowel cancer treatment is more successful. The national bowel cancer screening programme was introduced in 2009 with the aim to increase the proportion of bowel cancer diagnosed at any early stage. Patients between the ages of 60 and 74 are invited to perform faecal occult blood tests (FOBT) every two years. The soon-to-be-introduced faecal immunochemical test (FIT) will replace FOBT. It is hoped this simpler, more sensitive test will increase uptake in screening.

The vast majority of rectal cancers are adenocarcinomas. Signet ring and mucinous adenocarcinoma subtypes have a poorer prognosis. Patients with microsatellite instability/Lynch syndrome and medullary carcinoma often have a better prognosis. Less commonly, small cell carcinoma, carcinoid, lymphoma, sarcoma and squamous cell carcinoma may also arise within the rectum. Squamous cell carcinomas arising from the transitional area between the rectum and anal verge are classified and treated as anal cancer. Risk factors that have been linked with bowel cancer include inflammatory bowel disease, smoking, consumption of red/processed meats, and obesity.

Surgery is the mainstay of treatment and gives five-year overall survival rates of 97 per cent (Stage I), 72–85 per cent (Stage II), 44–83 per cent (Stage III) and 8 per cent (Stage IV). For early stage tumours (T1N0), resection of the rectum can be avoided with transanal endoscopic microsurgery (TEMS). Total mesorectal excision (TME), an en-bloc resection of the tumour, rectum, surrounding nodes/vessels and lymphatics encompassed within the mesorectal fascia has had a significant impact in reducing local recurrence. The quality of surgical resection (mesorectal, intramesorectal and muscularis propria resection plane) has been shown to correlate with local recurrence. Surgery with TME has reduced local recurrence rates compared to older surgical techniques. The most significant advancement in the surgical treatment of rectal cancer in recent times has been the identification of the importance of the circumferential resection margin (CRM). The status of the CRM is predictive of local recurrence and overall survival (OS). The presence of microscopic cells found within 1 mm of the CRM confers a positive status and will predict a poorer outcome for the patient. Surgical resection of liver metastases is possible in some patients with stage IV disease following primary treatment, with five-year survival of 36 per cent.

Curative Radiotherapy

For patients with early stage (T1N0) disease who decline or are not suitable for TEMS, contact brachytherapy using 50 kV photons can be considered. Low-energy contact X-ray brachytherapy (CXB), commonly referred to as the Papillon technique, uses a 50 kV X-ray tube which is placed in the rectum after dilation of the anus with GTN. The Papillon technique can treat low tumours up to 10 cm from the anal verge. The low energy of the tube limits the treatment depth to only a few millimetres. Judicious selection of patients is critical in the use of Papillon and requires MDT input. Papillon represents an attractive

DOI: 10.1201/9781315171562-26

treatment option for the aging population. CXB can be used to avoid surgical intervention both as a sole modality and in combination with EBRT. In cases of recurrence or poor response following CXB, surgery can still be used as a salvage option.

Neoadjuvant Radiotherapy

Patients whose CRM is involved or threatened (<1 mm) are most likely to benefit from neoadjuvant radiotherapy and can be identified using MRI. Treatment with radiotherapy can downstage a positive CRM identified on MRI and reduce the risk of a positive resection margin and in turn the risk of local recurrence. In a case series of 150 patients, 65 per cent of patients with a positive CRM on initial MRI staging were found to be CRM negative on histopathological review following treatment with neoadjuvant radiotherapy with concomitant chemotherapy and surgery.

The use of concomitant 5-fluorouracil (5-FU) with radiotherapy has a better response rate than radiotherapy alone. Oral capecitabine can be substituted for 5-FU with no loss in efficacy. Studies comparing the addition of a second agent, oxaliplatin, have shown an increase in pathological complete response (pCR) rates as well and an increase in associated toxicity but no improvement in the overall survival. The ARISTOTLE study is investigating the addition of irinotecan, the results of which are awaited. Currently, no recommendation can be made for the addition of further agents to capecitabine and radiotherapy. Neoadjuvant radiotherapy with concomitant chemotherapy is associated with a complete pathological response in 10–20 per cent of patients. If a complete radiological response is demonstrated on MRI following neoadjuvant radiotherapy with concomitant chemotherapy, there remains uncertainty on optimum management. In the UK, the current standard is to continue to surgery. There are currently trials investigating deferral of surgery, with strict follow-up with MRI and PET imaging and clinical examination, with the option to proceed to surgery when progression is detected.

Rectal cancers can be stratified into low, moderate and high-risk groups using MRI findings and the status of the CRM to predict the risk of local recurrence. This can help select which patients will benefit from neoadjuvant treatment (Table 26.1).

Moderate and high-risk patients are more likely to benefit from preoperative treatment and should be considered for neoadjuvant radiotherapy when considering management. In the UK, two courses of radiotherapy are commonly used: short course preoperative radiotherapy (SCPRT) and long course preoperative neoadjuvant radiotherapy with concomitant chemotherapy (LCPCRT).

SCPRT consists of 5 fractions of radiotherapy over one week. SCPRT aims to sterilise the surgical resection margins whilst allowing surgery to be performed before any radiation-related fibrosis forms.

LCPCRT consists of 25 fractions of radiotherapy over five weeks. Treatment is given concurrently with capecitabine chemotherapy.

SCPRT is a fast and effective treatment that reduces the risk of local recurrence when compared to TME alone. However, there is evidence to show that when the CRM is threatened or involved, LCPCRT provides superior local control. No difference in OS has been observed between SCPRT and LCPCRT. Current recommendations therefore suggest either SCPRT or LCPCRT in moderate risk patients, but LCPCRT in high-risk patients because of superior local control. Radiotherapy is not recommended in the

TABLE 26.1

Stratification of Risk of Local Recurrence Based on MRI (Based on the Results of the Mercury Study)

Risk of Local Recurrence	MRI Predictors
Low	• cT1 or cT2 or cT3a **and** • No lymph node involvement
Moderate	• Any cT3b or greater, in which the potential surgical margin is not threatened **or** • Any suspicious lymph node not threatening the surgical resection margin **or** • The presence of extramural vascular invasion (EMVI)
High	• A threatened (<1 mm) or breached resection margin **or** • Low tumours encroaching onto the inter-sphincteric plane **or** with levator involvement

low-risk patients because the potential benefit is low and is outweighed by the risks of long-term toxicity and secondary malignancy.

Adjuvant Radiotherapy

Postoperative radiotherapy is indicated where positive surgical margins are present, and no neoadjuvant radiotherapy has been administered. With the advent of neoadjuvant radiotherapy, the need for adjuvant radiotherapy is limited.

Palliative Radiotherapy

Palliation may be achieved for unresectable and locally advanced T4 tumours with radiotherapy alone. Alternatively, long course neoadjuvant radiotherapy with concomitant chemotherapy may be given to try to downstage a tumour for resection. Hypofractionated weekly radiotherapy may be used to palliate local symptoms in patients unfit for daily schedules.

Local recurrence is less common with the widespread use of TME and preoperative radiotherapy, but when it does arise it is a difficult and complex problem to manage. It may cause neuropathic sacral and sciatic pain with bladder and bowel dysfunction. In patients who have not been previously irradiated, radiotherapy with or without concomitant chemotherapy may offer effective short-term palliation. Patients who have received radiotherapy previously may be considered for re-irradiation, with either brachytherapy or external beam radiotherapy, but long-term toxicity data are lacking.

Sequencing of Multimodality Therapy

The sequencing of radiotherapy and surgery has been studied extensively, with preoperative radiotherapy showing better local control. The main RCTs that have influenced practice are shown in Table 26.2.

TABLE 26.2

Main RCTs Which Have Influenced Management of Rectal Cancer

Trial	Randomisation	Results
GTSG Study	Surgery	9-yr OS 27%, LR 25%
NEJM 1985	Surgery + POCRT	9-yr OS 54%*, LR 10%*
Mayo NCCTG	S + PORT	5-yr OS 40%, LR 25%
NEJM 1991	S + POCRT	5-yr OS 55%*, LR 15%*
Swedish Rectal Trial	Surgery	5-yr OS 48%, CSS 65%, LR 27%
NEJM 1997	Pre-Op SCRT + S (25 Gy/5#)	5-yr OS 58%*, CSS 74%*, LR 11%*
Dutch Rectal Trial	S (TME)	2-yr OS 81.8%, LR 8.2%
NEJM 2001	Pre-Op SCRT + S(TME) (25 Gy/5#)	2-yr OS 82.0%, LR 2.4%*
German Rectal Trial	Pre-Op LCCRT + S (TME)	5-yr OS 76%, LR 6%*
NEJM 2004	S (TME) + POCRT	5-yr OS 74%, LR 13%
CR07 Rectal Trial	Pre-Op SCRT + S (TME)	3-yr OS 80.8%, DFS 79.5%, LR 4.7%*
ASCO 2006	S (TME) + selective POCRT	3-yr OS 78.7%, DFS 74.5%, LR 11.1%
Polish Study	Pre-Op SCRT + S(TME)	4-yr OS 67.2%, DFS 58.4%, LR 9%
Br J Surg 2006	Pre-Op LCCRT + S(TME)	4-yr OS 66.2%, DFS 55.6%, LR 14.2%

Abbreviations: OS = overall survival, CSS = cause specific survival, DFS = disease free survival, LR = local recurrence, S = surgery, PORT = postoperative radiotherapy, POCRT = postoperative radiotherapy with concomitant chemotherapy, pre-op LCCRT = preoperative long course radiotherapy with concomitant chemotherapy, pre-op SCRT = preoperative short course radiotherapy, TME = total mesorectal excision.

* Significant p <0.05.

Surgery is carried out one week after SCPRT. Surgery takes place several weeks after LCPCRT surgery to allow recovery and to assess disease response. The optimal duration of this interval is currently under investigation. It has been suggested that the time between completion of radiotherapy and surgery may influence complete pathological response rates and is the subject of many ongoing trials such as the 6- vs 12-week trial.

Total neoadjuvant therapy (TNT) is a relatively new paradigm in the treatment of rectal cancer. It involves delivering the adjuvant phase of chemotherapy before radiotherapy with concomitant chemotherapy. The aims of this approach are to provide maximum downstaging where the primary tumour is borderline resectable or unresectable, but to also reduces the risk of metastatic spread where risk is thought to be increased by the presence of EMVI (Extra Mural Vascular Invasion) or local lymph nodes. The TNT approach has been added to the list of standard treatment regimens in the United States. Although not considered standard treatment in the UK, TNT should be considered on an individual basis for patients who may benefit.

Clinical and Radiological Anatomy

The rectum is the distal fifteen centimetres of the large bowel; it starts at the rectosigmoid junction and terminates at the external sphincter. The rectum can be considered as three sections based on distance from the anal verge. Upper third – 10 to 15 cm, middle third – 5 to10 cm, lower third – 0 to 5 cm (Figure 26.1). The distance of the tumour from the anal verge can be overestimated with flexible sigmoidoscopy so MRI is often a more accurate measure. The upper third of the rectum has a peritoneal covering over the anterior and lateral surfaces and is retroperitoneal posteriorly. At the level of the rectovesical/uterine pouch, the rectum becomes retroperitoneal. Inferiorly, the rectum enters the anal canal at the level of the levator ani having descended along the anterior surface of the sacrum. The rectum is relatively fixed compared to the colon above. It is encased in the mesorectum, a layer of fat containing nerves, blood vessels and lymphatic drainage. It is bounded by the mesorectal fascia, a distinct layer which separates the mesorectal fat from the surrounding pelvic fat.

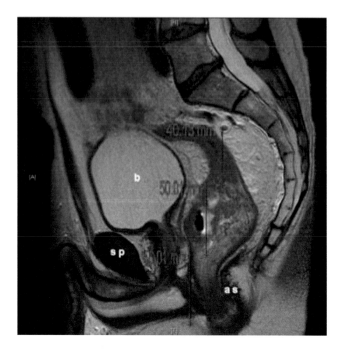

FIGURE 26.1 Sagittal T2-weighted MRI of a middle third rectal cancer showing division of the rectum into lower, middle and upper thirds. b, bladder; sp, symphysis pubis; as anal sphincter.

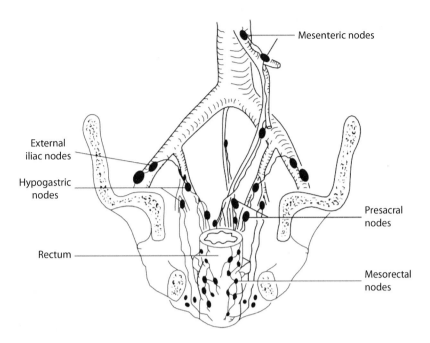

FIGURE 26.2 Lymphatic drainage of the rectum.

Rectal carcinomas arise in the mucosa and may be exophytic, ulcerated or annular. As tumours grow they extend through the wall of the serosa to invade surrounding organs such as the bladder, prostate and vagina, with direct extension into the presacral region in advanced cases. The lymphatic drainage of the rectum is to the mesorectal lymph nodes (within mesorectum), mesenteric lymph nodes (along inferior mesenteric artery), lateral lymph nodes (along with middle rectal, obturator and internal iliac vessels) and external iliac lymph nodes. There is also drainage to hypogastric and presacral lymph nodes (Figure 26.2). Tumours that are near or involve the anal margin may be associated with inguinal lymph node involvement. The proximal segment of the rectum and colon drain via the portal system into the liver, whilst the distal segment drainage bypasses the portal system. This difference in drainage accounts for the difference in metastatic patterns of spread between rectum and colon cancers, with rectal cancers twice as likely to metastasise to the thorax.

Assessment of Primary Disease

A clinical history and examination are performed routinely for all patients. Digital rectal examination findings should be recorded in detail including distance of tumour from the anal verge, any fixation and any involvement of the sphincters. Baseline blood work should include FBC, U&Es, LFTs and CEA. A significantly elevated CEA can be predictive of metastatic disease.

Up to 20 per cent of patients diagnosed with rectal cancer may have a synchronous primary colonic tumour. It is therefore important that the remaining colon is examined with colonoscopy or CT colonography. Radiological staging is useful to assess extent of local and distant disease. An MRI scan of the pelvis is used to assess the local extent of disease and detect the presence of pelvic nodal disease. Some centres use endorectal ultrasound, particularly when considering local surgical options such as TEMS. A CT scan of the thorax, abdomen and pelvis is used to detect the presence of any distant metastatic disease.

The radiological and clinical findings are used to stage patients. Clinical staging provides a guide to treatment options and prognosis. The TNM staging system is used to stage rectal cancer (AJCC 8th edition 2017). Following surgery, pathological staging will determine the need for adjuvant treatment. Nodal staging requires at least 12 lymph nodes to be examined.

Data Acquisition

Patients are scanned in the supine position, particularly if the patient has a stoma, as it is more comfortable and improves set-up reproducibility. In some situations, it may be preferable to scan the patient in the prone position. This is usually when the bowel needs to be displaced out of the pelvic cavity, with the aid of a bellyboard. When using a bellyboard, particular attention needs to be given to immobilisation at the ankles and knees as patient stability may be compromised. An anal marker can be placed at the anal verge before scanning to aid planning. The patient is scanned from the superior aspect of L5 to 4 cm inferior to the anal marker or the lowest edge of the tumour. A CT slice thickness of 2.5 mm is considered standard. Intravenous contrast is recommended, where appropriate, to aid in the identification and delineation of the pelvic blood vessels and differentiation of nodal structures.

Target Volume Definition

Preoperative Radiotherapy

Treatment is planned using CT defined target volumes. The same method of delineation applies to both SCPRT and LCPCRT. The target volumes are based on the known patterns of local recurrence in rectal cancer and includes the primary tumour, adjacent lymph nodes, the mesorectum and the presacral region. It has been shown that extension of the treatment volume above L5 increases late complications significantly and should only be considered on an individual patient basis.

In January 2021, the Royal College of Radiologists published national guidelines that provided a practical framework for the introduction of rectal IMRT planning into clinical practice. These new guidelines introduced a new set of planning target definitions, which are described later in the chapter.

Gross Tumour Volume (GTV)

GTVp – This volume should include all macroscopic primary tumour, areas of adjacent extramural vascular invasion or postoperative macroscopic disease identified on imaging. GTV should be delineated with reference to clinical findings and diagnostic MRI imaging. Where available, review of the GTV by a consultant GI radiologist should be considered. If the tumour can be confidently identified, the GTVp can include macroscopic disease only, without the whole lumen. Where this is not possible, it is accepted that the whole lumen can be delineated.

- GTVn – Include all lymph nodes suspected to be involved with tumour.
- GTVp_Boost – This label is used when the clinician wishes to boost the primary tumour to a higher dose. This is an optional target volume may be identical to GTVp.
- GTVn_Boost – This defines the areas of GTVn the clinician wishes to boost (which may be identical to GTVn). This is an optional target volume.

Internal Clinical Target Volume (ICTV)

The clinical target volume (CTV) aims to encompass potential microscopic extension of the tumour within the rectum, in the peri-rectal nodes, the mesorectum and the posterior pelvic nodes (pre-sacral, obturator, internal iliac). Inclusion of an ICTV is the most significant change to previous recommendations. Like a CTV, the ICTV includes regions of potential microscopic disease, but in addition to this includes a margin for motion (American Association of Physicists in Medicine (AAPM) and the International Commission on Radiation Units and Measurements [ICRU]).

ICTVp (primary ICTV) = GTVp + 10 mm in all directions except anteriorly, where 15 mm should be considered for tumours that may be more mobile anteriorly (e.g. upper rectal tumours above the peritoneal reflection). ICTVp is the GTVp with a margin to include both any potential microscopic disease and potential motion. The ICTVp should be edited off bone in all directions other than posteriorly towards the sacrum and edited off muscles unless there are obturator nodes, in which case the obturator internus muscle should be included on that side.

ICTVn (involved nodes) = GTVn + 5 mm in all directions. ICTVn is the GTVn with a margin for both potential microscopic disease and potential motion. The RCR guidelines suggests that 'although mesorectal nodes may move more than 5 mm, to limit the complexity of the guidelines and due to the fall-off dose that will be present in practice, a 5 mm margin' is acceptable. Like the ICTVp, ICTVn should be edited off bone in all directions other than posteriorly towards the sacrum, and edited off muscles unless there are obturator nodes, in which case the obturator internus muscle should be included on that side.

ICTV_elec = all elective nodal groups combined. This volume should always include the nodal compartments of mesorectum, presacral, obturator nodes and internal iliac nodes.

The clinician should ensure the ICTV_elec includes a 1-cm margin anterior to the mesorectum to account for any changes to the position of the anterior border of the mesorectum as the bladder changes in size over the course of treatment.

In cases where neoadjuvant chemotherapy has been used, the ICTV_elec should cover all compartments that contained nodal disease at the outset. The ICTV_elec should be at least 2 cm above the most superior node that was identified at the outset of neoadjuvant chemotherapy.

If there is radiological evidence of nonregional nodal involvement (for example, external iliac node or inguinal node) or disease in the ischio-rectal fossa, the entire compartment should be included. For guidance on delineation of these compartments, see the anal cancer chapter.

ICTV_final = ICTVp + ICTVn + ICTVpb (if present) + ICTV_elec.

Optional ICTV Volumes

- ICTV_Boost = GTVp_Boost + 10 mm in all directions except anteriorly where 15 mm can be considered for tumours that may be more mobile anteriorly (e.g. upper rectal tumours). In practice this is usually identical to the ICTVp.
- ICTVn_Boost = GTVn_Boost + 5 mm in all directions.
- ICTVsb = Area around surgical bed at risk for microscopic disease. This target volume is only used in the postoperative setting. ICTVsb should include all areas of disease present on preoperative imaging as well as all areas of potential microscopic disease postoperatively. Using surgical clips, if present, can be helpful to define the postoperative region at risk.
- ICTV_high = ICTVp_Boost + ICTVn_Boost. The ICTV_High is the region defined for boosting and includes a margin for microscopic disease and movement.

ICTV_elec Borders

Superior limit:

This starts at the S2/3 interspace with the internal iliac arteries or 2 cm above the superior extent of the GTV, whichever is higher.

Inferior limit:

The inferior limit is the superior aspect of the puborectalis. This is best identified on the slice where the mesorectum can no longer be seen on CT. The inferior limit may need to be extended in some situations so that the inferior extent is at least 2 cm below the inferior extent of the GTV.

Lateral limits are subdivided depending on the location within the pelvis:

- Upper pelvis – Internal iliac vessels are outlined; a 7-mm margin is applied. The lateral margin, once applied, extends vertically to the sacrum in the AP direction.
- Mid pelvis – The medial edge of obturator internus is used. The bony pelvic sidewall should be used in the presence of positive internal iliac nodes.
- Low pelvis – The outer border of the anorectal sphincter complex is used. Should there be levator or sphincter involvement, a 1-cm lateral margin is added to ICTV_elec.

The anterior limit is also subdivided:

- Upper pelvis – The anterior limit is determined by the internal iliac arteries, after a 7-mm margin is applied to the vessels. The most anterior aspect of the 7-mm margin forms the border. It is usual for one vessel to lie more anteriorly.
- Mid pelvis – The anterior border is 1 cm forward of the meso-rectal fascia or the internal iliac nodal compartment, whichever is the most anterior.
- Low pelvis – The anterior limit is placed at the border of the anorectal complex.

Posterior limit:

- The sacrum forms the posterior border throughout the volume. This applies at the level of the coccyx.

Planning Target Volumes (PTV)

As tumour motion is already included in the ICTV, the ICTV to PTV margin only needs to account for set-up error. The exact CTV to PTV margin to use will therefore depend on the centre-specific set-up error.

The RCR has recommended minimum CTV-PTV margins depending on which treatment verification technique is available.

With Daily Online CBCT

- PTV = ICTV_Final + 5 mm in all directions (in patients with one dose level only)
- PTV_High = ICTV_High + 5 mm in all directions
- PTV_Low = ICTV_Final + 5 mm in all directions (elective dose level for patients treated with SIB)

With Offline Imaging (Verification Protocol That Does Not Include Daily Online Imaging)

- PTV = ICTV_Final + 10 mm in all directions (in patients with one dose level only)
- PTV_High = ICTV_High + 10 mm in all directions
- PTV_Low ICTV_Final + 10 mm in all directions (elective dose level for patients treated with SIB)

Palliative Radiotherapy

Since the introduction of 3D conformal planning and IMRT, the use of bony landmarks to define field edges is no longer used in the UK. 3D conformal planning using three or four fields with modulation through static beams or IMRT/VMAT has taken over as standard practice. Historically, bony landmarks were used to define field borders and are only used now in rare emergency pallia-tive settings.

Bony landmarks can be used to define field borders:

Lateral: 1 cm outside bony pelvis.

Posterior: 1 cm behind sacrum to include sacral hollow and pre-sacral lymph nodes.

Superior: Sacral promontory, L5/S1 border as defined on lateral sagittal view.

Anterior: 2–3 cm anterior to sacral promontory and including the anterior vaginal wall in females. Care must be taken to include the whole rectum which may be more anteriorly placed. This can be seen on CT, at virtual simulation or on diagnostic MR scans.

Inferior: 3 cm below the inferior edge of the tumour. For lower third tumours the border should lie below the anal marker to cover the perineum.

Postoperative Radiotherapy

Postoperative radiotherapy is considered when a patient is upstaged on histopathology following sur-gery to a moderate or high-risk group. It is not given in all cases but should be considered when there is concern over whether a resection margin is clear or when there is residual. MDT discussion is vital as adjuvant chemotherapy, rather than radiotherapy, may be considered a more useful management option.

In the postoperative setting, there is often no GTV to delineate. The clinical target volume for post-operative radiotherapy should include all areas where disease was present on the pre-surgical scans, the tumour bed, elective lymph node compartments and any residual tumour. An additional 1-cm margin around the surgical bed may be applied if there are concerns over the surgical margin. Clinical examina-tion is used to localise the level of the anastomosis in patients after anterior resection or the perineal scar following abdominoperineal resection. Surgical procedures such as the reconstruction of the pelvic floor and absorbable mesh slings can be used to reduce the amount of small bowel in the pelvis.

Organs at Risk

The femoral necks, small bowel and bladder are the organs at risk when treating the rectum and should be delineated in all cases. For low rectal cancers, one should consider delineating the external genitalia. There is currently no consensus on the dose limitations for these organs, but it is agreed that the dose to these organs should be reduced as much as possible. Using IMRT appears to reduce the high dose exposure to organs at risk, at the cost of increased low dose exposure. It is unclear whether a relationship exists between the volume of small bowel irradiated and the risk of toxicity. A safe approach is to limit the volume of bowel receiving 45 Gy and to ensure that no bowel receives a dose in excess of 50 Gy.

Dose Solutions

Homogeneous dose distribution to the PTV is best achieved using IMRT (Figure 26.3). 3D conformal plans can also provide good solutions (Figure 26.4). This is usually achieved with three beams: two wedged lateral beams and a posterior beam. There are occasions where anterior coverage of the PTV will require an anterior beam. Lateral beam placement can reduce the anterior dose to normal tissues and allows a sharp cutoff in dose, where the oblique beam placement causes the dose to leak anteriorly. Overlapping of the oblique beams over the natal cleft must be avoided, as this increases the risk of skin toxicity.

For palliative treatment, a smaller volume can be used which covers the rectal tumour, sacrum, and involved soft tissue and local lymph nodes only to minimise the amount of small bowel treated. Treatment can be planned in the same way as described earlier using CT planning.

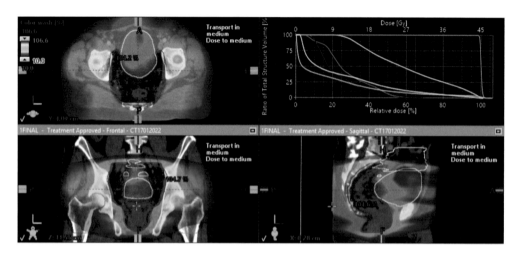

FIGURE 26.3 Preoperative rectum *IMRT plan*. (PTV_45: red, bladder: cyan, left femoral head: orange, right femoral head: brown and bowel: yellow).

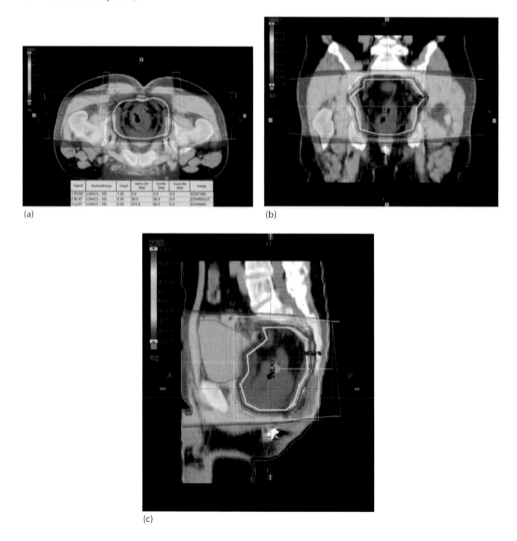

(a)

(b)

(c)

FIGURE 26.4 Conformal plan using direct posterior and lateral beams shown on CT slice: (a) axial, (b) coronal and (c) sagittal.

Dose Fractionation

Preoperative Radiotherapy

SCPRT: • 25 Gy in 5 daily fractions of 5 Gy given in one week
LCPCRT: • 45 Gy in 25 daily fractions of 1.8 Gy given in five weeks with concurrent capecitabine
• 50 Gy in 25 daily fractions SIB to sites of macroscopic disease

Postoperative Radiotherapy

45Gy in 25 daily fractions of 1.8Gy given in 5 weeks. If an R1 or R2 resection, consider SIB to total dose of 50Gy in 25 daily fractions.

Palliative Radiotherapy

Long course radiotherapy with concomitant chemotherapy may be used for maximal local control for inoperable rectal cancers where prolonged survival is expected.

• 45 Gy in 25 daily fractions of 1.8 Gy given in five weeks with concurrent capecitabine

or

• 30–36Gy in 5–6 fractions of 6 Gy once weekly given in five to six weeks

For patients with a limited prognosis, a shorter regimen may be more suitable

• 25 Gy in 5 daily fractions of 5 Gy in one week

or

• 20 Gy in 5 daily fraction of 4 Gy in one week

Treatment Delivery and Patient Care

Weekly patient review is performed to monitor toxicity. Erythema and desquamation of the skin can occur in the perineal and sacral areas. Nursing assessment, hydrocolloid dressings, nutritional support and analgesia are essential. Diarrhoea should be treated with loperamide hydrochloride. Abdominal pain and localised peritonism should prompt assessment for small bowel acute radiation toxicity; the patient should be rested from treatment and the radiotherapy plan and sites of small bowel reviewed. A minority of patients receiving short course preoperative radiotherapy develop an acute sensory neuropathy, which can be alleviated by a reduction in the treatment volume to the level of S2/3. Weekly FBC to monitor neutrophil and platelet counts are performed in patients who are undergoing chemotherapy. Patients receiving chemotherapy who have diarrhoea require medical review and a decision regarding suitability of treatment continuation.

Verification

Patients are set up daily, using anterior and lateral tattoos (over the iliac crests) and lasers to reduce lateral rotation. Set-up is then verified using the best available technique, such as cone beam CT (CBCT) or electronic portal imaging (EPI). EPI (both kV and mV) can be used daily to compare with the digital reconstructed radiographs to ensure the isocentre, beams and MLC-shielding configuration are correct. CBCT is now more frequently available in centres and can be used daily to ensure set-up is within departmental tolerance; this is usually 5 mm. In centres where CBCT has limited availability, daily EPI can be supplemented with CBCT in the first three fractions and then weekly after the systematic errors have been calculated.

Key Trials

Bujko K, Nowacki MP, Nasierowska-Guttmejer A, et al. Long-term results of a randomised trial comparing preoperative short-course radiotherapy with preoperative conventionally fractionated chemoradiation for rectal cancer. Br J Surg 2006;93(10):1215–1223.

Battersby NJ[1], How P, Moran B, et al.; Mercury II Study Group. Prospective validation of a low rectal cancer magnetic resonance imaging staging system and development of a local recurrence risk stratification model: The mercury II study. Ann Surg 2016 Apr;263(4):751–760.

Kapiteijn E, Marijnen CA, Nagtegaal ID, et al.; Dutch Colorectal Cancer Group. Preoperative radio therapy combined with total mesorectal excision for resectable rectal cancer. N Engl J Med 2001;345:638–646.

Sauer R, Becker H, Hohenberger W, et al.; German Rectal Cancer Study Group. Preoperative versus postoperative chemoradiotherapy for rectal cancer. N Engl J Med 2004;351:1731–1740.

Sebag-Montefiore D, Stephens RJ, Steele R, Monson J, Grieve R, Khanna S, et al. Preoperative radiotherapy versus selective postoperative chemoradiotherapy in patients with rectal cancer (MRC CR07 and NCIC-CTG C016): A multicentre, randomised trial. Lancet 2009;373(9666):811–820.

Swedish Rectal Cancer Trial. Improved survival with preoperative radiotherapy in resectable rectal cancer. N Engl J Med 1997;336:980–987.

INFORMATION SOURCES

Aristotle, A phase III trial comparing standard versus novel CRT as pre-operative treatment for MRI defined locally advance rectal cancer: Trial protocol. http://www.ctc.ucl.ac.uk/TrialDetails.aspx?Trial=82

Braendengen M, Tveit KM, Berglund A, et al. Randomized phase III study comparing preoperative radiotherapy with chemoradiotherapy in nonresectable rectal cancer. J Clin Oncol 2008;26:3687–3694.

Bujko K, Nowacki MP, Nasierowska-Guttmejer A, et al. Long-term results of a randomized trial comparing preoperative short-course radio- therapy with preoperative conventionally fractionated chemoradiation for rectal cancer. Br J Surg 2006;93:1215–1223.

Camma C, Giunta M, Fiorica F, Pagliaro L, Craxi A, Cottone M. Preoperative radiotherapy for resectable rectal cancer: A meta-analysis. JAMA 2000;284(8):1008–1015.

Cancer Research UK. http://www.cancerresearchuk.org/health-professional/cancer-statistics/statistics-by-cancer-type/bowel-cancer/incidence

Colorectal Cancer Collaborative Group. Adjuvant radiotherapy for rectal cancer: A systematic overview of 8,507 patients from 22 randomised trials. Lancet 2001;358(9290):1291–1304.

Contact Brachytherapy, the Papillon technique for early rectal cancer. https://www.nice.org.uk/guidance/ipg532/documents/lowenergy-contact-xray-brachytherapy-the-papillon-technique-for-earlystage-rectal-cancer-overview-2

Gerard JP, Conroy T, Bonnetain F, Bouche O, Chapet O, Closon-Dejardin MT, et al. Preoperative radiotherapy with or without concurrent fluorouracil and leucovorin in T3–4 rectal cancers: Results of FFCD 9203. J Clin Oncol 2006;24(28):4620–4625.

Jayne DG, Guillou PJ, Thorpe H, Quirke P, Copeland J, Smith AM, et al. Randomized trial of laparoscopic-assisted resection of colorectal carcinoma: 3-year results of the UK MRC CLASICC Trial Group. J Clin Oncol 2007;25(21):3061–3068.

Kapiteijn E, Marijnen CA, Nagtegaal ID, Putter H, Steup WH, Wiggers T, et al. Preoperative radiotherapy combined with total mesorectal excision for resectable rectal cancer. N Engl J Med 2001;345(9):638–646.

Marechal R, Vos B, Polus M, et al. Short course chemotherapy followed by concomitant chemoradiotherapy and surgery in locally advanced rectal cancer: A randomized multicentric phase II study. Ann Oncol 2012;23:1525–1530.

Mawdsley S, Glynne-Jones R, Grainger J, Richman P, Makris A, Harrison M, et al. Can histopathologic assessment of circumferential margin after preoperative pelvic chemoradiotherapy for T3-T4 rectal cancer predict for 3-year disease-free survival? Int J Radiat Oncol Biol Phys 2005;63(3):745–752.

Mercury Study Group. Diagnostic accuracy of preoperative magnetic resonance imaging in predicting curative resection of rectal cancer: Prospective observational study. BMJ 2006;333(7572):779.

Mercury Study Group. Extramural depth of tumor invasion at thin-section MR in patients with rectal cancer: Results of the mercury study. Radiology 2007;243(1):132–139.

Nagtegaal ID, Quirke P. What is the role for the circumferential margin in the modern treatment of rectal cancer? J Clin Oncol 2008;26(2):303–312.

Ngan SY, Burmeister B, Fisher RJ, et al. Randomized trial of short- course radiotherapy versus long-course chemoradiation comparing rates of local recurrence in patients with T3 rectal cancer: Trans-Tasman Radiation Oncology Group trial 01.04. J Clin Oncol 2012;31:3827–3833.

NICE, Colorectal cancer: Diagnosis and management. Clinical guideline [CG131] Published date: November 2011. Last updated: December 2014. https://www.nice.org.uk/guidance/cg131

Nogue M, Salud A, Vicente P, et al. Addition of bevacizumab to XELOX induction therapy plus concomitant capecitabine-based chemoradiotherapy in magnetic resonance imaging-defined poor- prognosis locally advanced rectal cancer: The AVACROSS study. Oncologist 2011;16:614–620.

Quirke P, Durdey, Dixon MF, Williams NS. Local recurrence of rectal adenocarcinoma due to inadequate surgical resection: Histopathological study of the lateral tumour spread and surgical excision. Lancet 1986;2:996–999.

Quirke P, Steel R, Monson J, Grieve R, Khanna S, Couture J, et al. Effect of the plane of surgery achieved on local recurrence in patients with operable rectal cancer: A prospective study using data from the MRC CR07 and NCIC-CTG CO16 randomised clinical trial. Lancet 2009;373(9666):821–828.

Riihimäki M, Hemminki A, Sundquist J, Hemminki K. Patterns of metastasis in colon and rectal cancer. Sci Rep 2016;6:29765.

Sauer R, Becker H, Hohenberger W, Rodel C, Wittekind C, Fietkau R, et al. Preoperative versus postoperative chemoradiotherapy for rectal cancer. N Engl J Med 2004;351(17):1731–1740.

Sebag-Montefiore D, Glynne-Jones R, Falk S, Meadows HM, Maughan T. A phase I/II study of oxaliplatin when added to 5-fluorouracil and leucovorin and pelvic radiation in locally advanced rectal cancer: A Colorectal Clinical Oncology Group (CCOG) study. Br J Cancer 2005;93(9):993–998.

Van Cutsem E, Twelves C, Cassidy J, Allman D, Bajetta E, Boyer M, et al. Oral Capecitabine compared with intravenous fluorouracil plus leucovorin in patients with metastatic colorectal cancer: Results of a large phase III study. J Clin Oncol 2001;19(21):4097–4106.

Wibe A, Rendedal PR, Svensson E, Norstein J, Eide TJ, Myrvold HE, et al. Prognostic significance of the circumferential resection margin following total mesorectal excision for rectal cancer. Br J Surg 2002;89(3):327–334.

27

Anus

Indications for Radiotherapy

Anal cancer is three times more common in women than men and its incidence is rising. Over the last decade, the incidence of anal cancer has doubled in the UK, with 1484 new cases in 2015 compared to 726 in 2005. Over this period, the incidence of anal cancer has remained stable in men, but rates in women have risen by more than 50 per cent. The peak incidence is in those aged between 85 and 89 years of age.

Eighty per cent of all anal cancers are epidermoid squamous cell carcinomas (SCC). The majority of these cases are preceded by high-grade anal intraepithelial neoplasia (AIN). Roughly 1 per cent of patients with AIN go on to develop invasive cancer every year. Tumours of the anal margin are often keratinising and well differentiated, while canal tumours are usually non-keratinising and poorly differentiated. Upper canal tumours may be mixed squamous cell and adenocarcinoma of transitional, basaloid or cloacogenic type. Rare types of primary anal cancer include adenocarcinomas, small cell carcinomas, melanoma, lymphoma and leiomyosarcoma.

Human papilloma virus (type 16 and 18) infection is associated with more than 90 per cent of cases of anal SCC. Other risks factors include immunosuppression, ano-receptive intercourse and tobacco smoking. Anal SCC is associated with HIV infection but is not correlated with the degree of immunosuppression, and it is not considered an AIDS defining illness.

Curative Radiotherapy with Concomitant Chemotherapy

Curative radical radiotherapy with concomitant chemotherapy remains the treatment of choice for both localised and locally advanced disease. The five-year survival rates are >90 per cent for T1, >80 per cent for T2, 45–55 per cent for T3/4 and 65–75 per cent overall.

The initial studies of Nigro in 1974 demonstrated the curative potential of radiotherapy with chemotherapy for anal cancer (RT 30 Gy and MMC/5 FU). Further studies confirmed the benefit of adding mitomycin C (MMC) and 5 FU to radiotherapy for anal cancer. Three of the larger randomised controlled trials in the1990s are listed in Table 27.1.

Although curative radical radiotherapy with concomitant chemotherapy should be considered for all patients with non-metastatic anal cancer who are fit for radical treatment it is associated with an increased risk of toxicity in patients with HIV infection, inflammatory bowel disease and after previous pelvic surgery or renal transplantation. Patients with HIV and immunosuppression with a CD4 count <200 develop significant toxicity and morbidity with radiotherapy and chemotherapy. Patients should be managed in partnership with the local HIV team to ensure toxicity and counts are managed in conjunction with antiviral medications. Outcomes in HIV patients on HARRT are the same as non-HIV patients. The dose of radiotherapy and chemotherapy can be modified in this group of patients but this may reduce control rates, so pre-emptive management of HIV is often best.

Patients with inflammatory bowel disease tolerate pelvic radiotherapy poorly with a high risk of late toxicity. Patients who have had previous pelvic surgery often have adhesions and risk increased dose to small bowel and late complications. The multidisciplinary team should carefully consider the risks and benefits of radical surgical resection versus radical radiotherapy.

DOI: 10.1201/9781315171562-27

TABLE 27.1

RCT of Radiotherapy for Anal Cancer

Trial	Randomisation	Results
UKCCR ACT1 (n=585)	RT alone	3-yr LC 39%, CSS 61%, OS 58%
	RT +5 FU/MMC	3-yr LC 61%, CSS 72%, OS 65%
EORTC (n=103)	RT alone	3-yr LC 55%, OS 65%
	RT+5 FU/MMC	3-yr LC 65%, OS 70%
RTOG (n=291)	RT alone	4-yr LC 64%, DFS 50%, OS 65%
	RT+5 FU/MMC	4-yr LC 83%, DFS 67%, OS 67%

Abbreviations: OS = overall survival, LC = local control, CSS = cause specific survival, DFS = disease free survival

Adjuvant Radiotherapy with Concomitant Chemotherapy

Surgery is now most commonly performed for failure after radiotherapy or in cases where radiotherapy is contraindicated. For early tumours of the anal margin local excision may be considered, where the tumour diameter measures less than 2 cm and no lymph nodes are involved, providing the tumour can be completely excised without damage to the sphincter. After incomplete excision, adjuvant radiotherapy with concomitant chemotherapy is advised. Excision margins less than or equal to 1 mm are eligible for participation in the ACT III trial, which is described later.

Palliative Radiotherapy

Palliative radiotherapy can be considered for patients who present with metastatic disease or for those with a poor performance status such that they will not tolerate radical treatment.

Clinical and Radiological Anatomy

The anal canal is 3–4 cm long and extends from the anorectal ring (top of 'surgical' anal canal), composed of upper fibres of the internal sphincter, to the anal margin as shown in Figure 27.1. The anal margin consists of the area of skin around the anal orifice. Tumours of the anal margin are slow growing and tend to infiltrate locally within the perineum, with late spread to lymph nodes. Tumours of the anal canal

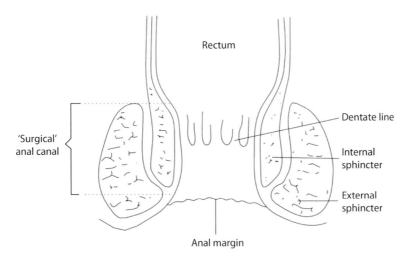

FIGURE 27.1 Anatomy of the anus.

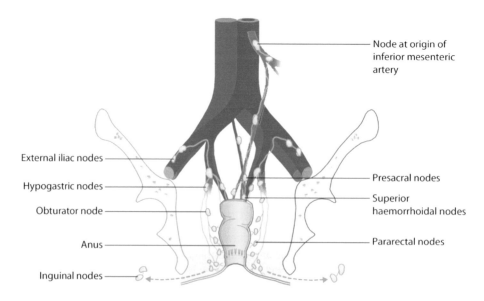

Node at origin of inferior mesenteric artery

External iliac nodes

Hypogastric nodes

Obturator node

Anus

Inguinal nodes

Presacral nodes

Superior haemorrhoidal nodes

Pararectal nodes

FIGURE 27.2   Lymphatic drainage of the anus.

most commonly arise in the transitional zone just above the dentate line, and tend to spread proximally in the submucosa to the distal rectum. Tumours invade anteriorly into the vagina and uncommonly to the prostate, laterally to the ischio-rectal fossa, and posteriorly along the ano-coccygeal ligament to the coccyx. Anterior spread to the prostate may be limited by Denonvilliers' fascia, and inferior spread may be limited by the suspensory ligaments.

Lymphatic drainage from the anal margin and peri-anal skin is to the superficial inguinal and femoral lymph nodes, and thence to the external iliac nodes. The lymphatic drainage of the anal canal, proximal to the dentate line, is to the superior rectal, superior haemorrhoidal, hypogastric, obturator, internal iliac and presacral lymph nodes (Figure 27.2). Tumours distal to the dentate line drain to superficial inguinal nodes as well as to pararectal nodes.

Sequencing of Multimodality Therapy

The RTOG-8704 trial was the first to show improved local control with the addition of mitomycin C (MMC) to 5-fluorouracil-based (5-FU) radiotherapy treatment: disease-free survival with the dual agents increased from 51 per cent to 79 per cent. ACT I – the first UK-based anal cancer trial, showed a 41 per cent reduction in local recurrence using the combination of MMC/5 FU with radiotherapy versus radiotherapy alone. ACT II, the second large UK-led study, looked at the use of cisplatin in place of MMC in combination with 5 FU. It used a 2×2 factorial trial design: it compared MMC/5-FU and cisplatin/5 FU, both when no maintenance chemotherapy was given, and also when maintenance chemotherapy was given consisting of a further two cycles of cisplatin/MMC. The ACT II trial showed no gain from maintenance chemotherapy or from the use of cisplatin, but showed improved outcomes in the MMC/5-FU group (no maintenance chemotherapy) when compared to that studied in ACT I. This has been attributed to the removal in ACT II of the radiotherapy treatment gap between phase I and phase II (which was in place in ACT I to allow for recovery from toxicity). ACT II confirmed that MMC and 5 FU given with radiotherapy should be standard of care in the UK. ESMO, ESSO, ESTRO and NCCN guidelines also endorse this combination of treatment.

UK standard radiotherapy protocols recommend that the first fraction of radiotherapy should be given after the commencement of an intravenous infusion of 5-fluorouracil chemotherapy. 5-FU is given in the first and last weeks of radiotherapy with mitomycin C on day 1 only. It is accepted that 5-fluorouracil can be replaced with capecitabine 825 mg/m^2, with no loss of efficacy in treatment. RTOG 98–11 randomised patients to radiotherapy with MMC/5-FU or cisplatin/5-FU in an attempt to improve outcome. No advantage of cisplatin-based therapy was shown; disease-free survival was better for mitomycin but was not significant. The rate of colostomy was significantly higher in the cisplatin-based group – 19 per cent vs 10 per cent, P = 0.02 – compared with those given MMC/5-FU + radiotherapy.

The ACCORD 03 trial investigated the role of induction chemotherapy and radiotherapy dose intensification. A 2 × 2 factorial trial studied the role of induction chemotherapy, using two cycles cisplatin/5 FU, and dose intensification (a 20–25 Gy or 15 Gy boost in phase II). No difference was seen with the use of induction chemotherapy or dose-intensified boost. Use of the most intense treatment, induction with increased boost, trended to improved colostomy-free survival p=0.067, but was not statistically significant.

Assessment of Primary Disease

A full history should elicit symptoms of local tumour, possible spread, and record comorbidities and performance status to determine fitness for radical treatment. Clinical examination includes inspection of the perineal skin, digital rectal examination (DRE) to assess the site and extent of the primary tumour and vaginal examination to detect involvement of the posterior vaginal wall. Due to the known associations with HPV, any concern of a coexisting cervix tumour requires referral to the gynaecology service as a matter of urgency.

Patients should have an examination under anaesthesia (EUA) to provide a detailed assessment of the primary tumour and biopsies of the tumour and of any enlarged inguinal lymph nodes >1 cm. Thirty per cent of patients have enlarged inguino-femoral lymph nodes at presentation, of which 50 per cent are involved and 50 per cent show reactive inflammatory change only. An endoscopy should also be performed to exclude a synchronous rectal or colonic tumour. Serum HIV testing is carried out in all patients.

Further local staging is performed with endorectal ultrasound and MRI scan of the pelvis. A CT scan of the chest and abdomen is performed to exclude distant metastases. FDG-PET scans are increasingly used to assess for metastatic disease, but there remains debate around their role.

Tumours of the anal canal and margin are staged according to the TNM and AJCC 8th, 2017 classification (Table 27.2). The terms 'anal margin' and 'perianal skin' are synonymous and cancers at this site are classified as skin tumours. Poor prognostic factors include metastases, lymph node spread, higher T stage, older age, poor performance status and anaemia (Hb <10 g/dL).

TABLE 27.2

AJCC TNM Staging 8th 2017 Classification

Primary Tumour – T	
Tx	Cannot be assessed
T0	No evidence of primary
Tis	Carcinoma in situ or anal intraepithelial neoplasia (AIN)
T1	2 cm or less in greatest dimension
T2	>2 cm but <5 cm
T3	>5 cm
T4	Invades adjacent organ: vagina, urethra, bladder
	Not: rectal wall, perirectal skin/subcutaneous tissue or sphincters
Nx	Lymph nodes cannot be assessed
N0	No evidence of cancer containing lymph nodes
N1a	Inguinal, mesorectal and or internal iliac
N1b	External iliac
N1c	External iliac AND inguinal, mesorectal AND/OR internal iliac
M1	Distant metastasis

Data Acquisition

Before the CT planning scan, assessment of the patient should answer the need for:

1. Defunctioning stoma (infiltrating into posterior vagina/significant faecal incontinence secondary to indication or sphincter dysfunction). Note that patients who are defunctioned have a poor reversal rate.
2. Bolus. Most patients will self-bolus with their buttocks but should there be less then 5 mm around the tumour and/or nodes in the inguinal/femoral region, wax or bolus sheet can be applied.

Patients are scanned in the supine position with an anal marker placed at the anal verge. They are immobilised at the feet and popliteal fossa. A comfortably full bladder is used to displace the small bowel. Intravenous contrast is used to aid identification and delineation of vessels. Any macroscopic disease can be marked with wire if more inferior than anal marker. If the patient's tumour has been excised, it is useful to mark the scar with wire. Oral contrast can be used to help identify bowel at the clinician's discretion. Tattoos are placed anteriorly and laterally. The scan limits are from the cranial aspect of L3 to 5 cm caudal to the lowest extent of disease or 10 cm below the lesser trochanter, whichever is lower.

Target Volume Definition

Since the relatively simple fields and parallel opposed treatment plans of ACT II, radiotherapy treatment has evolved and IMRT is now the standard of care in the UK. RTOG 05-29, a phase II trial evaluating IMRT dose painting in anal cancer treatment has showed IMRT to be feasible and reduce grade 3 toxicity compared to a historic cohort that received conventional radiotherapy. The shrinking fields of ACT II are no longer used but should still be known as they may be given if emergency/palliative treatment is needed in a time-sensitive situation. The National Guidance for IMRT in Anal Cancer consensus details the target volumes and the approach to delineation of these structures with contoured images that can be referred to (see information sources). These guidelines have formed the basis for the contouring recommendations in the PLATO trials.

When considering radiotherapy target volumes, anal cancer is divided into early and locally advanced disease. Early-stage disease is considered any T1 or T2 without any regional nodal spread. This group has a low risk of locoregional failure (10 per cent). This group includes post-surgical T1N0 with residual disease. For patients with good prognosis T1N0 disease it is at the clinician's discretion whether to offer prophylactic nodal irradiation. Disease that is node positive or T3/4 is described as locally advanced – this group has a higher risk or locoregional failure (30 per cent). Using the CT planning scan with MRI or PET fusion, where possible, the tumour is outlined according to the following.

Early – T1N0 and T2N0

- GTV_A = Gross primary disease (scar if tumour resected), limited to disease not lumen.
- CTV_A = GTV with 10-mm circumferential expansion, edited to ensure the entire anal canal including the outer boarder is included (internal/external anal sphincters to the anorectal junction, approximately 4 cm from anal verge/marker), editing off muscle and bone.
- CTV_E = Elective nodal regions – see following section Creation of CTV_E.
- PTV_Anus = CTV_A with 10-mm margin.
- PTV_E = CTV_E with 5-mm* margin.

Locally Advanced – T3/4N0 or T1-4N1

- GTV_A = Gross primary disease (scar if resected), limited to disease not lumen.
- GTV_N = Involved nodes.

- CTV_A = GTV with 15-mm circumferential expansion, edited to ensure the entire anal canal including the outer boarder is included (internal/external anal sphincters to the anorectal junction, approximately 4 cm from anal verge/marker). Note to edit muscle and bone.
- CTV_N = GTV_N with a 5-mm circumferential expansion.
- CTV_E = Elective nodes – see following section Creation of CTV_E.
- PTV_Anus = CTV_A with 10-mm expansion.
- PTV_N = CTV_N with 5-mm expansion.
- PTV_E = CTV_E with 5-mm* margin.

Creation of CTV_E

The CTV_E includes the internal iliac, external lilac, obturator, inguinal, presacral and mesorectal nodal groups. Where mesorectal nodes are involved, the whole mesorectum in included. If no mesorectal nodes are involved, then only the lower 50 mm is contoured. The nodal volumes are based around the vasculature. Start with the internal and external iliac vessels – 20 mm above the sacroiliac joints or 15 mm above the tumour, whichever is most superior. Follow this inferiorly to the external iliac artery until the slice showing the lesser trochanter. This volume must then be expanded by 7 mm. The resulting volume should be edited off bone and muscle. Then join the two volumes along the medial edges of iliopsoas and obturator internus, and anterior to the sacrum. As the volume extends inferiorly, the mesorectum is incorporated. The most inferior extent of the volume covers the inguinal nodes and femoral triangle. The ischio-rectal fossa is only included if there is infiltration into the levators, puborectalis, external anal sphincter, anal verge or ischio-rectal fossa.

Dose Solutions

All radical treatments are inversely planned to deliver simultaneous integrated boost IMRT with coplanar beams, arc delivery, VMAT or tomotherapy. The D95 per cent should be >95 per cent, the D50 per cent between 99 per cent and 101 per cent, the D5 per cent <10.5 per cent and the C2 per cent less than 107 per cent (see Figure 27.3). The organ at risk objectives should be easily met with IMRT, but all efforts should be used to reduce the dose to the organs at risk to a minimum (see Table 27.3).

The conventionally planned shrinking fields of ACT II are no longer used but may be of historical interest and may be considered in the urgent setting when awaiting the creation of an IMRT plan. Conventional fields are designed to include all potential nodal groups and should be substituted for

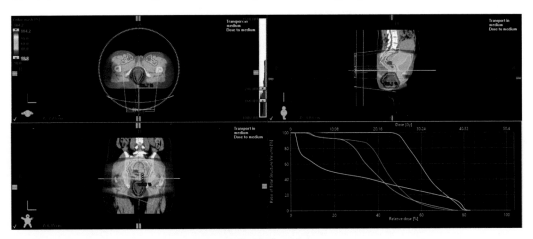

FIGURE 27.3   Example IMRT plan for anal cancer.

---

* Please note that this margin is thought to be acceptable only where daily online image correction is in place.

TABLE 27.3

Anal Cancer Organs at Risk Dose Constraints

Organ	OAR	Optimal	Mandatory
Small Bowel	D200 cc	<30 Gy	<35 Gy
	D150 cc	<35 Gy	<40 Gy
	D20 cc	<45 Gy	<50 Gy
	D_{max}	<50 Gy	<55 Gy
Femoral	D50%	<30 Gy	<45 Gy
Heads	D35%	<40 Gy	<50 Gy
	D5%	<50 Gy	<55 Gy
Genitalia	D50%	<20 Gy	<35 Gy
	D35%	<30 Gy	<40 Gy
	D5%	<40 Gy	<55 Gy
Bladder	D50%	<35 Gy	<45 Gy
	D35%	<40 Gy	<50 Gy
	D5%	<50 Gy	<58 Gy

Source: National Guidance for IMRT in Anal Cancer Version 3.

a radical IMRT plan as soon as possible. Anterior and posterior opposing beans are used with MLC shielding to normal tissue. This Phase 1 large field was treated to 30.6 Gy and then smaller phase 2 was defined by 3 cm around the GTV. High photon energies (10–20 MV) give more satisfactory dose distributions, especially for large patients. Bolus is used between the buttocks and over the perineum to ensure adequate dose to anal margin tumours and tumours within 2 cm of the anal verge. Superior-inferior dose compensation may be needed to improve dose homogeneity.

In ACT II, the borders for phase 1 were (see Figure 27.4):

Superior border: 2 cm above inferior aspect of the SI joints. A minimum margin of 3 cm above the upper extent of GTV-T or GTV-N.

Lateral border: To include both inguinal nodal regions – in practice this border lies lateral to the femoral head.

Inferior border: 3 cm below the anal margin or 3 cm below the most inferior extent of tumour (for anal margin tumours).

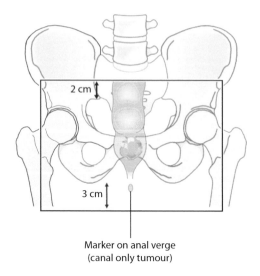

Marker on anal verge
(canal only tumour)

FIGURE 27.4 Phase 1 treatment borders for all anal tumours (from ACT II). (Reproduced with permission from Dr D Sebag-Montefiore on behalf of the ACT II trialists.)

Postoperative Radiotherapy

As discussed earlier, the need for postoperative treatment following surgery is now uncommon. In cases where there has been incomplete excision or involved circumferential margins and the patient has not received prior radiotherapy, the patient can be treated with radiotherapy with concomitant chemotherapy as outlined earlier.

Palliative Radiotherapy

In patients who present with metastatic disease, the initial treatment is with systemic chemotherapy if they are fit. Consider cisplatin/5-FU and carboplatin/paclitaxel, first and second line respectively. If however the volume of metastatic disease is small, many patients benefit from additional radiotherapy with concomitant chemotherapy to achieve local control in the pelvis. This can be planned as for curative radical radiotherapy, or smaller volume: GTV plus a margin of 3 cm. Depending on patient fitness, a more conventional palliative dose may be used.

Dose Fractionation

Curative Radiotherapy with Concomitant Chemotherapy

Early disease – T1/2 N0

- PTV_A = 50.4Gy in 28# (1.8Gy per #) in 5.5 weeks
- PTV_E = 40Gy in 28# (1.4Gy per #) in 5.5 weeks

Locally advanced - T3/4N0 or T1-4N1

- PTV_A = 53.2Gy in 28# (1.9Gy per #) in 5.5 weeks
- PTV_N with gross nodal disease >3 cm = 53.2Gy in 28# (1.9Gy per #) in 5.5 weeks
  with gross nodal disease <3 cm = 50.4Gy in 28# (1.8Gy per #) in 5.5 weeks
- PTV_E = 40Gy in 28# (1.4Gy per #) in 5.5 weeks

Chemotherapy

- Mitomycin C 12 mg/m^2 IV on day 1 (max. 20 mg)
- Capecitabine 825 mg/m^2 PO BD on days of radiotherapy

Or

- 5-Flurouracil 1000 mg/m^2 IV days 1–4 and D29–32.
- Consider dose adjustment on a case-by-case review if patient age is >70.

Postoperative Radiotherapy with Concomitant Chemotherapy

As described earlier in selected cases.

Palliative Radiotherapy

Low dose radiotherapy with concomitant chemotherapy

- 30 Gy 15# in three weeks to GTV + 3-cm margin with continuous 5FU

Palliative dose

- 8 Gy in 1#
- 20 Gy in 5# in one week

Treatment Delivery and Patient Care

Patients may lose weight/change shape during the planning and treatment phases so it is important to ensure the patients are still self-bolus with their buttocks, and if needed additional wax or bolus sheet is applied to guarantee the correct dosimetry. Treatment is delivered with a comfortably full bladder in the supine position.

The perineal and inguinal tissues are particularly sensitive to irradiation and skin reactions are often brisk and painful. Regular review and use of hydrocolloid dressings, nutritional support, analgesia and anti-diarrhoeal medication are essential.

During concomitant chemotherapy, patients should receive appropriate antiemetics, and prophylactic antibiotic cover is advised for the duration of treatment. Blood tests are monitored regularly for myelosuppression, and any sign of infection is treated promptly. Prior to commencing treatment, patients should be consented for infertility, sexual dysfunction. Female patients should be informed about vaginal dryness and the role of vaginal dilators.

Verification

Lasers and skin tattoos are used to align the patient each day and lateral tattoos over the iliac crests help to prevent lateral rotation. Daily cone beam CT (CBCT) imaging is used for verification. In some instances, CBCT is performed on the first three days of treatment and then weekly, provided there are no gross errors in alignment. Electronic portal imaging is used to verify the treatment set-up in the absence of cone beam imaging.

Upcoming Trials

The UK has launched the next series of trials into anal cancer with the PLATO study. This incorporates the next set of ACT trials: ACT 3, 4, and 5. PLATO has been set up to look at personalising radiotherapy for early and advanced anal cancer. Given the original trials of Nigra et al. showed a relatively low dose of radiation was able to achieve cure in a significant proportion of patients and the more recent and varying use of a boost dose, the study is aiming to look at both dose de-escalation and dose escalation, depending on the stage of disease.

ACT 3 investigates radiotherapy in T1 anal margin tumours with excision margins <1 mm. Randomising observation to radiotherapy 41.4 Gy 23# in four and a half weeks, in an attempt to improve control and reduce toxicity.

ACT 4 investigates if dose de-escalation in early-stage anal cancer can reduce toxicity. 50.4 Gy to tumour and 40 Gy to nodes in 28# randomised 41.4 Gy to tumour and 34.5 Gy in 23#.

ACT 5 investigates dose escalation using a simultaneous integrated boost with concurrent chemotherapy can reduce locoregional failure. Randomising three dose levels: 53.4 Gy, 58.8 Gy and 61.6 Gy all in 28# with 40 Gy to the elective nodes.

Key Trials

Ajani JA, Winter KA, Gunderson LL, et al. Fluorouracil, mitomycin, and radiotherapy vs fluorouracil, cisplatin, and radiotherapy for carcinoma of the anal canal: A randomised controlled trial. JAMA 2008;23:299(16):1914–1921.

Bartelink H, Roelofsen F, Eschwege F, et al. Concomitant radiotherapy and chemotherapy is superior to radiotherapy alone in the treatment of locally advanced anal cancer: Results of a phase III randomised trial of the European Organization for Research and Treatment of Cancer Radiotherapy and Gastrointestinal Cooperative Groups. J Clin Oncol 1997;15(5):2040–2049.

Flam M, John M, Pajak TF, et al. Role of mitomycin in combination with fluorouracil and radiotherapy, and of salvage chemoradiation in the definitive nonsurgical treatment of epidermoid carcinoma of the anal canal: Results of a phase III randomised intergroup study. J Clin Oncol 1996;14(9):2527–2539.

Glynne-Jones R, Meadows H, Wan S, et al. Extra—a multicenter phase II study of chemoradiation using a 5 day per week oral regimen of capecitabine and intravenous mitomycin C in anal cancer. Int J Radiat Oncol Biol Phys 2008;72(1):119–126.

Gunderson LL, et al. Long-term update of US GI intergroup RTOG 98-11 phase III trial for anal carcinoma: Survival, relapse, and colostomy failure with concurrent chemoradiation involving fluorouracil/mitomycin versus fluorouracil/cisplatin. J Clin Oncol 2012;30(35):4344–4351.

James R, Meadows H, Wan S. ACT II: The second UK phase III anal cancer trial. Clin Oncol 2005;17(5):364–366.

James RD[1], Glynne-Jones R, Meadows HM, et al. Mitomycin or cisplatin chemoradiation with or without maintenance chemotherapy for treatment of squamous-cell carcinoma of the anus (ACT II): A randomised, phase 3, open-label, 2 × 2 factorial trial. Lancet Oncol 2013 May;14(6):516–524.

Kachnic LA, et al. RTOG 0529: A phase 2 evaluation of dose-painted intensity modulated radiation therapy in combination with 5-fluorouracil and mitomycin-C for the reduction of acute morbidity in carcinoma of the anal canal. Int J Radiat Oncol Biol Phys 2013 May 1;86(1):27–33. doi: 10.1016/j.ijrobp.2012.09.023. Epub 2012 Nov 12.

Peiffert D, et al. Induction chemotherapy and dose intensification of the radiation boost in locally advanced anal canal carcinoma: Final analysis of the randomized UNICANCER ACCORD 03 trial. J Clin Oncol 2012;30:1941–1948.

UKCCCR Anal Cancer Trial Working Party. UK Co-ordinating Committee on Cancer Research. Epidermoid anal cancer: Results from the UKCCCR randomised trial of radiotherapy alone versus radiotherapy, 5-fluorouracil, and mitomycin. Lancet 1996;348(9034):1049–1054.

INFORMATION SOURCES

ACT II Trial. http://www.ucl.ac.uk/cancertrials/trials/actii/index.htm

Bhuva NJ, et al. To PET or not to PET? That is the question. Staging in anal cancer. Annals of Oncology 1 August 2012;23(8):2078–2082.

Charnley N, Choudhury A, Chesser P, et al. Effective treatment of anal cancer in the elderly with low-dose chemoradiotherapy. Br J Cancer 2005;92(7):1221–1225.

Nigro ND, Vaitkevicius VK, Considine B Jr., et al. Combined therapy for cancer of the anal canal: A preliminary report. Dis Colon Rectum 1974;17(3):354–356.

UK National Guidance for IMRT for Anal cancer. http://analimrtguidance.co.uk/National-Guidance-IMRT-Anal-Cancer-V4-Dec16.pdf

28

Prostate

Indications for Radiotherapy

Prostate cancer is now the most common cancer in men, accounting for 26 per cent of all new male cancer diagnoses, and it is the second most common cause of cancer-related death in men. The incidence of prostate cancer is projected to rise by 12 per cent in the UK between 2014 and 2035 and one in eight men will be diagnosed with prostate cancer during their lifetime. In 2014, there were 46,690 new cases and 11,287 deaths from prostate cancer that year in the UK. However, 84 per cent of men survive prostate cancer for ten or more years, most dying with their prostate cancer rather than from it. Management must balance the potential toxicity of active treatment with the chances of benefit in a disease with a long natural history.

Advances in diagnosis and screening policies with the use of PSA have led to a stage migration so that prostate cancer is now detected at earlier stages with better prognostic features.

The most common type of prostate cancer is adenocarcinoma (95 per cent). Tumours are graded using the Gleason scoring system, which evaluates architectural details of individual cancer glands and describes five distinct growth patterns, from Gleason 1 (well differentiated) to Gleason 5 (poorly differentiated). The pathologist then sums the pattern number of the primary and secondary grades to obtain the final Gleason score. Gleason scores of 2–5 are no longer used, and certain patterns that Gleason defined as a score of 6 are now graded as 7, meaning that contemporary Gleason 6 cancers have a better prognosis than historic cases. A new grade grouping has now been adopted by the 2016 WHO classification. The five-year biochemical recurrence-free progression probability following radical treatment for localised prostate cancer for the grade groups 1–5 are 96 per cent, 88 per cent, 63 per cent, 48 per cent and 26 per cent.

Prostate cancer is staged using the AJCC and TNM staging. Localised prostate cancer is stratified by T stage, GS and PSA into five prognostic groups (Table 28.1).

Patients with very high risk for locally advanced prostate cancer may have involvement of regional lymph nodes below the bifurcation of the common iliac arteries stage N1. Lymph nodes involved beyond this are staged as metastatic M1a nonregional lymph nodes. Bone metastases are staged as M1b, and other metastatic sites as M1c.

There are other rarer types of prostate carcinoma, such as ductal, intralobular acinar, small cell and clear cell. This chapter focuses on the treatment of the common adenocarcinoma. There is less evidence to guide treatment of other pathological subtypes.

Patients are offered appropriate treatment options by a multidisciplinary team, according to stage of disease, prognostic risk group and estimated survival, taking into account performance status and comorbidity.

Curative Radiotherapy

External Beam Radiotherapy (EBRT), interstitial brachytherapy and surgery are options for the curative treatment of localised prostate cancer, with equivalent outcomes but different side effects.

The options for treatment by risk group prostate cancer are listed in Table 28.1. Factors that influence the choice include performance status, other medical illnesses, likelihood of progression to symptomatic disease, life expectancy, morbidity of treatment (particularly on sexual function) and patient preference.

Watchful waiting is an option for all risk groups where other medical factors are a higher risk to the patient's mortality than their prostate cancer. Watchful waiting involves monitoring until symptoms develop or are imminent (e.g. PSA >100) when the patient then starts palliative androgen deprivation hormone therapy (ADT).

DOI: 10.1201/9781315171562-28

TABLE 28.1

Patient Risk Groups and Treatment Options

Risk Group	Clinical/Pathological Features			Treatment Options
Very Low	All of: T1c, G3+3, PSA <10 ng/mL, <3 biopsy cores positive, ≤50% cancer in each core, PSA density <0.15 ng/mL/g			Active surveillance is strongly recommended
Low	All of: T1/T2a, G3+3, PSA <10 ng/mL, but does not qualify for very low risk			Active surveillance recommended to avoid overtreatment LDR brachytherapy monotherapy Radical EBRT +/– 6 months ADT Radical prostatectomy
Intermediate	All of: No high risk group features No very high risk group features One or more intermediate risk factors (IRF):	Favourable Intermediate	Has all of the following: 1 IRF Gleason 3+3 or G3+4 <50% biopsy cores positive	LDR brachytherapy monotherapy Radical hypofractionated EBRT + 6 months ADT (+/– WPRT) Radical prostatectomy
	T2b/T2c G3+4 or G4+3 PSA 10–20 ng/mL	Unfavourable Intermediate	Has one or more of the following: 2 or 3 IRFs Gleason 4+3 ≥50% biopsy cores positive	LDR or HDR brachytherapy in combination with EBRT (+/– 6–12 months ADT, +/– WPRT) Radical hypofractionated EBRT + 6 months ADT (+/– WPRT) Radical prostatectomy
High	Has no very high-risk features and has at least one high risk feature: T3a G8–10 PSA >20 ng/mL			LDR or HDR brachytherapy in combination with EBRT with 1–3 years ADT (+/– WPRT) Radical EBRT with 2–3 years ADT (+/-WPRT) Radical prostatectomy (in [a]select patients) counseled on likely need for salvage radiotherapy
Very High	Has at least one of the following: T3b–T4 Primary Gleason pattern 5 2 or 3 high-risk features >4 cores with G8–10			Neoadjuvant ADT (+/– upfront Docetaxel or Abiraterone[b]): LDR or HDR brachytherapy in combination EBRT with 2–3 years or long-term ADT (+/– WPRT) Radical EBRT with 2–3 years or long-term ADT (+/-WPRT)

Abbreviations: ADT = Androgen deprivation hormone therapy; WPRT = whole pelvis radiotherapy.
Notes:
[a] Select patients younger, healthier, without tumour fixation to the pelvic side wall and counseled on the likely need for postoperative EBRT.
[b] Upfront Docetaxel or Abiraterone have been shown in men with high risk and very high risk non-metastatic prostate cancer to reduce treatment failure, but have not been shown to improve survival.

Hypofractionated radiotherapy has been shown to be noninferior to conventional fractionated radiotherapy and is now recommended for patients with low- and intermediate-risk prostate cancer. Extreme hypofractionation is now possible using SBRT techniques and it is an option for patients with low- to intermediate-risk prostate cancer, ideally within clinical trials.

Higher doses of radiotherapy, with dose-escalated EBRT or with brachytherapy as a boost to EBRT have been shown to improve long-term biochemical failure free survival. New imaging and treatment techniques have been shown to reduce the risks of toxicity. Patients are encouraged to join randomised clinical trials to help further improve outcomes and the quality of life for patients with prostate cancer.

In general, patients should have a life expectancy of greater than ten years before radical treatment is recommended. Men younger than 75 with other major illnesses such as ischaemic heart disease and diabetes may not live ten years and men over 75 with no other illnesses may live into their nineties. There is evidence that radical radiotherapy in fit men over 75 is very well tolerated and just as effective. It is the role of the multidisciplinary team to identify patients who will benefit from radical treatment and counsel the patient on the different options available. Radical treatments with surgery, EBRT or brachytherapy have similar outcomes, and the patient should be informed of the different side effects of each treatment. Factors that influence the final choice for an individual patient include lower urinary tract symptoms, sexual function, likelihood of infertility, and risks of anaesthesia and surgery. Contraindications to EBRT include prior pelvic irradiation, active inflammatory bowel disease and urinary obstruction. The benefits and risks of surgery, EBRT and brachytherapy are shown in Table 28.2.

TABLE 28.2

Benefits and Risks of Radical Treatment Options for Localised Disease

Treatment	Advantages	Disadvantages
EBRT	Curative	Daily treatment for 4 to 8 weeks
	No operation	Combined with hormone therapy
	No anaesthetic	Early side effects:
	No inpatient stay	Frequency, urgency, cystitis
	Carry on usual activities during treatment	Proctitis and diarrhoea
	PSA monitoring to detect recurrence (PSA more difficult to interpret than after surgery)	Fatigue
		Late side effects:
		Change in bowel habit
		Rectal bleeding
		Haematuria/frequency/urgency
		Erectile dysfunction
		Infertility
		Second malignancy
Brachytherapy (+/-EBRT)	Curative	Needs anaesthetic
	Brachytherapy day case	Early side effects:
	EBRT outpatient	Urine retention
	No hormone therapy in selected cases	Local discomfort
	PSA monitoring to detect recurrence (can take 2 years for PSA to fall)	Frequency, urgency, cystitis
		Proctitis and diarrhoea
		Fatigue
		Late side effects:
		Change in bowel habit
		Rectal bleeding
		Haematuria/frequency/urgency
		Urethral stricture
		Erectile dysfunction
		Infertility
		Second malignancy
Surgery	Curative	Risks of major surgery
	Also treats BPH and symptoms	3–7 days inpatient
	Pathological assessment of whole prostate	6 weeks recovery
	PSA falls quickly following surgery allowing monitoring	May leave cells that have breached the capsule
		Early side effects:
		Incontinence of urine
		Surgical risks of bleeding, infection, thrombo-embolism
		Mortality 0.16–0.66%
		Late side effects:
		Incontinence
		Erectile dysfunction
		Urethral stricture
		Infertility
Active Surveillance	Avoid unnecessary treatment	"Worry" while closely monitored
	No side effects	Treatment may be needed at later date
		Only an option for cancers with a low risk of progression

The results of radiotherapy are assessed by monitoring the PSA, DRE and symptoms and signs of metastases. A PSA nadir of <2 within two years is associated with long-term control. Biochemical failure is defined by a rise in PSA by 2.0 ng/mL above the nadir level following radiotherapy, according to the international RTOG-ASTRO Phoenix consensus. Published nomograms are very useful for assessing potential benefits from treatment.

Pelvic Lymph Node Radiotherapy

Selected patients with a risk of lymph node involvement between 15 and 35 per cent (LN risk = (2/3 PSA + [(GS-6) × 10] may benefit from radiotherapy to the pelvic lymph nodes in addition to the prostate and seminal vesicles. In prospective studies of the role of ADT in addition to EBRT, the majority of studies treated the pelvic lymph nodes. There are two randomised studies evaluating the role of treating the pelvic lymph nodes, one of which showed no benefit and one of which showed an improvement in progression free survival at four years, which was subsequently no longer significant at longer follow-up. There may be an interaction between the timing of ADT and the side of the radiation field used, with a trend towards improved PFS with neoadjuvant ADT and pelvic nodal radiotherapy.

The role of EBRT in patients with involved pelvic lymph nodes is also not clearly defined. The Stampede has shown in patients with N1M0 stage prostate cancer at trial entry who were treated in the control arm had an improvement in two-year failure free survival. Modern imaging such as multiparametric MRI and PSMA PET CT scanning can now pick up lymph node involvement in intermediate- and high-risk prostate cancer, which can be used to guide treatment and pelvic lymph node radiotherapy.

The possible benefits need to be balanced with the increased toxicity associated with treating the pelvic lymph nodes. Modern techniques, including IMRT and IGRT, reduce the risk of toxicity.

The pelvic lymph nodes are treated concomitantly with conventional fractionation and hypofractionation protocols. Clinical trials of treating pelvic lymph nodes with ultra-hypofractionated radiotherapy with 5 fractions are being carried out.

Adjuvant and Salvage Radiotherapy

Adjuvant radiotherapy is not given routinely when PSA levels are undetectable after surgery to avoid overtreatment of the majority of patients already cured. In patients who have an initial undetectable PSA and then subsequently develop biochemical recurrence (three rises in PSA with final level <0.1 ng/mL or two rises in PSA with final level >0.1 ng/mL) salvage prostate bed radiotherapy is recommended. If the PSA is persistently raised following surgery, it may indicate local or metastatic disease. If staging scans are negative and the PSA is <5.0 ng/mL salvage prostate bed radiotherapy can be considered. The margin status following radical prostatectomy does not correlate with the outcomes from salvage radiotherapy. Results are better with early salvage radiotherapy when the PSA is <0.2, and the results are poor when the PSA is >1.2 ng/mL.

Clinical trials of adjuvant radiotherapy may be appropriate for patients with high risk factors for local recurrence but undetectable PSA.

The role of pelvic radiotherapy in addition to prostate bed radiotherapy has not been fully investigated and the possible benefits need to be balanced with the risk of increased toxicity and discussed with the patient. The recent SPPORT RTOG 0534 randomised controlled trial has shown an improvement in five-year freedom from progression with the addition of pelvic radiotherapy to short-term ADT and prostate bed salvage radiotherapy.

Palliative Radiotherapy

Prostate and Pelvis

The Stampede trial has shown that radiotherapy to the prostate in addition to ADT and Docetaxel or Abiraterone in patients with newly diagnosed metastatic prostate cancer improved overall survival in selected patients with a low metastatic burden. A high metastatic burden is defined as four or more bone metastases with one or more outside the vertebral bodies or pelvis, or visceral metastases. All other patients have low metastatic burden. Radiotherapy to the prostate is planned in the same way as described later in the chapter for radical radiotherapy to the prostate.

Patients with extensive local disease in the prostate and pelvis may benefit from a course of palliative EBRT to relieve symptoms. Bleeding from the prostate may also be alleviated by EBRT.

Bone and Lymph Node Metastases

EBRT is an excellent treatment for palliation of pain from symptomatic bone metastasis. A single fraction of 8 Gy is very effective with few side effects. A fractionated course of EBRT may be used to treat spinal cord compression, and is given postoperatively following orthopaedic fixation of pathological fractures. Symptoms from lymph node and visceral metastases can also be relieved by EBRT. Solitary metastases or up to three small metastases may benefit from treatment with SBRT.

Breast Buds

Gynaecomastia is a major problem for patients on long-term antiandrogen and oestrogen therapy. Superficial X-ray or electron therapy (9–12 MeV) to the breast bud area using a 7–9-cm diameter circular field has been shown to reduce the incidence significantly when used prophylactically. In established cases, radiotherapy can reduce symptoms. The alternative is medical treatment with Tamoxifen.

Sequencing of Multimodality Therapy

EBRT and Hormone Therapy

Hormone therapy before, during and after EBRT (neoadjuvant, concurrent and adjuvant androgen deprivation [NCAD]) has been proven to increase local control, disease-free survival and overall survival for selected patients with prostate cancer. Androgen deprivation reduces the size of the prostate by 30 per cent and the number of tumour cells, possibly through synergistic apoptotic mechanisms.

Six months NCAD can be used with EBRT for low- and intermediate-risk disease to reduce the target volume and allow safer dose escalation. ADT is started at least two months before radiotherapy. Two to three years NCAD deprivation is beneficial for high-risk disease. There is evidence that starting radiotherapy after six months neoadjuvant hormone therapy may lead to improved results in patients with high-risk disease. In patients receiving a brachytherapy boost with EBRT 12 months NCAD is recommended in patients with high-risk disease.

Standard androgen deprivation is achieved with bicalutamide 50 mg once daily for three weeks starting one week before the first LH-releasing hormone agonist (LHRHa) injection. The LHRHa is continued either monthly or three monthly.

Two years of hormone therapy has been shown in two large RCT to improve overall survival when combined with salvage prostate bed radiotherapy.

EBRT and Brachytherapy

HDR and LDR brachytherapy may be used as a boost to EBRT to escalate dose to the prostate. It may be given prior to or after EBRT, depending on local protocols.

EBRT and Chemotherapy

Six cycles of Docetaxel or 24 months of Abiraterone have been shown in men with high risk, very high risk and stage N1 non-metastatic prostate cancer to reduce treatment failure, and is given with the neoadjuvant hormone prior to radiotherapy in high-risk cases.

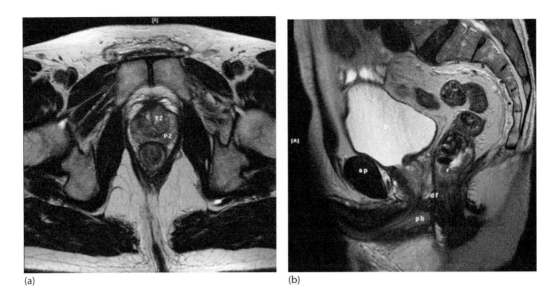

FIGURE 28.1 Anatomy of prostate shown on T2-weighted MRI. (a) Axial (TZ transitional zone, PZ peripheral zone). (b) Sagittal (pb, penile bulb; b, bladder; sp, symphysis pubis; r, rectum; df, Denonvilliers' fascia).

Clinical and Radiological Anatomy

The prostate gland lies between the pubic symphysis and the anterior rectal wall, and is closely applied to the bladder neck and seminal vesicles (Figure 28.1). The lymphatics drain from the prostate to the obturator, presacral, internal, external, common iliac and para-aortic lymph nodes (Figure 28.2).

Assessment of Primary Disease

Prostate cancer is confirmed by multiple biopsies, preferably by the transperineal route using a perineal template and image guidance to target dominant intra-prostatic lesions.

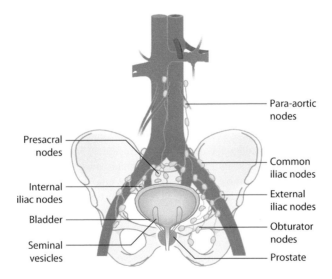

FIGURE 28.2 Lymphatic drainage of the prostate.

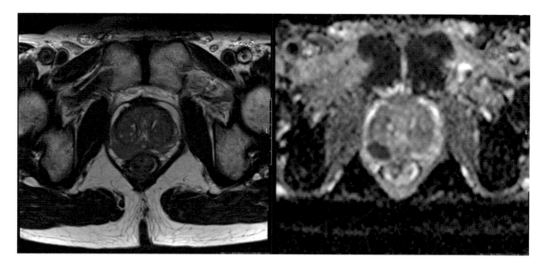

FIGURE 28.3   T2 and ADC MRI showing T3 prostate cancer with extraprostatic extension in right peripheral sector.

The extent of primary disease is assessed by multi-parametric MRI of the prostate and pelvis to detect locoregional and distant spread. Further staging with CT, bone scan and Choline or PSMA PET CT scans should be considered in high-risk cases. Prostate cancer can extend through the prostate capsule, especially posteriorly, at the apex, and at the junctions between the base and bladder neck and seminal vesicles. Denovilliers' fascia reduces spread towards the rectum. Extraprostatic extension is shown on MRI in Figure 28.3. Spread occurs to the seminal vesicles and lymph nodes with increasing tumour stage and histological grade. The risk of microscopic seminal vesicle and lymph node involvement can be assessed by nomograms or the Roach formula, which is based on the Partin data.

Roach Formula

- Percentage risk of seminal vesicle involvement = PSA + [(GS - 6) × 10]
- Percentage risk of LN involvement = 2/3 PSA + [(GS - 6) × 10]

Data Acquisition

Immobilisation

A planning CT scan is obtained in the treatment position. Patients are treated supine rather than prone as this has been shown to produce less prostate motion, reduce doses to normal organs at risk and is more comfortable for the patient.

A bladder filling protocol should be used to maintain a constant bladder filling – 'comfortably full'. Patients are asked to empty the bladder and drink 200 mL of water 20 to 40 minutes before the scan and before treatment each day. Bladder scanning during treatment can give helpful feedback to the patient and identify a personalised comfortable volume for the patient. A completely full bladder has been shown to displace small bowel away from the treated volume, but it also leads to greater variation in prostate position and is not recommended. The rectum should be empty for treatment, as a full rectum also leads to greater variation in prostate position. Patients should be advised on a low residue diet, and if they have a full rectum at the time of planning CT scan should receive further dietary advice before repeating the scan and some patients may require daily micro enemas.

An immobilisation system using a head pad combined with individually adjustable knee and ankle supports provides a high degree of accuracy without the need for further pelvic immobilisation (Figure 28.4).

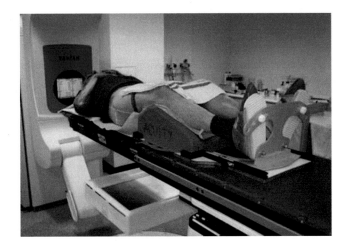

FIGURE 28.4   Immobilisation for treatment of prostate cancer.

Spacer Devices

Biodegradable substances (polyethylene glycol hydrogel, hyaluronic acid and human collagen) can be inserted into the space between the rectum and prostate to temporarily increase the distance between them to reduce the amount of radiation delivered to the rectum. An RCT of a hydrogel spacer has shown the spacer is safe and reduces the rectal dose, reduces toxicity and improves patient quality of life. NICE have recommended that the evidence supports the use of biodegradable spacer devices. The spacer is inserted trans-perineally under general anaesthetic two weeks prior to radiotherapy planning. At the time of the spacer insertion, fiducial markers can also be inserted into the prostate. Some spacers are not visible on CT and an MRI scan at the time of planning is needed to co-register with the planning CT for target volume and normal organ definition.

CT Scanning

With the patient immobilised in the treatment position following bladder and rectal preparation protocols, a radiotherapy planning CT scan is performed. Skin reference tattoos are placed anteriorly on the midline of the symphysis pubis and laterally over the hips and aligned with lasers to prevent lateral rotation. Radio-opaque markers are placed on the skin to locate the tattoos on the CT scans. The CT scan is taken with 3–5 mm slices from the mid sacroiliac joint to 1 cm below the anus/ischium to include the prostate, seminal vesicles, rectum and bladder, and is extended superiorly to L3 if the pelvic lymph nodes are to be treated. No oral or rectal contrast is used, but intravenous contrast is used to aid delineation of the pelvic lymph nodes. At the time of the planning CT scan, the size of the rectum and bladder should be assessed. If the bladder is empty or the rectum is >4 cm in AP diameter at the level of the prostate base, the scan should be repeated after implementing the bladder and rectal protocols until the desired parameters are met. Inappropriately large rectal volumes have been shown to reduce local control rates.

   CT data are then transferred to a radiotherapy planning computer for outlining and target volume definition. To improve target definition, MRI scans of the pelvis and PET CT scan images can be fused with CT and incorporated into radiotherapy planning protocols. Outlining studies have shown that the size of the prostate is overestimated on CT compared with MRI, which defines the apex of the prostate better and is associated with less image degradation with fiducial markers. Solutions to overcome the geometrical distortion and shift artefact seen with MRI are currently being investigated. CT-MRI image registration (Figure 28.5) is useful for defining the contour of the prostate, especially at the apex and for identifying hydrogel spacers.

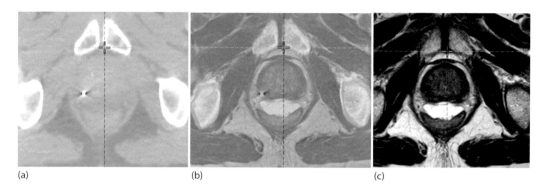

(a)   (b)   (c)

FIGURE 28.5 Co-registration of CT and MR images for target volume definition; (a) planning CT, (b) fused CT and MRI, (c) MRI T2.

Tumour and OAR Motion

Immobilisation, drinking and rectal emptying protocols as just described are used to position the patient accurately each day for treatment and to minimise the differences in bladder and rectum size and shape. Fiducial marker studies have shown significant inter-fraction prostate motion with average displacements of 6 mm in the posterior and inferior directions, and >30 per cent of patients have a displacement of >10 mm posteriorly, which standard planning margins would not encompass. Studies have also shown intra-fraction motion of the prostate of >2 mm over a treatment time of five to seven minutes, most frequently in the anterior posterior and superior inferior directions. There can also be rotational displacements, which can be difficult to correct for. Online correction using fiducial markers and daily soft tissue imaging improves the accuracy of treatment and reduces toxicity without any compromise of treatment outcomes.

Target Volume Definition

Prostate +/− Seminal Vesicles +/− Pelvic Nodes

It is standard practice to define a CTV that includes the whole prostate and any possible extracapsular extension, with either the base (proximal 1 cm), or the entire seminal vesicles. The risk of involvement of the seminal vesicles is defined using the Roach formula and target volume chosen accordingly.

- T1c or T2a/b and PSA +[(GS -6) × 10] <15 per cent risk of SV involvement CTV to include prostate + base of seminal vesicles
- T2c or T3a or (PSA + [(GS -6) × 10]) >15 per cent risk of SV involvement CTV to include prostate and seminal vesicles

Prostate outlining starts on the mid gland slice along the fat plane between the prostate and pelvic floor muscles and along Denovilliers' fascia posteriorly. Defining the apex can be difficult, and this can be aided with reference to diagnostic MR scans or by image registration as discussed earlier. The base of the seminal vesicles is included in the CTV for all patients. This is defined as 1 cm of central seminal vesicles proximal to the base of the prostate, often at the same level as the middle lobe that bulges into the bladder. Portions of the seminal vesicles visible on axial slices that also contain prostate can be counted within the proximal 1 cm. When the entire seminal vesicles are to be included in the CTV, the distal ends may have to be excluded if the seminal vesicles wrap around the prostate, to keep the rectal dose within safe limits. Studies have shown that only 7 per cent of patients have SV involvement beyond 1.0 cm, and 1 per cent beyond 2.0 cm. The whole SV can be defined as the proximal 2 cm using isotropic expansion of the prostate contour to exclude the distal tips.

The PTV is defined with a 3D margin around the CTV to include an internal margin accounting for physiological variations in the shape, position and size of the prostate, and a set-up margin to compensate for uncertainties in patient position and set-up during planning and treatment. The set-up margins can be measured with verification studies and quality assurance programmes. The CTV to PTV margins are grown isotropically around the CTV. To limit the dose to the rectum, the posterior margin is reduced if verification studies allow, and is reduced further for a phase 2 volume when needed, to keep within rectal dose constraints. If the rectal volume cannot be reduced to 4 cm in diameter at the base of the prostate, the margins from CTV to PTV may need to be increased posteriorly. Image guidance techniques discussed later will allow further safe reduction of these margins.

The pelvic lymph nodes should be outlined following the RTOG consensus guidelines and pelvic lymph node atlas. Examples are shown in Figure 28.6. In current protocols, the vessels are outlined from the L5/S1 vertebral interspace and proceed inferiorly. More recent consensus guidelines recommend commence the superior contours at the bifurcation of the aorta into the common iliac arteries or the proximal inferior vena cava to the common iliac veins whichever occurs more superiorly (typically at the level of L4-L5). The external iliac vessels are outlined until the top of the femoral head is reached, and at this point the vessel contour moves inside the bony pelvis to the obturator lymph nodes and stops 1 cm superior to the pubic symphysis. The vessel contours are expanded by a 7-mm margin in the lateral and anterior-posterior directions. The volume is then edited to add the presacral lymph node area, and to connect the internal and

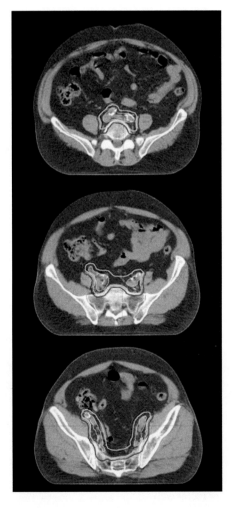

FIGURE 28.6 CTV and PTV for pelvic node irradiation shown on three level axial CT scans (blood vessels = yellow).

external iliac vessel volumes. A bowel avoidance volume (obtained by adding a 3-mm isotropic margin to the total bowel outline) may be used to reduce the bowel and planning target volume overlap.

The following are suggested CTV doses and PTV margins for planning treatment when using fiducial markers and daily imaging and online correction with soft tissue matching. The margins can be modified to individualise treatment and meet the organ at risk constraints if needed.

Hypofractionated Radiotherapy (60 Gy in 20 Fractions)

- CTVn_47 = Pelvic lymph nodes
- PTVn_47 = CTVn_47 = 5-mm uniform margin
- CTVpsv_47 = Prostate + SV (base only if SV risk <15%)
- PTVpsv_47 = CTVpsv_ 47 + 6 mm sup/inf/right/left/ant/post
- CTVp_60 = Prostate (+base SV if SV risk >15%, + any suspected SV involvement on MRI)
- PTVp_60 = CTVp 60 + 3 mm sup/inf/right/left/ant/post

Conventional Fractionated Radiotherapy (78 Gy in 39 Fractions)

- CTVn_55.8 = Pelvic lymph nodes
- PTVn_55.8 = CTVn_55.8 + 5-mm uniform margin
- CTVpsv_67 = Prostate + SV
- PTVpsv_67 = CTV 56 + 6 mm uniform margin
- CTVp_78 = Prostate + extracapsular extension + base of SV + involved SV if T3b
- PTVp_78 = CTV 78 + 3 mm sup/inf/right/left/ant/post

Ultra-Hypofractionated Radiotherapy (42.7 Gy in 7 Fractions)

- CTV_42.7 = Prostate only
- PTV_42.7 = CTV_42.7 + 6 mm sup/inf/right/left/ant and 4 mm post

SABR (36.25 Gy in 5 Fractions)

- CTV_36.25 = Prostate (+ base of SV if SV risk >15%)
- PTV_36.25 = CTV 36.25 + 4–5 mm sup/inf/right/left/ant and 3–5 mm post

Prostate Bed

After prostatectomy there is no GTV. The CTV is the prostate bed as best defined on the CT planning scan. The histopathology report of the prostatectomy specimen and preoperative MRI can be helpful. The CTV is based on an estimation of the location of the prostate preoperatively and is centred on the vesico-urethral junction. Surgical clips within the prostate bed are included in the CTV, but those in the anatomical position of vessels are not. The preoperative location of the seminal vesicles is included if pathologically involved or the risk of seminal vesicle involvement according to the Roach formula is >15 per cent.

The following guidance defines the prostate bed when contouring and gives a typical field size of between 8 and 12 cm.

- Inferior border = 5 mm cranial to superior border of the penile bulb
- Anterior border = posterior aspect of symphysis pubis (<2 cm above the vesico-urethral anastomosis). Posterior 1/3 of bladder wall (>2 cm above anastomosis)
- Posterior border = anterior rectal wall
- Lateral border = medial border of obturator internus and levator ani muscles

- Superior border = base of SV if uninvolved and risk <15 per cent. Distal ends of SV if involved or risk >15 per cent
  - CTV_52.8 = Pelvic lymph nodes
  - PTV_52.8 = CTV 52.8 + 5 mm uniform margin
  - CTV_66 = Prostate bed
  - PTV_66 = CTV 66 with 10 mm ant/post/right/left/sup/inf and 5–8 mm posterior

Organs at Risk (OAR)

The OAR are the rectum, bladder, nerves of the prostatic plexus lying adjacent to the penile bulb, small bowel and femoral heads. The rectum is outlined from the inferior level of the ischial tuberosities and at least 1 cm below the PTV to the recto-sigmoid junction above the PTV to give a length of approximately 12 cm. The small bowel, large bowel and sigmoid colon are contoured from 2 cm above the PTV down to the recto sigmoid junction. An isotropic margin of 3 mm can be added to create a PRV as an avoidance structure. Consideration of small bowel in the target volume is important when pelvic nodes are treated.

Dose Solutions

Complex

In the past, prostate cancer was treated with sequential two or three phase treatments. This has now been replaced by simultaneous integrated boost IMRT, VMAT or tomotherapy delivering simultaneously different dose levels in a single treatment session. These modern planning techniques ensure better coverage of the target volumes, sparing of the OAR, safer dose escalation, shorter treatment times and less monitor units. IMRT has significant advantages when irradiating the pelvic lymph nodes with the ability to conform to the nodes and spare normal bowel in the pelvis (Figure 28.7).

The dose is prescribed to the PTV and should meet the constraints shown in Table 28.3.

The dose to OAR is assessed by DVHs. Plans are reviewed to minimise hot-spots in OAR. The acceptable dose constraints for OAR are shown in Table 28.4. If the PTV overlaps with the OAR try to minimise the dose in the overlap region while maintaining PTV coverage.

Ultra-hypofractionated radiotherapy to the prostate is a new development. It has been shown to be noninferior to conventionally fractionated radiotherapy with more early toxicity but similar late toxicity in the HYPO-RT-PC phase 3 RCT. This study used 42.7 Gy in 7 fractions, three days per week over

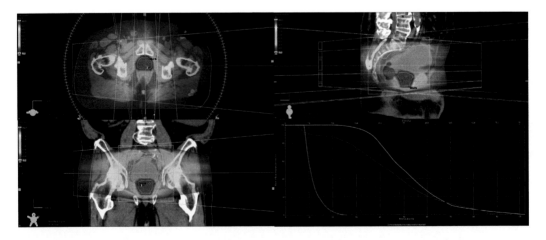

FIGURE 28.7 IMRT VMAT plan for prostate and pelvic nodes 78 Gy in 39 fractions (rectum = brown, bladder = yellow, penile bulb = dotted yellow, spacer = orange).

TABLE 28.3

Prostate Dose Constraints

Criteria	Dose-Volume Constraint	78 Gy/39f	60 Gy/20f
Minimum D98%, PTV	≥95% prescription dose	≥74.1 Gy	≥57 Gy
Median D50%, PTV	99% to 101% of prescriptions dose	77.2–78.78 GY	59.4–60.6 Gy
Maximum D2%, PTV	<105% prescription dose	81.9 GY	63 Gy

TABLE 28.4A

OAR Prostate

OAR	Prescription Dose		Optimum	Mandatory
	2 Gy/#	3 Gy/#	Max Vol % or cc	Max Vol % or cc
Bladder	V50 Gy	V40 Gy	<50%	-
	V60 Gy	V48 Gy	<25%	<50%
	V78 Gy	V56.8	<5%	-
		V60 Gy	<3%	<35%
Femoral Heads	V50 Gy	V40 Gy	<5%	<50%
Bowel	V45 Gy	V36 Gy	<78 cc	<158 cc
(Sigmoid, Large	V50 Gy	V40 Gy	<17 cc	<110 cc
& Small Bowel)	V55 Gy	V44 Gy	<14 cc	<28 cc
	V60 Gy	V48 Gy	<0.5 cc	<6 cc
	V65 Gy	V52 Gy	0 cc	<0 cc
Penile Bulb	V50Gy	V40 Gy	<50%	-
	V60 Gy	V48 Gy	<10%	-
Rectum	V30 Gy	V24 Gy	<70%	<80%
	V40 Gy	V32 Gy	<51%	<65%
	V50 Gy	V40 Gy	<38%	<50%
	V60 Gy	V48 Gy	<27%	<35%
	V70 Gy	V54 Gy	<15%	<20%
	V75 Gy	V57 Gy	<10%	<15%
	V78 Gy	V60Gy	<0.01%[a]	<3%
Rectum D$_{mean}$	≤45 Gy	≤35 Gy		

Note:

[a] The <0.01 constraint is a very small volume and care should be taken to ensure that this optimum constraint is achieved without compromising the PTV coverage.

TABLE 28.4B

OAR Prostate Bed

OAR	Prescription Dose	Optimum	Mandatory
	2 Gy/#	Max Vol % or cc	Max Vol % or cc
Rectum	30 Gy	<80%	<80%
	40 Gy	<65%	<65%
	50 GY	<50%	<60%
	60 GY	<35%	<50%
	66 GY	<30%[a]	<30%
Bladder	50 GY	<50%	<80%
	60 GY	<25%	<50%
Femoral heads	50 Gy	<5%	<25%
Penile Bulb	50 Gy	<50%	
	60 Gy	<10%	
Bowel	50 GY	<17 cc	110 cc

Note:

[a] As low as possible without compromise of PTV coverage.

TABLE 28.4C

OAR Prostate +/– Nodes with Brachytherapy Boost

OAR	Prescription Dose	Optimum	Mandatory
	2 Gy/#	Max Vol % or cc	Max Vol % or cc
Rectum	18 Gy	<80%	<80%
	24 Gy	<65%	<70%
	30 Gy	<38%	<50%
	35 Gy	<27%	<35%
	41 Gy	<15%	<20%
	46 Gy	<0.01%[a]	<3%
Bladder	30 Gy	<50%	<80%
	36 Gy	<25%	<50%
Femoral Heads	30 Gy	<5%	<25%
Penile Bulb	30 Gy	<50%	
	36 Gy	<10%	
Bowel	30 Gy	<17 cc	110 cc

Note:

[a] The <0.01 constraint is a very small volume and care should be taken to ensure that this optimum constraint is achieved without compromising the PTV coverage.

two and a half weeks and no hormone therapy. The CTV was defined as the prostate only. CTV to PTV margin was 6 mm (4 mm towards the rectum). Radiotherapy was planned and delivered with IMRT or VMAT with the use of fiducial markers. The OAR dose constraints used were rectum V38.4 Gy <15 per cent, V32 Gy <35 per cent and V28 Gy <45 per cent, bladder V41.4 Gy <5, V34.7 Gy <25 per cent, V29.9 Gy <50 per cent.

SABR

SABR differs significantly from conventional fractionation delivering much larger doses per fraction and real time IGRT. It is prescribed to the 60–80 per cent isodose, creating a steep internal dose gradient and can be planned for a homogenous or heterogenous dose distribution. The heterogenous dose distributions resemble those delivered by HDR brachytherapy. The prescription dose of 36.25 Gy in 5 fractions to the PTV should cover at least 95 per cent of the PTV and should be 65–85 per cent of D_{max}. A secondary dose of 40 Gy is delivered to the CTV. The recommended OAR constraints include rectum V36 Gy <1 cc, bladder V37 Gy <10 cc, urethra V47 Gy <20 per cent, penile bulb V29.5 Gy <50 per cent and, where visualised, the neurovascular bundle V38 Gy <50 per cent.

Simple or Conformal

Palliative treatment to the prostate may be given very simply using opposing anterior and posterior beams and MLC shielding, planned by CT virtual simulation. Or it may be planned conformally with an anterior and two wedged oblique beams with optimised weighting and wedging (Figure 28.8). In some cases, palliative radiotherapy is planned and delivered using IMRT, VMAT or tomotherapy with the advantages of sparing the OAR and reducing toxicity.

Dose Fractionation

Curative Radiotherapy

- Hypofractionated: 60 Gy in 20 fractions (+/– pelvic nodes) over four weeks
- Conventional: 78 Gy in 39 fractions (+/– pelvic nodes) over eight weeks

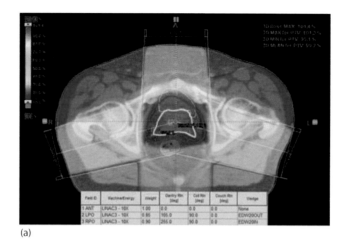

(a)

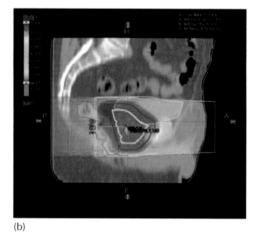

(b)

FIGURE 28.8 (a) Axial and (b) sagittal dose distributions of conformal treatment for prostate cancer (bladder = yellow, rectum = brown).

- Ultra-hypofractionated: 42.7 Gy in 7 fractions over two and a half weeks
- SBRT: 36.25 Gy in 5 fractions over five days
- Prostate bed: 66 Gy in 33 fractions given in six and a half weeks

Palliative Radiotherapy

- Prostate: low metastatic burden:
  - 55 Gy in 20 fractions or 60 GY in 20 fractions over four weeks
  - 36 Gy in 6 fractions weekly over six weeks
- High metastatic burden:
  - 30 Gy in 10 fractions given in two weeks
  - 36 Gy in six weekly fractions of 6 Gy given in six weeks
- Bone: 8 Gy single fraction
  - 20 Gy in 5 fractions in one week
- Other Metastases: 20 Gy in 5 fractions given in one week
  - 30 Gy in 10 fractions given in two weeks

Breast Bud Radiotherapy

- Prophylaxis: 8 Gy single fraction
- Palliation: 12 Gy in 2 fractions given in two days

Treatment Delivery and Patient Care

The patient is treated supine with a comfortably full bladder and after rectal voiding. Immobilisation systems are used with anterior and lateral laser lights to align midline and lateral skin tattoos to prevent lateral rotation. The isocentre is marked with reference to the anterior tattoo over the pubic symphysis. All patients treated with IMRT should be treated with IGRT protocols (see Verification section below).

Severe skin reactions are rare but may occur over the sacrum and natal cleft. If loose stools develop, a low residue diet is advised to prevent diarrhoea. Loperamide hydrochloride may be used for diarrhoea, with care to avoid constipation. Mild proctitis and tenesmus are common and, if severe, may be treated with steroid or local anaesthetic suppositories. Urinary symptoms of frequency, urgency and slow stream are common. Patients should remain well hydrated and a mid-stream urine should be examined to exclude infection. Patients with preexisting obstructive problems may be helped by α-blockers such as Tamsulosin. Cystitis may be helped by potassium citrate, cranberry juice or simple analgesia.

After radiotherapy, the incidence of grade 3 chronic intestinal sequelae requiring hospitalisation for diagnosis and/or minimal intervention is very low with modern radiotherapy. Most cases occur within three to four years of treatment. A gastroenterologist should investigate rectal bleeding, diarrhoea, urgency and tenesmus. Rectal biopsies are best avoided unless completely necessary. Rectal bleeding can be managed expectantly or Argon plasma coagulation (APC), a non-contact thermal coagulation technique, applied endoscopically, can be used for severe cases.

Verification

Electronic portal images are taken for the first three to five days of treatment to document the photon fields and compared with DRRs from the planning CT scan. All patients treated with IMRT, VMAT or tomotherapy should have daily image guidance prior to the delivery of radiotherapy. The transponder systems and autobeam hold can provide intra-fraction IGRT. Patients treated with SBRT also require IGRT that can correct for intra-fraction motion.

Various IGRT solutions are available:

- Implanted fiducial markers with KV imaging
- Implanted fiducial markers with KV imaging and Auto Beam Hold
- Ultrasound
- Cone Beam CT (KV or MV)
- Tomotherapy
- Transponder systems (e.g. Calypso)

Prostate Brachytherapy

Prostate brachytherapy may be used as monotherapy or as a boost to EBRT (see Table 28.1).

Randomised trials have shown that both LDR and HDR brachytherapy as a boost to external beam radiotherapy (EBRT) improves biochemical free survival compared to conventional hormone EBRT alone.

Selection criteria for brachytherapy:

- Life expectancy >10 years
- Biopsy-confirmed adenocarcinoma prostate

- Prostate volume 50 mL (dynamic techniques can treat up to 90 mL)
- IPSS score <12
- Urine flow Q max >15mL/s

It is important to select patients with no significant urinary outflow obstruction since they are at increased risk of urinary retention and morbidity following brachytherapy.

LDR Permanent Seed Brachytherapy

The most frequently used isotope is iodine-125. An alternative is palladium-103, which has a higher dose rate. The technique is most commonly carried out as a single stage procedure with intra operative planning under general or spinal anaesthesia. A transrectal ultrasound (TRUS) probe is inserted into the rectum attached to a stepping unit that can advance or retract the probe (Figure 28.9). Attached to the TRUS is a template, the coordinates of which are transposed onto the ultrasound images of the prostate. Needles are inserted into the prostate at 1 cm intervals with a peripheral:central ratio of 3:1. The needle position is registered on the planning software. Serial ultrasound sections with 5-mm slices of the prostate from the base to the apex are captured onto the planning computer. The prostate, urethra (identified with the aid of aerosolised jelly) and rectum are outlined on the ultrasound images. A margin of 2–3 mm is added in all directions except posteriorly to form the PTV. The computer generates a plan within 30 seconds. Advanced dynamic dose calculation can capture seed position in real time continuously updating dosimetry as seeds are inserted. Seeds can be inserted using a stranded or loose seed technique. Any deviations from the plan can be corrected in real time before the end of the procedure.

Current standard reporting of dose is based on dosimetry from a CT scan performed four weeks after seed implantation when oedema has settled. Doses to the prostate, rectum and urethra are calculated. The V100 is the percentage of the prostate volume that has received the 100 per cent prescription dose and should be >90 per cent. The D90 is the dose received by 90 per cent of the prostate volume and should be at least 90 per cent of the prescribed dose. The prostate V150 and V200 give a measure of the homogeneity

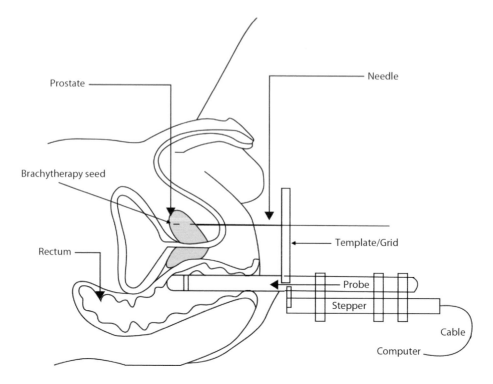

FIGURE 28.9   Technique for insertion of radioactive seeds into the prostate. (Courtesy of prostate cancer charity.)

of the dose distribution. The maximum rectal dose should be kept as low as possible. If it is less than 140 per cent of the treatment dose, the risk of proctitis is less than 1.2 per cent. The maximum urethral dose should be kept as low as possible, and should be less than 150 per cent of the treatment dose.

Using the same technique, LDR brachytherapy can be used for a boost treatment combined with EBRT to the prostate and pelvis. A randomised trial has shown this to be superior to standard 78 Gy/39f EBRT with patients twice as likely to be free of biochemical relapse at six and a half years, but at the expense of higher genitourinary morbidity. Modern brachytherapy techniques and better patient selection are important to reduce the toxicity of this treatment approach.

HDR Afterloading Brachytherapy

HDR afterloading brachytherapy is performed under general anaesthesia using a stepping iridium-192 HDR machine. In contrast to LDR permanent seed implants, there is no calculated pre- or post-implant dosimetry, and dosimetry is defined by catheter position and dwell times. Large fraction sizes can be delivered, which may have a biological advantage in prostate cancer. A randomised trial has shown that HDR brachytherapy as a boost to EBRT is superior to standard EBRT 55 GY/20f with a 31 per cent reduction in the risk of recurrence at four years. The technique reduces radiation exposure to the oncologist and other staff. Trials of monotherapy are underway. Afterloading catheters are inserted into the prostate through the perineum under TRUS guidance using a template that is sutured or fixed with adhesive to the patient. A CT scan is performed of the patient with the catheters in place and the dosimetry calculated on a 3D planning system. MRI scans can also be done and fused with the planning CT scan. Several high dose fractions are then delivered in the HDR afterloading room and the patient remains an inpatient with an indwelling urinary catheter until the end of treatment. HDR monotherapy is performed in exactly the same way but recent UK data shows suboptimal outcomes for single dose HDR in intermediate risk prostate cancer.

Dose Fractionation

Monotherapy

- LDR: 145 Gy (I-125), 125 Gy (Pa-103)
- HDR: 2×13 Gy, 3×10.5 Gy

Combination Therapy

- **LDR** LDR Brachytherapy boost 115 Gy (I-125)
- EBRT: Prostate +/- pelvis 46 Gy in 23 fractions of 2 Gy over four and a half weeks
- HDR EBRT: Prostate only: 35.75 Gy in 13 daily fractions over two and a half weeks
- Prostate + pelvis: 45 Gy in 25 daily fractions over five weeks
- HDR Brachytherapy: 2×8.5 Gy or 1×15 Gy

Key Trials

Bolla M, Collette L, Blank L, et al. Long-term results with immediate androgen suppression and external irradiation in patients with locally advanced prostate cancer (an EORTC study): A phase III randomised trial. Lancet 2002;360:103–106.

Bolla M, van Poppel H, Collette L, et al. Postoperative radiotherapy after radical prostatectomy: A randomised controlled trial (EORTC trial 22911). Lancet 2005;366:572–578.

Bruner DW, Moughan J, Prestidge BR, et al. Patient reported outcomes of NRG oncology/RTOG 0232: A phase III study comparing combined external beam radiation and transperineal interstitial permanent brachytherapy with brachytherapy alone in intermediate risk prostate cancer. Int J Radiat Oncol Biol Phys 2018 Nov 1;102(3) S2–S3.

D'Amico AV, Manola J, Loffredo M, et al. 6-month androgen suppression plus radiation therapy vs. radiation therapy alone for patients with clinically localised prostate cancer: A randomised controlled trial. JAMA 2004;292:821–827.

Dearnaley D, Syndikus I, Mossop H, et al. Conventional versus hypofractionated high-dose intensity-modulated radiotherapy for prostate cancer: 5-year outcomes of the randomised, non-inferiority, phase 3 CHHiP trial. Lancet Oncol 2016 Aug;17(8):1047–1060.

Dearnaley D, Griffin CL, Lewis R, et al. Toxicity and patient-reported outcomes of a phase 2 randomized trial of prostate and pelvic lymph node versus prostate only radiotherapy in advanced localised prostate cancer (PIVOTAL). Int J Radiat Oncol Biol Phys 2019 Mar 1;103(3):605–617.

Hamstra DA, Mariados N, Sylvester J, et al. Continued benefit to rectal separation for prostate radiation therapy: Final results of a phase III trial. Int J Radiat Oncol Biol Phys 2017 Apr 1;97(5):976–985.

Horwitz EM, Bae K, Hanks GE, et al. Ten-year follow-up of radiation therapy oncology group protocol 92–02: A phase III trial of the duration of elective androgen deprivation in locally advanced prostate cancer. J Clin Oncol 2008;26:2497–2504.

Hoskin PJ, Rojas AM, Bownes PJ, et al. Randomised trial of external beam radiotherapy alone or combined with high-dose-rate brachytherapy boost for localised prostate cancer. Radiother Oncol 2012 May;103(2):217–222.

James ND, Spears MR, Clarke NW, et al. Failure-free survival and radiotherapy in patients with newly diagnosed nonmetastatic prostate cancer: Data from patients in the control arm of the STAMPEDE trial. JAMA Oncol 2016 Mar;2(3):348–357.

King CR, et al. Stereotactic body radiotherapy for localized prostate cancer: Pooled analysis from a multi-institutional consortium of prospective phase II trials. Radiother Oncol 2013 Nov;109(2):217–221.

Lawton CA, DeSilvio M, Roach M 3rd, et al. An update of the phase III trial comparing whole pelvic to prostate only radiotherapy and neoadjuvant to adjuvant total androgen suppression: Updated analysis of RTOG 94–13, with emphasis on unexpected hormone/radiation interactions. Int J Radiat Oncol Biol Phys 2007;69:646–655.

Morris WJ, Tyldesley S, Rodda S, et al. Androgen suppression combined with elective nodal and dose escalated radiationtherapy (the ASCENDE-RT trial): An analysis of survival endpoints for a randomized trial comparing a low-dose-rate brachytherapy boost to a dose-escalated external beam boost for high- and intermediate-risk prostate cancer. Int J Radiat Oncol Biol Phys 2017 Jun 1;98(2):275–285.

Murray J, Griffin C, Gulliford S, et al. A randomised assessment of image guided radiotherapy within a phase 3 trial of conventional or hypofractionated high dose intensity modulated radiotherapy for prostate cancer. Radiother Oncol 2020;142:62–71. doi: 10.1016/j.radonc.2019.10.017

Parker CC, James ND, Brawley CD, et al. Radiotherapy to the primary tumour for newly diagnosed, metastatic prostate cancer (STAMPEDE): A randomised controlled phase 3 trial. Lancet 2018 Dec 1;392(10162):2353–2366.

Pollack A, et al. The addition of androgen deprivation therapy and pelvic lymph node treatment to prostate bed salvage radiotherapy (NRG Oncology/RTOG 0534 SPPORT): An international, multicentre, randomised phase 3 trial. The Lancet 2022 May 14;399(10338):1886–1901.

Pollack A, Zagars GK, Starkschall G, et al. Prostate cancer radiation dose response: Results of the MD anderson phase III randomised trial. Int J Radiat Oncol Biol Phys 2002;53:1097–1105.

Prestidge BR, Winter K, Sanda MG, et al. Initial report of NRG oncology/RTOG 0232: A phase 3 study comparing combined external beam radiation and transperineal interstitial permanent brachytherapy with brachytherapy alone for selected patients with intermediate-risk prostatic carcinoma. Int J Radiat Oncol Biol Phys 2016 Oct 1;96(2) Supplement page S4.

Widmark A, Gunnlaugsson A, Beckman L, et al. Ultra-hypofractionated versus conventionally fractionated radiotherapy for prostate cancer: 5-year outcomes of the HYPO-RT-PC randomised, non-inferiority, phase 3 trial. Lancet 2019 Aug 3;394(10196):385–395.

Wilkins A, Naismith O, Brand D, Fernandez K, Hall E, Dearnaley D, Gulliford S; CHHiP Trial Management Group. Derivation of dose/volume constraints for the anorectum from clinician and patient-reported outcomes in the CHHiP trial of radiotherapy fractionation. Int J Radiat Oncol Biol Phys 2020 Apr 1;106(5):928–938.

INFORMATION SOURCES

Chen RC, Clark JA, Talcott JA, et al. Individualizing quality-of-life outcomes reporting: How localized prostate cancer treatments affect patients with different levels of baseline urinary, bowel, and sexual function. J Clin Oncol 2009 Aug 20;27(24):3916–3922.

Epstein JI, Zelefsky MJ, Sjoberg DD, et al. A contemporary prostate cancer grading system: A validated alternative to the Gleason score. Eur Urol 2016 Mar;69(3):428–435.

Harris VA, Staffurth J, Naismith O, et al. Consensus guidelines and contouring atlas for pelvic node delineation in prostate and pelvic node intensity modulated radiation therapy. Int J Radiat Oncol Biol Phys 2015 Jul 15;92(4):874–883.

Hall WA, Paulson E, Davis BJ, et al. NRG oncology updated international consensus atlas on pelvic lymph node volumes for intact and postoperative prostate cancer. Int J Radiat Oncol Biol Phys 2021 Jan 1;109(1):174–185.

Jackson ASN, Sohaiby SA, Staffurth JN, et al. Distribution of lymph nodes in men with prostatic adenocarcinoma and lymphadenopathy at presentation: A retrospective radiological review and implications for prostate and pelvis radiotherapy. Clin Oncol 2006;18:109–116.

Kishan AU, Cook RR, Ciezki JP, et al. Radical prostatectomy, external beam radiotherapy, or external beam radiotherapy with brachytherapy boost and disease progression and mortality in patients with Gleason score 9–10 prostate cancer. JAMA 2018 Mar 6;319(9):896–905.

Memorial Sloan Kettering Prostate Cancer Nomogram. www.mskcc.org

O'Neill AG, Jain S, Hounsell AR, O'Sullivan JM. Fiducial marker guided prostate radiotherapy: A review. Br J Radiol 2016 Dec;89(1068):20160296.

Roach M 3rd, Hanks G, Thames H Jr, et al. Defining biochemical failure following radiotherapy with or without hormonal therapy in men with clinically localised prostate cancer: Recommendations of the RTOG-ASTRO Phoenix consensus conference. Int J Radiat Oncol Biol Phys 2006;65:965–974.

29

Bladder

Indications for Radiotherapy

In the UK there are approximately 10,000 new cases of bladder cancer a year, and 5000 deaths. Only 50 per cent of patients survive longer than ten years following a diagnosis of bladder cancer. Approximately 49 per cent of bladder cancers are preventable, the majority of these being smoking related.

Non-muscle invasive 'superficial' tumours account for 75 per cent of cases. Their behaviour depends on their grade, size, multifocality and whether they are confined to the mucosal layer or have invaded the lamina propria. Carcinoma in situ lies at the aggressive end of the spectrum. Post resection, five-year recurrence rates for non-muscle invasive bladder cancer (NMIBC) range from 30–80 per cent, with progression to muscle invasive disease ranging from 1–45 per cent. Intravesical therapies with mitomycin and/or BCG are used to reduce the rates of recurrence and progression respectively. Radical cystectomy and urinary diversion is the definitive management for recurrent high risk NMIBC, refractory to intravesical therapy. Radical radiotherapy has not been found to have efficacy in this setting.

The overall survival for muscle invasive bladder cancer (MIBC) is poor, with less than 50 per cent of patients surviving five years. Ninety per cent of these high-grade tumours are transitional cell (urothelial) carcinomas; the remaining histological types are squamous cell carcinoma (5 per cent), small cell carcinoma, adenocarcinoma, sarcoma, carcinosarcoma, lymphoma or melanoma. For operable T2–4 N0–1 transitional cell tumours, the combination of neoadjuvant chemotherapy, radical cystectomy and urinary diversion is considered definitive management. Five-year survival rates range from 30–45 per cent for T2 N0 tumours to 15–30 per cent for T3 N0 tumours. In selected patients, keen to preserve their bladder, multimodality nonsurgical treatment based on radical radiotherapy can result in comparable survival rates – although approximately 15 per cent of patients subsequently require a cystectomy due to local recurrence or development of a new bladder primary tumour.

More than 50 per cent of patients with MIBC either present with metastatic disease or subsequently develop metastatic disease. Palliative treatment options include best supportive care, palliative radiotherapy, palliative systemic therapy and palliative surgery (e.g. cystectomy for persistent significant haematuria, orthopaedic fixation of fractures). Multi-agent cytotoxic regimens have been used to treat metastatic bladder cancer since the 1980s. Cisplatin-based regimens are the standard of care, and studies have been aimed at increasing the efficacy of combination therapy (by increasing dose density) whilst reducing the toxicity (with supportive medication and alterations in the dosing of accompanying non-platinum cytotoxic agents). Second-line agents with modest activity include paclitaxel and vinflunine. There is a growing interest in the use of immunotherapy to treat metastatic transitional cell carcinoma. Pembrolizumab (a humanised antibody targeting PD-1) has demonstrated efficacy in the second-line setting post platinum-containing chemotherapy, and studies are underway across all clinical settings (including NMIBC) to determine the future role of immunotherapy.

Curative Radiotherapy

Radiotherapy is an effective treatment modality for bladder cancer. The aim for patients treated with curative radical radiotherapy is to achieve local tumour control whilst preserving normal bladder function and minimising the toxicity to neighbouring structures. Patients with T2–4b N0–3 M0 tumours may be considered for radical treatment. Active inflammatory bowel disease, bowel adhesions, poor bladder function, bilateral hip

DOI: 10.1201/9781315171562-29

prostheses, previous pelvic radiotherapy, preexisting hydronephrosis, multifocal disease, large volume tumours (>7 cm maximum diameter), tumour within a diverticulum, the presence of non-adjacent CIS and nontransitional cell carcinoma histology (unless small cell carcinoma) all favour surgery as the treatment of choice.

Palliative Radiotherapy

Palliative radiotherapy is an effective treatment as high dose palliation for locally advanced tumours to prevent the development of uncontrolled pelvic disease. It is also is useful for the relief of symptoms such as haematuria and pain in patients with incurable bladder cancer. It can also treat symptoms due to nodal, bone and lung metastases. In patients with poor performance status, multiple unstable comorbidities, hypofractionated radiotherapy may be considered for T2/3 tumours for local control. The intention is to prevent the development of pain and bleeding due to local tumour progression.

Sequencing of Multimodality Radical Therapy

A TURBT is performed initially to obtain the histological diagnosis of MIBC. In patients who may be considered for a bladder preservation strategy, a maximal resection of the macroscopic tumour should be performed. This may require a repeat TURBT.

Neoadjuvant chemotherapy should be considered for all suitable patients with muscle-invasive bladder cancer prior to radical local therapy (surgery or radiotherapy). This is based on an 11 trial meta-analysis which demonstrated a 5 per cent absolute improvement in overall survival at five years for platinum-based combination therapy. Most patients in this meta-analysis received three cycles of neoadjuvant chemotherapy (range two to four cycles). Patients should have good performance status (PS0–1; PS2 in selected cases), adequate renal function, no hydronephrosis, no persistent frank haematuria and transitional cell histology. For patients with impaired renal function, a 'split dose' cisplatin regimen should be considered rather than using carboplatin. Caution is required if considering neoadjuvant chemotherapy for patients with transitional cell carcinoma with extensive variant histology (e.g. micropapillary, squamous, sarcomatoid) due to a lack of evidence for the efficacy of chemotherapy in these histological subtypes. Biomarkers for transitional cell carcinoma chemosensitivity (ATM, RB1, FANCC, ERCC2) and chemoresistance (p53-like) are being investigated to determine whether they can reliably predict which patients will benefit from neoadjuvant chemotherapy.

Definitive local therapy involves a radical cystectomy and urinary diversion, or radical radiotherapy with radiosensitisation. Radical cystectomy involves the en bloc removal of the pelvic organs anterior to the rectum; bladder, urachus, prostate, and seminal vesicles in men; bladder, urachus, ovaries, fallopian tubes, uterus, cervix, and vaginal cuff in women. In addition, the pelvic lymph nodes groups are removed, at a minimum to the level of the iliac bifurcation. Urinary diversion can be continent or incontinent. Incontinent diversion classically involves an ileal conduit, with urine collecting in a urostomy bag attached to the anterior abdominal wall. However, alternative continent urinary diversions are possible in highly motivated patients keen to avoid an ileal conduit. These include an orthotopic neo-bladder, a Mitroffanoff continent urinary diversion and a Mainz-II urinary diversion. New surgical techniques, including robot-assisted radical cystectomy, have been shown to reduce intraoperative blood loss and wound-related complications with equivalent oncological outcomes. Currently, it remains to be seen whether the reduction in postoperative length of stay and complication rates make this technique cost-effective.

Adjuvant chemotherapy (post cystectomy) has less supporting evidence than it's neoadjuvant counterpart. Potential advantages include basing treatment decisions on a complete assessment of pathological risk factors, and that it doesn't delay definitive local therapy in patients subsequently found to have chemoresistant disease. However, it does delay the treatment of micrometastatic disease, and patients may not be well enough to receive chemotherapy post cystectomy within an effective therapeutic window (three months post cystectomy). A meta-analysis from 2005 suggested a 25 per cent survival advantage for patients with pathological T3, T4 or lymph node involvement, but concluded the study was insufficiently powered to make treatment recommendations. A subsequent analysis, including three further trials, but only published in abstract form, detected a similar survival advantage for four cycles of platinum-based chemotherapy.

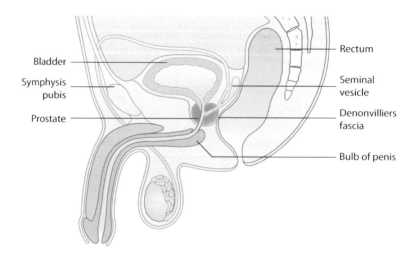

FIGURE 29.1   Sagittal section through pelvic to show prostate and bladder anatomy.

Adjuvant chemotherapy should not be viewed as an equivalent alternative to neoadjuvant chemotherapy. However, it remains an option for select patients who did not receive neoadjuvant chemotherapy (e.g. due to significant haematuria) but are found to have locally advanced disease on post-op histology.

Clinical and Radiological Anatomy

The bladder occupies the anterior portion of the pelvic cavity just superior and posterior to the pubic bone (Figure 29.1). The base of the bladder is posterior and separated from the rectum by the vas deferens, seminal vesicles and ureters in men, and by the uterus and vagina in females. As the bladder distends the neck remains fixed and the superior part rises into the pelvic cavity. The bladder mucosa is lined with transitional epithelium and appears smooth when full and has numerous folds when empty.

Assessment of Primary Disease

Bladder cancer is staged using the AJCC TNM staging system. Tumours originate in the epithelium lining the bladder, and progress by invading through the muscle layers into perivesical fat and adjacent pelvic organs. Lymphatic spread is to paravesical, obturator, internal iliac, external iliac, pre-sciatic, presacral and common iliac nodes, then to para-aortic nodes and beyond. Haematogenous spread most commonly occurs to bone, liver and lung.

   Bladder cancer can present with haematuria, urinary frequency, urinary urgency, as an incidental finding on imaging, or with symptoms from metastatic/locally advanced disease. Initial outpatient assessment includes sending urine for cytological analysis and performing a flexible cystoscopy to visualise the inside of the bladder wall. If an abnormality is seen, a definitive diagnosis requires a rigid cystoscopy, biopsy (transurethral resection of bladder tumour: TURBT) and bimanual pelvic examination under general anaesthetic. It is important that the TURBT specimen includes muscle from the bladder wall to determine if this has been invaded. A bladder map is drawn at the time to document the findings.

   When a bladder cancer is found, a CT-IVU or USS of the urinary tract is performed to screen the remaining urothelium for tumours, and to rule out hydronephrosis. With muscle-invasive bladder tumours, a CT scan is required to stage the chest and abdomen, and either a CT or MRI can be used to stage the pelvis. If the tumour appears to be muscle-invasive at the time of flexible cystoscopy, it is preferable to perform the pelvic staging before the TURBT as invasion through the bladder wall is difficult to assess post-resection. FDG-PET-CT can be used to help resolve staging uncertainty (e.g. equivocal lymph nodes).

Data Acquisition

Patients should be scanned with an empty bladder. They should be advised not to drink fluids during the 30 minutes prior to the planning CT scan, and to void immediately before the scan is performed. Patients with difficulty voiding require re-assessment by the clinical team to determine whether urinary catheterisation is required for the planning CT scan and throughout treatment. Patients should also be encouraged to open their bowels prior to the planning CT scan, to minimise rectal distension from flatus and faeces.

Patient positioning should be the same for the planning CT scan as for treatment. They should lie supine, with their arms folded across their chest away from the radiotherapy fields. Immobilisation techniques should include a knee-and-ankle support system, and a head-rest, fixed onto a flat-top couch. A free-breathing CT scan is performed, using at least 2.5 cm slices, from the top of the iliac crests to 2 cm below the ischial tuberosities. A skin tattoo is placed over the pubic symphysis and two additional lateral tattoos are placed over the iliac crests to prevent lateral rotation. The locations of the tattoos are marked on the planning scan using radio opaque markers. IV contrast should be considered if treating the pelvic lymph nodes.

Target Volume Definition

The bladder GTV is the primary bladder tumour, which may be difficult to define on CT alone. Voluming should be performed with reference to the bladder map from cystoscopy. MRI, fiducial markers or lipiodol injections may also be used to guide GTV definition.

The standard approach is to define the bladder CTV as the whole bladder, including the primary tumour. Any extravesical spread should be encompassed with a 5-mm margin. In patients with tumours located at the bladder base, or with distant CIS, the proximal urethra should also be included: 15 mm in men, 10 mm in women (see Figure 29.2).

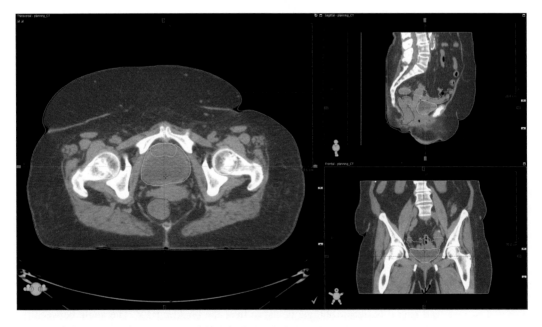

FIGURE 29.2 CT orthogonal views showing GTV, CTV and OAR outlines.

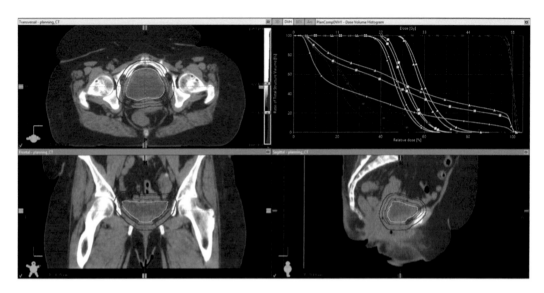

FIGURE 29.3   CT orthogonal views showing adaptive radiotherapy PTVs.

For patients with pelvic lymph node involvement, the nodal CTV encompasses the obturator, external iliac, internal iliac, pre-sciatic, presacral and lower common iliac lymph nodes. It can be formed by voluming the pelvic blood vessels with a 7-mm margin, excluding bone and muscle. The superior limit is usually at the level of the L5/S1 intervertebral space.

The bladder PTV has traditionally been the bladder CTV with a 15-mm margin in all directions. Studies have shown that the largest variation in bladder outline occurs due to bladder volume changes in the superior-inferior and anterior-posterior directions, which has led some centres to adopt nonuniform expansion margins.

As experience with image guidance techniques grows, particularly pretreatment verification CT imaging (cone-beam CT, MV CT imaging), adaptive radiotherapy has become feasible for bladder cancer. Variable CTV-PTV margins are applied to the bladder CTV to create 'small', 'medium' and 'large' PTVs (see Figure 29.3). Daily online pretreatment imaging is used to determine which plan to use, based on the smallest PTV that encompasses the bladder volume that day with a small margin (e.g. 5 mm). The aim is to reduce the total radiotherapy dose to surrounding normal tissue (reducing toxicity) while minimising the risk of a geographical miss. This approach is currently being assessed in the Cancer Research UK RAIDER Study (CRUK/14/016).

The organs at risk are the femoral heads, rectum and bowel. Each femoral head is volumed to the inferior extent of its curvature, excluding the femoral neck. The full circumference of the rectum is outlined, from the recto-sigmoid junction (the level where the bowel turns anteriorly – best seen on sagittal views) to the lowest level of the ischial tuberosities. This should result in a length of 10–12 cm. The small and large bowel should be volumed as a single structure ('other bowel'), the superior extent of the volume being 2 cm above the superior border of the PTV.

Dose Solutions

Conformal

Traditional 3D conformal radiotherapy (3D CRT) planning techniques generated a three-field plan (anterior and two wedged lateral/posterior oblique fields) to treat the bladder PTV. The angle between the posterior oblique fields was usually 110°, to spare the rectum. MLCs were used to minimise the dose to normal tissue, with high energy photons (10–15 MV) depending on patient size.

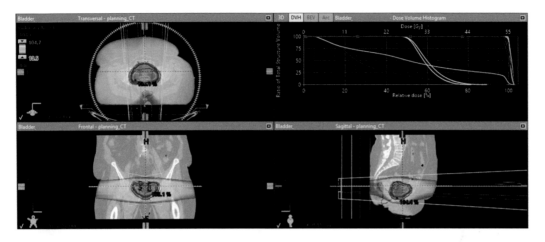

FIGURE 29.4 IMRT plan and DVH constraints.

Complex

With the increasing availability of tomotherapy or volumetric modulated arc therapy (VMAT) IMRT, and the speed of modern planning systems, radical bladder radiotherapy now frequently employs these techniques (see Figure 29.4). They are also the preferred option for pelvic nodal irradiation. IMRT produces better conformity indices compared to 3D CRT, reducing the dose to normal tissues. VMAT uses shorter treatment times and less monitor units to deliver an equivalent dose.

For an IMRT plan, the dose is prescribed to the PTV, which should be encompassed by the 95 per cent isodose. The optimal PTV dose constraints are shown in Table 29.1.

The dose delivered to the femoral heads, rectum and other bowel (small and large bowel volumes combined) should be kept as low as possible. The optimal and mandatory OAR dose constraints are shown in Table 29.2.

TABLE 29.1

Optimal PTV Dose Constraints

PTV Dose Constraint	Terminology	Optimal
Dose covering 98% of the PTV	$D_{98\%}$	$\geq$ 95% prescription dose
Dose covering 50% of the PTV	$D_{50\%}$	+/- 1% prescription dose
Dose covering 2% of the PTV	$D_{2\%}$	< 105% prescription dose

TABLE 29.2

Radical Bladder Cancer Radiotherapy OAR Dose Constraints

Organ at Risk	Dose Constraint (Gy)		Max Vol % or cc	
	64 Gy 32#	55 Gy 20#	Optimal	Mandatory
Rectum	V30	V28	50%	80%
	V50	V43.2	20%	60%
	V60	V52	15%	50%
	V65	V56	5%	30%
Femoral Heads	V50	V43.2	<50%	
Other Bowel (Large and Small Bowel)	V30	V28	149 cc	178 cc
	V45	V39.8	116 cc	139 cc
	V50	V43.2	104 cc	127 cc
	V55	V48	91 cc	115 cc
	V60	V52	73 cc	98 cc
	V65	V56	23 cc	40 cc

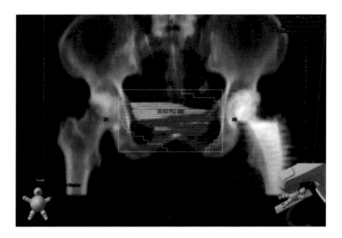

FIGURE 29.5   Virtual CT simulation of a palliative bladder field.

When planning palliative bladder radiotherapy, the patient preparation, immobilisation, set-up, and CT acquisition are the same as for radical treatment. A range of planning techniques are available, ranging from virtual simulation (with or without voluming the bladder CTV to guide field and MLC placement) to 3D-CRT planning (see Figure 29.5). The choice of schedule and planning technique depend on whether the treatment is required to start urgently, and whether the patient is likely to experience reduced toxicity with attempts to minimise the dose delivered to adjacent normal tissue.

A common hypofractionated regimen, that results in good local control, is 36 Gy in 6 fractions over six weeks. It is also an option for patients with localised disease who are not fit for radical radiotherapy. Radiobiologically, it is very close to a radical dose when it comes to tumour kill, and should be delivered with a 3D-CRT plan to minimise side effects. Centres may even employ VMAT techniques if their familiarity with this planning approach makes generation of the plan quicker than a 3D-CRT plan. The OAR dose constraints are outlined in Table 29.3.

Dose Fractionation

Curative Radiotherapy

- PTV_Bladder: 64 Gy in 32 fractions over six and a half weeks
- 55 Gy in 20 fractions over four weeks

TABLE 29.3

Palliative Bladder Cancer Radiotherapy OAR Dose Constraints

	Dose Constraint (Gy)	Max Vol % or cc	
Organ at Risk	**36 Gy 6#**	**Optimal**	**Mandatory**
Rectum	V17	50%	80%
	V28	20%	60%
	V33	15%	50%
	V36	5%	30%
Femoral Heads	V28	<50%	
Other Bowel (Large	V25	139 cc	208 cc
and Small Bowel)	V28	122 cc	183 cc
	V31	105 cc	157 cc
	V33	84 cc	126 cc
	V36	26 cc	39 cc

Palliative Radiotherapy

- PTV_Bladder: 36 Gy in 6 weekly fractions over six weeks
- 21 Gy in 3 alternate day fractions over one week
- 8 Gy in 1 single fraction
- 20 Gy in 5 fractions over one week

Treatment Delivery and Patient Care

All patients receiving radical daily radiotherapy to the bladder alone should be considered for a concomitant radiosensitiser. The three radiosensitisers in common use are outlined here. Note, this is outside their licensed indications.

- At least 10 per cent of bladder tumours contain regions of hypoxia, which predicts for radio-resistance and reduced survival. Breathing carbogen (98 per cent oxygen 2 per cent carbon dioxide) before and during each fraction, in combination with nicotinamide (60 mg/kg) taken two hours beforehand, was found in a phase 3 study to improve three-year overall survival in MIBC by 15 per cent (58 per cent versus 43 per cent). It may be most effective in tumours featuring necrosis but cannot be used in patients taking ACE-inhibitors, or with unstable ischaemic heart disease.
- Another phase 3 study assessed the use of concomitant chemotherapy with Mitomycin C (12 mg/m^2: pre fraction 1) and 5-FU (500 mg/m^2/day continuous infusion: fractions 1–5 and 16–20). This regimen was used with both 20 fraction and 32 fraction radiotherapy regimens. Long-term follow-up demonstrated an improvement in locoregional control rate, and a 6 per cent reduction in two-year salvage cystectomy rate.
- Phase 2 data also supports the use of weekly Gemcitabine with radiotherapy, with 88 per cent achieving a complete endoscopic response with acceptable toxicity.

Patients should give their informed consent undergoing bladder radiotherapy, to ensure they are aware of both the potential acute and late side effects. They should be reviewed during their radiotherapy schedule to assess, record and manage any acute toxicities (see Table 29.4). Radiation cystitis

TABLE 29.4

Acute and Late Side Effects of Bladder Radiotherapy

Organ	Acute Side Effects	Late Side Effects
Bladder	Dysuria	Haematuria
	Frequency	Pain
	Urgency	Frequency
	Incontinence	
Rectum	Mucous discharge	Bleeding
	Flatulence	Flatulence
	Diarrhoea	Mucous Discharge
	Urgency	Urgency
Prostate		Dry Ejaculation
		Urethral Stricture
Vagina		Stenosis
		Dryness
Nerves / Blood Vessels		Impotence
Pelvis		Secondary Malignancy

is common towards the end of a radiotherapy schedule. Infection should be excluded by urine dipstick, and a high fluid intake advised. Catheterisation should be avoided as the resultant change in local anatomy requires replanning, and it also increases the risk of infection. Mild proctitis and lethargy are also common.

Verification

All radical bladder patients should have their daily set-up verified pretreatment using cone beam CT (CBCT) imaging or equivalent. After CBCT acquisition, a bone match is performed by appropriately trained personnel. The region of interest should include the true pelvis, medial edge of femoral heads, sacrum and symphysis pubis. Prior to each treatment fraction, translational errors are corrected, and daily shifts applied. Once bone match is confirmed, the treatment radiographers verify that the bladder lies within the PTV (or selects the appropriate PTV plan if delivering adaptive radiotherapy). If the bladder is too full, the patient is asked to re-void before being re-set-up for treatment. The radiographers also monitor the small bowel within the PTV and will notify the clinical team if a particular bowel loop is consistently within the PTV.

Key Trials

Advanced Bladder Cancer (ABC) Meta-analysis Collaboration. Neoadjuvant chemotherapy in invasive bladder cancer: A systematic review and meta-analysis of individual patient data: Advanced bladder cancer (ABC) meta-analysis collaboration. Eur Urol 2005 Aug;48(2):202–205 (discussion 205–6).

Advanced Bladder Cancer (ABC) Meta-analysis Collaboration. Adjuvant chemotherapy in invasive bladder cancer: A systematic review and meta-analysis of individual patient data: Advanced bladder cancer (ABC) meta-analysis collaboration. Eur Urol 2005 Aug;48(2):189–199 (discussion 199–201).

British Uro-Oncology Group/British Association of Urological Surgeons Section of Oncology/ Action of Bladder Cancer. MDT (Multi-Disciplinary Team) Guidance for Managing Bladder Cancer, 2nd ed, 2013. https://www.baus.org.uk/professionals/baus_business/publications/11/ bladder_cancer_mdt/.

Bellmunt J, de Wit R, Vaughn DJ, et al. Therapy for advanced urothelial carcinoma. NEJM 2017 Mar;376:1015–1026.

Hall E, Hussain SA, Porta N, et al. BC2001 long-term outcomes: A phase III randomized trial of chemoradiotherapy versus radiotherapy (RT) alone and standard RT versus reduced high-dose volume RT in muscle-invasive bladder cancer. JCO 2017 Feb;35(Sup_6):280.

Harland SJ, Kynaston H, Grigor K, et al. A randomized trial of radical radiotherapy for the management of pT1G3 NXM0 transitional cell carcinoma of the bladder. J Urol 2007 Sep;178(3 Pt 1):807–813.

Hoskin PJ, Rojas AM, Bentzen SM, Saunders MI. Radiotherapy with concurrent carbogen and nicotinamide in bladder carcinoma. JCO 2010 Nov;28(33):4912–4918.

James ND, Hussain SA, Hall E, et al. Radiotherapy with or without chemotherapy in muscle-invasive bladder cancer. NEJM 2012 Apr;366:1477–1488.

Tjokrowidjaja A, Lee C, Stockler MR. Does chemotherapy improve survival in muscle-invasive bladder cancer (MIBC)? A systematic review and meta-analysis (MA) of randomised controlled trials (RCT). JCO 2013 May;31(15 Sup):4544.

Von der Maase H, Sengelov L, Roberts JT, et al. Long-term survival results of a randomized trial comparing gemcitabine plus cisplatin, with methotrexate, vinblastine, doxorubicin, plus cisplatin in patients with bladder cancer. JCO 2005 Jul;23(21):4602–4608.

INFORMATION SOURCES

Action Bladder Cancer. www.actionbladdercanceruk.org.

British Uro-oncology Group. https://www.bug.uk.com.

Bladder Cancer WebCafé. www.blcwebcafe.org.

Cancer Research UK. https://www.cancerresearchuk.org/health-professional/cancer-statistics/statistics-by-cancer-type/bladder-cancer.

Choudhury A, Swindell R, Logue JP, et al. Phase II study of conformal hypofractionated radiotherapy with concurrent gemcitabine in muscle-invasive bladder cancer. JCO 2011 Feb;29(6):733–738.

Duchesne GM, Bolger JJ, Griffiths GO, et al. A randomized trial of hypofractionated schedules of palliative radiotherapy in the management of bladder carcinoma: Results of medical research council trial BA09. Int J Radiat Oncol Biol Phys 2000 May 1;47(2):379–388.

Goodfellow H, Viney Z, Hughes P, et al. Role of fluorodeoxyglucose positron emission tomography (FDG-PET) - computed tomography (CT) in the staging of bladder cancer. BJUI 2014;114:389–395.

NCRI trials portfolio. http://csg.ncri.org.uk/portfolio/portfolio-maps/.

Rodel C, Grabenbauer G, Kuhn R, et al. Combined-modality treatment and selective organ preservation in invasive bladder cancer: Long-term results. J Clin Oncol 2002;20:3061–3071.

Sternberg CN, de Mulder P, Schornagel JH, et al. Seven year update of an EORTC phase III trial of high-dose intensity M-VAC chemotherapy and G-CSF versus classic M-VAC in advanced urothelial tract tumours. Eur J Cancer 2006 Jan;42(1):50–54.

30

Testis

Indications for Radiotherapy

Testicular cancer is the most common malignancy in young men, with approximately 2300 cases a year in the UK. More than 90 per cent are germ cell tumours, consisting of seminoma and non-seminomatous germ cell tumours (NSGCTs). NSGCTs are usually a mixture of teratoma, embryonal carcinoma, yolk sac tumour and choriocarcinoma. Other rare testicular tumours include Leydig, Sertoli and granulosa cell tumours. Ninety per cent of patients with testicular germ cell tumour have stage I–IIB disease at presentation. In stage I seminoma, the risk factors for metastatic relapse are tumour size >4 cm and rete testis invasion, whereas in stage I NSGCT it is vascular invasion.

Seminoma

There are three options for the management of stage I seminoma following radical orchidectomy:

- Surveillance
- Single cycle of carboplatin chemotherapy
- Para-aortic nodal radiotherapy (consider 'dog leg' radiotherapy to include the ipsilateral iliac nodes in patients who had previous inguinal/scrotal/pelvic surgery or distortion of the lymphatic pathways)

Surveillance studies have shown that approximately 15–20 per cent of patients with stage I seminoma have occult metastatic disease, mainly in the retroperitoneum and para-aortic nodes. Using the prognostic factors of rete testis involvement and tumour size >4 cm, the relapse rate is 32 per cent in patients with both risk factors, 15 per cent in patients with one risk factor and 12 per cent in those with no risk factors. Adjuvant para-aortic nodal radiotherapy or a single cycle of carboplatin can reduce the risk of relapse to 1–3 per cent. Surveillance involves more intensive follow-ups and restaging investigations and is reliant on patient compliance. It is recommended especially for patients at very low risk of metastatic relapse.

The following trials have influenced clinical practice:

- *MRC TE10:* This trial randomised patients between treatment with para-aortic nodal radiotherapy or a 'dog leg' field with both arms receiving a dose of 30 Gy in 15 fractions. There were no significant differences in disease-free or overall survival.
- *MRC TE18:* This trial randomised patients undergoing para-aortic nodal radiotherapy to receive a dose of 30 Gy in 15 fractions or 20 Gy in 10 fractions. There were no significant differences in relapse-free or overall survival, but acute toxicity, such as lethargy, was less with the lower dose.
- *MRC TE19:* This trial randomised patients to receive one cycle of carboplatin (area under curve 7) or para-aortic nodal radiotherapy, with no significant differences with regard to the rate of recurrence, time to recurrence and survival.

DOI: 10.1201/9781315171562-30

In the UK, adjuvant carboplatin is preferred over para-aortic nodal radiotherapy. Due to concerns over the increased risk of second malignancies, adjuvant radiotherapy is not recommended in patients under the age of 40. The risk of cardiovascular disease beyond 15 years is also increased at least twofold by infradiaphragmatic radiotherapy.

In stage IIA seminoma, radiotherapy offers a high cure rate of 85–90 per cent. The current guidelines recommend radiotherapy to the para-aortic and ipsilateral iliac nodes to a dose of 30 Gy in 15 fractions as a treatment option. In stage IIB seminoma, most patients receive chemotherapy, but current guidelines also consider the option of radiotherapy with a dose of 30 Gy in 15 fractions to the para-aortic and ipsilateral iliac field, and an additional boost of 6 Gy in 3 fractions to the enlarged lymph nodes. The alternative is three cycles of bleomycin, etoposide and cisplatin chemotherapy, especially in the presence of a horseshoe kidney or inflammatory bowel disease. There have been no randomised studies comparing the efficacy of radiotherapy versus chemotherapy in stage IIA/B seminoma.

The incidence of relapse after chemotherapy alone is low and radiotherapy may have a role in patients with small localised relapses. Radiotherapy may also be used palliatively in those with chemoresistant disease.

In the UK, patients with testicular intraepithelial neoplasia (TIN) are managed with close surveillance or orchidectomy. In Europe, radiotherapy to a dose of 16–20 Gy in fractions of 2 Gy is also used in patients with a solitary testis. This approach will result in infertility and an increased long-term risk of Leydig cell insufficiency.

Nonseminomatous Germ Cell Tumours

The management options for stage I NSGCT following radical orchidectomy include surveillance, adjuvant chemotherapy and nerve-sparing retroperitoneal lymph node dissection. Patients with more advanced or relapsed disease are treated with chemotherapy. Radiotherapy may have a palliative role in chemoresistant cases for those with inoperable bulky disease, or cerebral, bone or lymph node metastases.

Sequencing of Multimodality Therapy

If adjuvant chemotherapy or radiotherapy is indicated, it should ideally commence within six to eight weeks after radical orchidectomy.

Clinical and Radiological Anatomy

Regional spread is predominantly lymphatic. From the testis, it follows the testicular arteries to the para-aortic, renal hilar and retro-crural lymph nodes with involvement of the contralateral nodes occurring in 15–20 per cent of cases. The typical 'landing zone' of left-sided tumours is the left renal hilar and para-aortic nodes, while it is the inter-aortocaval nodes for right-sided tumours (Figure 30.1).

The lymphatics from the scrotum drain to the inguinal lymph nodes. This may be distorted by hernia repair, orchidopexy, scrotal surgery or pelvic infection.

Malignant teratomas also have a propensity for early vascular spread to the lungs and liver.

Assessment of Primary Disease

The standard assessment includes a clinical examination of the contralateral testis, lymph node areas (especially the abdomen and supraclavicular nodes) and breasts to exclude gynaecomastia. Routine tests should include tumour markers alpha-fetoprotein, human chorionic gonadotrophin and lactate dehydrogenase, baseline luteinising hormone, follicle-stimulating hormone and testosterone, and CT scan of the chest, abdomen and pelvis with intravenous contrast. MRI is equally sensitive but less commonly used

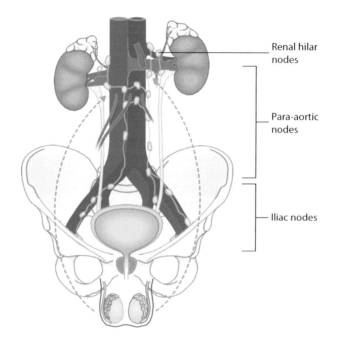

FIGURE 30.1 Lymphatic drainage of the testis.

except for imaging of brain metastases. [18F] 2-fluoro-2-deoxy-D-glucose PET is useful for assessing the significance of residual masses shown on CT following treatment. Patients should be given advice on sperm cryopreservation.

Data Acquisition

A CT scan of the abdomen is acquired with the patient lying supine in the treatment position, using head rest and knee supports. Midline and lateral tattoos are used, together with laser lights, to align the patient and prevent lateral rotation. Patients can also be planned conventionally in a simulator.

Target Volume Definition

CT Scanning

For stage I seminoma, the CTV includes lymph node areas at high risk of microscopic involvement; they are the para-aortic, renal hilar and retro-crural nodes bilaterally. These lymph node regions can be encompassed through a 1.2-cm expansion on the inferior vena cava and a 1.9-cm expansion on the aorta to form the CTV. An isotropic margin of 0.5 cm is then applied around this CTV to create the PTV. If there has been previous scrotal/pelvic surgery, the target volume should also include the ipsilateral pelvic and inguinal lymph nodes and the ipsilateral scrotal sac.

For stage II disease, the GTV is defined by outlining the enlarged (>1 cm in short axis dimension) lymph nodes. The CTV should include the same nodal areas as for stage I plus the ipsilateral iliac nodes (1.2-cm expansion on the ipsilateral common, external and proximal internal iliac veins and arteries) and an isotropic margin of at least 0.8 cm around the GTV. The same 0.5 cm PTV margin is used as per stage I seminoma. Both kidneys must be identified and outlined as critical normal structures, taking care to exclude a horseshoe kidney. Figure 30.2 shows how virtual CT simulation can be used for accurate targeting of the lymph node areas, while shaping the fields to avoid the normal kidneys.

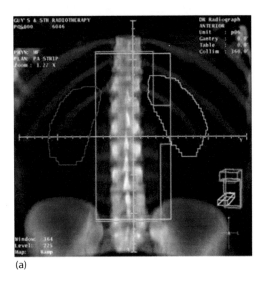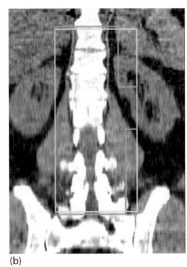

(a) (b)

FIGURE 30.2 Virtual simulation for para-aortic nodal irradiation for seminoma of the left testis. (a) Anterior DRR with the kidneys outlined. (b) Coronal multiplanar reconstruction with MLC shielding of the kidneys.

Conventional Simulation

Conventionally, the target volume for para-aortic nodal radiotherapy as defined by standard field sizes on a simulator is as follows:

- Superior: Upper border of T11
- Inferior: Lower border of L5
- Lateral: To include the transverse processes of vertebrae, approximately 9–11 cm wide

These field margins will ensure inclusion of the para-aortic, renal hilar and retro-crural lymph nodes. The kidneys must be identified at the time of simulation by an IVU, and a horseshoe kidney excluded. As much normal kidney as possible should be excluded from the treatment field using shielding.

In patients where the ipsilateral iliac nodes or the ipsilateral iliac and inguinal nodes are to be treated, a larger 'dog leg' field is defined with shielding added to protect the kidneys, bladder and bowel as shown in Figure 30.3. It is important to ensure adequate inclusion of the lymph nodes lying

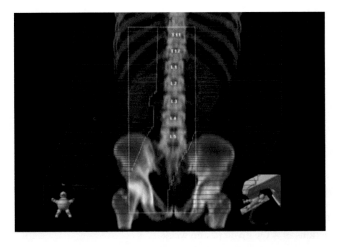

FIGURE 30.3 Virtual simulation for para-aortic, iliac and inguinal 'dog leg' irradiation for seminoma of the right testis.

at the mid-level of the fifth lumbar vertebra between the para-aortic and the pelvic nodes. For the lower part of the 'dog leg' field, the lateral border runs from the tip of the ipsilateral transverse process of L5 to the superolateral border of the ipsilateral acetabulum while the medial border extends from the tip of the contralateral transverse process of L5 to the medial border of the ipsilateral obturator foramen. The inferior border is at the top of the ipsilateral acetabulum. A 2-cm margin is required from gross disease to the edge of the treatment fields. Lead shields 1 cm thick are used to protect the remaining testis from scattered radiation to preserve fertility. Measurements using TLDs have shown that the radiation dose to the testis can be reduced to 0.5–0.7 Gy. If scrotal irradiation is necessary because of previous scrotal surgery, a scrotal field using electron therapy is used to treat the scrotal sac and the lower inguinal nodes on the affected side. This field is matched to a tattoo on the inferior border of the 'dog leg' field at the top of the acetabulum. A lead cut-out is made to shield the penis and remaining testis.

Dose Solutions

CT-based fields with their vessel-based target volumes tend to be wider than traditional simulator-based fields and provide improved dosimetry. In practice, opposing anterior and posterior beams with individual shielding of the renal parenchyma by MLC may provide the best target volume coverage with the lowest integral dose.

The conventional simulator-based technique involves anterior and posterior opposed fields, using Perspex templates to define shielding to critical structures when 'dog leg' fields are used. Calculations of the dose distributions for 'dog leg' fields are made as for other irregular fields.

Dose Fractionation

Seminoma Stage I

- 20 Gy in 10 fractions of 2 Gy given in two weeks

Seminoma Stage IIA

- 30 Gy in 15 fractions of 2 Gy given in three weeks

Seminoma Stage IIB

- Phase I 'dog leg'
- 30 Gy in 15 fractions of 2 Gy given in three weeks
- Phase II boost to gross tumour
- 6 Gy in 3 fractions of 2 Gy given in half a week

TIN

- 20 Gy in 10 fractions of 2 Gy given in two weeks

Palliative Radiotherapy

- 8 Gy as a single fraction
- 20 Gy in 5 fractions of 4 Gy given in one week
- 30 Gy in 10 fractions of 3 Gy given in two weeks

Treatment Delivery and Patient Care

The patient lies supine on the treatment couch and lasers are used to align the anterior and lateral tattoos. In the case of 'dog leg' irradiation, a template is required to place lead shielding, or this is done more commonly now with MLC. Nausea and vomiting are common side effects and they can be reduced with prophylactic antiemetics such as ondansetron. Patients should be offered sperm cryopreservation prior to treatment. They can be reassured that the para-aortic treatment does not result in any significant radiation dose to the testis nor does it impair fertility in the long term. 'Dog leg' fields and scrotal irradiation using testicular shielding, however, do result in some radiation dose to the testis (0.7 Gy and 1.5 Gy respectively) and patients should be counselled accordingly.

Verification

Daily portal imaging or cone beam CT.

Key Trials

Fossa SD, Horwich A, Russell JM, et al. Optimal planning target volume for stage I testicular seminoma: A Medical Research Council randomized trial. J Clin Oncol 1999;17:1146–1154.

Jones WG, Fossa SD, Mead GM, et al. Randomized trial of 30 versus 20Gy in the adjuvant treatment of stage I testicular seminoma: A report on Medical Research Council trial TE18, European Organisation for the Research and Treatment of Cancer trial 30942 (ISRCTN18525328). J Clin Oncol 2005;23:1200–1208.

Oliver RTD, Mason MD, Mead GM, et al. Radiotherapy versus single-dose carboplatin in adjuvant treatment of stage I seminoma: A randomised trial. Lancet 2005;366:293–300.

INFORMATION SOURCES

Albers P, Albrecht W, Algaba F, et al. Guidelines on testicular cancer: 2015 update. Eur Urol 2015;68:1054–1068.

Aparicio J, Maroto P, Garcia del Muro X, et al. Prognostic factors for relapse in stage I seminoma: A new nomogram derived from three consecutive, risk-adapted studies from the Spanish Germ Cell Cancer Group (SGCCG). Ann Oncol 2014;25:2173–2178.

Martin JM, Joon DL, Ng N, et al. Towards individualised radiotherapy for stage I seminoma. Radiother Oncol 2005;76:251–256.

Oldenburg J, Fossa SD, Nuver J, et al. Testicular seminoma and non-seminoma: ESMO clinical practice guidelines for diagnosis, treatment and follow-up. Ann Oncol 2013;24(Suppl 6):vi125–vi132.

Paly JJ, Efstathiou JA, Hedgire SS, et al. Mapping patterns of nodal metastases in seminoma: Rethinking radiotherapy fields. Radiother Oncol 2013;106:64–68.

Warde P, Specht L, Horwich A, et al. Prognostic factors for relapse in stage I seminoma managed by surveillance: A pooled analysis. J Clin Oncol 2002;20:4448–4452.

Wilder RB, Buyyounouski MK, Efstathiou JA, et al. Radiotherapy treatment planning for testicular seminoma. Int J Radiat Oncol Biol Phys 2012;83:e445–e452.

31

Penis

Indications for Radiotherapy

Penis cancer is rare, with approximately 700 new cases per year in the UK, and should be treated in specialised centres. Over 95 per cent of tumours are SCCs. Penile cancer is staged by the AJCC TNM 7 classification (see Table 31.1). This chapter describes the management of SCC of the penis. There are other rare cancers that can involve the penis and tumour histology specific advice should be sought, e.g. Kaposi sarcoma (see Chapter 7).

With advances in reconstructive surgical techniques, all patients who are fit for an operation should be treated with penile preserving surgery. The overall five-year survival is 52 per cent, ranging from 66 per cent to 29 per cent in lymph node negative and positive disease, respectively. The local control rate with radical surgery is >90 per cent. Radiotherapy for the primary tumour is largely used palliatively in advanced inoperable cases.

Palpable mobile inguinal nodes are found in 30–50 per cent of patients at presentation, but half of these are due to infection rather than tumour. If tumour is confirmed by cytology or histology, an ipsilateral modified radical inguinal node dissection is performed with a dynamic sentinel node study on the contralateral side. If no lymph nodes are palpable then a bilateral sentinel node procedure should be done to stratify patients to full lymph node dissection or not. Patients with two or more inguinal nodes or any extracapsular spread in the groin should be considered for an ipsilateral pelvic lymph node dissection.

Curative Radiotherapy

Historically, electron beam radiotherapy and interstitial brachytherapy have been used. Electron beam radiotherapy can be used for very small stage I superficial tumours. Interstitial brachytherapy has been used for selected early stage I and II tumours <4 cm in size, and where there is invasion of the corpora cavernosa <1 cm. With the advances in surgery, radiotherapy to the primary penile tumour is now only used for palliation.

Adjuvant Radiotherapy

Although some guidelines do not support the use of adjuvant radiotherapy, many UK centres offer adjuvant radiotherapy to nodal basins at high risk of local recurrence. Adjuvant nodal radiotherapy can be used to

TABLE 31.1

Adapted from AJCC TNM 7 Staging System for Invasive Penile Cancer

Stage	Characteristics
T1	T1a tumour invades subepithelial connective tissue without LVI, not poorly differentiated
	T1b tumour invades subepithelial connective tissue with LVI or is poorly differentiated
T2	Tumour invades corpus spongiosum with or without urethral invasion
T3	Tumour invades corpus cavernosum with or without urethral invasion
T4	Tumour invades other adjacent structures
pN1	Metastasis in one or two groin nodes (both in the same groin)
pN2	Metastasis in more than two or bilateral groin nodes
pN3	Extracapsular spread in a groin node or any pelvic nodes
pM1	Metastatic spread outside the groin or pelvic nodes

DOI: 10.1201/9781315171562-31

reduce the risk of local recurrence after nodal dissection. Contemporary UK data shows that after adjuvant radiotherapy for N3 disease, five-year overall survival is over 40 per cent, which compares favourably with other series (Ager et al., in preparation). Each nodal basin (left vs right groin and left vs right pelvis) should be considered for radiation on their own individual merits, acknowledging that the nodal spread of penile cancer is stepwise and ipsilateral i.e. if the left groin is negative, there is no need to stage or irradiate the left pelvis.

The indication for irradiating a nodal basin is extracapsular spread or patients with pelvic lymph node positivity. For patients who have had inguinal surgery but are not fit for pelvic surgery, adjuvant radiotherapy can be considered to the unoperated pelvis, if the groin is sufficiently high risk.

Currently the InPACT trial is open in the UK and the United States, looking at the role of definitive radiotherapy and concomitant chemotherapy and the role of adjuvant chemotherapy. The trial has associated with it radiotherapy contouring guidelines, based on a vascular expansion method, which are helpful to follow.

Palliative Radiotherapy

Palliative radiotherapy and chemotherapy can be used for advanced inoperable primary tumours or to treat fixed or fungating inguinal nodes or distant metastases.

Clinical and Radiological Anatomy

The penis is composed of two corpora cavernosa and the corpus spongiosum. Distally the corpus spongiosum expands into the glans penis, which is covered by a skin fold known as the prepuce. The prepuce and skin of the penis drain to the superficial inguinal lymph nodes. The glans penis and corpora have a very rich lymphatic supply, which drains to the deep inguinal and external iliac lymph nodes as shown in Figure 31.1.

Assessment of Primary Disease

After histological confirmation of primary +/- nodal disease, patients should have a full assessment including endoscopic examination of the urethra, cystoscopy, CT scan of the chest, abdomen and pelvis. In advanced cases, MRI of the penis may be useful to delineate the target. FDG-PET can be used for staging, in lieu of CT, particularly where there are indeterminate findings.

CT Planning

Patients are treated supine with arms folded comfortably across the chest. Treatment is planned using a planning CT scan with intravenous contrast to delineate the inguinal and pelvic lymph node regions. Scans are taken from the mid lumbar spine to at least 5 cm inferior to the ischial tuberosities.

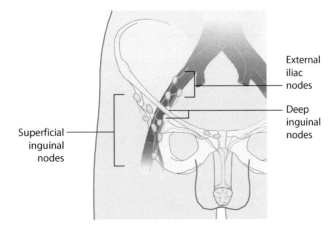

FIGURE 31.1 Lymphatic drainage of the penis.

Target Volume Definition and Dose Solutions

Adjuvant Radiotherapy

For inguinal and pelvic node adjuvant radiotherapy, pelvic blood vessels shown on a contrast-enhanced planning CT scan are used to define the nodal CTV. The technique for defining the pelvic nodal volume mirrors that of prostate pelvic nodal definition, with the exception of the presacral nodes which are not at risk in penile cancer. See Harris et al. (2015) for a description of the prostate nodal contouring technique, describing the 0.7-cm vascular expansion method. In addition, for penile cancer patients with positive pelvic nodal dissection, the volume should be extended to include the common iliac nodes. The common iliac nodes are a bilateral structure, hence are bilaterally at risk even if the pelvis is negative on one side. Hence, when included, the common iliacs should be contoured bilaterally.

For the definition of the inguinal CTV, the vessels should be contoured from the border of the pelvic nodes (top of femoral head level) down to the level at the bottom of the ischial tuberosity. A margin of 1 cm should be applied except anteriorly and medially where a 3-cm margin is applied. The CTV should then be cropped off muscle and bone. A further PTV margin should be added as per local guidelines.

- CTV_57 = residual/macroscopic disease
- CTV_54 = inguinal lymph nodes
- CTV_45 = pelvic lymph nodes

The pelvic and inguinal lymph nodes are treated with IMRT using tomotherapy or VMAT. The normal tissue organs at risk are the same as for treating the pelvic nodes for prostate cancer and the same organ at risk dose constraints should be applied.

Palliative Radiotherapy to the Primary

For locally advanced inoperable primary tumours, the external (skin) extent of the invasion should be marked so that it is visible on CT, and the target defined on CT. However, for palliative cases it is sufficient to create a customised lead cut-out and apply a single anterior field, or parallel pair, depending on the depth of disease. This technique is only suitable for palliative fractionations such as 20 Gy in 5 fractions. In advanced cases, radiotherapy can be used to palliate pain and bleeding with a simple beam arrangement to the affected area, including superficial energies for bleeding subcutaneous metastases.

Dose Fractionation

Adjuvant Radiotherapy

- 54 Gy in 25 fractions over five weeks to the inguinal lymph nodes
- 45 Gy in 25 fractions over five weeks to the pelvic lymph nodes
- Boost sites of residual/macroscopic disease to 57 Gy in 25 fractions over five weeks

Palliative Radiotherapy to the Primary

- 30 Gy in 10 daily fractions given in two weeks
- 20 Gy in 5 fractions over one week
- 8 Gy in 1 fraction

Treatment Delivery and Patient Care

At a minimum, set-up should be verified with CBCT days 1–3 and weekly. Patients often have postoperative seromas at the site of nodal dissection, and these can alter set-up during radiotherapy.

Complications of radiotherapy include tissue swelling, moist desquamation, secondary infection, alteration in bladder and bowel function (if treating the pelvis). There is a risk of worsening lymphoedema, which can already be present in patients after surgery but can be worsened by radiotherapy.

INFORMATION SOURCES

Cancer Research UK Cancer stats. https://www.cancerresearchuk.org/health-professional/cancer-statistics/statistics-by-cancer-type/penile-cancer/incidence#heading-Zero.

Hadway P, Smith YC, Corbishley C, et al. Evaluation of dynamic lymphoscintigraphy and sentinel lymph-node biopsy for detecting occult metastases in patients with penile squamous cell carcinoma. BJU Int 2007;100:561–565.

Harris VA, Staffurth J, Naismith O, Esmail A, Gulliford S, Khoo V, et al. Consensus guidelines and contouring atlas for pelvic node delineation in prostate and pelvic node intensity modulated radiation therapy. Int J Radiat Oncol Biol Phys [Internet] 2015;92(4):874–883. http://dx.doi.org/10.1016/j.ijrobp.2015.03.021.

Mistry T, Jones RWA, Dannatt E, et al. A 10-year retrospective audit of penile cancer management in the UK. BJU Int 2007;100:1277–1281.

Radiographics. Imaging of penile neoplasms. http://radiographics.rsnajnls.org/cgi/content/full/25/6/1629 (accessed 15 December 2008).

Sarin R, Norman AR, Steel GG, et al. Treatment results and prognostic factors in 101 men treated for squamous carcinoma of the penis. Int J Radiat Oncol Biol Phys 1997;38:713–722.

Smith Y, Hadway P, Biedrzycki O, et al. Reconstructive surgery for invasive squamous carcinoma of the glans penis. Eur Urol 2007;52:1179–1185.

Sri D, Sujenthiran A, Lam W, Minter J, Tinwell BE, Corbishley CM, et al. A study into the association between local recurrence rates and surgical resection margins in organ-sparing surgery for penile squamous cell cancer. BJU Int 2018;122(4):576–582.

32

Cervix

Indications for Radiotherapy

Cervical cancer is the second most common female malignancy worldwide and occurs predominantly in developing countries. Following the introduction of a national screening programme, there has been a significant reduction in the incidence of cervical cancer in the UK. Its pathogenesis is associated with persistent human papillomavirus (HPV) infection, smoking, multiple sexual partners, low socioeconomic status and early coitus. HPV vaccination is now offered to all girls aged 12 years and above, and this should reduce their risk of developing invasive cervical cancer. The vast majority of cervical cancers are HPV-induced squamous cell carcinomas arising from the squamo-columnar junction. Adenocarcinomas are commonly of endocervical type. Anaplastic small cell tumours are aggressive. Direct spread from uterine malignancies are also seen.

The choice of treatment for carcinoma of the cervix depends on the disease stage at presentation (FIGO), tumour size and volume, histology, lymph node status and the likelihood of lymph node involvement, age, comorbidities and the performance status of the patient. Cervical intraepithelial squamous or glandular neoplasia is managed with local excision or superficial ablative techniques. Microinvasive stage IA1 disease (no greater than 3 mm in depth of stromal invasion and no greater than 7 mm in diameter) is treated with total hysterectomy or excisional cone biopsy in patients who wish to retain their fertility. Adenocarcinomas are managed in the same way as squamous cell carcinomas.

Early-Stage Disease

Stage IA2 (3–5 mm depth of stromal invasion and no greater than 7 mm in diameter) and IB1 (4 cm or less in greatest dimension) tumours are managed with radical hysterectomy and bilateral pelvic lymphadenectomy. In selected patients with tumour of 2 cm or less in dimension who are keen to preserve fertility, radical vaginal trachelectomy and laparoscopic pelvic lymphadenectomy may be carried out.

Stage IB1 and IIA1 tumours are managed equally effectively with either radical surgery or combined curative external-beam radiotherapy and concomitant chemotherapy (CRT) followed by intrauterine brachytherapy. Both treatments provide five-year survival rates of 80–90 per cent. Surgery is preferred in younger women as it enables preservation of ovarian function.

The treatment of choice for patients with stage IB2 and IIA2 disease is primary CRT. This avoids the increased morbidity observed when surgery is combined with postoperative radiotherapy. Primary radiotherapy may also be considered for patients deemed unsuitable for radical surgery.

Absolute indications for postoperative CRT (only one factor required)

- Residual macroscopic disease
- Involved resection margins
- Parametrial involvement
- More than one lymph node with metastatic involvement
- Incidental discovery of cervical cancer at simple hysterectomy

DOI: 10.1201/9781315171562-32

Relative indications for postoperative CRT (more than one factor required)

- Resection margins of less than 5 mm
- Poorly differentiated tumour
- Lymphovascular space invasion (LVSI)
- Deep stromal invasion
- One lymph node with metastatic involvement

Locally Advanced Disease

Primary CRT followed by intrauterine image-based brachytherapy is the treatment of choice for locoregionally advanced disease. Studies of CRT with concomitant cisplatin +/- 5FU have shown a 30–50 per cent reduction in the risk of death from cervical cancer compared with radiotherapy alone. Radiotherapy alone is considered in patients with poor performance status, impaired renal function or significant comorbidities. Where a vesico- or recto-vaginal fistula is present, a urinary diversion procedure or defunctioning colostomy should be performed prior to commencing primary CRT.

Stage IVB Metastatic Disease

Patients with stage IVB tumour are managed primarily with palliative systemic therapy. Short course palliative pelvic radiotherapy can be useful in relieving bleeding and pelvic pain in patients with metastatic disease and those unfit for curative treatment. Palliative radiotherapy may also relieve pain from bone secondaries.

Occult Disease

Patients who have invasive cervical cancer (stage IA2 and above) detected as an incidental finding at simple hysterectomy performed for a presumed benign condition are usually treated postoperatively with CRT and vault brachytherapy. In some cases, further surgery including lymph node dissection can be considered.

Recurrent Disease

CRT is the treatment of choice in patients with pelvic recurrent disease who have not received previous radiotherapy to the pelvis. Pelvic exenterative surgery performed with curative intent can be considered in those with central locally recurrent disease who have received previous pelvic radiotherapy. Highly conformal reirradiation can be considered in selected patients who have received previous pelvic radiotherapy in whom surgical resection is not feasible.

Sequencing of Multimodality Therapy

CRT with concomitant chemotherapy (such as weekly cisplatin 40 mg/m^2) is the treatment of choice for both high-risk early-stage disease and locally advanced tumours unless medically unfit for chemotherapy. Overall treatment time, including subsequent intracavitary brachytherapy, should ideally be 49 days or less and it should not exceed 56 days. If primary surgery is used and adjuvant radiotherapy is indicated, radiation should begin four to six weeks postoperatively or when adequate wound healing has taken place.

Clinical and Radiological Anatomy

Cervical cancer arises at the junction of the columnar epithelium of the endocervix and the squamous epithelium of the ectocervix. It spreads directly into the cervical stroma, presenting either as an exophytic tumour protruding into the vagina or an endocervical tumour expanding the cervix. It can infiltrate superiorly into the lower uterine segment, inferiorly into the vagina and laterally from the paracervical spaces into the parametrium, broad and utero-sacral ligaments and pelvic side-walls. This can in turn result in hydronephrosis through involvement of the distal ureters. Rectal and bladder mucosal involvement is uncommon at presentation. The cervix has a rich lymphatic plexus, connecting with those of the lower uterine segment and draining laterally into the paracervical, para-metrial, obturator, internal and external iliac nodes. Posterior tumours may spread to the presacral, common iliac and para-aortic nodes along the ovarian vessels. The inguinal nodes may be involved in tumours affecting the lower third of the vagina. Lymph node spread is common in cervical cancer and can be noncontiguous. Stage 1B tumours have a 15–25 per cent risk of pelvic, and a 5–15 per cent risk of para-aortic nodal involvement, depending on tumour size, depth of stromal invasion and presence of LVSI. Blood-borne spread occurs late, with metastases seen in the lungs, extra-pelvic nodes, liver and bone.

Assessment of Primary Disease

Clinical assessment includes colposcopy and vaginal examination to inspect and palpate the tumour extent in the cervix and vagina, and a bimanual examination to determine mobility and enlargement of the uterus. Vaginal spread can also be visualised using a speculum and a rectal examination may be required. Examination under anaesthesia is sometimes necessary for accurate assessment of the lesion according to the FIGO staging system. Cystoscopy is performed to look for invasion of the bladder mucosa, and sigmoidoscopy where rectal invasion is suspected. CT scanning of the chest and abdomen is performed for staging, to assess the renal tract, and to detect ureteric obstruction or hydronephrosis, which may require stent placement prior to treatment. MRI of the pelvis is the imaging modality of choice for assessing the depth of cervical stromal invasion, uterine extension and parametrial involvement. CT and MRI detection of pelvic and para-aortic nodal involvement has a low sensitivity, as nodes are usually designated involved when their short axis diameter is greater than 1 cm. FDG PET-CT has a higher sensitivity for detecting nodal and distant metastases. It is now used in place of CT in locally advanced tumours to evaluate the extent of nodal involvement and exclude distant metastases. PET-CT and MRI of the pelvis should also be performed prior to curative CRT for recurrent disease.

Data Acquisition

Patients are immobilised supine using knee supports and ankle brace. Anterior and lateral skin tattoos, marked with radio-opaque material, are aligned with lasers to prevent lateral rotation. For obese patients, a prone bellyboard immobilisation system may be used to allow the small bowel to fall anteriorly away from the target volume. This is however a difficult position for patients to maintain and this may in turn lead to greater daily setup uncertainties. Clinical examination is performed, with the patient in the treatment position, and the inferior tumour extent within the vagina is marked with radio-opaque material. A protocol is used to maintain constant bladder filling – 'comfortably full' – as variations in bladder volume can affect the position of the uterus and cervix. It will also help to reduce the volume of small bowel and bladder irradiated. For example, patients are asked to empty their bladder and drink 250 mL of fluid 30 minutes before planning CT acquisition and treatment each day. Daily bladder ultrasound may be used to ensure consistent bladder volumes. Patients are also encouraged to empty their bowels before CT scanning and each treatment, and this may require the use of enemas/laxatives. The rectal diameter should be less than 4 cm.

CT scans are acquired from the superior border of the first lumbar vertebra to 5 cm below the vaginal introitus. The superior scan limit should be extended to the junction between T10 and T11 if para-aortic nodal irradiation is required. Intravenous contrast is used to enhance visualisation of the pelvic blood vessels as they act as surrogates for the pelvic nodes during CTV-N delineation. Intravenous contrast may also enhance the primary tumour and uterus. In addition, oral contrast may be given to outline the small bowel.

EUA findings along with diagnostic MRI and PET-CT are used to localise the tumour during target volume delineation. MRI fusion, using T2-weighted axial images, is helpful due to difficulties in distinguishing soft tissue components on planning CT scans.

Target Volume Definition

Primary Radiotherapy

Two planning CT scans are performed: one with an empty bladder and the other with a 'comfortably full' bladder. These are used to assess internal organ motion. Target volume and OAR definition are performed using the 'comfortably full' bladder planning CT images. The GTV-T comprises the full extent of the primary cervix tumour and it is defined using information from clinical examination, T2-weighted MRI and FDG PET-CT. The high-risk (HR) CTV-T consists of the GTV-T and any remaining cervix not infiltrated by tumour. The low-risk (LR) CTV-T includes the CTV-T HR with anterior and posterior margins of 5 mm towards the bladder and rectum (excluding uninvolved walls), the entire uterus and parametria bilaterally and 20 mm of uninvolved vagina measured from the most inferior extent of CTV-T HR along the axis of the vagina. Where there is involvement of the pelvic sidewall, meso-rectum or uterosacral ligaments, the CTV-T LR will be extended to include a 20-mm margin from the CTV-T HR into these structures. The CTV-T LR is then expanded using margins of 10 mm anteroposteriorly and superoinferiorly and 5 mm laterally to form the ITV-T LR (Figure 32.1). An extra 5-mm isotropic margin from the uterine body should be

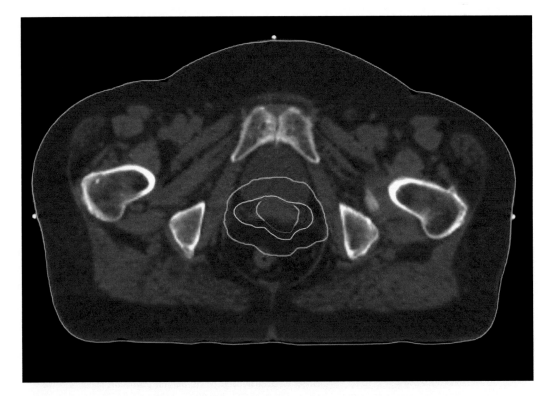

FIGURE 32.1 Axial planning CT scan showing the GTV-T (cyan), the HR CTV-T (red), the CTV-T LR (yellow) edited to exclude the uninvolved bladder wall and the ITV-T LR (green).

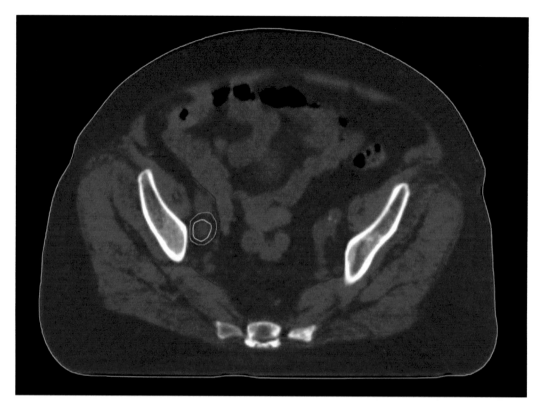

FIGURE 32.2   Axial planning CT scan showing the GTV-N (green), the CTV-N (pink) and the CTV-E (blue).

added to the ITV-T LR if there is tumour involvement of the upper uterus. The ITV-T LR is then displayed onto the co-registered empty bladder planning CT images to ensure that the CTV-T LR structures are still encompassed. Adaptations may be required. The GTV-N should include all FDG-avid nodes on PET-CT along with nodes measuring 1 cm or more in short-axis dimension on CT or MRI. A margin of 0–3 mm may be added to GTV-N to form CTV-N to take into account extracapsular nodal extension and possible nodal progression between planning CT acquisition and radiotherapy commencement (Figure 32.2). The elective nodal regions (CTV-E) to be irradiated are shown in Table 32.1.

TABLE 32.1

Lymph Node Regions for CTV-E

Risk Group	Definition	Lymph Node Regions to Be Included in CTV-E
Low Risk	Tumour size 4 cm or less AND stage IA/IB1/IIA1 AND no pathological nodes AND squamous cell carcinoma AND no uterine invasion	'Small pelvis' Internal iliac External iliac Obturator Presacral
Intermediate Risk	Not low risk No high-risk features	'Large pelvis' Nodes included in 'small pelvis' plus common iliac including the aortic bifurcation Inguinal nodes should be included if there is distal vaginal involvement Mesorectal space should be included if there are involved mesorectal nodes and advanced local disease
High Risk	Pathological nodes at common iliac or above OR three or more pathological nodes	'Large pelvis + para-aortic' Nodes included in 'large pelvis' plus the para-aortic region with the upper border of CTV-E at the level of the renal veins (usually including L2) and at least 3 cm cranial of the highest pathological node

The CTV-E is delineated by identifying the contrast-enhanced pelvic blood vessels on each CT slice and using a 7-mm circumferential margin around these vessels to create a 3D CTV-E. Muscles and bones are edited off the CTV-E. It is then extended to include the area between the vertebral body and psoas muscle and the 10-mm wide presacral strip by connecting the nodal areas on either side of S1 and S2 (the sacral foramina do not need to be included). The medial border around the external iliac vessels is continued posteriorly and parallel to the pelvic sidewall until it joins the medial contour of the internal iliac vessels to create an 18-mm-wide strip medial to the pelvic sidewall in order to encompass the obturator and infra-iliac nodes. The CTV-E is also extended to include all visible nodes and lymphoceles. The inguinal nodes are irradiated only if there is tumour involvement of the lower third of the vagina.

- ITV45 = ITV-T LR + CTV-N + CTV-E
- PTV45 = ITV45 + 5 mm
- PTV55 = CTV-N + 5 mm (for pathological nodes below the common iliac bifurcation, likely 3–4 Gy from intracavitary brachytherapy)
- PTV57.5 = CTV-N + 5 mm (for pathological nodes above the common iliac bifurcation, negligible dose from intracavitary brachytherapy)
- PTV60 = CTV-T HR + 5 mm (for patients not suitable for intracavitary brachytherapy)

Adjuvant Radiotherapy

The GTV has been resected at surgery, so the CTV-T comprises the surgical tumour bed including the vaginal vault and parametrial/paravaginal tissues. CTV-N contains the obturator, internal, external and common iliac nodes. CTV-T is delineated using preoperative MRI, operative diagrams and histological findings to include sites at high risk of recurrence. CTV-N is delineated using CT contrast-enhanced blood vessels with a 7-mm margin. A CTV-PTV margin of 10–15 mm is used for CTV-T and a 7–10 mm margin for CTV-N to allow for organ motion and setup uncertainties.

Para-aortic Radiotherapy

Indications for para-aortic radiotherapy include positive para-aortic nodes on lymph node dissection, involved nodes at the aortic bifurcation or at the level of the common iliac vessels on histology and radiologically abnormal para-aortic or common iliac nodes. CT scanning is performed with intravenous contrast to enhance the blood vessels and kidneys and to locate the para-aortic nodes. The CTV is defined by adding a 5–7-mm margin around the aorta and medial half of the inferior vena cava to cover the para-aortic, aorto-caval and retro-caval nodes with the most superior CTV extent at the level of the renal hilum or at least 2 cm above the highest involved lymph node region. PTV margin is 5–7 mm. Virtual simulation can be used to design anterior and posterior beams, with the superior border at the upper level of L1. The width of the treatment fields is approximately 8 cm, avoiding the kidneys laterally with MLC shielding. The inferior border is matched to the top of the pelvic beams. Additional organs at risk include the kidneys and spinal cord. 3D volume outlining allows the use of IMRT or VMAT.

Organs at Risk

Organs at risk to be contoured include the small and large bowel, rectum, sigmoid, bladder, femoral heads down to the level of the lesser trochanter and kidneys if para-aortic nodal irradiation is required. Organs at risk should be contoured to at least 2 cm beyond the PTV. The normal tissue dose constraints are shown in Table 32.2.

Simulator Planning

The patient is examined in the treatment position and a radio-opaque marker is used to indicate the most inferior tumour extent within the vagina. Anteroposterior and lateral simulator films are taken.

TABLE 32.2

Normal Tissue Dose Constraints for IMRT in Cervix Cancer

	No Lymph Node Involvement		Involved Lymph Nodes	
	Hard Dose Constraints	**Soft Dose Constraints**	**Hard Dose Constraints**	**Soft Dose Constraints**
Bowel	D_{max} <105%	V40 Gy <250 cm^3 V30 Gy <500 cm^3	D_{max} <105% in regions outside 10–15 mm from PTV-N	When no para-aortic irradiation: V40 Gy <250 cm^3 V30 Gy <500 cm^3 For para-aortic irradiation: V40 Gy <300 cm^3 V30 Gy <650 cm^3
Sigmoid	D_{max} <105%		D_{max} <105% in regions outside 10–15 mm from PTV-N	
Bladder	D_{max} <105%	V40 Gy <60% V30 Gy <80%	D_{max} <105% in regions outside 10–15 mm from PTV-N	V40 Gy <60% V30 Gy <80%
Rectum	D_{max} <105%	V40 Gy <75% V30 Gy <95%	D_{max} <105% in regions outside 10–15 mm from PTV-N	V40 Gy <75% V30 Gy <95%
Spinal Cord	D_{max} <48 Gy		D_{max} <48 Gy	
Femoral Heads	D_{max} <50 Gy		D_{max} <50 Gy	
Kidney	D_{mean} <15 Gy	D_{mean} <10 Gy	D_{mean} <15 Gy	D_{mean} <10 Gy

All clinical, surgical and histological data are used to define the treatment fields, along with diagnostic MRI or PET-CT information showing the tumour extent and position of the kidneys.

The superior border of the treatment beam is placed at the lower edge of L4 to include the distal common iliac nodes. The inferior border is placed at least 3 cm below the most inferior disease extent within the vagina as palpated or seen on MRI, which is usually the lower border of the obturator fossae. Lateral borders are 2 cm outside the bony pelvic sidewalls. The anterior border must encompass the GTV-T, uterine body and common iliac nodes and is usually placed through the anterior third of the symphysis pubis. The posterior border should include the proximal utero-sacral ligaments, internal iliac and upper presacral nodes. It is commonly situated 0.5 cm posterior to the anterior border of the S2/3 junction. Individualised shielding is employed to the superior corners of the anterior and posterior beams to exclude small bowel. Shielding to the inferior corners to protect the femoral heads may mask the external iliac nodes and should be used sparingly. Lateral beams have shielding to the sacral nerve roots posteriorly.

Palliative Radiotherapy

Symptoms of bleeding or pain from locally advanced cervical cancer can be alleviated with short-course radiotherapy. CT planning is used as just described. The macroscopic tumour alone is encompassed to minimise the treatment volume and toxicity. The PTV is created by adding a 1.5–2-cm margin around the GTV.

Dose Solutions

Complex

IMRT or VMAT techniques will significantly reduce the radiation dose to the small bowel, rectum and bladder (Figure 32.3). This may in turn lead to lower rates of acute and late toxicities. Organ motion studies have shown that the position of the cervix and uterus can vary by up to 30 mm as a result of changes

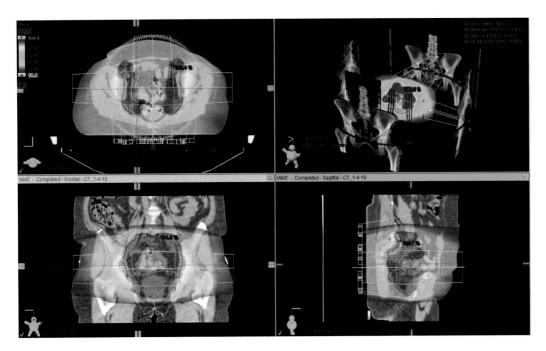

FIGURE 32.3 VMAT plan of a low risk FIGO stage IB1 node-negative squamous cell carcinoma of the cervix.

in bladder and rectal filling. Daily image-guided radiotherapy (IGRT) should therefore be employed to localise the target volume to ensure that IMRT or VMAT is delivered accurately and safely.

Conformal

An anterior, a posterior and two lateral wedged beams are used. The rectum is spared through a low weighting of the posterior beam. Using 3D planning, multi-leaf collimators are shaped to the target volumes to spare normal tissues. The four-field technique can also be used to cover the para-aortic nodal volume with low weighting of the lateral fields to spare the kidneys.

Brachytherapy

Brachytherapy allows delivery of a very high radiation dose to the tumour volume for maximal local control without exceeding the tolerance doses of the surrounding normal tissues. This is feasible because the normal uterus and vaginal vault are relatively radio-resistant and there is rapid dose fall-off from the cervix to the adjacent rectum, sigmoid colon, bladder and small bowel. Gynaecological brachytherapy can be delivered at low, medium or high dose rates, or as pulsed brachytherapy where many, closely spaced radiation fractions or pulses are delivered to mimic continuous low dose rate treatment.

Image-based 3D Brachytherapy

This method relies on CT and MR imaging. Doses are prescribed to volumes rather than reference points. The GEC-ESTRO group has published recommendations on the target volume concepts and plan evaluation using dose-volume histograms in image-based 3D brachytherapy. An MRI scan is performed during the final week of external-beam radiotherapy (EBRT) to assess the tumour response to treatment and to plan subsequent brachytherapy. A central intrauterine tube and vaginal ovoids are inserted to treat

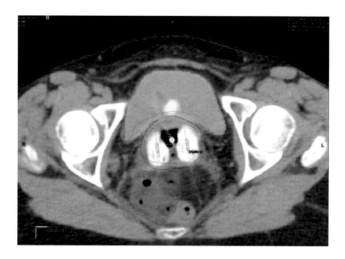

FIGURE 32.4   CT scan of a patient with HDR brachytherapy applicators in situ and isodoses; HR (high-risk) CTV cyan, IR (intermediate-risk) CTV magenta.

the primary tumour and its surrounding area. Following the first insertion, an MRI scan is performed with the applicator in situ and this is co-registered with the planning CT scan to guide target delineation. The planning CT scan should include the entire applicator with at least 5-cm margin above the most superior extent of the uterus. The treatment targets are defined primarily on the para-axial sequences, although the para-coronal and sagittal sequences should also be inspected to ensure target consistency. The GEC-ESTRO recommendations on target volume definition and normal tissue delineation are followed. The GTV, high-risk (HR) CTV and intermediate-risk (IR) CTV are defined alongside the bladder, rectum, sigmoid colon and small bowel (Figure 32.4). The GTV comprises the macroscopic tumour at the time of brachytherapy as defined by clinical examination and as visualised on MRI. The HR CTV should include the GTV and entire cervix at the time of brachytherapy taking into account the tumour extent at diagnosis. The IR CTV comprises the HR CTV with an isotropic margin of 10 mm excluding organs at risk. The magnitude of this margin is dependent on the tumour size, location, its potential spread and the degree of tumour regression following EBRT. The total dose, including that from the EBRT phase of treatment, should be isoequivalent to 85–95 Gy in 2 Gy fractions for the HR CTV, and 60 Gy for the IR CTV. The organs at risk are contoured from 2 cm above the uterus to at least 2 cm below the IR CTV. They include the bladder, rectum, sigmoid colon and bowel loops. In cases where there is significant tumour involvement of the vagina, the urethra should be contoured to enable assessment of the dose to this structure. Doses to 2 mL of tissue volume (D2 cc) for the OARs are calculated at 2 Gy per fraction. Isoequivalent doses of 80–90 Gy for the bladder and 65–75 Gy for the rectum and sigmoid colon are generally accepted (Table 32.3).

TABLE 32.3

Target Dose Aims and Normal Tissue Dose Constraints for Image-Based 3D Brachytherapy

Target	D98 GTV EQD2	D90 HR CTV EQD2	D98 HR CTV EQD2	D98 IR CTV EQD2	Point A EQD2
Planning Aims	>95 Gy	>90 Gy <95 Gy	>75 Gy	>60 Gy	>65 Gy
OAR	Bladder D2 cc EQD2	Rectum D2 cc EQD2	Sigmoid D2 cc EQD2	Bowel D2 cc EQD2	
Planning Aims	<80 Gy	<65 Gy	<70 Gy	<70 Gy	

The Manchester System for Gynaecological Brachytherapy

This system relies on prescribed doses to defined reference points. Manchester point A is defined as a point 2 cm lateral to the central uterine canal and 2 cm superior to the lateral fornix in the plane of the uterus. It lies within the paracervical tissues near the uterine artery and ureter, and was chosen to take into account the tolerances of adjacent dose-limiting normal structures. In practice, the prescribed dose is specified at a point 2 cm above and 2 cm lateral to the flange of the intrauterine tube at the external os. This point is taken to be equivalent to Manchester point A. Point B is defined as 3 cm lateral to point A, i.e. 5 cm from the midline on the lateral axis, and it is used to provide an indication of dose to the distal parametria. The ICRU Report No. 38 specifies reference points for the bladder and rectum. The bladder point is posterior to the catheter balloon filled with 7 mL of contrast solution. The rectal point is 0.5 cm posterior to the most posterior packing or the posterior surface of the ovoids.

Applicators Used in Gynaecological Brachytherapy

A number of different applicators are available for use with an intact uterus. A central intrauterine tube is used together with a vaginal applicator, which can consist of ovoids or a ring. Applicators have been developed that contain holes for interstitial needles, which can be used to produce better coverage of the parametrium.

Vaginal vault brachytherapy can be delivered using a cylindrical vaginal applicator or vaginal ovoids. Both are available in various diameters/sizes. Ovoids produce a better dose distribution if coverage of the parametrial soft tissues is required, whereas cylindrical applicators mainly treat the vaginal mucosa. Doses are prescribed to 0.5 cm from the surface of the applicator.

Applicator Insertion Technique

After an examination under general or spinal anaesthesia and urinary catheter insertion, the uterine cavity is measured with a sound. The cervical canal is dilated and a central uterine tube of appropriate length is inserted. The vaginal applicators are then positioned and fixed to the tube. Vaginal packing is used to distance the OARs from the applicator and to prevent applicator rotation. A Schmidt's sleeve may be placed or sutured into the cervical canal, which can facilitate reinsertion of the applicators without anaesthesia for subsequent fractions. A rectal retractor can be used instead of or along with vaginal packing to create distance between the applicator and rectum. 3D imaging is then performed.

Dose Fractionation

Primary Radiotherapy

EBRT followed by intracavitary brachytherapy aiming for an isoeffective dose of 85–95 Gy to the HR-CTV

EBRT

- 45 Gy in 25 daily fractions of 1.8 Gy given in five weeks
- 50.4 Gy in 28 daily fractions of 1.8 Gy given in five and a half weeks

Intracavitary Brachytherapy

HDR

- 6–7.5 Gy per fraction for 3–5 fractions
- 21 Gy in 3 fractions twice a week
- 28 Gy in 4 fractions twice a week

SIB-IMRT for node-positive disease, dose to macroscopic nodes

- 55–60 Gy in 25–28 daily fractions given in five to five and a half weeks

SIB-IMRT for parametrial disease that can't be encompassed by brachytherapy

- 57–60 Gy in 25–28 daily fractions given in five to five and a half weeks

SIB-IMRT to cervix tumour when intracavitary brachytherapy is not feasible

- 60–63 Gy in 25 daily fractions given in five weeks

Phase II EBRT boost to cervix tumour when intracavitary brachytherapy is not feasible and SIB-IMRT not available

- 16–20 Gy in 8–10 daily fractions given in one and a half to two weeks

Phase II EBRT boost to macroscopic nodes or parametrial disease if SIB-IMRT not available

- 5.4 Gy in 3 daily fractions given in three days
- 10.8 Gy in 6 daily fractions given in one and a half weeks

Adjuvant Radiotherapy

EBRT

- 45 Gy in 25 daily fractions of 1.8 Gy given in five weeks
- 50.4 Gy in 28 daily fractions of 1.8 Gy given in five and a half weeks

Vault Brachytherapy

HDR

- 8–11 Gy to 0.5 cm from the applicator surface in 2 fractions
- 12 Gy to 0.5 cm from the applicator surface in 3 fractions

Palliative Radiotherapy

- 8–10 Gy in 1 fraction
- 20 Gy in 5 daily fractions given in one week
- 30 Gy in 10 daily fractions given in two weeks

Treatment Delivery and Patient Care

Patients are aligned with skin tattoos and laser lights in a setup identical to that used for localisation in the CT scanner. When using CRT, radiotherapy is delivered within an hour of chemotherapy completion. Overall treatment time should be as short as possible, as protracted treatment duration is associated with reduced survival. The overall treatment time, including brachytherapy, should not exceed 49 days. These are category 1 patients and any unscheduled gaps in treatment are rectified by treating at the weekend or by using 2 fractions in one day with a minimal inter-fraction interval of six hours. Intracavitary brachytherapy should follow external beam radiotherapy without delay.

Patients are reminded to follow the bladder filling protocol. Acute side effects may increase when radiotherapy is combined with concomitant chemotherapy. Patients should be reviewed weekly during the course of treatment. Diarrhoea may occur during pelvic external beam radiotherapy, and is treated with loperamide hydrochloride and a low residue diet. If diarrhoea worsens and/or abdominal pain occurs, treatment may need to be interrupted. Urinary frequency and dysuria may occur, and a urine specimen should be taken to exclude infection. Rectal bleeding and painful defecation may also occur. Prophylactic antiemetics can be used to prevent nausea and vomiting. A good fluid intake should be encouraged, and patients should avoid smoking. Skin care advice is given as erythema may develop within the treatment area. Severe skin reactions are treated with 1 per cent hydrocortisone cream. Premenopausal patients will lose ovarian function, and hormone replacement therapy may be given following treatment completion to improve menopausal symptoms and prevent osteoporosis. Vaginal hydration gels and dilators are used to help reduce vaginal shortening and stenosis. Psychosexual counseling may be helpful.

Verification

Volumetric imaging with cone-beam CT for bone and soft tissue matching with daily online position verification and couch correction. Cone-beam CT will also allow daily monitoring of uterus movement. For patients with bilateral hip replacements, 2D-2D kV matching to bone is used instead, with daily online correction, as imaging artefacts from the hip prostheses will prevent any useful information being obtained from cone-beam CTs. However, in patients with single hip prostheses, cone-beam CT may still provide useful volumetric information about target volumes, bladder and rectum.

Key Trials

Keys HM, Bundy BN, Stehman FB, et al. Cisplatin, radiation, and adjuvant hysterectomy compared with radiation and adjuvant hysterectomy for bulky stage IB cervical carcinoma. N Engl J Med 1999;340:1154–1161.

Landoni F, Maneo A, Colombo A, et al. Randomised study of radical surgery versus radiotherapy for stage Ib-IIa cervical cancer. Lancet 1997;350:535–540.

Morris M, Eifel PJ, Lu J, et al. Pelvic radiation with concurrent chemotherapy compared with pelvic and para-aortic radiation for high-risk cervical cancer. N Engl J Med 1999;340:1137–1143.

Peters WA III, Liu PY, Barrett RJ II, et al. Concurrent chemotherapy and pelvic radiation therapy compared with pelvic radiation therapy alone as adjuvant therapy after radical surgery in high-risk early-stage cancer of the cervix. J Clin Oncol 2000;18:1606–1613.

Rose PG, Bundy BN, Watkins EB, et al. Concurrent cisplatin-based radiotherapy and chemotherapy for locally advanced cervical cancer. N Engl J Med 1999;340:1144–1153.

Whitney CW, Sause W, Bundy BN, et al. Randomized comparison of fluorouracil plus cisplatin versus hydroxyurea as an adjunct to radiation therapy in stage IIB-IVA carcinoma of the cervix with negative para-aortic lymph nodes: A Gynecologic Oncology Group and Southwest Oncology Group study. J Clin Oncol 1999;17:1339–1348.

INFORMATION SOURCES

Dimopoulos JCA, Petrow P, Tanderup K, et al. Recommendations from gynaecological (GYN) GEC-ESTRO working group (IV): Basic principles and parameters for MR imaging within the frame of image based adaptive cervix cancer brachytherapy. Radiother Oncol 2012;103:113–122.

Eminowicz G, Hall-Craggs M, Diez P, et al. Improving target volume delineation in intact cervical carcinoma: Literature review and step-by-step pictorial atlas to aid contouring. Pract Radiat Oncol 2016;6:e203–e213.

Green JA, Kirwan JM, Tierney JF, et al. Survival and recurrence after concomitant chemotherapy and radiotherapy for cancer of the uterine cervix: A systematic review and meta-analysis. Lancet 2001;358:781–786.

Haie-Meder C, Potter R, Van Limbergen E, et al. Recommendations from gynaecological (GYN) GEC-ESTRO working group (I): Concepts and terms in 3D image based 3D treatment planning in cervix cancer brachytherapy with emphasis on MRI assessment of GTV and CTV. Radiother Oncol 2005;74:235–245.

Huh SJ, Park W, Han Y. Interfractional variation in position of the uterus during radical radiotherapy for cervical cancer. Radiother Oncol 2004;71:73–79.

Lim K, Small W Jr., Portelance L, et al. Consensus guidelines for delineation of clinical target volume for intensity-modulated pelvic radiotherapy for the definitive treatment of cervix cancer. Int J Radiat Oncol Biol Phys 2011;79:348–355.

Potter R, Haie-Meder C, Van Limbergen E, et al. Recommendations from gynaecological (GYN) GEC ESTRO working group (II): Concepts and terms in 3D image-based treatment planning in cervix cancer brachytherapy – 3D dose volume parameters and aspects of 3D image-based anatomy, radiation physics, radiobiology. Radiother Oncol 2006;78:67–77.

Salem A, Salem AF, Al-Ibraheem A, et al. Evidence for the use PET for radiation therapy planning in patients with cervical cancer: A systematic review. Hematol Oncol Stem Cell Ther 2011;4:173–181.

Sedlis A, Bundy BN, Rotman MZ, et al. A randomized trial of pelvic radiation therapy versus no further therapy in selected patients with stage IB carcinoma of the cervix after radical hysterectomy and pelvic lymphadenectomy: A Gynecologic Oncology Group study. Gynecol Oncol 1999;73:177–183.

Small W Jr, Mell LK, Anderson P, et al. Consensus guidelines for the delineation of the clinical target volume for intensity modulated pelvic radiotherapy in the postoperative treatment of endometrial and cervical cancer. Int J Radiat Oncol Biol Phys 2008;71:428–434.

Stock RG, Chen AS, Flickinger JC, et al. Node-positive cervical cancer: Impact of pelvic irradiation and patterns of failure. Int J Radiat Oncol Biol Phys 1995;31:31–36.

33

Uterus

Indications for Radiotherapy

Uterine cancer is the fourth most common malignancy in women. The majority of cases are endometrioid adenocarcinomas. Risk factors include obesity, especially in postmenopausal women, polycystic ovary syndrome, tamoxifen and Lynch syndrome. Serous carcinomas have a greater propensity for peritoneal spread, whereas clear cell carcinoma, carcinosarcoma and the rare squamous cell carcinoma behave more aggressively than endometrioid adenocarcinoma and are associated with a worse prognosis.

Surgery is the mainstay of treatment for all tumours of the corpus uteri. It involves inspection of the abdominal/pelvic cavity and retroperitoneum, total hysterectomy, bilateral salpingo-oophorectomy and peritoneal washings. Any suspicious nodes identified on preoperative imaging or during surgery are removed and omentectomy is performed in patients with carcinosarcoma, serous and clear cell carcinoma or extrauterine disease. Although it permits assessment of nodal status, the MRC ASTEC study showed no overall and recurrence-free survival benefit with pelvic lymphadenectomy in patients with early endometrial cancer. Histological staging and prognostic factors, such as age, cell type, grade of tumour, lymphovascular space invasion (LVSI), depth of myometrial invasion and lymph node status, are used to guide adjuvant treatment. Risk factors for local recurrence include poorly differentiated adenocarcinoma, clear cell and serous carcinoma, carcinosarcoma, invasion of the outer half of the myometrium, presence of LVSI, cervix involvement and age greater than 60 years.

More than 80 per cent of endometrial cancer presents as stage I disease. For low-risk patients (stage IA, grade 1–2, endometrioid histology, no LVSI) relapse-free survival is 95 per cent with surgery alone; no adjuvant therapy is required. These patients are managed with observation, with an absolute risk of recurrence of less than 5 per cent. Adjuvant therapy is also not required in those with no residual disease in the hysterectomy specimen despite positive biopsy.

For intermediate-risk patients (stage I with at least one poor prognostic risk factor for recurrence) there is a 15–25 per cent risk of locoregional relapse following surgery. This risk can be reduced to 5 per cent with postoperative pelvic radiotherapy, although it does not confer any survival benefit. The current recommendation is vaginal vault brachytherapy, especially in those who have undergone comprehensive nodal assessment.

For high-risk stage I patients (stage IB, grade 3, or stage IB, grade 2 with LVSI or stage IA, grade 3 with LVSI) the risk of pelvic nodal involvement is 35 per cent. The current recommendation for this group of patients is external-beam radiotherapy (EBRT) treating the pelvic nodes, upper vagina and parametrium. Adjuvant pelvic EBRT is also indicated for carcinosarcomas. In patients with no evidence of nodal metastases following adequate lymph node dissection, vaginal vault brachytherapy is an alternative option to EBRT, which minimises the risk of lymphoedema. Vaginal vault brachytherapy is generally not required following pelvic EBRT unless risk factors for vaginal recurrence are present such as cervical stroma involvement. Patients with stage II disease are therefore managed with EBRT followed by vaginal vault brachytherapy irrespective of LVSI or tumour grade.

The randomised PORTEC-3 trial included patients with stage I grade 3 endometrioid cancer and deep myometrial invasion or LVSI, stage I–III endometrial cancer with serous or clear cell histology and those with stage II or III disease. It showed a significant improvement in five-year overall and failure-free survival with the addition of adjuvant chemotherapy during and after EBRT in this group of patients. The absolute survival benefit was greatest in those with stage III or serous cancers. Distant metastases were the first site of recurrence in the majority of patients with a relapse. Isolated pelvic or vaginal recurrences were uncommon.

Adjuvant pelvic EBRT has not been shown to improve survival in uterine leiomyosarcoma and endometrial stromal sarcoma. It may however improve locoregional control in those with locally advanced disease.

Radiotherapy may be used as a primary treatment for inoperable endometrial cancer and in the rare instance when the patient is unfit for surgery. Five-year survival rates of 70–75 per cent are obtained for stage II, 50 per cent for stage III and 25 per cent for stage IV disease. In stage I disease, two-thirds of recurrences occur in the vaginal vault. Such recurrences can be successfully salvaged with EBRT followed by vaginal vault brachytherapy if detected early. Radiotherapy is also the treatment of choice for localised pelvic recurrences not previously treated with EBRT. In addition, palliative radiotherapy can help with pelvic pain and bleeding.

Sequencing of Multimodality Therapy

If primary surgery is used and adjuvant radiotherapy is indicated, radiation should begin four to six weeks postoperatively or when adequate wound healing has taken place. If required, vaginal vault brachytherapy should be given within 10–14 days of EBRT completion. Patients treated according to the PORTEC-3 chemoradiotherapy protocol will receive two cycles of intravenous cisplatin in the first and fourth week of EBRT, followed by four cycles of intravenous carboplatin and paclitaxel at 21-day intervals starting three weeks after EBRT completion.

Clinical and Radiological Anatomy

The uterus is supported by the levator ani muscles and is commonly anteverted and inclined forwards at an angle of 90° to the axis of the vagina (Figure 33.1). The myometrial wall of the uterine body is lined by endometrium and covered externally by a reflection of the peritoneum. The base of the bladder is closely applied to the anteroinferior part of the uterus, and posteriorly the pouch of Douglas lies between the posterior fornix and rectum. Loops of small bowel may lie in the pouch of Douglas, limiting the dose of radiation that can be given.

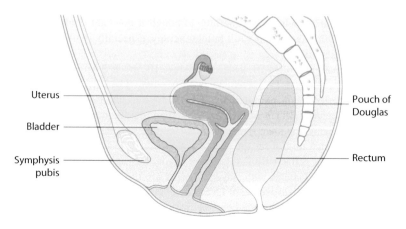

FIGURE 33.1   Regional anatomy of the uterus.

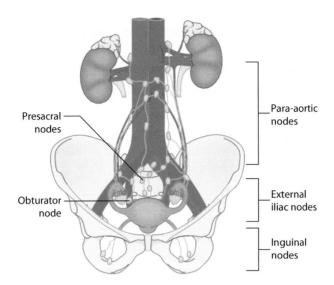

FIGURE 33.2 Lymphatic drainage of the uterus.

Tumours may infiltrate locally through the myometrium and parametrium to involve other pelvic organs and the peritoneal cavity, or it may extend inferiorly into the endocervix and vagina. Lymphatic drainage from the corpus passes through the broad ligament to the obturator, external iliac and presacral lymph nodes (Figure 33.2). Spread may also occur along the ovarian vessels to the para-aortic nodes. If the endocervix is involved, lymphatic spread occurs through paracervical and parametrial pathways to the pelvic lymph nodes. The risk of lymph node metastases increases with depth of invasion and tumour grade. Serous tumours spread like ovarian tumours transcoelomically. The most common sites for distant metastases are the lungs and liver.

Assessment of nodal involvement by CT and MRI are dependent on size criteria (usually a short axis lymph node diameter of greater than 1 cm), but the sensitivity is only 40–70 per cent. MRI with intravenous contrast agent USPIO (ultra-small particles of iron oxide) improves the sensitivity of detecting pelvic nodal metastases to 3 mm with maintained specificity. PET has a high sensitivity for detecting both nodal and distant metastases.

Assessment of Primary Disease

Patients commonly present with postmenopausal bleeding. They first undergo a pelvic examination and transvaginal ultrasound to assess endometrial thickness. Subsequent investigation involves hysteroscopy for endometrial assessment and biopsy for histological diagnosis (endometrial thickness of 5 mm or more on ultrasound or persistent symptoms). MRI of the pelvis is more sensitive than CT at identifying the presence and depth of myometrial invasion (Figure 33.3), extrauterine disease and pelvic lymph node and cervical involvement for accurate preoperative staging. CT scan of the chest and abdomen is performed if distant metastases are suspected. Assessment of patients for adjuvant radiotherapy should take into account all surgical and histological information including stage, grade, histological subtype, presence of LVSI, positive lymph nodes or positive washings collected at surgery. Inguinal lymph nodes are assessed by palpation, although the involvement of enlarged nodes can only be proved through histological or cytological examination. Inguinal lymph node involvement is uncommon and related to invasion of the lower third of the vagina.

CT scan of the chest and abdomen is routinely performed for all cases of high-grade uterine sarcoma to exclude distant metastases due to the risk of early haematogenous spread.

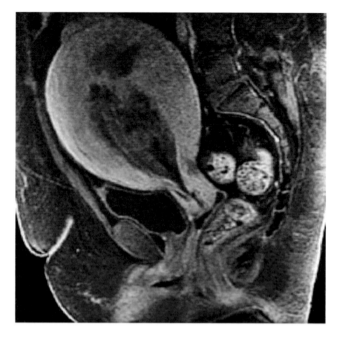

FIGURE 33.3   Sagittal T1-weighted MR scans showing an endometrial carcinoma infiltrating into the outer half of the myometrium.

Data Acquisition

CT Scanning

Patients are scanned in the treatment position supine with arms on the chest, knees and lower legs immobilised. Anterior and lateral tattoos are aligned with lasers to prevent lateral rotation and marked with radio-opaque material. For obese patients, a prone bellyboard may be used to allow the small bowel to fall anteriorly away from the target volume. A protocol is used to maintain constant bladder filling 'comfortably full' to push the small bowel superiorly. For example, patients may be asked to empty their bladder and drink 200 mL of water 20 minutes before the scan and treatment each day. Patients are also encouraged to empty their bowels before CT scanning and each treatment, and this may require the use of enemas/laxatives. The introitus is marked with radio-opaque material.

CT scans are acquired from the superior border of L3 to 5 cm beyond the vaginal introitus or ischial tuberosities. Intravenous contrast can be used to visualise the primary tumour and uterus if still in situ and to enhance visualisation of the pelvic blood vessels to aid CTV-N delineation. Image registration with diagnostic MRI is useful to localise the gross tumour in the uterus and/or involved nodes. Oral contrast can be given to outline the small bowel. The planning CT scan will need to be repeated if there is excessive rectal distension (rectal diameter greater than 4 cm).

Conventional

Conventionally, the simulator is used to acquire data with the patient supine, arms on the chest and knee and lower leg immobilisation or alpha cradles to prevent pelvic rotation. The patient is aligned using orthogonal laser beams with anterior and lateral tattoos marked with radio-opaque material. For obese patients, a prone bellyboard immobilisation system may be used to allow the small bowel to fall anteriorly away from the target volume. A protocol is used to maintain constant bladder filling 'comfortably full' as described earlier.

The vaginal vault is marked with a radio-opaque tampon for adjuvant treatment. In rare cases where surgery is not feasible, palpation of the primary tumour is carried out with the patient in the treatment position and the inferior border is marked with radio-opaque material.

AP and lateral simulator films are taken. All clinical, surgical and histological data must be used, together with diagnostic CT or MRI information, to design individually placed beam borders. Standard borders using bony anatomical landmarks have been shown to include unnecessary normal tissue and may miss the primary tumour or lymph nodes.

Target Volume Definition

Adjuvant Radiotherapy

There is no GTV postoperatively, and CTV-T includes the vaginal cuff/vault, upper 3 cm of vagina inferior to the cuff and parametrial/paravaginal soft tissues (to the medial edge of the internal obturator muscle/ischial ramus on each side). CTV-N includes the obturator, external, internal and distal common iliac nodes up to the L5/S1 level. For endometrial cancer with cervical stromal invasion, the presacral nodal region should also be included. CTV-T and CTV-N are delineated using information from preoperative CT and MRI, operative diagrams and histological findings to include sites at high risk of recurrence. There are published guidelines on pelvic nodal CTV delineation using CT scans with contrast-enhanced pelvic blood vessels (as surrogate for nodal regions). For CTV-N, a uniform contour with 7-mm margin is drawn around the pelvic blood vessels and extended to include all adjacent visible, enlarged or suspicious lymph nodes, lymphocoeles and surgical clips. Bones and muscles are excluded. The superior border of CTV-N is 1.5–2 cm below the aortic bifurcation. In cases where the pelvic nodes are involved, the common iliac nodes should be included up to the aortic bifurcation or 2 cm above the known disease, whichever is higher. The lateral border of CTV-N is at the pelvic sidewall and psoas muscle. This contour is extended anterolaterally along the iliopsoas muscle and around the external iliac artery to encompass all lateral external iliac nodes. This will create a strip medial to the pelvic sidewall that is at least 18 mm wide, encompassing the obturator, internal and external iliac nodes. If the presacral nodes are to be included, the nodal volumes on each side of the pelvis are connected using a 10–15-mm strip over the anterior sacrum at the level of S1-3, excluding the sacral foramina (Figure 33.4).

A typical CTV-PTV margin of 10–15 mm for CTV-T and 7 mm for CTV-N is added to allow for organ motion and setup uncertainties. Normal tissues to be contoured include bladder, rectum, small bowel and femoral heads.

Primary Radiotherapy

Nonsurgical patients with stage I and II disease may have multiple comorbidities which may limit the volume that can be treated radically. The GTV for uterine tumours is defined on clinical examination and with MRI. The CTV-T includes the primary tumour, entire uterus, cervix, ovaries, parametrium and upper half of vagina. The CTV-N comprises the common, external and internal iliac, obturator and subaortic presacral nodes. Involved nodes are detected by CT, MRI or MRI with USPIO. If the whole vagina is involved, the inguinal nodes may need to be included in the CTV-N. A CTV-PTV margin of 10–15 mm is commonly used to allow for setup uncertainty and physiological movement of the corpus and bladder. Macroscopic disease will receive a higher dose through either intrauterine brachytherapy or a second phase of EBRT. The simultaneous integrated boost (SIB) technique may also be used in those with involved nodes or whose primary tumour is not suitable for brachytherapy boost. In such cases, a 5–10-mm margin is added to the GTV to create the boost PTV.

Para-aortic Radiotherapy

See Chapter 32.

Conventional

The superior border is usually at the L5/S1 junction to include the external and internal iliac nodes. If these nodes are positive, then the superior border should be at the lower margin of L4, individualised to

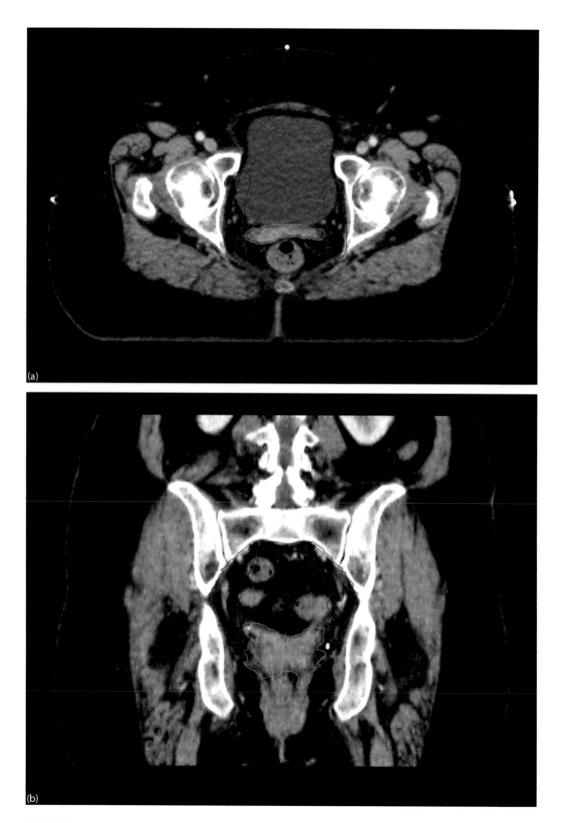

FIGURE 33.4 Planning CT showing the CTV-T (orange) and CTV-N (red), (a) axial and (b) coronal views.

include the distal common iliac nodes. The inferior border is placed at the lower border of the obturator foramen to include the upper half of the vagina for adjuvant treatment, or 3 cm below the most inferior disease extent in the vagina as palpated or seen on MRI. Lateral borders are 2 cm outside the bony pelvic sidewalls. The anterior border must encompass the CTV-N as well as GTV-T (if present) and is placed through the anterior third of the symphysis pubis. The posterior border is commonly situated 0.5 cm posterior to the anterior border of the S2/3 vertebral junction, varied according to surgical and histological findings. Individualised shielding is employed in the anterior beam to the superior corners to exclude small bowel. Shielding to the inferior corners to protect the femoral heads may mask the external iliac nodes and should be used sparingly. Lateral beams have shielding to the sacral nerve roots posteriorly.

A tattoo is placed at the center of the volume with two lateral pelvic tattoos to aid alignment and reproducibility of the treatment position.

Palliative Radiotherapy

For patients with locally advanced inoperable stage III/IV disease, the treatment intent is often palliative. Primary chemotherapy may be considered followed by EBRT individualised to the gross tumour in the uterus, cervix, parametrial tissues, any vaginal extension and involved lymph nodes with a 2-cm margin.

Organs at Risk

Organs at risk include the bladder, rectum, femoral heads down to the level of the greater trochanter, small bowel and pelvic kidney if present. The sigmoid colon is also included if intracavitary brachytherapy is to be used. Organs at risk should be contoured to at least 2 cm beyond the PTV. The rectum should be outlined from the anal verge (usually at the level of the ischial tuberosities) to the recto-sigmoid junction (where the bowel turns anteriorly and to the left). Dose constraints are shown in Table 33.1.

TABLE 33.1

Dose Constraints for IMRT in Uterine Cancers

	No Lymph Node Involvement		Involved Lymph Nodes	
	Hard Dose Constraints	**Soft Dose Constraints**	**Hard Dose Constraints**	**Soft Dose Constraints**
PTV45	V42.75 Gy >95% D_{max} <107%	V42.75 Gy = 95%	V42.75 Gy >95% D_{max} <107%	V42.75 Gy = 95%
PTV Boost			D_{min} >95%	
Bowel	D_{max} <105%	V40 Gy <250 cm³ V30 Gy <500 cm³	D_{max} <105% in regions outside 10–15 mm from PTV-N	When no para-aortic irradiation: V40 Gy <250 cm³ V30 Gy <500 cm³ For para-aortic irradiation: V40 Gy <300 cm³ V30 Gy <650 cm³
Sigmoid	D_{max} <105%		D_{max} <105% in regions outside 10–15 mm from PTV-N	
Bladder	D_{max} <105%	V40 Gy <60% V30 Gy <80%	D_{max} <105% in regions outside 10–15 mm from PTV-N	V40 Gy <60% V30 Gy <80%
Rectum	D_{max} <105%	V40 Gy <75% V30 Gy <95%	D_{max} <105% in regions outside 10–15 mm from PTV-N	V40 Gy <75% V30 Gy <95%
Spinal Cord	D_{max} <48 Gy		D_{max} <48 Gy	
Femoral Heads	D_{max} <50 Gy		D_{max} <50 Gy	
Kidney	D_{mean} <15 Gy	D_{mean} <10 Gy	D_{mean} <15 Gy	D_{mean} <10 Gy

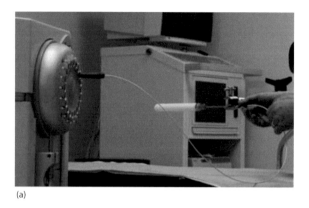

(a)

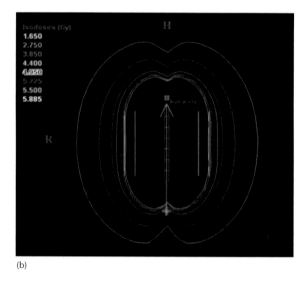

(b)

FIGURE 33.5   (a) Vaginal cylinder applicator for HDR brachytherapy with (b) dose distribution from an applicator 3 cm (W) × 3 cm (dwell length) prescribed to 0.5 cm from the applicator surface.

Brachytherapy

Vaginal vault brachytherapy can be delivered using a vaginal cylindrical applicator (Figure 33.5), with the reference isodose covering at least the proximal 4 cm of the vagina. It is available in varying diameters and sizes. Cylindrical applicators can be loaded to treat any length of vagina required. Vaginal examination is performed to determine the size of the vaginal cylinder. The patient then undergoes a CT scan with the cylinder in situ to confirm optimal placement of the vaginal device and to identify any anatomical challenges. Subsequent insertions may be performed without image guidance.

A central uterine tube +/- vaginal applicator is commonly used to treat the primary tumour in the unoperated patient.

Dose Solutions

Conformal

With 3D target volume localisation, 3D dose planning can be used with individual shaping of each beam using MLC to spare normal tissues. One anterior, two lateral opposing and one partially weighted posterior beam are commonly used (Figure 33.6). Conformal radiotherapy significantly reduces the

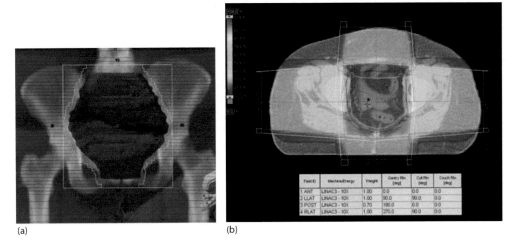

(a)   (b)

FIGURE 33.6 Postoperative radiotherapy for endometrial carcinoma. (a) DRR with anterior BEV. (b) Axial slice colour wash of the dose distribution using four-beam arrangement.

radiation dose to the rectum and bladder compared with conventional solutions, as well as avoiding geographical miss.

Complex

Pelvic IMRT or VMAT (Figure 33.7) has been shown to reduce the radiation dose to bladder, rectum and small bowel. This is especially important in the postoperative setting, with a reduction in acute and

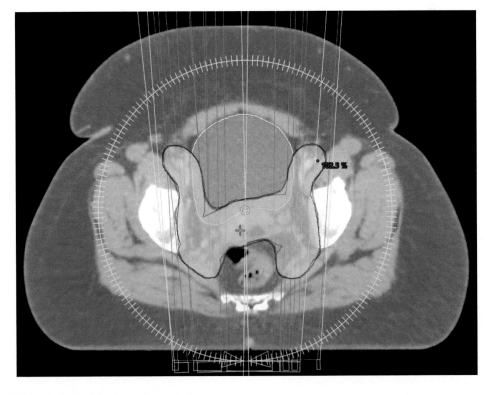

FIGURE 33.7 VMAT plan for postoperative EBRT.

late toxicity. It may also help to limit the dose to the pelvic bone marrow in patients undergoing radiotherapy with concomitant chemotherapy.

Simple

A 'brick' arrangement with four beams is commonly chosen (anterior, posterior and lateral opposing wedged beams), or, where possible, the posterior beam is omitted to reduce rectal dose. Higher energy photons (10–15 MV) are commonly employed and individual shielding used in the superior corners of the anterior beam to exclude small bowel and reduce normal tissue dose. Care should be taken to ensure that any shielding of the inferior corners to exclude femoral heads does not also shield the external iliac nodes. Shielding to the sacral nerve roots may be used posteriorly in the lateral beams.

Dose Fractionation

Adjuvant Radiotherapy

EBRT

- 45 Gy in 25 daily fractions of 1.8 Gy given in five weeks
- 50.4 Gy in 28 daily fractions of 1.8 Gy given in five and a half weeks

Vaginal vault brachytherapy as boost following EBRT for patients with cervical involvement. Brachytherapy should be delivered within 10–14 days of EBRT completion.

HDR

- 8–11 Gy to 0.5 cm from the applicator surface in 2 fractions

Vaginal vault brachytherapy as sole adjuvant treatment for selected intermediate risk patients:

HDR

- 21 Gy to 0.5 cm from the applicator surface in 3 fractions
- 22 Gy to 0.5 cm from the applicator surface in 4 fractions
- 12–30 Gy to 0.5 cm from the applicator surface in 3–8 fractions

Primary Radiotherapy

EBRT

- 45 Gy in 25 daily fractions of 1.8 Gy given in five weeks followed by intracavitary brachytherapy
- 50 Gy in 25 daily fractions of 2 Gy given in five weeks followed by intracavitary brachytherapy
- 50.4 Gy in 28 daily fractions of 1.8 Gy given in five and a half weeks followed by intracavitary brachytherapy

Simultaneous integrated boost to involved nodes using IMRT:

- 55–60 Gy in 25 daily fractions given in five weeks
- 57–60 Gy in 28 daily fractions given in five and a half weeks

Intracavitary brachytherapy following EBRT:

HDR

- 21 Gy in 3 fractions prescribed to the uterine serosa
- 25 Gy in 5 fractions prescribed to the uterine serosa
- 28 Gy in 4 fractions prescribed to the uterine serosa

EBRT Boost to Primary Tumour

Rarely, if intracavitary brachytherapy is not possible, EBRT may be followed by a second phase of treatment delivering an additional dose to the GTV using a conformal plan.

- 16–20 Gy in 8–10 daily fractions

Intracavitary brachytherapy alone in patients unfit for EBRT:

HDR

- 36 Gy in 5 fractions prescribed to the uterine serosa
- 37.5–42 Gy in 6 fractions prescribed to the uterine serosa

Para-aortic Radiotherapy

- 45 Gy in 25 daily fractions of 1.8 Gy given in five weeks

Vaginal Vault Recurrence

EBRT

- 45 Gy in 25 daily fractions of 1.8 Gy given in five weeks
- 50.4 Gy in 28 daily fractions of 1.8 Gy given in five and a half weeks

Vaginal vault brachytherapy boost:

HDR

- 15 Gy in 3 fractions to 0.5 cm from the applicator surface or to the depth of gross tumour

Palliative Radiotherapy

- 8–10 Gy as a single fraction
- 20 Gy in 5 fractions given in one week
- 30 Gy in 10 fractions given in two weeks

Treatment Delivery and Patient Care

Acute side effects may increase when radiotherapy is combined with concomitant chemotherapy. Diarrhoea or abdominal discomfort may occur during EBRT, and is usually managed with a low residue diet and loperamide hydrochloride. If these symptoms are severe, treatment may need to be interrupted to allow recovery. Care of the perineal skin is advised, but erythema and desquamation are now uncommon with 10–15 MV beams, unless the lower vagina is involved. Severe perineal or natal cleft skin reactions are treated with 1 per cent hydrocortisone cream and Intrasite gel. Less commonly, rectal discomfort or bleeding and urinary frequency or dysuria may occur, and a urinary specimen should be taken to exclude infection. A good fluid intake should be encouraged.

The risk of lymphedema is increased when EBRT is given to patients who have undergone pelvic lymphadenectomy. Premenopausal patients will lose ovarian function, and hormone replacement therapy may be given to improve menopausal symptoms and prevent osteoporosis. Psychosexual counseling may be helpful, as well as vaginal hydration gels and dilators to improve vaginal function. Chronic fatigue, pelvic pain and urinary or faecal urgency or incontinence are uncommon late effects of pelvic radiotherapy.

Verification

For conformal radiotherapy and IMRT, daily image guidance is recommended with cone beam CT for bone and soft tissue matching and online correction.

Key Trials

ASTEC Study Group, Kitchener H, Swart AM, et al. Efficacy of systematic lymphadenectomy in endometrial cancer (MRC ASTEC trial): A randomised study. Lancet 2009;373:125–136.

ASTEC/EN.5 Study Group, Blake P, Swart AM, et al. Adjuvant external beam radiotherapy in the treatment of endometrial cancer (MRC ASTEC and NCIC CTG EN.5 randomised trials): Pooled trial results, systematic review, and meta-analysis. Lancet 2009;373:137–146.

Creutzberg CL, Nout RA, Lybeert MLM, et al. Fifteen-year radiotherapy outcomes of the randomized PORTEC-1 trial for endometrial carcinoma. Int J Radiat Oncol Biol Phys 2011;81:e631–e638.

De Boer SM, Powell ME, Mileshkin LR, et al. Final results of the international randomized PORTEC-3 trial of adjuvant chemotherapy and radiation therapy (RT) versus RT alone for women with high-risk endometrial cancer. J Clin Oncol 2017;35:5502.

Hogberg T, Signorelli M, de Oliveira CF, et al. Sequential adjuvant chemotherapy and radiotherapy in endometrial cancer – results from two randomised studies. Eur J Cancer 2010;46:2422–2431.

Nout RA, Smit VT, Putter H, et al. Vaginal brachytherapy versus pelvic external beam radiotherapy for patients with endometrial cancer of high-intermediate risk (PORTEC-2): An open-label, non-inferiority, randomised trial. Lancet 2010;375:816–823.

Nout RA, van de Poll-Franse LV, Lybeert MLM, et al. Long-term outcome and quality of life of patients with endometrial carcinoma treated with or without pelvic radiotherapy in the post operative radiation therapy in endometrial carcinoma 1 (PORTEC-1) trial. J Clin Oncol 2011;29:1692–1700.

Reed NS, Mangioni C, Malmstrom H, et al. Phase III randomised study to evaluate the role of adjuvant pelvic radiotherapy in the treatment of uterine sarcomas stages I and II: An European Organisation for Research and Treatment of Cancer Gynaecological Cancer Group study (protocol 55874). Eur J Cancer 2008;44:808–818.

INFORMATION SOURCES

Klopp A, Smith BD, Alektiar K, et al. The role of postoperative radiation therapy for endometrial cancer: Executive summary of an American Society for Radiation Oncology evidence-based guideline. Pract Radiat Oncol 2014;4:137–144.

Meyer LA, Bohlke K, Powell MA, et al. Postoperative radiation therapy for endometrial cancer: American Society of Clinical Oncology clinical practice guideline endorsement of the American Society for Radiation Oncology evidence-based guideline. J Clin Oncol 2015;33:2908–2913.

Small W Jr, Mell LK, Anderson P, et al. Consensus guidelines for the delineation of the clinical target volume for intensity modulated pelvic radiotherapy in the postoperative treatment of endometrial and cervical cancer. Int J Radiat Oncol Biol Phys 2008;71:428–434.

34

Vagina

Indications for Radiotherapy

Primary carcinomas of the vagina are rare, accounting for less than 2 per cent of all cancers of the female genital tract. The majority are squamous cell carcinomas (SCCs) occurring in women over 60 years of age. Less common histologies include adenocarcinoma, melanoma and sarcoma. Clear cell adenocarcinomas of the vagina are seen in young women exposed to diethylstilbestrol in utero, the majority of which are stage I at diagnosis. More commonly, tumours found in the vagina are an extension from preexisting primary cervical, vulva or urethral malignancies or local spread from the rectum or bladder. Surgery is the mainstay of treatment for malignant melanomas of the vagina. These tumours have a high incidence of distant metastases and poor overall survival rates.

Vaginal intra-epithelial neoplasia (VAIN) may be multifocal, and most commonly involves the upper vagina. Untreated, VAIN3 may progress to invasive SCC of the vagina. VAIN can be treated with local ablation using carbon dioxide laser or diathermy, surgical excision or brachytherapy. Surgery is the preferred option, as it permits histological diagnosis, since invasive disease can be detected in up to a third of specimens. Vaginal brachytherapy is an effective treatment for patients with extensive multifocal disease along with those who have failed previous therapies or are unsuitable for organ-preserving surgery.

Surgery has a role in the management of selected patients with stage I and II disease, primarily lesions located at the apex, upper posterior or upper lateral third of the vagina. This usually involves a radical upper vaginectomy and bilateral pelvic lymphadenectomy with radical hysterectomy if the uterus has not previously been removed. An inguino-femoral lymphadenectomy is required for tumours involving the lower third of the vagina. Adjuvant radiotherapy should be considered if the surgical margins are positive for tumour. Surgery is the treatment of choice for patients with vesico-vaginal or recto-vaginal fistula at diagnosis. Pelvic exenteration with vaginal reconstruction is sometimes performed in those with locally advanced, residual or recurrent disease. Ovarian transposition before radiotherapy can help to preserve ovarian function in the premenopausal patient.

Radiotherapy is the treatment of choice for most patients with invasive vaginal tumours, especially those with lesions greater than 2 cm in diameter or involving the mid to lower vagina, as radical surgery may not achieve adequate margins without compromising bladder and/or rectal function. Small, well-differentiated, superficial (less than 5 mm thick), stage I lesions can be treated with intracavitary brachytherapy alone. All other disease stages require either combined external beam radiotherapy (EBRT) and brachytherapy or EBRT alone to treat the primary tumour and regional lymph nodes. Interstitial brachytherapy can be considered for lesions with depth of invasion greater than 5 mm. In addition, concomitant chemotherapy with cisplatin is used with EBRT for locally advanced disease.

Radiotherapy gives overall survival rates of 44–77 per cent, 34–48 per cent, 14–42 per cent and 0–18 per cent for stage I, II, III and IV disease, respectively. Most relapses after radiotherapy occur locally and cure rates are dose dependent. Palliative EBRT is given to control bleeding or pain from advanced primary tumours or vaginal metastases. Intracavitary or interstitial brachytherapy can also be used for palliation of vaginal mucosal disease.

Sequencing of Multimodality Therapy

If primary surgery is used and adjuvant radiotherapy is indicated, radiation should begin four to six weeks postoperatively or when adequate wound healing has taken place. Locally advanced non-metastatic tumours are managed with curative EBRT and concomitant chemotherapy with cisplatin followed by HDR brachytherapy boost.

Clinical and Radiological Anatomy

More than 50 per cent of vaginal tumours arise from the posterior wall of the upper third of the vagina and spread laterally into the paravaginal tissues (Figure 34.1). They can also invade directly into the adjacent bladder and rectum. Lymphatic spread from the upper part of the vagina is to the obturator nodes, from the posterior wall to the presacral nodes, and from the anterior wall to the lateral pelvic wall nodes. The lymphatics of the lower third of the vagina drain via the vulval lymphatics to the inguino-femoral and iliac nodes. Lower-third tumours can also directly invade the urethra and anus. Positive pelvic nodes are present in 25–30 per cent of patients with stage II disease, necessitating EBRT along with brachytherapy.

Assessment of Primary Disease

Clinical examination of the entire vaginal mucosa and cervix is made by colposcopy and multiple biopsies are taken from the primary tumour and any suspicious areas. For patients with invasive carcinoma, staging and assessment must include bimanual pelvic and rectovaginal examination, cervical biopsy and examination under anaesthesia, cystoscopy and sigmoidoscopy where indicated. The inguino-femoral region is examined for lymphadenopathy and needle aspiration of palpable nodes performed to obtain cytology. CT or MRI can be used to assess for lymph node involvement along with the size and extent of the primary tumour and to exclude distant metastases. [18F] 2-fluoro-2-deoxy-D-glucose PET-CT has a high sensitivity and specificity for detecting nodal and distant metastases. It can be used in place of CT prior to curative radiotherapy in locally advanced tumours to evaluate the extent of nodal involvement, and this can in turn facilitate radiotherapy target volume delineation and selection.

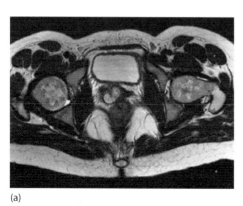
(a)

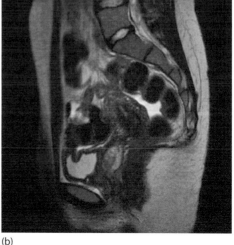
(b)

FIGURE 34.1   T2-weighted MR images of a patient with stage II clear cell adenocarcinoma of the vagina arising from the right posterior wall of the upper third. (a) Axial and (b) sagittal views.

Data Acquisition

Patients are scanned supine. Movement is limited by leg immobilisation with anterior and lateral tattoos to prevent lateral rotation. With patient in the treatment position, radio-opaque markers are placed at the inferior extent of the vaginal tumour and at the introitus. Variations in bladder volume have been shown to influence mobility and position of the uterus, cervix and vagina, and a protocol should be used to maintain constant bladder filling. Patients are asked to empty their bladder and drink 200 mL of water 20 minutes before their scan and treatment each day. Patients are also encouraged to empty their bowels before CT scanning and each treatment, and this may require the use of enemas/laxatives. Intravenous contrast is used to enhance the pelvic blood vessels, which are used as surrogates for the pelvic lymph nodes when delineating the CTV-N. CT scans are acquired from the superior border of L3 to 5 cm below the introitus.

Target Volume Definition

CT Planning

GTV-T is the primary vaginal tumour as defined by clinical examination, EUA, CT and co-registered MRI scan. CTV-T includes the entire vagina, cervix and paravaginal tissues with a 20-mm isotropic margin around the GTV-T, edited to exclude uninvolved anorectum, bladder, bones and pelvic muscles. For tumours of the lower third of the vagina, the introitus is also included. CTV-N encompasses different lymph node regions, depending on the site of the primary tumour:

- For tumours of the upper two-thirds of the vagina – obturator, external, internal and common iliacs and presacral lymph nodes
- For tumours of the lower third of the vagina – inguino-femoral and distal external iliac nodes
- For tumours involving the posterior vaginal wall – presacral nodes in addition to the preceding

These are delineated by identifying the contrast-enhanced pelvic blood vessels on each CT slice and using a 7-mm margin to create a 3D CTV-N.

A CTV to PTV margin of 10–15 mm is used around the CTV-T to allow for organ motion of the cervix and vagina and setup uncertainties. For CTV-N, organ motion occurs to a lesser extent and a 7-mm CTV to PTV margin is usually sufficient for setup variations. The simultaneous integrated boost technique may be used in those with involved nodes or whose primary tumour is not suitable for brachytherapy boost. In such cases, a 5–10-mm margin is added to the GTV to create the boost PTV. Bladder, rectum, small bowel and femoral heads are outlined as organs at risk.

Brachytherapy for well-defined tumours: CTV-T = GTV-T + 2 cm margin along the vaginal wall.

Brachytherapy for large/multicentric tumours: CTV = entire vaginal cavity.

After EBRT, brachytherapy is used to deliver a further localised high-dose boost. When the volume of residual tumour precludes brachytherapy, further EBRT is delivered using a conformal plan with a 10-mm margin around macroscopic disease to create the PTV.

Conventional Planning

Where CT is not available for planning, all clinical, surgical, histological and radiological data must be used to define the tumour extent before determining the beam borders using a simulator. Palpation of the primary tumour is performed with the patient in the treatment position and the inferior tumour extent and introitus are marked with radio-opaque material. AP and lateral simulator films are taken.

For tumours of the upper two-thirds of the vagina, the CTV should include the entire vagina, paravaginal tissues, cervix and the obturator, external and internal iliac and presacral lymph nodes. The superior border of the treatment beam is at the L5/S1 junction, lateral borders are 20 mm lateral to the bony pelvic sidewall and the inferior border is at the introitus or at least 3–4 cm below the most caudal aspect of the primary tumour. The anterior border should encompass the GTV-T and iliac nodes superiorly and is usually at the anterior one-third of the symphysis pubis. The posterior border is 20 mm from the GTV-T and internal iliac nodes and is commonly situated 5 mm posterior to the anterior border of the S2/3 vertebral junction. When tumours involve the posterior wall of the vagina, the presacral nodes are included, and the border should be placed posterior to these nodes and the GTV.

For tumours of the lower third of the vagina, the volume should include the entire vagina, introitus, paravaginal tissues, inguino-femoral and distal external iliac nodes. The superior border is at the upper acetabulum to include the inguinal nodes, inferior border is 30 mm below the introitus and the lateral borders should cover the femoral heads to include the femoral nodes.

Dose Solutions

Conformal

For all tumours of the vagina, a conformal plan is used with MLCs to avoid normal organs, especially small bowel. IMRT will provide the best solution for pelvic nodal treatments; it is also of value to patients with prosthetic hips. The simultaneous integrated boost or concomitant boost technique is recommended for those with involved nodes and/or tumour not amenable to subsequent brachytherapy.

Simple

For conventional treatment of upper vaginal tumours, four mega-voltage photon beams are commonly used (anterior, posterior and two laterals); for lower-third tumours, where CTV-N includes inguinal nodes, anterior and posterior opposing beams can be used, unequally weighted to spare the rectum and increase dose anteriorly to the inguino-femoral regions.

Brachytherapy

Cylindrical vaginal applicators can be used to deliver intracavitary brachytherapy for VAIN or superficial tumours that are less than 5 mm deep. Where tumours are more than 5 mm deep, interstitial brachytherapy is required. Interstitial implants using the Paris system are described in Chapter 5. Needles are placed approximately 1 cm apart with the aim of encompassing the tumour volume with margins of 1 cm. Brachytherapy for tumours of the upper third of the vagina is delivered using the same technique as for cervical carcinomas, with a central intrauterine tube and vaginal applicators, as discussed in Chapter 32. For HDR vaginal brachytherapy, patients will also undergo MRI and CT scans with applicators in situ to confirm optimal placement of device and to identify gross tumour post-EBRT.

Palliation

For palliation of locally advanced fixed and fungating, bleeding or recurrent vaginal tumours, either EBRT or, when technically feasible, brachytherapy can be given. Radiotherapy is limited to the GTV with a 15-mm PTV margin to reduce toxicity using conformal planning where possible or CT-simulated anterior and posterior opposing beams. Bony landmarks can also be used to define the treatment beams with the superior border at the bottom of the sacroiliac joints, inferior border at the introitus and lateral borders at the pelvic sidewalls.

Dose Fractionation

EBRT

- 45 Gy in 25 daily fractions of 1.8 Gy given in five weeks
- 50 Gy in 25 daily fractions of 2 Gy given in five weeks
- 50.4 Gy in 28 daily fractions of 1.8 Gy given in five and a half weeks

Simultaneous integrated boost (SIB) IMRT to involved nodes:

- 55–60 Gy in 25 daily fractions given in five weeks
- 57–60 Gy in 28 daily fractions given in five and a half weeks

SIB-IMRT to primary tumour if brachytherapy is not feasible:

- 55–63 Gy in 25 daily fractions given in five weeks
- 57–65 Gy in 28 daily fractions given in five and a half weeks

Sequential external beam boost to primary tumour if brachytherapy not feasible:

- 16–20 Gy in 8–10 daily fractions of 2 Gy given in one and a half to two weeks

Sequential external beam boost to macroscopic nodes if SIB-IMRT not available:

- 5.4 Gy in 3 daily fractions given in three days
- 10.8 Gy in 6 daily fractions given in one and a half weeks

HDR Brachytherapy Boost After EBRT

- $3–4 \times 7$ Gy or $3–6 \times 5$ Gy twice weekly (25–40 Gy EQD2)

Brachytherapy Alone for Stage I Tumours

HDR brachytherapy:

- 6×7 Gy or 8×5 Gy twice weekly (50–60 Gy EQD2) to GTV + 10–20-mm margin along the vaginal wall or entire vagina for multicentric tumours

If insufficient tumour regression, an additional boost to the GTV may be given:

- $1–2 \times 7$ Gy or $3–4 \times 5$ Gy twice weekly (10–25 Gy EQD2)

Palliative Radiotherapy

- 8–10 Gy as a single fraction
- 20 Gy in 5 daily fractions given in one week
- 30 Gy in 10 daily fractions given in two weeks

Treatment Delivery and Patient Care

These are category one patients when treated with curative intent. Treatment duration must not be prolonged by more than two days over the original prescription.

Patients are treated with the same bladder and bowel protocol and immobilisation devices as at CT scanning or simulation and aligned using three tattoos and laser lights to avoid lateral pelvic rotation. Care must be taken to ensure that the inferior border of the treatment fields encompass the distal extent of the tumour.

Acute perineal and natal cleft skin reactions are common and can be severe, and are treated with 1 per cent hydrocortisone cream. If moist desquamation occurs, treatment may need to be suspended and Intrasite gel used to promote healing, with morphine for pain control. Diarrhoea, abdominal pain, cystitis, proctitis and rectal bleeding may occur. Infections are excluded, loperamide hydrochloride prescribed and a low residue diet advised, as appropriate. Patients should be warned in advance of the 4–10 per cent risk of vesico-vaginal or recto-vaginal fistulae formation, which may occur especially with more advanced tumours invading the bladder or rectal wall. Patients should be encouraged to use vaginal rehydration gels and dilators to maintain vaginal function once treatment is completed and the acute reaction has settled, as vaginal fibrosis can lead to narrowing and shortening of the vagina and sexual dysfunction. There is an 11 per cent risk of necrosis of the femoral heads at five years when opposing anterior and posterior beams are used in an elderly population to treat inguinal nodes.

Verification

Daily image guidance is recommended with cone beam CT for bone and soft tissue matching.

INFORMATION SOURCES

Chyle V, Zagars GK, Wheeler JA, et al. Definitive radiotherapy for carcinoma of the vagina: Outcome and prognostic factors. Int J Radiat Oncol Biol Phys 1996;35:891–905.

Lee WR, Marcus RB Jr, Sombeck MD, et al. Radiotherapy alone for carcinoma of the vagina: The importance of overall treatment time. Int J Radiat Oncol Biol Phys 1994;29:983–988.

Mock U, Kucera H, Fellner C, et al. High-dose-rate (HDR) brachytherapy with or without external beam radiotherapy in the treatment of primary vaginal carcinoma: Long-term results and side effects. Int J Radiat Oncol Biol Phys 2003;56:950–957.

Perez CA, Grigsby PW, Garipagaoglu M, et al. Factors affecting long-term outcome of irradiation in carcinoma of the vagina. Int J Radiat Oncol Biol Phys 1999;44:37–45.

Pingley S, Shrivastava SK, Sarin R, et al. Primary carcinoma of the vagina: Tata Memorial Hospital experience. Int J Radiat Oncol Biol Phys 2000;46:101–108.

35

Vulva

Indications for Radiotherapy

Vulva cancer is a relatively uncommon neoplasm, constituting 5 per cent of malignancies arising from the female genital tract. The vast majority of cases are squamous cell carcinomas (SCCs), typically affecting older women. Vulva SCC is primarily a surgical disease. The goals of management are to treat the primary tumour and sites of potential lymph node metastasis.

Early Stage Disease

Patients with SCC of the vulva commonly present with early-stage T1, T2, N0 disease. Surgery is the mainstay of treatment with radical excision of the primary lesion. This can be achieved with wide local excision for early-stage disease and radical vulvectomy for larger or multicentric lesions. If microscopic residual disease is present in the vulva following initial surgery, a re-excision is recommended to obtain complete clearance. If re-excision is not possible, postoperative radiotherapy is administered with or without concomitant chemotherapy. In cases of close but uninvolved surgical margins, adjuvant vulva radiotherapy or re-excision may be considered to reduce the risk of local tumour recurrence. There is a lack of consensus on the margin threshold below which adjuvant vulva radiotherapy should be advised. A retrospective study has revealed a recurrence risk of 47 per cent with surgical margins of less than 8 mm and 0 per cent with surgical margins of 8 mm and greater. Adjuvant radiotherapy reduced the rate of local tumour recurrence to 16 per cent for patients with involved or close surgical margins. The two-year survival rate after developing a local recurrence is poor, at 25 per cent.

Inguino-femoral lymph node dissection (LND), with the removal of the superficial inguinal and deep femoral nodes, should be performed if the primary tumour is greater than 2 cm in maximum diameter or has a depth of invasion of greater than 1 mm. LND is not required for verrucous tumours or FIGO stage 1A SCCs. Sentinel lymph node biopsy (SLNB) can be performed in place of LND in unifocal vulva SCC with a maximum diameter of less than 4 cm and no clinical or radiological suspicion of lymph node involvement. Unilateral LND will suffice for lateral lesions with medial borders greater than 1 cm from the midline. Contralateral LND or nodal radiotherapy is required if the ipsilateral nodes are subsequently found to be involved by cancer. Indications for postoperative nodal radiotherapy with or without concomitant chemotherapy include metastases in two or more lymph nodes, extracapsular nodal extension and complete tumour replacement of any node. Primary nodal radiotherapy is used if upfront surgery is not possible due to fixed or ulcerated groin nodes. Fine-needle aspiration cytology should be obtained from clinically palpable inguinal nodes to confirm malignant involvement prior to primary nodal radiotherapy. Lymph node metastasis is the single most important prognostic factor in vulva cancer. Primary radiotherapy is also used in medically inoperable patients.

Locoregionally Advanced Tumours

Primary radiotherapy with concomitant chemotherapy can be used to 'downstage' locoregionally advanced vulva cancer to facilitate curative surgery. It can be employed as part of a sphincter preservation approach in cases where upfront surgery risks sphincter damage, urinary and faecal incontinence. Primary radiotherapy with concomitant chemotherapy is also the treatment of choice for patients with unresectable disease. Surgery can be considered in these cases if there is resectable residual disease following primary chemoradiotherapy. Patients with good performance status and involved inguino-femoral, external iliac, internal iliac or obturator nodes should be offered curative radiotherapy with concomitant chemotherapy. Curative radiotherapy with concomitant chemotherapy may be offered to those with involved common iliac or lower para-aortic nodes in highly selected cases.

Locoregional Recurrence

The preferred treatment for local/regional nodal recurrence is surgical excision followed by postoperative radiotherapy with concomitant chemotherapy where possible. Primary radiotherapy with concomitant chemotherapy can be considered if the recurrent tumour is not surgically resectable.

Palliative Radiotherapy

Palliative radiotherapy can be used to treat locally advanced fixed, fungating or bleeding tumours in patients not fit for curative radiotherapy with concomitant chemotherapy.

Sequencing of Multimodality Therapy

Postoperative radiotherapy should commence as soon as possible, ideally within four to six weeks of surgery. For those with stage III and IVA disease, primary radiotherapy with concomitant chemotherapy is recommended. If primary radiotherapy is used to downstage locoregionally advanced tumours, surgery should follow four to six weeks after treatment completion.

Clinical and Radiological Anatomy

The vulva forms part of the female external genitalia and consists of the mons pubis, labia majora, labia minora, clitoris, vestibule, vaginal introitus and Bartholin's glands. Most tumours of the vulva involve the labia majora. Lymphatics from the majority of the vulva drain initially into the superficial inguinal nodes followed by the deep femoral nodes. Regional lymph node metastases occur early. The superficial inguinal nodes are involved in 20–30 per cent of patients with early-stage disease. Tumour involvement of the midline structures of the vulva, such as the clitoris, may lead to bilateral groin node involvement; this is also present in 25–30 per cent of patients with a positive ipsilateral groin node. Occasionally, there is direct tumour spread to the pelvic nodes via the internal pudendal vessels. Direct tumour extension into the adjacent structures such as the vagina, urethra, anus, bladder and rectum are less common than lymph node spread. Blood-borne metastases are uncommon in the absence of lymph node involvement and occur late in the course of the disease.

Assessment of Primary Disease

Careful clinical examination of the vulva and the entire pelvis and perineum is essential, with biopsies taken from any suspicious areas along with a deep biopsy of the primary tumour for histological confirmation of invasive disease and assessment of the depth of invasion. Cervical cytology and inspection of the cervix, vulva, vagina and anus should also be performed.

The extent of the primary tumour is assessed by clinical examination, with anatomic drawings of the tumour location and extent, together with an MRI scan of the pelvis (Figure 35.1). Examination under anaesthesia, cystoscopy and proctoscopy may be required for locally advanced tumours. The inguino-femoral region is examined for lymphadenopathy. Fine needle aspiration of palpable nodes is performed to distinguish malignancy from infection. SLNB can be performed instead of LND in selected patients with stage IB or II tumours. FDG PET-CT may aid radiotherapy treatment planning and nodal selection for radiotherapy in locally advanced disease. Patients are assessed for their ability to tolerate curative treatment.

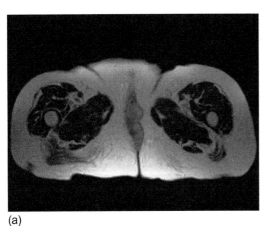

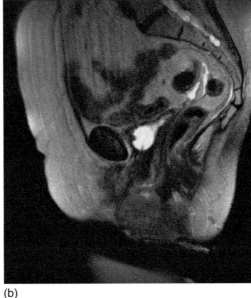

(a)   (b)

FIGURE 35.1   Stage III carcinoma of the vulva showing disease around the urethral catheter suggestive of urethral involvement. (a) Axial and (b) sagittal T2-weighted MR scans.

Data Acquisition

Patients are immobilised supine on a CT scanner with anterior and lateral tattoos to prevent pelvic rotation. The vulva tumour and surgical scars are wired. Bowel preparation is recommended to ensure that the rectum is not distended. Intravenous contrast is administered to outline the pelvic blood vessels.

When using a simulator, clinical examination in the treatment position is essential, with radio-opaque material marking the extent of the macroscopic tumour and lymph nodes. The introitus should also be marked with radio-opaque material to aid localisation of the inferior border of the CTV and treatment field.

Target Volume Definition

Primary Radiotherapy

Phase I

The CTV-T (primary tumour CTV) consists of the entire vulva with a margin of at least 2–3 cm around the GTV. The entire vagina should be included if there is uncertainty over the proximal extent of the vaginal involvement. Similarly, the entire urethra and bladder neck should be included in tumours involving the mid or proximal urethra. The CTV-N (nodal CTV) comprises all involved lymph node regions plus the echelon above the highest involved node. It should also include the inguinofemoral, obturator, internal and external iliac nodes. The pelvic blood vessels are used as surrogates for nodes and a 7-mm margin is created around these vessels to define the CTV-N. The inguinal region is contoured as a compartment (laterally – the medial border of the iliopsoas; medially – the lateral border of the adductor longus and the medial end of the pectineus; posteriorly – the iliopsoas muscle and the anterior aspect of the pectineus muscle; anteriorly – 20-mm margin on the inguinal vessels). The following nodes are also included in specific circumstances: presacral nodes from S1–3 for tumours involving the proximal half of the posterior vaginal wall or anal canal and perirectal nodes if the GTV involves the anus. If bilateral nodal irradiation is required, the CTV should include the same lymph node regions on both sides of the pelvis.

Phase II

A 'boost' dose is delivered to the primary tumour and macroscopically involved nodes. The boost PTV comprises the GTV with margins of 2–3 cm. Interstitial brachytherapy may be used to deliver this boost in selected patients, especially if the tumour involves the lower vagina.

Adjuvant Radiotherapy

Radiotherapy is given to the vulva alone for close or involved resection margins if re-excision is not possible and bilateral inguinofemoral LND are negative. Surgical findings and histopathology results are used to define the target volume. The CTV should include the entire surgical bed and excision scar with a 2-cm margin around areas of microscopic residual disease. For adjuvant nodal irradiation, the CTV should comprise the inguinofemoral, obturator, internal and external iliac nodal regions.

The CTV-PTV margin for both primary and adjuvant radiotherapy will be 10–15 mm, depending on measured setup errors within each department.

If the simulator is used, the superior field border is placed above the acetabulum to include the distal external and internal iliac nodes, the inferior field border is 2 cm below the vulva marker, and the lateral field borders are placed to cover the femoral heads/greater trochanters. This can be followed by smaller anterior and posterior opposing photon beams to deliver a 'boost' dose to areas of gross disease. The inguinofemoral nodes lie at a depth of 5–8 cm from the skin surface and a direct electron beam can be used as 'boost' treatment with the electron energy selected using information from CT scans.

Organs at Risk

Dose Constraints

- Bladder – V40 <60%, V30 <80%
- Bowel – V40 <250 cm^3, V30 <500 cm^3
- Femoral heads – D$_{max}$ <50 Gy
- Rectum – V40 <75 %, V30 <95 %

Dose Solutions

Conformal/Complex

For photon therapy to the vulva and lymph nodes, the target volume is irregular, lying anteriorly at the inguinal nodes, with deep extension to the femoral and pelvic lymph nodes. Treatment is usually delivered using 3-dimensional conformal radiotherapy (Figure 35.2) or IMRT. IMRT is particularly useful in patients with prosthetic hips to minimise rectal dose. Adaptive radiotherapy may be necessary if there is substantial tumour shrinkage or vulva oedema from treatment. Bolus may be required over the primary tumour and vulva to ensure adequate dose to the gross tumour or areas of involved surgical margins, especially with the skin-sparing effect of higher energy beams. It should also be used where there is skin involvement by tumour or superficially located lymph nodes.

Simple

If anterior and posterior opposing fields are used, unequal weighting, such as 2:1 anterior to posterior, may be helpful to increase the dose to the anterior structures.

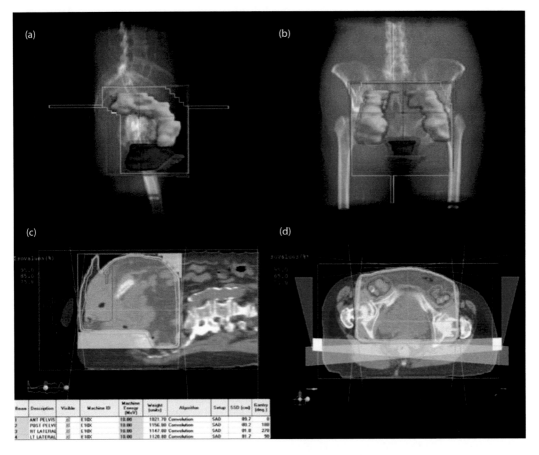

FIGURE 35.2 Treatment of T3N2G2 locally invasive carcinoma of the vulva and inguino-femoral and pelvic nodes showing GTV, CTV and PTV with bolus (pink), on (a) lateral and (b) anterior DRRs and (c) sagittal and (d) axial CT scans with four-beam configuration. (Courtesy of Dr Frances Calman and Marium Naeem.)

Dose Fractionation

Primary Radiotherapy

Phase I Dose

- 45 Gy in 25 daily fractions of 1.8 Gy given in five weeks
- 50 Gy in 25 daily fractions of 2 Gy given in five weeks
- 50.4 Gy in 28 daily fractions of 1.8 Gy given in five and a half weeks

Subsequent surgery is performed where possible or, alternatively, further radiotherapy to the primary tumour and involved nodes is given.

Phase II 'Boost' to the Primary Tumour and Involved Nodes

- 15–20 Gy in 8–10 fractions given in one and a half to two weeks aiming for a total dose of 60–65 Gy

Adjuvant Radiotherapy

- 45 Gy in 25 daily fractions of 1.8 Gy given in five weeks
- 50 Gy in 25 daily fractions of 2 Gy given in five weeks
- 50.4 Gy in 28 daily fractions of 1.8 Gy given in five and a half weeks

'Boost' to areas of residual gross disease

- 15–20 Gy in 8–10 daily fractions given in one and a half to two weeks

Palliative Radiotherapy

- 8 Gy in a single fraction
- 20 Gy in 5 fractions over one week
- 30 Gy in 10 fractions over two weeks

Treatment Delivery and Patient Care

Acute reactions of the vulva skin are common and can be severe. They should be managed with 1 per cent hydrocortisone cream. If moist desquamation occurs, treatment may need to be interrupted and Intrasite gel used to promote healing with morphine given for pain relief. Urinary frequency, dysuria, proctitis and diarrhoea are other possible side effects, which should be treated symptomatically. Late vulva fibrosis and atrophy may occur. Lymphoedema can occur in up to 30 per cent of patients when both inguinofemoral surgery and radiotherapy are used.

Verification

For conformal radiotherapy and IMRT, daily image guidance is recommended with cone beam CT for bone and soft tissue matching.

INFORMATION SOURCES

Beriwal S, Coon D, Heron DE, et al. Preoperative intensity-modulated radiotherapy and chemotherapy for locally advanced vulvar carcinoma. Gynecol Oncol 2008;109:291–295.

Beriwal S, Heron DE, Kim H, et al. Intensity-modulated radiotherapy for the treatment of vulvar carcinoma: A comparative dosimetric study with early clinical outcome. Int J Radiat Oncol Biol Phys 2006;64:1395–1400.

Faul CM, Mirmow D, Huang Q, et al. Adjuvant radiation for vulvar carcinoma: Improved local control. Int J Radiat Oncol Biol Phys 1997;38:381–389.

Gaffney DK, King B, Viswanathan AN, et al. Consensus recommendations for radiation therapy contouring and treatment of vulvar carcinoma. Int J Radiat Oncol Biol Phys 2016;95:1191–1200.

Glaser S, Olawaiye A, Huang M, et al. Inguinal nodal region radiotherapy for vulvar cancer: Are we missing the target again? Gynecol Oncol 2014;135:583–585.

Heaps JM, Fu YS, Montz FJ, et al. Surgical-pathologic variables predictive of local recurrence in squamous cell carcinoma of the vulva. Gynecol Oncol 1990;38:309–314.

Kim CH, Olson AC, Kim H, et al. Contouring inguinal and femoral nodes; How much margin is needed around the vessels? Pract Radiat Oncol 2012;2:274–278.

Montana GS, Thomas GM, Moore DH, et al. Preoperative chemo-radiation for carcinoma of the vulva with N2/N3 nodes: A Gynecologic Oncology Group study. Int J Radiat Oncol Biol Phys 2000;48:1007–1013.

Moore DH, Thomas GM, Montana GS, et al. Preoperative chemoradiation for advanced vulvar cancer: A phase II study of the Gynecologic Oncology Group. Int J Radiat Oncol Biol Phys 1998;42:79–85.

Rao YJ, Chundury A, Schwarz JK, et al. Intensity modulated radiation therapy for squamous cell carcinoma of the vulva: Treatment technique and outcomes. Adv Radiat Oncol 2017;2:148–158.

Van der Zee AG, Oonk MH, De Hullu JA, et al. Sentinel node dissection is safe in the treatment of early-stage vulvar cancer. J Clin Oncol 2008;26:884–889.

36

Sarcoma

Indications for Radiotherapy

Bone and soft tissue sarcomas are a heterogenous group of rare tumours of mesenchymal origin, accounting for less than 1 per cent of all cancers. More than 50 per cent of cases occur in the extremities; 35 per cent in the trunk, abdomen and retroperitoneum; and 10–15 per cent in other miscellaneous sites.

There are more than 50 different subtypes of soft tissue sarcomas, identified through histological examination, immunocytochemistry, cytogenetics and molecular pathology. The most significant prognostic factors are tumour size and grade. Recurrence following previous complete excision also confers a worse prognosis.

Surgery is the main treatment modality for soft tissue sarcoma, aiming for margins of 1–2 cm without sacrificing critical structures such as bone and the neurovascular bundle. The wider the surgical margins, the lower the risk of local failure. Following R1 resection, re-excision should be considered. The alternative to re-excision is adjuvant radiotherapy. The local recurrence rate following limb-sparing surgery alone for soft tissue sarcoma is approximately 30–50 per cent. Predictors of local recurrence include positive or close resection margins, high-grade tumours, unfavourable histology and tumour size greater than 5 cm. The addition of postoperative external-beam radiotherapy to limb-sparing surgery results in an improvement in local tumour control. With postoperative radiotherapy, no difference in local control and overall survival is detected between limb-sparing surgery and amputation. Thus, combined modality treatment is recommended for most cases of extremity soft tissue sarcoma, as it helps to preserve limb function by negating the need for amputation. Indications for postoperative radiotherapy include:

- Grade 2 or 3 tumours
- Tumours located in the deep muscle compartment
- Tumours greater than 5 cm in size
- Any grade tumour following marginal excision with margins of less than 1 mm where further surgery is either not possible or will likely result in functional defect

Postoperative radiotherapy can be omitted for low-grade tumours excised with histological margins of greater than 1 cm. For low-grade tumours excised with close margins, either re-excision or postoperative radiotherapy is required, depending on the impact of further surgery on limb function; surveillance may be an option if the tumour is superficial. All patients with locally recurrent disease or whose initial excision was performed without proper staging/imaging will require postoperative radiotherapy. Preoperative radiotherapy is preferred for tumours located close to neurovascular bundles where upfront surgery is likely to result in close or positive margins. Preoperative radiotherapy may not significantly reduce the tumour size; however, it may facilitate R0 resections and reduce the risk of intra-operative tumour rupture. Inoperable tumours are treated with initial radiotherapy, with subsequent surgery undertaken if marked tumour shrinkage makes this possible. In some sites, surgery may never be feasible and definitive radiotherapy is the treatment of choice.

The main treatment modality for osteosarcoma, chondrosarcoma and chordoma is surgery. In the case of osteosarcoma, peri-operative chemotherapy is used in addition to surgery. Indications for radiotherapy in osteosarcoma include unresectable tumours and positive resection margins where further surgery is not possible. Chondrosarcoma and chordoma are relatively radio-resistant tumours, and if surgery is not possible, referral to an appropriate centre for consideration of proton beam therapy should be made. If radiotherapy is to be used, high doses of at least 65 Gy are required for local control, and the best results are achieved in patients with small-volume residual disease following surgery.

Sequencing of Multimodality Therapy

The timing of radiotherapy in relation to definitive surgery in extremity soft tissue sarcoma has been studied in a randomised trial. The primary end-point of this trial was the presence or absence of major wound complications. There was no difference in local tumour control, progression-free survival and overall survival between preoperative and postoperative radiotherapy, although the trial was not powered to evaluate these end-points. Acute wound healing complications were twice as common with preoperative radiotherapy (35 per cent versus 17 per cent) and these were confined to patients with tumours in the thigh. However, preoperative radiotherapy resulted in lower rates of late toxicities and better long-term limb function, with less fibrosis (31.5 per cent versus 48.2 per cent), oedema (15.5 per cent versus 23.2 per cent) and joint stiffness (17.8 per cent versus 23.2 per cent). This was due to the lower radiation doses and smaller treatment volumes with preoperative radiotherapy. Preoperative radiotherapy also has the advantage of a tumour volume which is easier and more accurate to define with no risk of tumour spillage or surgical contamination, which would have required wider treatment margins. Moreover, acute wound complications are transient and manageable, whereas late toxicities tend to be chronic and irreversible. For retroperitoneal tumours, preoperative radiotherapy may result in less toxicity to the small bowel, as it is displaced by the gross tumour away from the radiation volume. Such small bowel commonly falls back into the radiotherapy target area following tumour resection.

Following preoperative radiotherapy, surgery should ideally take place four to six weeks after treatment completion to minimise wound complications. If postoperative radiotherapy is required, it should commence within 12 weeks of surgery.

The radical treatment of osteosarcoma consists of induction combination chemotherapy followed four to six weeks later by surgery or radiotherapy if the tumour is unresectable for technical or medical reasons. Adjuvant chemotherapy usually commences within 12 weeks of surgery.

Clinical and Radiological Anatomy

As soft tissue sarcomas may occur in any part of the body, treatment must take into account site-specific factors as well as sarcoma-related ones. Relevant anatomical details can be found in the various other chapters of this book. In the extremities, soft tissue sarcoma tends to spread in a longitudinal fashion within muscle groups. They tend not to breach barriers such as bone and fascia. Distant spread is frequently haematogenous to the lungs and, less commonly, through lymphatics to the regional lymph nodes.

Assessment of Primary Disease

Careful clinical examination is followed by plain X-ray for bone sarcomas to localise the tumour and assess the stability of the bone. For all patients with sarcoma, the tumour is imaged using ultrasound, CT and/or MRI, and a biopsy is performed at the same time under image guidance. CT and MRI are used to assess the relation of the tumour to bone and other soft tissues, most importantly the nerves and blood vessels (Figure 36.1). CT scan is also used to rule out metastases in the lungs, which are the commonest sites for metastatic spread except in epithelioid sarcoma (regional nodes), and angiosarcoma

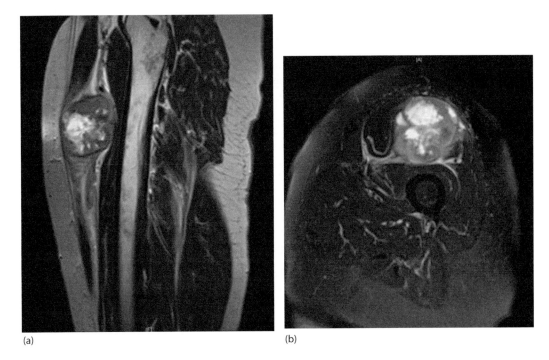

(a)   (b)

FIGURE 36.1 Preoperative MR scan of pleomorphic sarcoma in left vastus lateralis in (a) coronal and (b) axial views.

where subdermal spread makes treatment volume definition difficult. Sperm cryopreservation should be offered to male patients with tumour in the pelvis or thigh who wish to preserve their fertility. Ovary cryopreservation should also be considered for young women receiving pelvic radiotherapy. A spacer may be inserted prior to radiotherapy to displace bowel away from the treatment area for retroperitoneal sarcomas. For patients requiring postoperative radiotherapy, a preoperative MRI scan performed ideally not more than four weeks prior to surgery will aid radiotherapy treatment planning.

Data Acquisition

Immobilisation

Patient positioning and immobilisation technique are individualised based on the anatomical site and location of the primary tumour. Patients are discussed at pre-planning meeting with the radiographers and physicists to determine optimal patient positioning and immobilisation. Treatment position is usually supine, although the prone position may be preferred for tumours of the posterior trunk. Customised and comfortable immobilisation devices are required to ensure stable and reproducible positioning and to minimise setup uncertainties. For tumours of the upper or lower limbs, shoulder girdle, head and neck or trunk, individually prepared vacuum-formed polystyrene bags or Perspex shells are employed. Laser lights are used to minimise rotational movement, and cranio-caudal movement is prevented through the use of appropriate foot or hand restraints.

CT Planning

If possible, preoperative and pre-radiotherapy diagnostic imaging, such as gadolinium-enhanced MRI, should be acquired in the same position as the planning CT in order to facilitate co-registration or fusion of these images for radiotherapy treatment planning (aids GTV delineation and reconstruction).

The planning CT scan should cover the entire tumour region, surgical bed and scar (marked with a wire). For soft tissue sarcoma of the limbs, the entire adjacent bone should be included in the planning CT for organ at risk delineation. The use of intravenous contrast may aid GTV definition in patients undergoing preoperative radiotherapy. Changes in the anatomy and muscle configuration following surgery need to be taken into consideration, and it is important for both the surgeon and radiation oncologist to plan such treatments jointly.

Target Volume Definition

Preoperative Radiotherapy for Soft Tissue Sarcoma

The GTV is contoured using information from gadolinium-enhanced T1-weighted diagnostic MRI images. The CTV comprises the GTV with 3–4 cm longitudinal margins and 2–3 cm radial margins (Figure 36.2). For non-limb sites, the CTV is created by adding a 2–3-cm isotropic margin around the GTV. The CTV should include peri-tumoural oedema, identified on T2-weighted MRI images, as they may contain satellite tumour cells (except in cases of generalised oedema of the extremity secondary to tumour compression of the lymphatics). The CTV should not extend beyond muscle compartments and anatomical boundaries to tumour spread such as intact fascial barriers and uninvolved bone, joints and skin surface.

Postoperative Radiotherapy for Soft Tissue Sarcoma

The preoperative GTV is reconstructed on the planning CT with the help of the preoperative diagnostic MRI images, paying particular attention to the location and extent of the primary tumour before surgical resection. It should also take into account information obtained from the operation notes, resection histology, clinical photographs, postoperative anatomical changes, position of all visible surgical clips and possible tumour growth between preoperative imaging and surgery. The postoperative seroma should not be used as a surrogate for GTV reconstruction. Two CTVs are defined: the elective CTV and the boost CTV. The longitudinal margins for the elective CTV are 5 cm from the preoperative GTV or 0.5–1 cm from the scar, whichever is longer. Axial margins are 2–3 cm from the preoperative GTV or 0.5 cm over fascial or bone boundary if the GTV abuts these structures. For non-limb sites, the elective CTV is created by adding a 2–3-cm isotropic margin around the GTV. The elective CTV should include all surgically disturbed tissues, flaps, seroma, surgical scars and clips along with biopsy and drain sites, especially in high-risk, large (>5 cm) and high-grade tumours. It may be reasonable to omit drain site coverage in selected lower-risk cases such as low-grade tumours resected with generous margins or if the increase in treatment volume significantly enhances the anticipated risk of late radiation toxicity. Likewise, in some cases, it may not be feasible to include the entire length of the scar within the elective CTV if it extends the treatment volume significantly. If lymphocele or haematoma are present, a discussion with the surgeon is required to determine whether these should be included in the elective CTV. The CTV should not extend beyond anatomical boundaries to tumour spread such as intact fascial barriers and uninvolved bone, joints and skin surface. The boost CTV is defined in the same way as the elective CTV except for the longitudinal/craniocaudal extent where 2 cm margins are used. There is therefore no need to include the surgical scar, biopsy and drain sites in the boost CTV. For non-limb sites, aim to achieve a volume reduction for the boost CTV if feasible, although commonly this is not possible. Very large tumours (which may be 15–20 cm long in the extremities) may render the CTV, defined using the aforementioned method, prohibitively large. Thus, it may not be possible to encompass the scars and surgically disturbed tissues in full. In this situation, radiotherapy target volumes may be restricted to high-risk areas, for example around the neurovascular bundle. A normal tissue corridor of un-irradiated tissue should be maintained for limb tumours to minimise the risk of lymphoedema. This should be as large as feasible and no smaller than 1 cm in width.

CTV-PTV isotropic margins of 7–10 mm are added, depending on positional stability, the type of immobilisation and image guidance used and the reproducibility of setup. Larger PTV margins may be

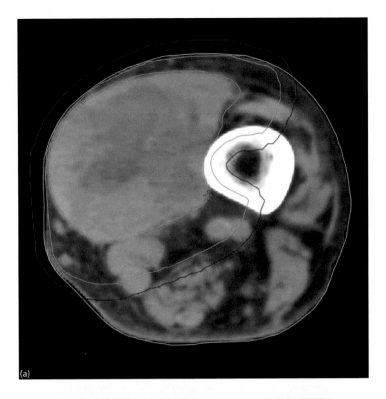

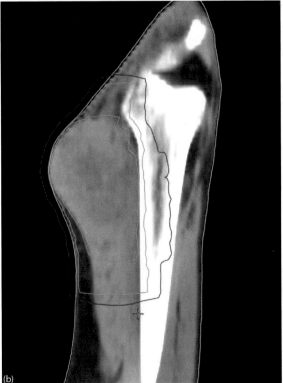

FIGURE 36.2 Preoperative radiotherapy of a pleomorphic sarcoma of the lower limb showing the GTV (orange), CTV (pink) and PTV (red) in (a) axial and (b) coronal views.

required for chest, abdominal trunk wall or shoulder girdle tumours. OARs will vary according to the location of the primary tumour.

Mandatory constraints include:

- Normal tissue limb corridor (longitudinal strip of skin and soft tissue from 2 cm above to 2 cm below the PTV as an avoidance structure to limit the radiation dose to a proportion of the limb outside of the treatment target volumes to allow sparing of lymphatic drainage and to minimise the risk of lymphoedema as a late toxicity) – V20 <50 per cent
- Brachial plexus – mean dose <60 Gy, maximum (D0.1 cc) dose <65 Gy

Optional constraints include:

- Bone within the treatment field (entire cross-section of the bone on the same CT slices as the PTV) – V50 ≤50 per cent.
- Whole bone adjacent to the tumour – mean dose ≤40 Gy, V40 ≤64 per cent.
- Femoral head and neck (from the top of the femoral head to the inferior aspect of the lesser trochanter) – mean dose ≤40 Gy.
- Joint – V50 ≤50 per cent (dose to be kept as low as possible).
- The genitalia should also be contoured as an organ at risk and avoided as much as possible. In males, it should be moved away from the treatment area and sperm cryopreservation should be offered if the testes are at risk of receiving a radiation dose.

The UK randomised phase III VORTEX study is designed to assess whether a reduction in the volume of tissue irradiated postoperatively improves limb function without compromising local tumour control in patients with extremity soft tissue sarcoma.

For simple palliative radiotherapy, the GTV is contoured. Margins of 10 mm axially and 10–20 mm cranio-caudally are added to the GTV to create the PTV.

Definitive Radiotherapy for Osteosarcoma

The GTV is the visible tumour extent on diagnostic imaging, with the CTV comprising the GTV + 2–3-cm margins, edited to take into account barriers to tumour spread.

Postoperative Radiotherapy for Osteosarcoma

The GTV is reconstructed using information from preoperative imaging, operation note and resection histology. The CTV comprises the GTV + 2–3-cm margins. The longitudinal CTV extent may need to be increased if scar + 0.5–1 cm is longer.

CTV-PTV margins of 7–10 mm are added, depending on positional stability, the type of immobilisation and image guidance used and the reproducibility of setup.

Dose Solutions

Conventional

Treatment plans are individualised, although simple arrangements of parallel opposing pairs of angled beams may be used for limb lesions. If possible, the exit beams should avoid the contralateral limb. Care should also be taken to leave a corridor of skin and subcutaneous tissues unirradiated to maintain lymphatic drainage of the distal limb and to minimise the risk of lymphoedema. Bolus should not be used except where there is skin involvement by tumour.

Conformal

As long as 3D imaging and planning are available, all treatments should be planned conformally, even though in some cases, beam arrangements may still be simple (Figure 36.3). If possible, part of the circumference of the limb should be treated to a lower dose to minimise the risk of lymphoedema. More complex beam arrangements may be necessary in cases where a reduction of radiation doses to normal structures or improved dose homogeneity is required. Patients requiring urgent radiotherapy may be treated using plans to mid-plane dose for up to 5 fractions before moving on to an optimised plan.

Complex

The use of IMRT in soft tissue sarcoma of the extremities is safe and results in excellent local tumour control. IMRT is particularly useful for sarcomas arising in sites such as the retroperitoneum or spine where a steep dose gradient between the tumour and adjacent OARs is required, or where a concave or convex dose distribution will help spare vital tissues such as the spinal cord. There is trial evidence to

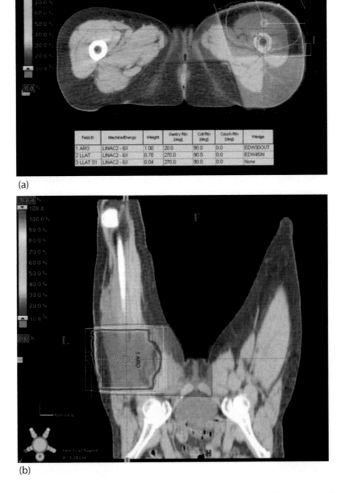

(a)

(b)

FIGURE 36.3 (a) Axial and (b) sagittal dose distribution for treatment of pleomorphic sarcoma of the left vastus lateralis.

show that IMRT results in significantly less late toxicities and morbidities compared with 3D conformal radiotherapy. If respiratory motion is significant, 4D-CT as well as some form of respiratory control such as gating, abdominal compression or breath-hold should be considered.

Brachytherapy

Postoperative brachytherapy alone without external-beam radiotherapy should not be used in the presence of R1 resection, skin involvement by tumour and inadequate CTV coverage due to suboptimal implant geometry.

Catheters are inserted into the tumour bed at the time of surgery and the target volume is determined intra-operatively using preoperative MRI. This usually consists of the tumour bed with 2-cm lateral margins and 2–5-cm longitudinal margins using the Paris system. The catheters are not loaded until the sixth postoperative day to permit wound healing.

Dose Fractionation

Preoperative Radiotherapy for Soft Tissue Sarcoma

- 50 Gy in 25 daily fractions given in five weeks

In cases of positive resection margins following preoperative radiotherapy, retrospective studies have shown high rates of local control even in the absence of postoperative boost and no improvement in local control with the addition of postoperative boost.

Postoperative Conformal Radiotherapy for Soft Tissue Sarcoma, Clear Resection Margins R0

- Elective PTV: 50 Gy in 25 daily fractions given in five weeks
- Boost PTV: 10 Gy in 5 daily fractions given in one week
- Total dose: 60 Gy in 30 daily fractions given in six weeks

In cases where the spinal cord, brachial or lumbar plexus or clinically significant amounts of bowel are within the PTV, the dose per fraction may be reduced to 1.8 Gy using the following fractionations:

- 50.4 Gy in 28 daily fractions given in five and a half weeks
- 59.4 Gy in 33 daily fractions given in six and a half weeks

For elderly patients and those with poor performance status:

- 55 Gy in 20 daily fractions given in four weeks
- 36 Gy in 6 once weekly fractions given in six weeks

Postoperative Conformal Radiotherapy for Soft Tissue Sarcoma, Positive Resection Margins R1

- Elective PTV: 50 Gy in 25 daily fractions given in five weeks
- Boost PTV: 16 Gy in 8 daily fractions given in one and a half weeks
- Total dose: 66 Gy in 33 daily fractions given in six and a half weeks

Postoperative IMRT for Soft Tissue Sarcoma, Clear Resection Margins R0

- Elective PTV: 52.2 Gy in 30 daily fractions given in six weeks
- Boost PTV: 60 Gy in 30 daily fractions given in six weeks

Postoperative IMRT for Soft Tissue Sarcoma, Positive Resection Margins R1

- Elective PTV: 53.5 Gy in 33 daily fractions given in six and a half weeks
- Boost PTV: 66 Gy in 33 daily fractions given in six and a half weeks

Definitive Radiotherapy for Inoperable Soft Tissue Sarcoma

- 66 Gy in 33 daily fractions given in six and a half weeks
- 50 Gy in 20 daily fractions given in four weeks
- 36 Gy in 6 once weekly fractions given in six weeks

Postoperative Radiotherapy for Osteosarcoma

- 60 Gy in 30 daily fractions given in six weeks

Definitive Radiotherapy for Inoperable Osteosarcoma

- 66–70 Gy in 33–35 daily fractions given in six and a half to seven weeks

Palliative Radiotherapy

- 40 Gy in 15 daily fractions given in three weeks
- 30–36 Gy in 5–6 once weekly fractions given in five to six weeks
- 30 Gy in 10 daily fractions given in two weeks
- 20 Gy in 5 daily fractions given in one week
- 8 Gy as a single fraction

Treatment Delivery and Patient Care

Skin reactions are common. This can be prevented through good skin care and reactions are treated with aqueous or 1 per cent hydrocortisone cream. Late effects of muscle fibrosis can be reduced through physiotherapy to encourage movement during treatment and for six to eight weeks thereafter. Other late effects include skin colour changes and telangiectasia, joint stiffness, lymphoedema which may affect limb function and an increased risk of bone fracture within the radiotherapy treatment area.

Verification

Daily KV portal imaging or cone beam CT depending on tumour site.

Key Trials

O'Sullivan B, Davis AM, Turcotte R, et al. Preoperative versus postoperative radiotherapy in soft-tissue sarcoma of the limbs: A randomised trial. Lancet 2002;359:2235–2241.

Pisters PWT, Harrison LB, Leung DH, et al. Long-term results of a prospective randomized trial of adjuvant brachytherapy in soft tissue sarcoma. J Clin Oncol 1996;14:859–868.

Rosenberg SA, Tepper J, Glatstein E, et al. The treatment of soft-tissue sarcomas of the extremities: Prospective randomized evaluations of (1) limb-sparing surgery plus radiation therapy compared with amputation and (2) the role of adjuvant chemotherapy. Ann Surg 1982;196:305–315.

Yang JC, Chang AE, Baker AR, et al. Randomized prospective study of the benefit of adjuvant radiation therapy in the treatment of soft tissue sarcomas of the extremity. J Clin Oncol 1998;16:197–203.

INFORMATION SOURCES

Al Yami A, Griffin AM, Ferguson PC, et al. Positive surgical margins in soft tissue sarcoma treated with pre-operative radiation: Is a postoperative boost necessary? Int J Radiat Oncol Biol Phys 2010;77:1191–1197.

Alektiar KM, Brennan MF, Healey JH, et al. Impact of intensity-modulated radiation therapy on local control in primary soft-tissue sarcoma of the extremity. J Clin Oncol 2008;26:3440–3444.

Dickie CI, Griffin AM, Parent AL, et al. The relationship between local recurrence and radiotherapy treatment volume for soft tissue sarcomas treated with external beam radiotherapy and function preservation surgery. Int J Radiat Oncol Biol Phys 2012;82:1528–1534.

Haas RLM, DeLaney TF, O'Sullivan B, et al. Radiotherapy for management of extremity soft tissue sarcomas: Why, when, and where? Int J Radiat Oncol Biol Phys 2012;84:572–580.

Tiong SS, Dickie C, Haas RL, et al. The role of radiotherapy in the management of localized soft tissue sarcomas. Cancer Biol Med 2016;13:373–383.

Wang D, Bosch W, Roberge D, et al. RTOG sarcoma radiation oncologists reach consensus on gross tumor volume and clinical target volume on computed tomographic images for preoperative radiotherapy of primary soft tissue sarcoma of extremity in Radiation Therapy Oncology Group studies. Int J Radiat Oncol Biol Phys 2011;81:e525–e528.

Wang D, Zhang Q, Eisenberg BL, et al. Significant reduction of late toxicities in patients with extremity sarcoma treated with image-guided radiation therapy to a reduced target volume: Results of Radiation Therapy Oncology Group RTOG-0630 trial. J Clin Oncol 2015;33:2231–2238.

37

Paediatric Tumours

General Considerations

Indications for Radiotherapy

Children who are cured of cancer have a long life expectancy, and treatment-related complications may be more severe than in adults. Although many paediatric tumours are very radiosensitive, current management protocols are designed to try to reduce the toxicity of treatment for those who can be cured and to increase the intensity of chemotherapy for those with poor outcome. Radiotherapy is therefore only used where it cannot effectively be replaced by surgery and chemotherapy. In very young children, even when radiotherapy will improve cure rates, it is often now deferred until the child is older as toxicity will be reduced because of greater maturity of organs and tissues.

Normal tissues in the period of development are more radiosensitive than adult normal tissues, and the relative sparing effect of low dose per fraction for late morbidity is therefore exploited using doses per fraction of 1.2–1.8 Gy. Sequential studies in various tumour types have led to reductions in total dose and target volumes. Nevertheless, radiotherapy is still an important component of curative therapy for many tumour types, and remains a valuable tool for easy and effective palliation.

Clinical trials have played a fundamental role in improving paediatric oncology outcomes. Patient enrolment into relevant clinical trials or registries is highly encouraged.

Sequencing of Multimodality Treatment

Depending on the tumour type and protocol, radiotherapy may be delivered before or after chemotherapy and/or surgery.

Assessment of Primary Disease

All patients must be treated at specialist centres with diagnostic and treatment expertise along with provisions for allied health professional care. Management should be based on agreed national or international protocols and must be discussed at an appropriate multidisciplinary team meeting. For certain tumour types, there are national advisory panels to provide support for the management of challenging and complex cases drawing expertise from experienced colleagues from various disciplines.

Data Acquisition

Immobilisation

Play specialists, specialist nurses and radiographers are essential for the preparation of all children for radiotherapy. Close collaboration is needed between paediatric and radiation oncologists. For very young children, adequate immobilisation may be difficult to achieve without anaesthesia, which increases the complexity of organising treatment. Anaesthesia needs to be provided by experienced paediatric anaesthetists who are familiar with the radiotherapy process to assure that treatments can be given safely and at the appropriate times. With adequate preparation and distraction, most children older than three years will learn to cope with the treatment satisfactorily without anaesthesia. Play specialists may help experienced mould room staff in making adjustments to normal practice to allow children who were initially apprehensive to become more at ease with the process. The final decision to deliver radiotherapy under anaesthesia is made on an individual basis depending on the need for immobilisation masks, complexity of treatment, maturity of the child and clinical status, irrespective of age.

Immobilisation may be achieved with thermoplastic masks and appropriate neck rests for the head and neck region or vacuum-moulded bags for the body. Limb positioning and immobilisation may require more thought, taking into consideration the likelihood of reproducibility, radiotherapy fields and technique used (for example irradiation of the lower limb requiring two lateral opposed fields may require the contralateral limb to be raised on a bridge).

CT Scanning

With the patient immobilised in the treatment position, CT scans are acquired through the region of interest (typically with 1–3 mm slice thickness). Appropriate diagnostic CT, MRI or functional imaging may be co-registered with planning scans and should include not only the whole tumour but the whole of any relevant organs at risk (OAR).

Dose Solutions

Treatment should always be as conformal as possible. Various modalities are now available with rapidly advancing technology, each with its own advantages and disadvantages. Therefore, the best modality should be carefully selected for the individual patient.

Three-dimensional conformal radiotherapy using MLC shaped beams, wedges, or field-in-field segments for dosimetric optimisation has largely replaced virtually simulated parallel opposed fields with midplane dose prescription, except in the palliative setting or urgent situations. IMRT solutions may produce better dose distributions with greater conformality of the high dose target volume and better sparing of OAR. However, they may result in increased low doses to larger volumes. There is concern about the potential risk of further increasing the incidence of second malignancies.

Proton therapy has the main advantage of having a finite range within tissue due to its unique Bragg Peak properties. As there is no exit dose, further sparing of healthy normal tissues can be achieved (Figure 37.1), resulting in the reduction of late effects (such as neurocognitive effects for young children with brain tumours) and risk of second malignancies. It is important to note that if an OAR is included within the target volume, the risk of late effects will be very similar to that of photons. The main disadvantage of proton therapy is that its dosimetry may be significantly affected by range uncertainties at the distal end of the beam due to radiobiological uncertainties, contour changes, density changes and interplay effects from respiratory motion. This could potentially result in unintended underdose to the target

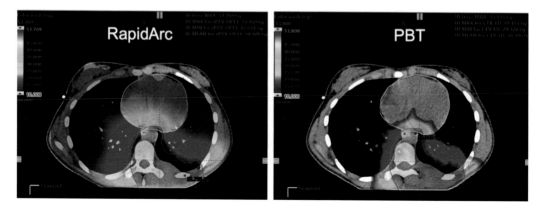

FIGURE 37.1 Intensity modulated radiotherapy plan using rapid arc technology versus pencil beam scanning proton beam therapy (PBT) plan at the low-dose (10 Gy) colour wash demonstrating the reduction of low-dose spill to the cardiac, lung and breast tissues with PBT.

volume or overdose to the OAR. Great care therefore must be taken in ensuring the selection of suitable patients, production of robust plans, avoidance of the distal beam ranging out into critical structures and employment of adaptive planning treatment pathways. Until recently, patients were referred abroad for proton therapy, but patients can now be referred to the two high-energy national proton beam centres in the UK – Manchester and London, both equipped with spot scanning technology.

Brachytherapy can be used in select cases where the tumour is small, localised, well defined and accessible. The most common indication is pelvic rhabdomyosarcomas (typically prostate/bladder neck), which have responded well to induction chemotherapy.

Dose Fractionation

Children should be treated by specialist teams working in collaboration with larger international and national groups. Details of treatment prescriptions are given in constantly revised protocols of the UK, European and American collaborative groups, which should always be consulted.

Treatment Delivery and Patient Care

If anaesthesia is needed, treatment should be given early in the morning to ensure that the necessary period of fasting before general anaesthesia happens during the night to avoid mealtimes. Attention must be paid to maintaining good nutritional status, especially if the treatment causes anorexia, nausea or vomiting. Central line access is needed. Medication for specific side effects for each tumour site is detailed in relevant chapters. Appropriate adjustments in dosage are made according to the weight of the child. The radiation oncologist should be involved in the follow-up of any child treated with radiotherapy to document late toxicity, the expression of which may be modified by continuing changes in chemotherapy practice.

Verification

On treatment position verification imaging (see Chapter 2) is usually performed for the first 3 fractions and sometimes weekly throughout treatment to ensure reproducibility, especially if the child is awake during treatment. There may be a necessity to utilise imaging modalities which allow accurate visualisation of soft tissues if complex, very conformal techniques are used.

The importance of radiotherapy quality assurance is increasingly recognised and is now a standard requirement for most paediatric multicentre clinical studies.

Special Considerations and Dose Constraints

It is important to maintain symmetry of growth of the spine by treating the vertebrae adjacent to the target volume homogenously across their whole width. The European consensus recommends that dose gradients to the adjacent vertebrae should be limited to <3 Gy for those under the age of two years or <5 Gy from two years until the end of pubertal acceleration phase. For dose prescriptions of more than 40 Gy, higher gradients may be allowed. For craniospinal irradiation, if the prescription is <25 Gy a posterior-anterior vertebrae gradient of <5 Gy is recommended; for prescriptions of >25 Gy, 20 Gy or more should be delivered to the vertebrae, or, alternatively, the dose gradient of a conventional photon plan can be mimicked.

Irradiation of the joints and unfused epiphyseal plates should be avoided wherever possible. Whilst these structures are traditionally shielded in conventional parallel opposed beam arrangements, with newer advanced complex techniques, the dose constraint is confined to V10 Gy <10 per cent.

For extremities, a strip of normal tissue corridor along the length of the limb should be spared to reduce the risk of lymphoedema.

Other commonly used paediatric specific dose constraints:

- Whole lungs – Mean ≤15–18 Gy, V20 Gy ≤25–30 per cent
- Heart – Mean ≤15 Gy, V25 Gy ≤10 per cent
- Liver – D50 per cent <20 Gy
- Spleen – Mean ≤10 Gy

- Combined kidneys – V20 ≤ 30 per cent, D_{mean} ≤15–18 Gy
- If only one kidney remaining – V14 Gy ≤10 per cent, D_{mean} ≤12–15 Gy

Baseline assessment of any normal organ function that may be affected by treatment must be undertaken to be used in monitoring of long-term effects. Fertility preservation options should be offered to patients and families where appropriate.

Certain chemotherapeutic agents may have potential synergistic or additive effects with radiotherapy. Actinomycin-D and doxorubicin should be omitted during radiotherapy and held for one to three weeks prior to and after radiotherapy, depending on the site treated and dose prescriptions. If high dose chemotherapy such as Busulfan and Melphalan (BuMel) regimen is used, radiation doses may need to be reduced for safety to maintain dose constraints to a maximum of:

- <45 Gy to gastrointestinal tract and rectum
- <50 Gy to bladder
- <30 Gy to spinal cord
- <36 Gy to cauda equina including sacrum and nerve roots
- Minimise any dose to the lung and avoid whole lung radiotherapy

EXTRACRANIAL SOLID TUMOURS

Wilms' Tumour

Indications for Radiotherapy

Wilms' tumour occurs in about eight per million children (80–90 cases per year in the UK), 70 per cent before the age of four and 90 per cent before age seven. The majority of Wilms' cases are sporadic but there is a strong association between Wilms', aniridia, genitourinary malformation and mental retardation in the WAGR (Wilms' tumour, aniridia, genitourinary abnormalities and mental retardation) syndrome, and in overgrowth syndromes such as Beckwith–Wiedemann and hemihypertrophy. Results of a series of randomised studies in Europe and the United States confirmed that:

- Preoperative radiotherapy reduces the risk of tumour rupture with increase in disease-free survival, but not overall survival.
- Preoperative chemotherapy is as effective as preoperative radiotherapy.
- Two drugs (vincristine and actinomycin) are better than one.
- Addition of a third drug (doxorubicin) improves outcome for high-risk and metastatic disease.

Treatment of this tumour is multimodal with surgery and chemotherapy, and in some cases radiotherapy. Actual sequencing of treatment varies between American and European studies, which have also used slightly different staging systems. The risk of biopsy tract seeding led the European groups to advocate chemotherapy without biopsy, but American groups are concerned about the 10 per cent incidence of misdiagnosis based on imaging alone.

Treatments are stratified by stage, histological subtype, tumour volume and treatment response into low-, intermediate- and high-risk groups. Majority of patients will be treated with induction chemotherapy followed by surgery. Postoperative radiotherapy is indicated based on histological subtype – low risk (completely necrotic), intermediate risk (all others), high risk (blastemal and diffuse anaplastic subtype) – and stage:

- Stage I – Limited to kidney, completely excised
- Stage II – Viable tumour extends beyond kidney capsule, completely excised

- Stage III – Residual disease after surgery, positive lymph nodes, positive margins, tumour rupture
- Stage IV – Haematogenous metastases
- Stage V – Bilateral kidney disease

Localised flank radiotherapy is recommended at two to four weeks post-nephrectomy (from week 7). The indications for radiotherapy are:

- Stage II high-risk (except blastemal subtype)
- Stage III intermediate and high-risk
- Stage IV, according to local stage

A boost is indicated if there is residual macroscopic disease after surgery.

Radiotherapy to the whole abdomen and pelvis is recommended if there is diffuse intra-abdominal tumour or gross tumour rupture.

In patients with pulmonary metastatic disease, whole lung radiotherapy should be given if there is still residual metastases after chemotherapy on the reassessment CT chest at week 10 or viable tumour at metastatic surgical clearance, or for any patient with high-risk histology regardless of metastatic response.

Metastases to other sites are rare. Radiotherapy may be used to treat liver metastases which are unresectable or show incomplete response to chemotherapy. Bone and brain metastases are irradiated regardless of chemotherapy response.

Survival rates are high – 90 per cent for stages I and II and 80 per cent for stage IV, so there has been a major emphasis on reducing treatment and its toxicity with a risk-stratified approach.

Assessment of Primary Disease

The most common presentation is with an asymptomatic abdominal mass (75 per cent), with pain (44 per cent), fever and haematuria occurring less commonly. The diagnosis must be differentiated from neuroblastoma by measurement of catecholamines, ultrasound and MRI. Staging includes chest X-ray and/or CT scan of the chest and measurement of renal function by DMSA scan. Biopsy is not always required unless there are unusual features.

Target Volume Definition

Flank Radiotherapy

GTV is defined as the tumour volume after chemotherapy but before surgery using co-registered MR-CT scans where available (Figure 37.2). The CTV is the GTV + 10 mm. PTV is individualised, taking into account departmental measurements of systematic errors. Care is taken to irradiate the vertebrae symmetrically, taking the volume across the midline to the lateral extent of the vertebral body and taking precautions to spare the remaining contralateral kidney.

If there were positive lymph nodes (stage III), the entire length of the para-aortic chain should be included (T10/11 interspace to aortic bifurcation).

Boost

GTV is based on the postoperative CT/MRI scan with a 10-mm margin for the CTV.

Whole Lung Radiotherapy

The CTV is both the lungs including apices and costo-diaphragmatic recesses. Humeral heads should be excluded.

Whole Abdomen and Pelvic Radiotherapy

The CTV volume should include peritoneal surfaces from the diaphragm superiorly to the level of the obturator foramen inferiorly. Dose to the acetabulum and femoral heads should be minimised.

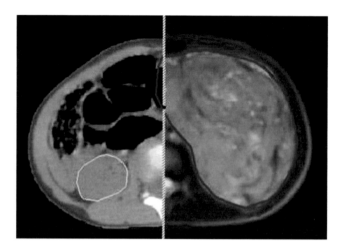

FIGURE 37.2   Fused CT/MR images of Wilms' tumour of left kidney. (Images courtesy of Dr M Gaze).

Dose Solutions

Flank Radiotherapy

Conventional optimised AP/PA beam arrangements with MLC shaping are often still appropriate to produce symmetrical irradiation of the vertebrae, avoid the contralateral kidney and minimise whole body doses (Figure 37.3). There is growing interest in a reduced-volume IMRT technique, but careful planning with long-term follow-up evaluation is required to ensure there is no detriment to locoregional control.

Whole Lung Radiotherapy

Conventional AP/PA beam arrangements are still used at most centres. There may be opportunity for improved cardiac sparing with IMRT techniques. Figure 37.4 illustrates whole lung irradiation.

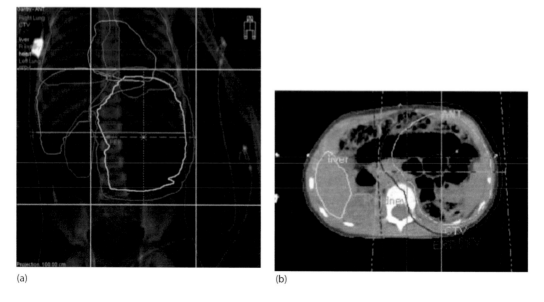

(a)   (b)

FIGURE 37.3   (a) Coronal DRR showing target volume and OAR for treatment of Wilms' tumour of the left kidney. (b) Axial CT scan showing AP/PA beam arrangement. (Images courtesy of Dr M Gaze).

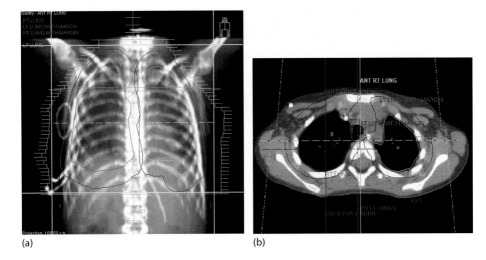

(a)   (b)

FIGURE 37.4   Whole lung irradiation. (a) Coronal DRR. (b) Axial CT scan showing AP/PA beam arrangement. (Images courtesy of Dr M Gaze).

Whole Abdomen and Pelvic Radiotherapy

Conventional AP/PA beam arrangements can be used with shielding of the kidney at 12 Gy. Rotational arc therapy techniques are being increasingly utilised, as the central dose to the kidney, liver and spleen may be further reduced. Figure 37.5 illustrates whole abdominal and pelvic radiotherapy dose distribution.

Dose Fractionation

The recommended dose fractionations are shown in Table 37.1. For very young children or extremely large volumes, individualised decisions may be made to reduce the dose per fraction to 1.2–1.5 Gy.

TABLE 37.1

Risk Adapted Radiotherapy Dose Fractionations for Localised and Metastatic Wilms' Tumour According to the CCLG Clinical Management Guidelines for Renal Tumours (Umbrella Study Protocol).

Localised

	Stage II	Stage III	Stage III (Major Rupture)
Intermediate Risk	No radiotherapy	Flank 14.4 Gy/8# +/- Boost 10.8 Gy/6#	WAPRT 15 Gy/10# +/- Boost 10.8 Gy/6#
High Risk *Diffuse Anaplastic*	Flank 14.4 Gy/8# +/- Boost 10.8 Gy/6#	Flank 25.2 Gy/14# +/- Boost 10.8 Gy/6#	WAPRT 19.5 Gy/13# +/- Boost 10.8 Gy/6#
High Risk *Blastemal Subtype*	No radiotherapy	Flank 25.2 Gy/14# +/- Boost 10.8 Gy/6#	WAPRT 19.5 Gy/13# +/- Boost 10.8 Gy/6#

Metastatic

	Whole Lung	Liver	Brain
Intermediate Risk	12 Gy/8#	Whole liver 14.4 Gy/8# +/- Boost 10.8 Gy/6#	WBRT 15 Gy/10# +/- Boost 10.5 Gy/7#
High Risk	15 Gy/10#	Whole liver 20–25.2 Gy/11–14# +/- Boost 10.8 Gy/6#	WBRT 25.2 Gy/14# +/- Boost 10.5 Gy/7#

Note: These are all given as daily fractions. *Abbreviations:* WAPRT = whole abdominal and pelvic radiotherapy, WBRT = whole brain radiotherapy.

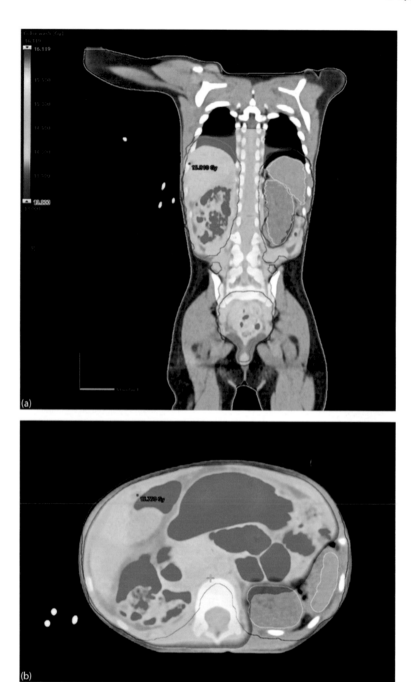

FIGURE 37.5   Whole abdominal and pelvic radiotherapy dose distribution using IMAT (intensity modulated arc therapy) technique in the (a) coronal and (b) axial sections. The prescribed dose was 15 Gy in 10 fractions. OAR constraints: remaining left kidney (light blue) mean 12 Gy and spleen (pink) mean 10 Gy.

Bone metastases may be irradiated to 30 Gy in 10 fractions or 30.6 Gy in 17 fractions.

If multiple areas need to be treated (i.e. flank plus lungs and/or liver) the treatments should be simultaneous to avoid the overlap of fields which would occur if the different areas were to be treated sequentially. For large radiotherapy fields, monitoring and supportive management of bone marrow suppression is required.

Neuroblastoma

Neuroblastoma is the most common extracranial solid tumour in children, with 80 per cent presenting before the age of four and 90 per cent before age ten, with a median of 22 months.

Indications for Radiotherapy

Tumours are now grouped by image-defined risk factors and histology, and survival is influenced by age and stage, with overall five-year survival rates of 44 per cent. Histology ranges from ganglioneuroma, which resembles normal organ architecture and requires little if any treatment, to undifferentiated neuroblastoma with MYCN amplification, which carries a poor prognosis. Neuroblasts are known to be radiosensitive in vitro but show variable sensitivity in vivo. There is little well-controlled trial data to define the role of radiotherapy, but review of studies undertaken showed reduction of risk of local relapse of between 22 per cent and 81 per cent. A study of chemotherapy alone versus chemotherapy and radiotherapy has shown improved overall survival rates when both modalities are used (41 per cent vs. 73 per cent).

Radiotherapy to the primary tumour or tumour bed is indicated in patients with high-risk disease and select intermediate risk disease. In general, these include patients aged over 18 months with stage M (metastatic) disease, undifferentiated or poorly differentiated localised disease or patients with MYCN amplification.

As these tumours may arise from a number of different sites, individualised planning must take into account all relevant normal tissue tolerances and possible late side effects.

Sequencing of Multimodality Treatment

Multimodality treatment includes initial chemotherapy followed by surgery, often high-dose chemotherapy and consideration of radiotherapy, finishing with immunotherapy with anti-GD2 monoclonal antibody and retinoic acid.

Assessment of Disease

Thirty-five per cent of neuroblastomas arise in the adrenal gland, 30 per cent from paraspinal ganglia, 19 per cent from the posterior mediastinal sympathetic chain and the rest in the neck or other sites. They originate from the primitive adrenergic neuroblast of neural crest tissues. Prognosis depends on histological type and differentiation, measurement of MYCN amplification and loss of heterozygosity (LOH) on chromosome 1p and 11q. Diagnosis is made on the basis of tumour imaging (MRI/CT scan) and measurement of urinary catecholamines, with biopsy to confirm histological subtype and for estimation of molecular markers of prognosis. MYCN is not just a marker of prognosis; it also determines risk stratification and therefore influences the selection of treatment. Meta-iodobenzylguanidine (^{123}I-MIBG) scans are used for staging and assessment of treatment response.

Target Volume Definition

Planning CT with intravenous contrast is recommended to allow for easier identification of the great vessels and its branches.

The GTV is defined as the post-chemotherapy, pre-surgical primary tumour volume and any immediately adjacent persistently enlarged lymph nodes as shown by MRI or CT imaging. Neuroblastoma tumours may lose MRI signal after responding to chemotherapy; therefore, CT imaging may be more helpful for tumour delineation, particularly in demonstrating abnormal calcification. Operation notes and histopathology reports should be taken into consideration to ensure adequate coverage of disease, which might not be apparent on imaging, usually at areas along the great vessels. The final volume should be edited off uninvolved normal organs such as the liver or kidneys, which have returned to their normal position after surgery.

CTV = GTV + 5 mm. This margin may include adjacent soft tissues (liver, kidney, vessels) where there is a risk of subclinical tumour spread. If a 4DCT is performed, internal motion may be considered on the ITV.

PTV = CTV/ITV + 5 mm or according to departmental protocols.

Consideration of potential growth impairment may require volumes to extend across the midline to preserve symmetry.

Dose Solutions

Simple opposing beam arrangements can be used but are usually limited by OAR tolerances of the liver and kidneys, resulting in an underdose of the target volume in some cases. IMRT techniques are now more commonly utilised to achieve an optimal plan. Proton therapy may be acceptable in carefully selected cases, which can be treated on plans with posterior fields to minimise uncertainties caused by passing through bowels which may vary in density during treatment.

Dose Fractionation

- 21.6 Gy in 12 daily fractions of 1.8 Gy given in two and a half weeks
- 21 Gy in 14 daily fractions of 1.5 Gy given in two and a half weeks

The benefits of dose escalation to 36 Gy in the context of macroscopic residual disease is currently under investigation.

Molecular Radiotherapy

Radioactive-labelled mIBG can be a useful treatment if scanning shows good uptake in tumour; 4 Gy to the whole body is given in two doses, the first determined by body weight (444 MBq/kg). The actual whole-body dose (WBD) achieved is then measured and the second dose adjusted to achieve the final desired WBD of 4 Gy. This can be administered with topotecan as a radiosensitiser. ^{131}I-mIBG therapy is usually used in relapsed disease but is now being investigated as an option for poorly responding disease.

Rhabdomyosarcoma

Indications for Radiotherapy

Seventy per cent of rhabdomyosarcomas occur before the age of ten with the peak incidence at two to five years of age. Radiotherapy improves local control rates compared with chemotherapy alone and is still necessary for cure in many patients. Radiotherapy plays an important role for local control of tumours with unfavourable histology, unfavourable site, those larger than 5 cm or those with regional nodal disease.

Local control is usually attained with surgery and/or radiotherapy. Only in very rare circumstances is induction chemotherapy sufficient (for example a fusion negative rhabdomyosarcoma of the vagina achieving complete remission with induction chemotherapy). Surgery may be used for easily resectable disease. Adjuvant radiotherapy is required if the planned surgical resection is marginal. If complete remission cannot be achieved by cosmetically and functionally satisfactory surgical excision after chemotherapy, definitive radiotherapy may be given instead. Radiotherapy is usually delivered after the fourth cycle of induction chemotherapy at week 13. Treatment decisions are always influenced by the need to minimise effects on normal tissues, and studies are underway to refine the indications for each component of the multimodality treatment.

In the metastatic setting, local therapy is considered after re-evaluation post six cycles of chemotherapy. Whole lung radiotherapy can be offered to patients with lung metastases only and whole abdomen and pelvic radiotherapy can be considered for patients with diffuse peritoneal involvement or malignant ascites. The role of systematically irradiating all sites of metastases where feasible is uncertain and is currently under investigation.

Sequencing of Multimodality Treatment

Patients are assigned to different treatment strategies according to known prognostic risk factors. Various combinations of induction chemotherapy are used either in the neoadjuvant or adjuvant setting.

Assessment of Primary Disease

These tumours may arise from many different sites in the body. Site of origin is a significant prognostic factor. Favourable sites include the orbit, genitourinary (bladder/prostate, paratesticular, vagina, uterus), head and neck (non-parameningeal) and biliary tumours. Unfavourable sites are parameningeal, extremities, abdomen, pelvis, retroperitoneum and trunk.

The two main histological subtypes are embryonal rhabdomyosarcoma (eRMS), which typically occurs in early childhood, and alveolar rhabdomyosarcoma (aRMS), which occurs mainly in the adolescent population. aRMS cases are associated with worse prognosis and majority demonstrate FOX01 gene fusion with PAX3 or PAX7. The use of gene fusion status is anticipated to replace traditional histopathology for risk stratification purposes.

Staging is according to the American Intergroup Rhabdomyosarcoma Study (IRS) definition:

1. Completely resected localised disease
2. Gross resection with microscopic residual and/or regional lymph node involvement
3. Incomplete resection, gross residual disease
4. Metastatic disease

MRI imaging is required to establish the locoregional extent of the primary tumour. [18]FDG-PET and CT chest are considered standard staging modalities for distant disease. CSF histology is required to exclude leptomeningeal disease in parameningeal cases.

Patients are categorised into low, standard, high and very high risk groups based on staging, site, size, age and histological (or biological) subtype.

Data Acquisition, Target Volume Definition and Dose Solutions

General principles of planning are applied depending on the site involved (see relevant chapters).

For treatment of the primary site after complete chemotherapy response or resection, the GTV includes the gross extent of the primary tumour at presentation. CTV = GTV + 10-mm expansion. The volume can be edited to take into account tumours that had shrunk after 'pushing' into a body cavity without invasion (e.g. chest wall lesion extending into pleural cavity displacing lung). For extremity tumours, a larger proximal and distal margin for CTV at 20 mm may be indicated.

In the case of residual macroscopic disease, a boost is indicated. The GTV boost volume is the extent of tumour after induction chemotherapy. CTV boost = GTV boost + 5 mm.

For nodal disease, the GTV includes the gross extent of nodal involvement at presentation. A 20–30-mm margin in the cranial and caudal direction following the nodal drainage should be applied to form the CTV.

Whole lung radiotherapy and whole abdominal radiotherapy volumes have been described earlier (see Wilms' section).

The most appropriate treatment technique should be chosen. Proton therapy and IMRT solutions are now commonly utilised to achieve highly conformal external radiotherapy plans. Brachytherapy may be considered for selected children with small tumours that have responded well to induction chemotherapy at implant-assessable sites such as the bladder/prostate or vagina.

Dose Fractionation

Adjuvant Radiotherapy to Primary Disease After R0/1 Resection

- 41.4 Gy in 23 daily fractions of 1.8 Gy given in four and a half weeks.

Definitive Radiotherapy After Complete Response

- 41.4 Gy in 23 daily fractions of 1.8 Gy given in four and a half weeks.

Definitive Radiotherapy with Residual Disease or R2 Resection

- 50.4 Gy in 28 daily fractions of 1.8 Gy given in five and a half weeks given at two dose levels.

- In two phases:
  - Phase 1: 41.4 Gy in 23 fractions (disease at presentation)
  - Phase 2: 9 Gy in 5 fractions (residual disease)
- As simultaneous integrated boost:
  - 42.5 Gy in 28 fractions (disease at presentation)
  - 50.4 Gy in 28 fractions (residual disease)

Nodal Disease

- 41.4 Gy in 23 daily fractions of 1.8 Gy given in four and a half weeks.

Boost is indicated for bulky residual disease – 9 Gy in 5 daily fractions of 1.8 Gy given in one week.

Whole Lung Radiotherapy

- 15 Gy in 10 daily fractions of 1.5 Gy given in two weeks.

Whole Abdomen and Pelvic Radiotherapy

- 24 Gy in 16 daily fractions of 1.5 Gy given in three and a half weeks.

Non-Rhabdomyosarcoma Soft Tissue Sarcoma

This is a highly heterogeneous group of patients. Surgery is the main treatment modality. Radiotherapy is indicated for synovial sarcomas and 'adult type' soft tissue sarcomas, depending on size, resection margins, grade and the age of the patient. A margin of 1–2 cm is usually required from GTV (disease at presentation) to CTV. Radiotherapy can be given preoperatively (50.4 Gy), postoperatively (50.4–54 Gy) or definitively (54–59.4 Gy) in 1.8 Gy daily fractions.

Desmoplastic Small Round Blue Cell Tumours

This is a rare and aggressive malignancy which commonly occurs in adolescent boys, typically presenting with large intra-abdominal mass with metastatic peritoneal dissemination. It is characterised by the EWS-WT1 gene fusion transcript associated with (t11; 22) (p13; q12) translocation. Treatment strategies include intensive induction chemotherapy, followed by radical surgical debulking where feasible. Consolidation with hyperthermic intraperitoneal chemoperfusion and/or whole abdominal and pelvic radiotherapy has been used although there is significant morbidity. Doses up to 30 Gy in 1.5 Gy daily fractions for whole abdominal and pelvic radiotherapy can be considered with simultaneous integrated boost to at-risk areas up to 36–40 Gy.

Ewing's Sarcoma

Indications for Radiotherapy

Chemotherapy is essential for control of systemic disease, which is the most common cause of treatment failure. All patients are treated within national or international protocols which use primary multi-agent induction chemotherapy, followed by local control strategy with maintenance chemotherapy concurrently or shortly thereafter.

The goal of achieving local control at initial therapy is important, as patients who relapse locally have a poor outcome, with survival of less than 25 per cent. Local control options are surgery alone, radiotherapy combined with surgery or definitive radiotherapy. The local therapy decision is usually complex, as the fine balance between the optimal chance of tumour control and the significant long-term treatment morbidity affecting function needs to be achieved.

- Surgery is preferred for selected sites where complete excision of all tissues involved at time of presentation is feasible. Intralesional excisions should be avoided as much as possible.
- Radiotherapy is used in conjunction with surgery if there is a marginal excision, positive margins (<1 mm), poor histological response (<90 per cent necrosis) or fracture at presentation. The decision on the timing of radiotherapy (preoperative or postoperative) very much depends on the anatomical site, type of surgical reconstruction required and the centre's experience.
- Definitive radiotherapy is indicated for unresectable tumours or in situations where surgery is extremely morbid (usually large pelvic tumours).

In the context of metastatic disease, whole lung radiotherapy should be offered to patients with lung metastases if it is the only site of distant disease. Chest wall tumours that present with an ipsilateral pleural effusion will require hemithorax radiotherapy, regardless of cytology. The decision to irradiate other metastatic sites in the oligometastatic setting is done on an individual basis depending on the chemotherapy response, symptoms and potential toxicity.

Assessment of Disease

Ewing's sarcoma in bone and soft tissue are characterised by a diagnostic (t11; 22) (q24; q12) chromosomal translocation associated with EWSR1/FLI1 gene fusion. They occur most commonly at the diaphysis of the long bones, followed by the pelvis, spine and chest wall (formerly known as Askin tumours). Most present with pain, swelling and sometimes systemic symptoms of fever and weight loss. They are diagnosed, as other sarcomas, by MRI (which clearly demonstrates the extent of soft tissue involvement which is a common finding), CT scanning and biopsy. Staging investigations must rule out metastases in bone, lungs, bone marrow, lymph nodes and other soft tissues. Lesions at a distance from the primary tumour may be found (skip lesions); therefore the entire long bone needs to be imaged.

Volume of primary tumour (>200 ml) and site (axial) are important prognostic factors, with bulky pelvic lesions carrying the worst prognosis. Patients with lung-only metastases have a better prognosis than those with bone metastases.

Data Acquisition, Target Volume Definition and Dose Solutions

Planning is carried out using the relevant principles outlined in site-specific chapters. MRI co-registered with CT scans gives the best definition of tumour extent.

Preoperative and Definitive Radiotherapy

GTV is defined as the pre-chemotherapy extent of disease. For pelvic and chest wall tumours where there are 'pushing margins', the GTV may need to be modified to reflect the new position of the surrounding organs such as the lungs and bladder returning to their normal positions after chemotherapy.

CTV is created by adding an isotropic 1.5–2-cm margin, encompassing any site of potential microscopic extension. The volume should be edited to consider barriers to tumour spread such as bone and fascial boundaries.

Postoperative Radiotherapy

A 'virtual' GTV is constructed as per the pre-chemotherapy extent of disease.

This is usually treated in two phases:

- The CTV1 is created by adding a margin of at least 1.5–2 cm around the virtual GTV. Since extension is primarily along the marrow cavity, it may be appropriate to create anisotropic margins with the greatest expansion in the long axis of the bone. If feasible, encompassing any potential contamination sites such as surgical scars, drain sites and metallic prosthesis is recommended. The decision to include the entire prosthesis or scar within the volume needs to be balanced with the anticipated morbidity of radiotherapy.
- The CTV2 is defined as the virtual GTV with a 1–2-cm margin, but does not need to include scars, drain sites or prosthesis.

Suitability of radiotherapy techniques is dependent on the site treated. Distal limb tumours are usually treated with 3D conformal plans to spare a strip of tissue along the limb to prevent lymphoedema. Pelvic tumours are better treated with proton therapy, as there is the potential of minimising toxicity to the bowel, bladder and genitalia.

Whole lung radiotherapy volumes and concepts have been described earlier (see Wilms' section).

Dose Fractionation

Radiotherapy in Combination with Surgery

Preoperative

- 50.4 Gy in 28 daily fractions of 1.8 Gy given in five and a half weeks

Postoperative

- PTV1 = 45 Gy in 25 daily fractions of 1.8 Gy given in five weeks
- PTV2 = 9 Gy in 5 daily fractions of 1.8 Gy given in one week

Definitive Radiotherapy

- 54 Gy in 30 daily fractions of 1.8 Gy given in five weeks

Boost (May Be Considered)

- 5.4 Gy in 3 daily fractions of 1.8 Gy given in half a week

Whole Lung Radiotherapy

- 15 Gy in 10 daily fractions of 1.5 Gy given in two weeks (<14 years)
- 18 Gy in 12 daily fractions of 1.5 Gy given in two and a half weeks (≥14 years)

Treatment Delivery and Patient Care

Principles are discussed in relevant site-specific chapters. Careful multidisciplinary surveillance is important during treatment. Diarrhoea and frequency of micturition may occur with pelvic irradiation. Gentle exercise should be encouraged during treatment of limb lesions to minimise fibrosis.

Osteosarcoma

Osteosarcoma most commonly arises from the long bones at the metaphyses, with its peak incidence in the teenage population. It is regarded as a radioresistant tumour and radiotherapy is rarely indicated. Chemotherapy and surgery are generally the mainstays of treatment. Radiotherapy is occasionally indicated in the adjuvant setting where there are positive margins (with no scope for re-resection) or contaminated margins such as a pathological fracture, or if the tumour is unresectable. Doses of >60 Gy at 1.8–2 Gy daily fractions are required.

HAEMATOLOGICAL MALIGNANCIES AND CONDITIONS

Hodgkin's Lymphoma

Indications for Radiotherapy

There has been a gradual reduction in the use of radiotherapy for lymphomas in childhood with the development of new effective chemotherapy combinations. The high rates of survival in children with Hodgkin's lymphoma has dictated recent treatment strategies which are aimed at reducing late effects. Given the risk of second tumours and morbidity with radiotherapy, the need and volume of radiotherapy required has been investigated. The EuroNet-PHL-C1 trial has confirmed that an interim PET-CT assessment scan can be used to safely omit radiotherapy. The EuroNet-PHL-C2 trial aims to assess if radiotherapy can be further reduced for a proportion of children with intensification of chemotherapy with the DECOPDAC regimen.

Patients are stratified into treatment risk groups (TL1, TL2 and TL3) dependent on their clinical stage and risk factors such as disease bulk, ESR and extranodal sites. All patients are treated with two cycles of OEPA (vincristine, etoposide, prednisolone and doxorubicin) followed by an early response assessment (ERA) PET-CT scan. No radiotherapy is required if the PET scan is negative. If the PET scan is positive, involved site radiotherapy (ISRT) to the disease at the time of presentation is recommended. In TL2 and TL3 groups, a boost is required if there is still residual disease at the late response assessment (LRA) PET scan at the end of chemotherapy.

In the C2 trial for which results are awaited, patients in the DECOPDAC arm receive radiotherapy only if the LRA PET scan at the end of chemotherapy is positive. An involved node radiotherapy (INRT) concept is used where only the PET-positive sites of ≥10 mm are irradiated.

Radiotherapy may also be given for palliation or as salvage therapy after chemotherapy failure.

Target Volume Definition

The GTV is the pre-chemotherapy extent of involved nodes at presentation. A 5-mm margin is applied to the CTV. This volume is edited to post-chemotherapy borders such as the mediastinum. If a boost is required, the GTV boost includes all LRA PET positive lesions of ≥10 mm. A 5-mm margin is applied for the CTV.

For patients with organ involvement (stage IV), radiotherapy is only required if these sites are still positive on the ERA PET. Please refer to the C2 trial protocol for further details on individual organ irradiation.

Dose Solutions

Plans with optimised AP/PA opposing beams are still used as the low dose bath of IMRT is a concern for children. Optimised IMRT plans with partial arcs or proton therapy may be preferable for some cases decided on an individual basis.

Dose Fractionation

Standard

19.8 Gy in 11 daily fractions of 1.8 Gy given in two and a half weeks. (1.5 Gy fractions may be used for very young children or very large volumes).

Boost

- 10 Gy in 5 daily fractions of 2 Gy given in one week.

INRT (If Received DECOPDAC Intensification)

- 28.8 Gy in 16 fractions of 1.8 Gy given in three and a half weeks.

Langerhans' Cell Histiocytosis

This is a disease in which it is believed that a common, as yet unidentified, pathogen triggers an aberrant immune response leading to lesions in single sites, or in multiple sites in the same system (for example bone) or several systems (skin, bone, lung, brain, etc.). These lesions are known to be radiosensitive, but immune modulating systemic treatment is now preferred to radiotherapy, which has a minor role for palliation of severe pain. For localised disease requiring treatment where surgery is impossible, or to abort severe functional deficits, as in the treatment of spinal cord compression, doses of 6–10 Gy in 1.5 Gy per fraction have been recommended.

Other indications for radiotherapy for haematological conditions such as total body irradiation +/- cranial or testicular boost and central nervous system irradiation are discussed in other chapters.

INFORMATION SOURCES

Botterberg T, Dieckmann K, Gaze M. Radiotherapy in Practice: Radiotherapy and the Cancers of Children, Teenagers and Young Adults, 1st ed. Oxford University Press, Oxford, 2021.

Children's Cancer and Leukaemia Group (CCLG) (UK). www.cclg.org.uk.

Children's Oncology Group (COG). www.childrensoncologygroup.org.

Euro Ewing Consortium (EEC). https://www.ucl.ac.uk/cancer/research/centres-and-networks/home-euro-ewing-consortium.

European Paediatric Soft Tissue Sarcoma Study Group (EPSSG). https://www.epssgassociation.it/en/.

European Society for Paediatric Oncology (SIOPE). https://siope.eu/.

Hoeben BA, et al. Management of vertebral radiotherapy dose in paediatric patients with cancer: Consensus recommendations from the SIOPE radiotherapy working group. Lancet Oncol 2019;20(3):e155–e166.

International Society of Paediatric Oncology (SIOP). https://siop-online.org/.

Pinkerton R, Matthay K, Shankar AG (eds). Evidence-Based Pediatric Oncology, 2nd ed. Blackwell Publishing, Oxford, 2007.

Quality and Excellence in Radiotherapy and Imaging for Children and Adolescents with Cancer across Europe in Clinical Trials (QUARTET). https://siope.eu/activities/joint-projects/quartet/.

Royal College of Radiologists. Good Practice Guide for Paediatric Radiotherapy, 2nd ed. The Royal College of Radiologists, London, 2018.

38

Radiotherapy for Benign Disease

The anti-proliferative and anti-inflammatory effects of radiotherapy can be exploited to provide symptomatic relief in a variety of benign diseases. Widely used in Germany, EBRT for benign disease is much less used elsewhere in the world. This may reflect concerns over the risk of radiation-induced malignancy, the lack of RCT evidence and an understandable focus on treating cancer. Most benign disease protocols use a relatively low dose applied with simple techniques to a small treated volume, and have a very small risk of causing malignant change in irradiated tissues, especially in older adults. Large case series provide evidence for considerable benefit in conditions that are often difficult to treat with drugs or surgery. Treatments for a number of conditions where radiotherapy is used in UK centres are described here.

Thyroid Eye Disease

Indications for Radiotherapy

Thyroid eye disease is an autoimmune-mediated inflammation of the extra-ocular muscles and retro-orbital tissues. It can be mild and self-limiting but can also threaten sight. Treatment to make the patient euthyroid is important. Steroids are the main therapy for moderate to severe disease, defined as two or more of the following: lid retraction ≥2 mm, moderate or severe soft-tissue involvement, exophthalmos ≥3 mm above normal for race and gender, inconstant or constant diplopia. Several small, randomized controlled trials have assessed the role of radiotherapy, but in patients with different severity of disease and with various other treatments. A European consensus group guideline recommends considering radiotherapy in moderate to severe disease that remains active after a course of intravenous steroids. Other options at this stage include immunosuppressive drugs such as cyclosporine or rituximab.

Technique

The patient is immobilized in a thermoplastic mask. The CTV is the bilateral extra-ocular muscles and retro-orbital tissues. There is no real dosimetric advantage to using anything more complicated than small bilateral opposed fields angled 5° posteriorly to avoid exit dose through the contralateral lens. Beam borders are specified by the 50 percent isodose at the front of the pituitary fossa and the 10 percent isodose at the posterior lens edge if virtual simulation is used. 20 Gy in 10 fractions is given over two weeks. Concomitant steroids reduce the risk of oedema or acute inflammation – e.g. prednisolone 20 mg daily for the duration of radiotherapy. Radiotherapy is contraindicated in people with diabetic retinopathy or severe hypertension. There is a small risk of causing a cataract even with low doses (Figure 38.1).

Dupytren's Disease and Ledderhose Disease

Indications for Radiotherapy

Palmar fibromatosis (Dupytren's) and plantar fibromatosis (Ledderhose) are benign proliferative disorders of the fascia of the hand and foot respectively. They present as subcutaneous nodules, cords and skin thickening and can progress to cause a flexion deformity. They are incurable but can progress very slowly.

DOI: 10.1201/9781315171562-38

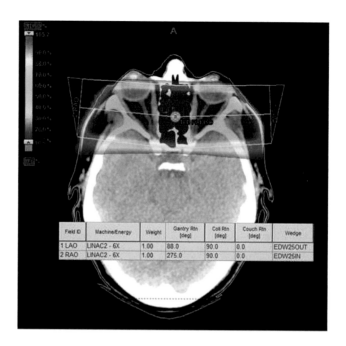

FIGURE 38.1   Beam arrangement and dose distribution for treatment of the retro-orbital tissues in thyroid eye disease.

In some patients they cause pain or interfere with function. Surgery (fasciectomy) is not that effective. Radiotherapy probably affects the development and growth rate of fibroblasts in the fascia. It should be considered in people with symptomatic disease which is progressing over the previous 12 months and in whom there is no fixed contracture or a contracture of less than 10 degrees. It probably provides benefit in about 80 percent of patients but with the caveats of a lack of randomized controlled trial data and a disease which can progress at a very variable pace with no treatment.

Technique

Treatment is with superficial Xrays (120–150 KV), though electrons can be used. The target volume is the palpable nodules and cord, treating from the skin surface to the periosteum (approx. 10 mm deep). Palpable disease is marked on the skin in pen and a 5–10 mm lateral and 10–20 mm longitudinal margin added to form the field border. A custom-made lead cutout is constructed. 15 Gy in 5 fractions are delivered over one week, with treatment repeated 6–12 weeks later to give a total dose of 30 Gy. Acute side effects are uncommon and second malignancy rates are estimated to be much lower than 1 percent (Figure 38.2).

Keloid Scarring

Indications for Radiotherapy

Keloid scars are an abnormal healing response to injury characterized by raised dermal fibroproliferative growths which can be disfiguring and painful. They can occur with relatively minor trauma (e.g. piercing) and are more common in young people. Intralesional steroids can be used, but for larger, symptomatic lesions, surgical excision is recommended, and this risks causing a further keloid which may be worse than the original one. Radiotherapy given after surgery can reduce the risk of subsequent keloid formation from 70 percent to approximately 15 percent at five years.

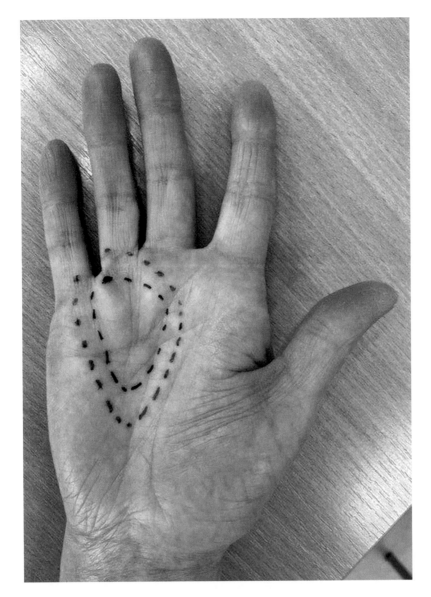

FIGURE 38.2 Radiotherapy for early Dupuytren's contracture. The palpable disease is defined (blue) and a margin added (red). A lead cutout will be made corresponding to the red shape.

Technique

Superficial X-rays or electrons can be used. The CTV is the scar produced by surgery with a 5 mm margin to PTV. A custom-made lead cutout is created. Various dose-fractionation protocols have been used, including 9–12 Gy in 1 fraction, 10 Gy in 2 fractions over two days or 12–15 Gy in 3 fractions over three days, depending on the site and risk of recurrence. Where the keloid is excised and sutured with primary closure, radiation should ideally start within 24 hours of surgery but up to 72 hours is acceptable. In some cases, the keloid is too large for primary closure and the wound is closed by secondary intention, and radiotherapy is given four weeks later as the wound starts to granulate. For inoperable keloids, radiotherapy alone can be used; schedules of 20 Gy in five monthly fractions are used.

Heterotopic Ossification

Indications for Radiotherapy

Heterotopic ossification (HO) is the abnormal formation of new bone within soft tissues following trauma, most often planned surgery. It is most commonly described after a hip replacement, but other joints can be affected. In most patients, it is asymptomatic but can cause pain, swelling or reduced movement. As the treatment for severe symptoms is surgery, which would then cause more HO, treatment is considered at this point to prevent recurrence. Radiotherapy given immediately pre- or postoperatively, and nonsteroidal anti-inflammatory drugs (NSAIDs) are equally effective. Choice depends on patient age and risks of NSAIDs. Radiotherapy is thought to inhibit the osteo-progenitor cells.

Technique

Anterior-posterior opposed fields are defined to encompass the regions that are mostly likely to form heterotopic bone – the neck of the femur, the tip of the greater trochanter, between the greater trochanter and the ilium, and between the lesser trochanter and the ischial ramus. 7 Gy is prescribed in a single fraction. It can be given within four hours prior to surgery or up to 72 hours after, but it is usually more practical to treat prior to surgery when the patient is likely to be more mobile (Figure 38.3).

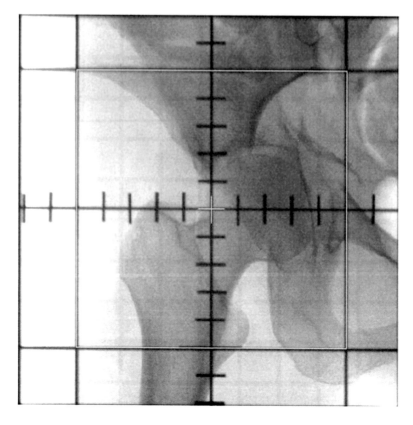

FIGURE 38.3 Anterior fields for treating heterotopic ossification of the hip.

Vestibular Schwannomas

Indications for Radiotherapy

These are benign tumours originating in the Schwann cells in the vestibular portion of the vestibulo-cochlea nerve. They can cause unilateral deafness or tinnitus. Many patients have observation with serial MRI scans. Surgery is the main treatment and is recommended in tumours that are growing in order to preserve facial nerve function or hearing, or when there are compressive symptoms. Fractionated stereo-tactic radiotherapy should be considered as an alternative to surgery, particularly in larger tumours or in patients with high operative risks. Local control rates are 95 percent at five years, with hearing preserved in 75 percent.

Technique

The patient is immobilized in a stereotactic frame. The tumour is easily visible on MRI so planning CT images are co-registered with T1-weighted, gadolinium-enhanced MRI. The GTV is the tumour as seen on MRI. There is no expansion to CTV. A standard department isotropic PTV expansion is made. Three-beam conformal, IMRT or VMAT plans can be used to deliver 50 Gy in 30 fractions over six weeks.

Pleomorphic Adenoma

Indications for Radiotherapy

These are benign salivary gland tumours usually occurring in the superficial parotid glands and often found incidentally or presenting as a painless lump. There is a 10 percent risk of malignant transformation over 15 years if left untreated. Surgery is usually recommended but pleomorphic adenomas can recur locally and multifocally. Re-resection is usually recommended, but there is a risk of facial nerve damage. EBRT should be considered for a second recurrence, particularly if there is a short interval between recurrences relative to the life expectancy of the patient, or when re-resection is not possible without significant risk of neuropraxia. Ten-year local control rates of 80–90 percent are reported.

Technique

Treatment is similar to other parotid tumours (see Chapter 15). The CTV is the visible disease on imaging and the adjacent surgical bed, as recurrence can occur in this whole region. A 3–5 mm margin to PTV is added. 50 Gy in 25 fractions is recommended, usually delivered by IMRT or VMAT as for other head and neck sites.

Head and Neck Paraganglioma

Indication for Radiotherapy

These are very slow-growing tumours arising in the neuroendocrine paraganglial cells. They can present with local symptoms, cranial nerve palsies or as incidental findings. They are usually, but not always, benign. Common sites include the carotid bifurcation (carotid body tumours), jugular bulb or vagus. The risks of surgery include bleeding and nerve damage and are higher with larger tumours. EBRT is an option for symptomatic, progressive disease if the risks are thought to be lower than those of surgery. Ten-year local control rates are 95 percent but with no randomized comparison to observation.

Technique

The tumour is contoured as GTV and expanded by a small margin (3–5 mm) to form a PTV based on department setup errors. 45 Gy in 25 fractions are prescribed, usually delivered by IMRT or VMAT similar to other head and neck cancers. Stereotactic radiotherapy (12–15 Gy) has also been used (Figure 38.4).

Cardiac SABR

Indications for Radiotherapy

Cardiac SABR, also known as stereotactic arrhythmia ablation (STAR) or cardiac radiosurgery, is a new technique devised to treat cardiac arrhythmias. Arrhythmias can be atrial or ventricular in origin and arise because of electrical signalling malfunction. The most common ventricular arrhythmia is monomorphic ventricular tachycardia (VT). It often occurs in patients with long-standing ischaemic heart disease.

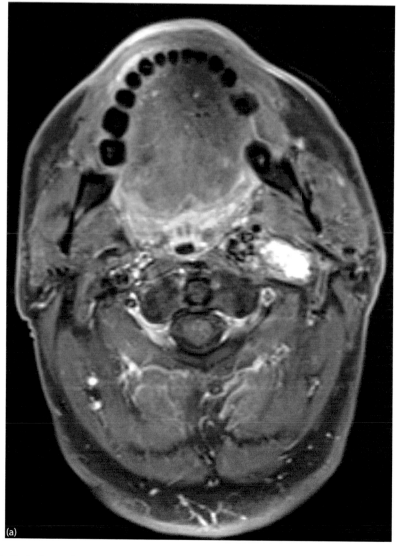

FIGURE 38.4 Radiotherapy for left carotid space paraganglioma. (a) Axial T1 + contrast MRI. (*Continued*)

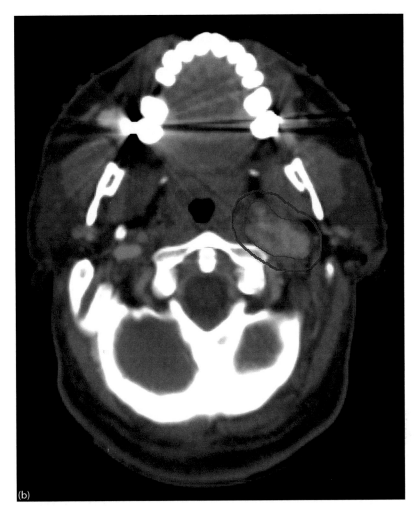

FIGURE 38.4 (*Continued*) Radiotherapy for left carotid space paraganglioma. (b) target volumes – GTV (blue) and PTV (red). Note there is no CTV defined in this benign tumour.

Ischaemic damage can cause myocardial fibrosis or scarring, which can instigate an electrical re-entry and subsequent arrhythmia. Treatment of VT includes drug management with anti-arrhythmic agents, trans-catheter ablation techniques with radiofrequency or cryoablation and implantable defibrillating devices.

Cardiac SABR has been explored as a treatment for VT in patients with disease that is refractory to currently available treatments.

Technique

A dose of 25 Gy in a single fraction is delivered to a predetermined target called the substrate. The substrate is identified using ECGs and electrophysiological mapping data along with cardiac CT and MRI. This is often a joint process conducted with the clinical oncologist and cardiologist. The substrate is volumed on a 4D radiotherapy planning CT. The substrate is edited over the 4D phases to create an ITV allowing for cardio-respiratory motion and a final ITV-PTV margin added isotropically. Patients are treated with IMRT taking particular care over OAR doses. Typically, patients will have oral and intravenous contrast in order to best visualize the substrate. Patients may also require abdominal compression.

The preliminary data for this treatment has proved encouraging. It remains an experimental treatment which requires further study and research but may become part of the treatment of VT in the future.

INFORMATION SOURCES

Bartalenaa L, Baldeschib L, Boboridis K, et al. The 2016 European Thyroid Association/European Group on Graves' orbitopathy guidelines for the management of Graves' orbitopathy. Eur Thyroid J 2016;5:9–26.

Kriz J, Seegenschmiedt HM, Barlets A, et al. Updated strategies in the treatment of benign diseases—a patterns of care study of the German cooperative group on benign diseases. Advances in Radiation Oncology 2018;3:240–244.

Muzevic D, Legcevic J, Splavski B, et al. Stereotactic radiotherapy for vestibular schwannoma. Cochrane Database of Systematic Reviews 2014;(12). Art. No.: CD009897. DOI: 10.1002/14651858.CD009897.pub2. Accessed 26 March 2023.

Ogawa R, Tosa M, Dohi T, et al. Surgical excision and postoperative radiotherapy for keloids. Scars, Burns & Healing 2019;5:1–11.

Radiation therapy for early Dupuytren's disease. (NICE Interventional procedures guidance [IPG573] Published: 21 December 2016. https://www.nice.org.uk/guidance/ipg573.

The Royal College of Radiologists. Recommendations for Using Radiotherapy for Benign Disease in the UK. London: The Royal College of Radiologists, 2023.

Index

Note: Locators in *italics* represent figures and **bold** indicate tables in the text.

A

Abdominal compression, 9, 12, 223, 288, 303, 412, 437
Accelerated dose fractionation for breast radiotherapy, 240
Accelerated hyperfractionation (CHART), **34**
Active breathing control (ABC), 9
Adaptive radiotherapy (ART), 11
Adenoid cystic carcinomas, 163–164, 170
AIN, *see* Anal intraepithelial neoplasia
Alpha-fetoprotein (AFP), 61
Alveolar rhabdomyosarcoma (aRMS), 425
Anal intraepithelial neoplasia (AIN), 318
Antiemetics, 190, 279, 294, 301, 326, 363, 379
Antioxidants, 5
Anus/anal cancer, 318–326
APC, *see* Argon plasma coagulation
Argon plasma coagulation (APC), 343
ARMS, *see* Alveolar rhabdomyosarcoma
As low as reasonably practicable (ALARP), 55
Astrocytoma, 186
Ataxia telangiectasia, 39
Atypical teratoid/rhabdoid tumours (ATRT), 199
Autoimmune connective tissue diseases, 46
Autologous stem cell transplantation (ASCT), 260

B

Backscatter Factors Table, 70
Basal cell carcinoma (BCC), 66–73
Basal dose (BD) rate point, *52*
BCC, *see* Basal cell carcinoma
Beam junctions, 16–17
Beam penumbra, 96
Benign disease, 431–436
Biologically effective dose (BED), 29–30, 42
Bladder/bladder cancer, 350–356
Bloom's syndrome, 39
Bone metastases, 62–63
Brachytherapy, 49, 88, 112
    cervix/cervical cancer, 375–377
    delivery systems, 49–50
    dose reporting, 54–55
    dosimetry, 50–51
    legislation pertaining, 55
    Manchester System for Interstitial
        Implants, 51–52
    of oral cavity tumours, *120*
    paediatric tumours, 417, 425
    Paris System for Iridium Wire Implants and
        Afterloading Techniques, 52–54
    prostate, 343–345

uterine cancer, 388, *388*
    vagina, 393, 396–397
Breast, 240–257

C

Calibration checks, 25
Cardiac devices, 46
Cardiac SABR, 436–437
Cell survival curves, 27–28
Central nervous system (CNS), 186–203
Cervical intraepithelial squamous/glandular neoplasia, 368
Cervix/cervical cancer, 4, 368–379
Choroidal melanoma, 179
Choroidal metastasis, palliative radiotherapy for, *182*
Colorectal cancer, 305; *see also* Rectum/rectal cancer
Commissioning Through Evaluation (CTE), 64
Compton scattering, 12
Conformity index, 10
Conjunctiva, 180
Conjunctival lymphomas, 179
Contact X-ray brachytherapy (CXB), 305–306
Craniospinal radiotherapy (CSRT), 199–202
Cutaneous angiosarcoma, 78–79
Cutaneous lymphoma, 72–78

D

Deep inspiratory breath-hold (DIBH) position, 242, 245
Desmoplastic small round blue cell tumours, 426
Diffuse intrinsic pontine glioma (DIPG), 203
Diffuse large B-cell lymphoma (DLBCL), 260
Diffuse midline gliomas (DMG), 203, *203*
DNA damage, 27
Dose–cure relationship, 32
Dose reporting, 54–55
Dose-response relationship, 28, *32*
Dose specification, 21–23
Dose–volume histogram (DVH) assessment, 10, 42, 262
Double trouble, 35
Ductal carcinoma in situ (DCIS), 240
Dupuytren's disease, 431–432

E

Ear, squamous cell cancers of, 105–108
EBV-associated NPC, 145
Eclipse electron Monte Carlo Algorithm, 71
Electronic patient record systems, 25
Electronic portal images (EPIs), 13
Electronic portal imaging devices (EPIDs), 9

Embryonal rhabdomyosarcoma (eRMS), 425
Embryonal tumour with multilayered rosettes (ETMR), 199
Emergency and palliative radiotherapy, 62–63
Ependymomas, 202
Epidermal growth factor receptor (EGFR), 87
Equivalent pulse dose rate, 121
Equivalent uniform dose (EUD), 42
ERMS, *see* Embryonal rhabdomyosarcoma
Ewing's sarcoma, 427–428
Extended-field radiotherapy, 264
Extraocular tumours, 182–184
Eye, anatomy of, *180*

F

Faecal immunochemical test (FIT), 305
Faecal occult blood test (FOBT), 305
Fanconi's anaemia, 39
Focus skin distance (FSD), 15

G

Gaps during treatment, avoidance of, 33–34
Gastric cancer, postoperative radiotherapy in, 289–290
Gastric MALT lymphoma, 261
Germ cell tumours, 186, 202
Glioblastoma (GBM), 186
Glioma
    in children, 202–203
    high-grade (HGG), 186
    low-grade (LGG), 191

H

HCC, *see* Hepatocellular carcinoma
HDR brachytherapy, 74
Head and neck cancers, 81–100
Head and neck paraganglioma, 435
Hepatocellular carcinoma (HCC), 303
Heterotopic ossification (HO), 434
High-grade glioma, *see* Glioma, high-grade
Hodgkin's lymphoma, 38, 46, 260, 264
    classical, 268–269
    grades, 269
    nodular lymphocyte predominant Hodgkin lymphoma
        (NLPHL), 260, 269
Hyperfractionation, **34**, 85
Hypofractionation, 46, 74
Hypopharynx, 136–144
Hypothalamic gliomas, 202
Hypoxic cell sensitizers, 87

I

Image guided radiotherapy (IGRT), 9
[131]I-mIBG therapy, 424
Inhomogeneity corrections, 15
International Commission on Radiation Units (ICRU), 40
Intracavitary brachytherapy, 49
Intraluminal brachytherapy, 50
Intraocular tumours, 179, 181–183
Involved field radiotherapy (IFRT), 264

Involved node radiotherapy (INRT), 264, 430
Involved site radiotherapy (ISRT), 264–265, 429
Ionising Radiation (Medical Exposures) Regulations, 38

K

Kallman-relative seriality model, 41
Kaposi Sarcoma, 78
Keloid scars, 433

L

Langerhans' cell histiocytosis, 430
Larynx, 154–162
Late-responding tissues, 28–29
Lead eye shield, *68*
Lead mask, *67*
Lead shielding, 67
Ledderhose disease, 431–432
Lentigo maligna, 74–75
Linear quadratic (LQ) model, 21
Lip, squamous cell cancers of, 103–105
Liver tumours, 302–303
Low dose rate (LDR) brachytherapy, 49
Low-grade glioma, *see* Glioma, low-grade
Lung cancer, 214–232
Lyman-probit model, 41
Lymphoma, 260–270
    non-Hodgkin, 260–262
        grades, 269

M

Malignant melanomas (MM), 65, 74–75, 171
Malignant phyllodes tumours, 240
Manchester System, 51
Masaoka clinical staging system, **210**
Maxillary tumours, 171
Maximum heart distance (MHD), 245
Medulloblastoma, 199
Meningiomas, 186, 192–195
Merkel cell carcinoma (MCC), 79
Mesothelioma, 230, 234–239
Meta-iodobenzylguanidine (^{123}I-MIBG) scans, 423
Mohs micrographic surgery, 66
Monte Carlo algorithm, 15
Mould brachytherapy, 50
Multi-leaf collimation (MLC), 10, 14, 17
Muscle invasive bladder cancer (MIBC), 348–349, 355
Mycosis fungoides (MF), 76

N

Nasopharyngeal cancer (NPC), 145–153
Non-germinomatous germ cell tumours (NGGCTs), 202
Non-Hodgkin lymphoma, *see* Lymphoma, non-Hodgkin
Non-seminomatous germ cell tumours (NSGCTs),
        358–359
Non-small cell lung cancer (NSCLC), 214–216
Normal tissue complication probability (NTCP), 30, 34
Nose, squamous cell cancers of, 108–110
NTCP (normal tissue complication probability), 38

O

Oesophageal cancer, 283–294
Olfactory neuroblastomas, 170, 172, *174*
Optic nerves and orbital tissues, 43–44
Oral cavity, 112–121, 169
Oral contrast medium, 12
Orbit, 179–184
Organ motion/internal margin, 7–9
Organ tolerance doses, 41–42
Oropharynx cancer, 122–135, 169
Osteosarcoma, 428–429

P

Paediatric and rare adult brain tumours, 198
Paediatric tumours, 415–430
Palmar fibromatosis, *see* Dupuytren's disease
Pancreas/pancreatic cancer, 296–302
Papillon technique, 305
Paranasal sinuses excluding sinonasal melanoma, **170**
Paris System for Iridium Wire Implants and Afterloading
        Techniques, 52–54
Parotid tumours, 164
Patient-reported outcome measures (PROMs), 3–4, 47
Penis/penile cancer, 364–367
Pituitary adenoma, 195–197
Plantar fibromatosis, *see* Ledderhose disease
Plasma cell neoplasms, 270–271
Poisson model, 32
Primitive neuroendocrine tumours (PNET), 186
Prostate/prostate cancer, 328–345
Protons, 20–21, 87

Q

Quality assurance, 24
Quality-of-life measures, 5
QUANTEC initiative, 42–43

R

Radiation dose and tumour cure probability, 30–33
Radiation-induced cancer, 5
Radio-opaque clips, 92
Radio-opaque material, 12
Rectum/rectal cancer, 305–316
Recursive partitioning analysis (RPA), 75

S

Sarcoma, 405–414
Scleroderma, 46
Screen-detected cancers, 4
Sealed source radiotherapy, *see* Brachytherapy
Second malignancies, 38, 46
Selective internal radiotherapy (SIRT), 302
Seminoma, 358
Sentinel lymph node biopsy (SLNB), 399–400
Set-up variations/set-up margin, 9–10
Shielding, 67
Simultaneous modulated accelerated radiation therapy
        (SMART), 234

Sinuses, 170–178
SIRT, *see* Selective internal radiotherapy
Skin, 65–80, 100–101
Solitary plasmacytoma and multiple myeloma, 270–273
Spinal cord compression, 56, *57*, 59
Splenic irradiation, 269–270
Stereotactic arrhythmia ablation (STAR), *see* Cardiac SABR
Stereotactic body radiotherapy (SABR), 19–20, 56, 75
Stereotactic radiosurgery/radiotherapy (SRS/SRT),
        19–20, 197
Strontium-90, 49
Superficial/orthovoltage radiotherapy, 68–69
Superior vena cava obstruction (SVCO), 60–61
Surviving fraction (SF), *28*
Systemic irradiation, 273–281

T

Tattoos, 73, 247
TCP (tumour control probability), 38
TEMS, *see* Transanal endoscopic microsurgery
Testis/testicular cancer, 358–363
Thermoluminescent dosimeters (TLDs), 24, 279, *280*
Thermoplastic shells, 11, *89*, 157, 197
Thymus, 211
Thyroid, 205–213
Thyroid eye disease, 431, *432*
Tolerance doses, 30, 41–42
Total reference air kerma (TRAK), 54
Transanal endoscopic microsurgery (TEMS), rectal
        cancer, 305
Trans-arterial chemoembolisation (TACE), 302
Transoral robotic surgery (TORS), 123
Transurethral resection of bladder tumour (TURBT),
        349–350
Treated volume, 10
    double trouble, 35
Tumour control probability (TCP), 34

U

Uterus/uterine cancer, 381–392

V

Vagina, 393–398
Vaginal intra-epithelial neoplasia (VAIN), 393
Vaginal vault brachytherapy, 377, 388, 391
VAIN, *see* Vaginal intra-epithelial neoplasia
Ventricular tachycardia (VT), 436–437
VMAT, *see* Volumetric modulated arc therapy
Volumetric–modulated arc therapy (VMAT), 19, 20, **84**,
        88, 95, 107, 111, 118, 142, 151, 153, 161, 167,
        188, 193, 195, 199, 254–255, 263, 268, 272,
        278, 312, 323, 339, 341, 343, 353–354, 366, 373,
        374–375, 389, 435, 436
VT, *see* Ventricular tachycardia
Vulva/vulva cancer, 399–404

Y

Yttrium-90 radio-embolisation, 302